SEVENTH
EDITION

Interpersonal Relationships

Professional Communication Skills for Nurses

Elizabeth C. Arnold, PhD, RN, PMHCNS-BC

Associate Professor, Retired
University of Maryland School of Nursing
Baltimore, Maryland

Family Nurse Psychotherapist
Montgomery Village, Maryland

Kathleen Underman Boggs, PhD, FNP-CS

Family Nurse Practitioner
Associate Professor Emeritus
College of Health and Human Services
University of North Carolina Charlotte
Charlotte, North Carolina

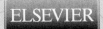

ELSEVIER

3251 Riverport Lane
St. Louis, Missouri 63043

INTERPERSONAL RELATIONSHIPS: PROFESSIONAL
COMMUNICATION SKILLS FOR NURSES, SEVENTH EDITION   ISBN: 978-0-323-24281-3

Notices

Knowledge and best practice in this field are constantly changing. As new research and experience broaden
our understanding, changes in research methods, professional practices, or medical treatment may become
necessary.

Practitioners and researchers must always rely on their own experience and knowledge in evaluating and
using any information, methods, compounds, or experiments described herein. In using such information or
methods they should be mindful of their own safety and the safety of others, including parties for whom they
have a professional responsibility.

With respect to any drug or pharmaceutical products identified, readers are advised to check the most
current information provided (i) on procedures featured or (ii) by the manufacturer of each product to be
administered, to verify the recommended dose or formula, the method and duration of administration, and
contraindications. It is the responsibility of practitioners, relying on their own experience and knowledge of
their patients, to make diagnoses, to determine dosages and the best treatment for each individual patient, and
to take all appropriate safety precautions.

To the fullest extent of the law, neither the Publisher nor the authors, contributors, or editors, assume any
liability for any injury and/or damage to persons or property as a matter of products liability, negligence or
otherwise, or from any use or operation of any methods, products, instructions, or ideas contained in the
material herein.

Previous editions copyrighted 2011, 2007, 2003, 1999, 1995, and 1989.

International Standard Book Number: 978-0-323-24281-3

Content Strategist: Jamie Randall
Content Development Manager: Jean Fornango
Associate Content Development Specialist: Melissa Rawe
Publishing Services Manager: Julie Eddy
Senior Project Manager: Marquita Parker
Designer: Julia Dummitt

Printed in the United States of America

Last digit is the print number: 9   8   7   6   5   4   3   2   1

**Working together
to grow libraries in
developing countries**

www.elsevier.com • www.bookaid.org

To the memory of my husband George Arnold who believed in me
and supported me unconditionally,
and to all the students I have had the privilege of teaching.

Elizabeth C. Arnold

To Sydney Lavarnway, may you find strong mentors.

Kathleen Underman Boggs

REVIEWERS

Amy Ellsworth, AND
Nursing Instructor
Kirkwood Community College
Cedar Rapids, Iowa

Cindy Carter, MSN, RN, IBCLC, RLC, ICCE
Nursing Instructor
Colorado Christian University
Indiana Wesleyan University
Texas Health Resources
Nocona, Texas

Kim Clevenger, EdD, MSN, RN, BC
Baccalaureate & RN-BSN Program Coordinator
Associate Professor of Nursing
Morehead State University
Morehead, Kentucky

Dr. Bonnie DeSimone, EdD, RN, BC
Professor of Nursing
Coordinator of the ABSN Weekday
Division of Nursing
Dominican College of Blauvelt
Orangeburg, New York

Linda Finch, PhD, ANP-BC
Associate Professor/Associate Dean-Retired
Loewenberg School of Nursing
University of Memphis
Memphis, Tennessee

Shari Kist, PhD, RN, CNE
Assistant Professor
Goldfarb School of Nursing at Barnes-Jewish
 College
St. Louis, Missouri

Robyn C. Leo, MS, RN
Associate Professor Nursing
Worcester State University
Putnam, Connecticut

Scott A. Davis
Police Officer
Crisis Intervention Team (CIT) Coordinator
Montgomery County Police Department,
Gaithersburg, Maryland

Danette Yolanda Wall, DNP, MSN, MBA, ACRN, RN, CPHQ, LNC
Chief Operating Officer
Odot, LLC
Clinical Advisor Quality Improvement
Humana CarePlus, Inc.
Tampa, Florida

Brian Zager, MA
PhD Candidate
Department of Speech Communication
Southern Illinois University
Carbondale, Illinois

CONTRIBUTOR

Shari Kist, PhD, RN, CNE
Assistant Professor
Goldfarb School of Nursing
Barnes-Jewish College
St. Louis, Missouri

ACKNOWLEDGMENTS

Elizabeth C. Arnold
Kathleen Underman Boggs

The seventh edition of *Interpersonal Relationships: Professional Communication Skills for Nurses* continues to reflect the ideas and commitment of our students, valued colleagues, clients, and the editorial staff at Elsevier. The first edition, aligned with an interpersonal relationship communication seminar developed at the University of Maryland School of Nursing, was published 25 years ago. Developing effective communication was important then and it remains central to effective clinical practice in contemporary health care. The text was originally designed by faculty to facilitate nursing students' understanding of therapeutic communication in clinical settings, using case examples and experiential simulations. At this point in time, professional nursing role relationships and the use of relational communication in health care is more complex and multi-layered.

The scope of content in the seventh edition reflects a markedly different contemporary health care landscape, one which is open-ended, client-activated and interdisciplinary in function and skill development. The vitality of its contents reflects the commitment of faculty and students from many nursing programs and the clinical nurses who have deepened the understanding of the materials presented in this text through their positive support, ideas, and constructive feedback. In particular, the voices of the following faculty and professional nurses have contributed directly and indirectly to the development of this text: Verna Carson, PhD, RN, PCNS; Judith W. Ryan, PhD, RN, CRNP; Michelle Michael, PhD, APRN, PNP; Barbara Harrison, RN, PMH-NP; Ann O'Mara, PhD, RN, AOCN, FAAN; Barbara Dobish, MS, RN; Anne Marie Spellbring, PhD, RN, FAAN; Kristin Bussell, MS, RN, CS-P; Patricia Harris, MS, APRN, NP; and Jacqueline Conrad, BS, RN, from the University of Maryland; Ann Mabe Newman, DSN, RN, CS and David R. Langford, RN, DSNc, from the University of North Carolina Charlotte, and Dr. Bonnie DeSimone from Dominican College of Blauvelt. Nurses in the community: Luwana Cameron, RN; Nancy Pashby, RN; Mary Jane Joseph, RN; and Dr. Stephanie Wright provided valuable input related to their clinical expertise. We are indebted to Dr. Shari Kist of the Goldfarb School of Nursing at the Barnes-Jewish College for her thoughtful revision of Chapter 12.

We acknowledge with deep gratitude the unique Elsevier team efforts of Melissa Rawe, Associate Content Development Specialist, Jamie Randall, Content Strategist, and Marquita Parker, Senior Project Manager-book production. Their dedicated commitment to the completion of this text and expertise were notable in making the revision process for this seventh edition a seamless and timely developmental experience.

Finally, we acknowledge the loving support of our families and Michael J. Boggs for their unflagging support and encouragement.

PREFACE

Elizabeth C. Arnold
Kathleen Underman Boggs

Recognition of the importance of therapeutic communication and professional relationships with clients and families as a primary means of achieving treatment goals in health care continues to be the underlying theme in *Interpersonal Relationships: Professional Communication Skills for Nurses.* This seventh edition has been thoroughly revised, rewritten, and updated to meet the challenge of serving as a primary communication resource for nursing students and professional nurses.

While maintaining the integrity of previous text versions, the seventh edition introduces a broadened interprofessional perspective on communication, occasioned by historical transformational changes currently occurring in contemporary health care delivery. Expanded content is competency based and draws from many different sources: Joint Commission Standards, the Institute of Medicine (IOM) reports, QSEN, communication theory, Essentials of Baccalaureate Education, systems thinking and interprofessional team-based communication, as advocated by AHRQ's TeamSTEPPS program. The content, exercises, and case examples are intentionally integrated to support students in developing the interpersonal and technical communication skills required in contemporary health care environments. Examples provide students with opportunities to apply new research and new technologies to their practice.

Content in this text, as in previous editions' can be used as individual teaching modules, as a primary text, or as a communication resource integrated across the curriculum. New subject matter related to interprofessional team communication and nursing leadership reflect the latest applications of communication in contemporary health care delivery across clinical settings. Knowledge and skills related to spirituality, health literacy promotion, interdisciplinary thinking, advocacy and social responsibility are expanded in this edition. These topics are addressed as relevant components of interprofessional and client-centered relationships of health care.

Although the seventh edition is divided into six sections, using a similar format to that of previous editions, the organization of the chapters has been significantly revised based on reviewer comments. *Part I, Conceptual Foundations of Interpersonal Relationships and Professional Communication Skills*, provides a theory-based approach to therapeutic relationships and communication in nursing practice and identifies professional, legal, and ethical standards guiding professional actions. Chapters describe the relevance of critical thinking to clinical reasoning and key linkages between communication clarity and client safety in health care situations. *Part II, Essential Communication Skills*, focuses on development of therapeutic communication skills. Chapters in this second section also address variations in communication styles, intercultural communication diversity, and group communication strategies.

Part III, Therapeutic Interpersonal Relationship Skills begins with a chapter on the role of self-concept and measurable personal characteristics, as a key influencer of communication in therapeutic relationships. The chapter on therapeutic communication presents a structured approach to the competency skills nurses need for effective communication in health care settings. Chapters on client-centered and family-centered relationships explore basic concepts of therapeutic communication and applications of strategies nurses can use with individuals and families. Bridges and barriers to the development and maintenance of therapeutic relationships highlight key relational elements in professional interactions with clients and families. The final chapter in Part III addresses conflict resolution strategies in nurse-client relationships.

Part IV, Communicating to Foster Health Literacy, Health Promotion, and Prevention of Disease among Diverse Populations, provides students with the necessary background and communication approaches to effectively cope with the unique complexities of client/family health care needs across clinical settings, including cultural and language diversity. This section also focuses on strategies to enhance health literacy, the nature and scope of health teaching, and communication with clients in stressful situations.

Part V, Accommodating Clients with Special Communication Needs provides students with a basic understanding of the communication accommodations needed by clients with specialized communication needs. Specific chapters offer communication strategies nurses and other health providers can use to respond effectively with children and older adults. Content on communicating with clients in crisis situations and in palliative care complete Part V.

Contemporary nurses are living and practicing in a rapidly changing collaborative interprofessional health care environment in which they are expected to take an active leadership role. The professional health care landscape remains still generally uncharted and open to interpretation.

Part VI, Collaborative and Professional Communication, proactively prepares students to develop competence and self assurance as professional nurses. Chapters address the major behavioral elements, habits of thinking, and feeling deemed essential to developing productive collegial working relationships within the nursing profession and interprofessionally with team members of other disciplines. Part VI discusses role relationships and speaks to the significance of nursing leadership and collaborative team communication strategies. The importance of communicating for continuity of care, electronic documentation, application of e-health information technologies, and technology integrated applications at point of care are also addressed.

Each chapter is designed to illuminate the connection between theory and practice by presenting basic concepts, followed by clinical applications, using updated references and instructive case examples. *Developing an Evidence-Based Practice* boxes offer a summary of a current research article related to each chapter subject and are intended to stimulate awareness of the essential links between research and practice. The *Ethical Dilemmas* presented in each chapter offer the student an opportunity to reflect on common ethical situations, which occur on a regular basis in health care relationships. New to the seventh edition are *Discussion Questions* at the end of each chapter. References have been chosen and suitably updated to align with the content in each chapter.

Experiential exercises provide students with the opportunity to practice, observe, and critically evaluate their professional communication skills in a safe learning environment. Learning exercises are designed to encourage self-reflection about how one's personal practice fits with the larger picture of contemporary nursing, health practice models, and interdisciplinary team communication. Through active experiential involvement with relationship-based communication principles, students can develop confidence and skill with using patient-centered communication in real-life team-based clinical settings. The comments and reflections of other students provide a unique, enriching perspective on the wider implications of communication in clinical practice.

Communication is thought of as the primary medium for moving quality care in our health system forward. This text gives voice to the centrality of communication as the basis for helping clients, families, and communities make sense of relevant health issues and develop effective ways of coping with them. Our hope is that the seventh edition will continue to serve as a primary reference source for nurses seeking to improve their communication and relationship skills across traditional and nontraditional health care settings. As the most consistent health care provider in many clients' lives, the nurse bears an awesome responsibility to provide communication that is professional, honest, empathetic, and knowledgeable in a person-to-person relationship that is without equal in health care. As nurses, we are answerable to our clients, our profession, and ourselves to communicate with clients in a therapeutic manner and to advocate for their health care and well-being within the larger sociopolitical community. We invite you as students, practicing nurses, and faculty to interact with the material in this text, learning from the content and experiential exercises but also seeking your own truth and understanding as professional health care providers.

Instructor Resources are available on the textbook's Evolve web site. New PowerPoint presentations include audience response questions, teaching tips and lecture ideas, instructor-focused exercises, and case studies. A revised Test Bank reflecting the updated content in the text is also included. Instructors are encouraged to contact their Elsevier sales representative to gain access to these valuable teaching tools.

Theory Based Perspectives and Contemporary Dynamics

Elizabeth C. Arnold

OBJECTIVES

At the end of the chapter, the reader will be able to:

1. Identify essential characteristics of the nursing discipline.
2. Describe the art and science of nursing.
3. Discuss the core constructs of professional nursing's metaparadigm.
4. Compare and contrast different models of communication.
5. Identify relevant theoretical frameworks used in nursing relationships.
6. Explain the role of systems thinking in contemporary health care.
7. Identify issues related to health care reform.
8. Apply Institute of Medicine (IOM) recommendations as a framework for the study of relationships and communication skills in nursing practice.
9. Discuss implications for the future of nursing.

Chapter 1 identifies selected conceptual frameworks relevant to the study of client-centered communication, and professional relationships in a contemporary health care system. Socioeconomic factors related to health care reform and the driving forces of Institute of Medicine (IOM) reports outline some of the changes required to transform the health care system.

BASIC CONCEPTS

Historically, nursing is as old as humankind. Originally nursing was practiced informally by religious orders dedicated to care of the sick, and later in the home by female caregivers with no formal education (Egenes, 2009). Nursing was not identifiable as a distinct occupation until the 1854 Crimean War when Florence Nightingale's *Notes on Nursing* (1860, 2010) introduced the world to the functional roles of professional nursing, and the need for formal education (D'Antonio, 2010). Her use of statistical data to document the need for hand washing in preventing infection marks her as the profession's first nurse researcher. An early advocate for high-quality care, Nightingale viewed nursing as both a science and an art form (Alligood, 2014).

Over the next 150 years, nursing evolved into a recognizable highly respected profession. The discipline's unique body of knowledge and theoretical perspectives help define the nursing discipline, and strengthen its voice in effectively responding to the current global health care crisis (Smith and McCarthy, 2010). The profession's next step is to solidly position professional nursing practice as having a key role within a larger collaborative health care team paradigm.

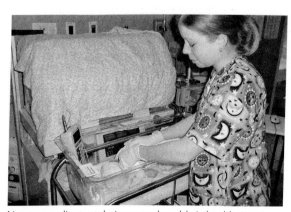

Nurses see clients at their most vulnerable in health situations.

THE DISCIPLINE OF NURSING

Litchfield and Jonsdottir (2008) contend that our "discipline is relational and creative in practice" (p. 79). Professional nursing is a "practice" discipline, which combines specialized knowledge and skills with prudent clinical judgment to meet client, family, and community health care needs. Donaldson and Crowley (1978) characterize the discipline of nursing as having a specialized perspective related to

- "Principles and laws that govern the life processes, well-being, and optimum functioning of human beings, sick or well;
- Patterning of human behavior in interaction with the environment in critical life situations; and
- Processes by which positive changes in health status are affected." (p. 113).

As the discipline of nursing evolved, apprentice-type training was replaced with a higher level of nursing education provided at the college level. Today, professional nursing education begins at the undergraduate level, with a growing number of nurses choosing graduate studies to support differentiated advanced practice roles and/or research opportunities. Nurses with advanced preparation are prepared to function as nurse practitioners, clinical specialists, administrators, and educators. Today nurses represent the largest group of health care professionals in the United States (IOM, 2010; Pelletier and Stichler, 2013). The scope of practice for professional nurses has increased exponentially, and is increasingly practiced within the context of supportive collaborative interdisciplinary health care teams.

THE SCIENCE OF NURSING

Nursing theory represents the basis for science of nursing. Theory development is essential to maintaining the truth of any discipline (Reed and Shearer, 2007). Nursing theory emerged as a serious form of study in the 1940s and 1950s as a means to identify the unique specialized body of knowledge associated with the discipline of nursing. The intent was to examine the phenomenon of professional nursing in *systematic ways* as a means of clarifying its unique body of knowledge, making visible the nature of its domain, informing clinical practice, and forming a basis for research related to its practice domain.

Nursing theories and models, used to describe, explain, predict, and prescribe phenomena applicable to nursing practice, education, and research didn't really take hold until the 1950s (Alligood, 2014). Today, nursing frameworks serve as a contextual background for practice and research. Common conceptual threads enable nurses, and the general public, to have a clearer understanding of the domain of professional nursing. Theoretical constructs in nursing strengthen the focus of the discipline, and provide a foundation for generating hypotheses in research. As the profession positions itself to play a key role in a transformed health care system, there is a noticeable shift from theory development to a new era of theory applicability and utilization (Alligood, 2010).

Expectations for professional nursing practice in the twenty-first century are being recast within collaborative team care approaches rather than separated by discipline-specific care for clients (Ritter-Teitel, 2002). Nurses are expected to pool their expertise with other providers through a skilled network of team-based care for the benefit of clients and their families.

NURSING'S METAPARADIGM

Individual nursing theories represent different interpretations of the phenomenon of nursing, but central constructs: person, environment, health, and nursing are found in all theories and models (Karnick, 2013; Marrs and Lowry, 2006). They are referred to as nursing's *metaparadigm*. The four constructs continue to comprise the metalanguage about the primary emphasis of nursing practice (Jarrin, 2012).

Concept of Person

Person, is defined as the recipient of nursing care, having unique biopsychosocial and spiritual dimensions. The concept of "person" supersedes health diagnosis apart from, and before a specific health care problem is considered. Person factors "comprise features of the individual that are not part of a health condition or health states" (World Health Organization [WHO], 2001, p. 17). Gender, lifestyle, coping styles, habits, among others, are considered person attributes. The term is applied to individuals, family units, the community, and target populations such as the elderly or mentally ill—anyone in need of health care. In health care settings, and throughout this text, person may be referred to as "patient" or "client." The complexity of "person" is a holistic concept. It is evidenced in patient-centered care, "which honors patients' preferences, needs, and values; applies biopsychosocial perspectives… and forces a strong partnership between patient and clinician (Greene et al., 2012, p. 49).

Knowledge of the "client as a person" is the starting point in health care delivery, essential to both client safety and quality of care (Zolnierek, 2013). Client centered care considers the impact of an illness or injury on a person—not only physiologically, but mentally, spiritually, and socially. Client preferences, perceptions, beliefs, and values, combined with clinical facts, and the nurse's self-awareness (personal ways of knowing) form an essential understanding of each person's unique clinical situation. Protecting a client's basic integrity and health rights is an ethical responsibility of nurse to client, whether the person is a contributing member of society, a critically ill newborn, a comatose client, or a seriously mentally ill individual (Shaller, 2007).

Concept of Environment

Environment refers to the internal and external *context* of the client, as it shapes and is affected by a client's health care situation. Person and environment are so intertwined that to consider person as an isolated variable in a health care situation without considering environmental factors acting as barriers or supports to healing is impracticable (WHO, 2001). That clients cannot be successfully treated apart from their environments is a central thesis in Nightingale's nursing framework, and Martha Rogers's Science of Unitary Human Beings.

Environment plays a significant role in health promotion, disease prevention, and care of individuals with chronic conditions within the community. The concept of environment reflects multiple factors of cultural, developmental, and social determinants that influence a client's health perceptions and behavior. Examples of environmental factors include poverty, level of education, religious or spiritual beliefs, type of community (rural, or urban), family strengths and challenges, access to resources, and level of social support are examples of a client's environmental context. Even climate, space, pollution, and food choices are important dimensions of environment that nurses may need to consider in choosing appropriate nursing interventions.

Concept of Health

The word *health* derives from the word *whole*. Health is a multidimensional concept, having physical, psychological, sociocultural, developmental, and spiritual characteristics. WHO (1946) defines **health** as "a state of complete physical, mental, social well-being, not merely the absence of disease or infirmity" (p. 3). This definition has not been amended to date.

Nordstrom and colleagues (2013) describe the healthy person as the person who is able to "realize *his* or *her* vital goals, not vital goals in general" (p. 361). For example, an active 80-year-old woman can consider herself quite healthy, despite having osteoporosis and a controlled heart condition. **Wellness** is a dimension of health, evidenced in satisfaction with a person's quality of life and sense of well-being. Health is a value-laden concept, which includes both the general state of the person, *and* objective medical data. Culture and life experiences influence how people think about health, wellness, illness and treatment implications. Health is a social concern, particularly for people who do not have personal control over their health, or the necessary resources to enhance their health status. Contemporary concepts of health encompass disease prevention, chronic care self-management and promoting healthy lifestyle behaviors, such that nurses can anticipate and respond to the needs of those at greatest risk for adverse health situations.

During the last century, most professional care was delivered in acute care settings, based on a disease-focused medical model. Switching to today's community focus recognizes the fact that chronic medical conditions account for most of today's care, with most being treated in the community (Henley and colleagues, 2011). The environment and health ecology has emerged as an intertwined concept as health care is becoming a global enterprise. In fact, health care access is considered a social ecological determinant of health (McGibbon et al., 2008).

Healthy People 2020 (DHHS, 2010) considers quality of life to be a key outcome of disease prevention, health promotion and maintenance activities. **Quality of life** is defined as a subjective experience of well-being and general satisfaction with one's life that includes, but is not limited to, physical health. Nurses play a major role in assessing health behaviors, and negotiating lifestyle changes that allow individuals and families to achieve and maintain a healthy lifestyle. Exercise 1-1, The Meaning of Health as a Nursing Concept, provides an opportunity to explore the multidimensional meaning of health.

EXERCISE 1-1	The Meaning of Health as a Nursing Concept

Purpose: To help students understand the dimensions of health as a nursing concept.

Procedure
1. Think of a person whom you think is healthy. In a short report (1-2 paragraphs), identify characteristics that led you to your choice of this person.
2. In small groups of three or four, read your stories to each other. As you listen to other students' stories, write down themes that you note.
3. Compare themes, paying attention to similarities and differences, and developing a group definition of health derived from the stories.

4. In a larger group, share your definitions of health and defining characteristics of a healthy person.

Discussion
1. Were you surprised by any of your thoughts about being healthy?
2. Did your peers define health in similar ways?
3. Based on the themes that emerged, how is health determined?
4. Is illness the opposite of being healthy?
5. In what ways, if any did you find concepts of health to be culture or gender bound?
6. In what specific ways can you as a health care provider support the health of your client?

EXERCISE 1-2	What Is Professional Nursing?

Purpose: To help students develop an understanding of professional nursing.

Procedure
1. Interview a professional nurse who has been in practice for more than 12 months. Ask for descriptions of what he or she considers professional nursing to be today, in what ways he or she thinks nurses make a difference, and how the nurse feels the role might evolve within the next 10 years.

2. In small groups of three to five students, discuss findings and develop a group definition of professional nursing.

Discussion
1. What does nursing mean to you?
2. Is your understanding of nursing different from those of the nurse(s) you interviewed?
3. As a new nurse, how would you want to present yourself?

Concept of Nursing

Kim (2010) terms the nursing construct in nursing's *metaparadigm* as the practice domain of nursing. The overarching goal of nursing activities is to empower clients and strengthen their skill sets by providing them with the support they need to achieve optimal health and well-being. Nursing actions help clients achieve identifiable health goals through a continuum of services ranging from health promotion and health education, to direct care, rehabilitation, and research evaluation.

The International Council of Nurses' (ICN) definition of nursing states:
Nursing encompasses autonomous and collaborative care of individuals of all ages, families, groups and communities, sick or well and in all settings. Nursing includes the promotion of health, prevention of illness, and the care of ill, disabled and dying people. Advocacy, promotion of a safe environment, research,

participation in shaping health policy and in patient and health systems management, and education are also key nursing roles (ICN, 2014).

New specialty and advanced practice roles as nurse practitioners, doctors of nursing practice, clinical nurse leader roles in hospitals and clinics reinforce the complexity of the discipline. Nurses are increasingly involved in community advocacy. They are actively shaping public health policies and have assumed transformational roles in practice, research, and education. Mallock (2014) Exercise 1-2, What Is Professional Nursing?, can help you look at your philosophy of nursing.

Finkelman and Kenner (2009) differentiate between the science and art of nursing, stating that, "**knowledge** represents the science of nursing, and **caring** represents the art of nursing" (p. 54). Both are required for safe quality care. The science of nursing provides an essential knowledge base for professional nursing, but it is the art of nursing that takes into account the variations in unique client characteristics and life experiences, which influence client choices in health care.

THE ART OF NURSING

The "art of nursing" represents a seamless interactive process in which nurses blend their knowledge, skills, and scientific understandings with their individualized knowledge of each client as a unique human being with physical, cognitive, emotional, and spiritual needs. Individualized knowledge is assembled from each "nurse's mode of being, knowing, and responding" to each clients' unique care needs (Gramling, 2004, p. 394). Nurses use classic patterns of knowing to bridge the interpersonal space between science and client-centered needs to individualize client-centered care (Zander, 2007).

Patterns of Knowing

Knowledge rarely proceeds to understanding in a simple direct way. In clinical practice where so many dynamics are involved, a broad spectrum of knowledge is essential. In a seminal work, Carper (1978) maintains that nurses use multiple forms of knowledge to inform their praxis. She describes four patterns of knowing embedded in nursing practice: empirical, personal, aesthetic, and ethical. Although described as individual prototypes, Carper emphasizes that in practice, these patterns inform care as an integrated form of knowledge. Holtslander (2008) notes that "this integrated, inclusive, and eclectic approach is reflective of the goals of nursing, which are to provide effective, efficient, and compassionate care while considering individuality, context, and complexity" (p. 25). The four patterns (ways) of knowing consist of:

- **Empirical** ways of knowing: knowledge that is objective and observable. Empirical knowledge draws upon verifiable data from science. The process of empirical ways of knowing includes logical reasoning and problem solving. Nurses use empirical ways of knowing to provide scientific rationales when choosing appropriate nursing interventions.
- **Personal** ways of knowing: Personal knowledge is "characterized as subjective, concrete and existential" (Carper, 1978, p. 251). Personal knowing is relational. It is a pattern of knowing about self and other, which occurs when nurses connect with the humanness of the client experience. Personal knowledge develops when nurses intuitively understand and connect

with clients as unique human beings. Nurses may not be able to define why they intuitively believe something is true, but they trust this knowledge. They have experiential knowledge of their own responses, plus knowledge of professional experiences with other clients facing similar situations. Self-awareness provides nurses with a different authentic dimension of what it means to live through a particular health disruption.

- **Aesthetic** ways of knowing are sometimes referred to as the "art of nursing" because this knowledge links the humanistic components of care with its scientific application. There is a deeper appreciation of the whole person or situation, a moving beyond the superficial to see the experience as part of a larger whole. Esthetic knowledge enables nurses to experientially know about the fear behind a client's angry response, the courage of a client with stage four cancer offering her suffering up for her classmates, the pain of a father cutting off funds for a drug addicted son. Aesthetic ways of knowing can be enhanced with storytelling, in which nurses seek to understand the experience of the client's personalized journey through illness (Leight, 2002).
- **Ethical ways of knowing** refer to the moral aspects of nursing care (Altman, 2007; Porter et al., 2011). This knowledge helps nurses provide principled care when confronted with moral issues in health care. Ethical ways of knowing encompass knowledge of what is right and wrong, attention to standards and codes in making moral choices, responsibility for one's actions, and protection of the client's autonomy and rights.

Exercise 1-3, Patterns of Knowing in Clinical Practice, provides practice with using patterns or ways of knowing in clinical practice.

Chinn and Kramer (2011) introduced a fifth pattern, *emancipatory ways of knowing*, which includes the nurse's awareness of social problems and social justice support for issues affecting health care delivery to clients and populations. The concept of emancipatory knowing expands the nurse's praxis role within the larger health care arena. By recognizing, and acting upon the social, political, and economic determinants of health and well-being, nurses are in a better position to act as advocates in helping the nation identify and reduce the inequities in health care (Chinn and Kramer, 2011).

EXERCISE 1-3   Patterns of Knowing in Clinical Practice

Purpose: To help students understand how patterns of knowing can be used effectively in clinical practice.

Procedure
1. Break into smaller groups of three to four students. Identify a scribe for each student group.
2. Using the following case study, decide how you would use empirical, personal, ethical, and aesthetic patterns of knowing to see that Mrs. Jackson's holistic needs were addressed in the next 48 hours.

Case Study
Mrs. Jackson, an 86-year-old widow, was admitted to the hospital with a hip fracture. She has very poor eyesight because of macular degeneration and takes eye drops for the condition. Her husband died 5 years ago, and she subsequently moved into an assisted housing development. She had to give up driving because of her eyesight and sold her car to another resident

5 months ago. Although her daughter lives in the area, Mrs. Jackson has little contact with her. This distresses her greatly, as she describes being very close with her until 8 years ago. She feels safe in her new environment but complains that she is very lonely and is not interested in joining activities. She has a male friend in the complex, but recently he has been showing less interest. Her surgery is scheduled for tomorrow, but she has not yet signed her consent form. She does not have advance directives.

Discussion
1. In a large group, have each student share their findings.
2. For each pattern of knowing, write the suggestions on the board.
3. Compare and contrast the findings of the different groups.
4. Discuss how the patterns of knowing add to an understanding of the client in this case study.

Caring

The concept of caring is a characteristic of all helping professions. In nursing practice, caring is considered an *essential* functional construct and core value of nursing practice (Wagner and Whaite, 2010; Watson, 2005). Caring strengthens patient-centered knowledge and adds depth to nursing competencies that nurses bring to the clinical situation. Empathy serves as the connective caring bridge between health providers and clients. Clark (2010) describes empathetic understanding as consisting of a health provider's combined subjective experiencing of what it is like to be a client, an interpersonal understanding of what the client is currently experiencing in the moment, and an objective empathy related to a broader understanding of a client's situation from outside the client's frame of reference.

Crowe (2000) suggests, "Caring does not involve specific tasks, instead it involves the creation of a sustained relationship with the other" (p. 966). Caring is the component of care best remembered by clients and nurses. In a qualitative research study, graduate nurses described characteristics of professional caring in their practice as (a) giving of self, (b) involved presence, (c) intuitive knowing and empathy, (d) supporting the client's integrity, and (e) professional competence (Arnold, 1997).

The American Nurses Association (ANA, 2010) affirms that "the essence of nursing is caring" (p. 45).

As professional nurses assume broader leadership roles in health care, caring should be embodied as a visible component of relationships with all members of the health care team.

COMMUNICATION THEORY

Effective communication with clients, families, coworkers, and other health care professionals involved with the care of clients is an essential foundation of effective health care. Hargie (2011) asserts, "communication represents the very essence of the human condition" (p. 2). Communication is a human enterprise and a fundamental underpinning of all nurse-client interactions. Through purposeful communication, you can help clients and families make sense of their health needs, assist them in learning how to self-manage chronic health conditions, and provide therapeutic support for decision making.

Communication takes place intrapersonally (within the self) or interpersonally (with others). *Intrapersonal communication* occurs in the form of a person's inner thoughts and beliefs, colored by feelings that influence behavior. It often is a hidden component of the communication process related to either nurse or client's past experience and something within the current discussion. Understanding of intrapersonal meanings requires self-awareness and reflection as it usually is not a spoken part of the message. In addition, seeking frequent validation from the receiver incorporates client feedback to improve nurse/client collaboration and mutual understanding of the message and/or the process itself.

Interpersonal communication is defined as a reciprocal, interactive, dynamic process, having value, cultural, emotive, and cognitive variables that influence its transmission and reception. Interpersonal communication theories are concerned with the transmission of information *and* with how people create meaning. Through speech, touch, listening, and responding, people construct personal meanings and share them with others. Most of us take interpersonal communication for granted until we cannot engage in the process, or it is no longer a part of our lives. Human interpersonal communication is unique. Only human beings have large vocabularies and are capable of learning new languages as a means of sharing their ideas and feelings. Relational communication is an important source of personal expression and influence. Included in the concept are language, gestures, body movements, eye contact, and personal or cultural symbols. People combine words and nonverbal signals into a montage to convey intended meaning, exchange or strengthen ideas and feelings, and to share significant life experiences.

Communication has both content and relationship dimensions (Watzlawick et al., 1967). The **content dimension** of communication (verbal component) refers to shared verbal, written, or digitally delivered data. The relationship dimension (expressed nonverbally through metacommunication) helps the receiver interpret the meaning of the message. People tend to pay more attention to nonverbal communication than to words especially when they are not congruent with each other. Basic assumptions related to the concept of communication are presented in Box 1-1.

Channels of communication is the term used to designate one or more of the connectors through which a person receives a message. Primary channels of human communication include the five senses: sight, hearing, taste, touch, and smell. Technology has introduced secondary channels of communication in the form of media messaging.

In professional business settings, the term has a different connotation. Channels of communication describe the hierarchy of reporting relationships individuals need to respect when communicating with coworkers and authority figures. Each person is expected to answer to the person at the next higher

BOX 1-1	Basic Assumptions of Communication Theory

- All behavior is communication and it is impossible to not communicate.
- Every communication has a content and a relationship (metacommunication) aspect.
- We only know about ourselves and others through communication.
- Faulty communication results in flawed feeling and acting.
- Feedback is the only way we know that our perceptions about meanings are valid.
- Silence is a form of communication.
- All parts of a communication system are interrelated and affect one another.
- People communicate through words (digital communication) and through nonverbal behaviors and analog-verbal modalities; both forms are needed to interpret a message appropriately.

(Adapted from Bateson G, 1979 *Mind and nature* Dutton: New York; Watzlawick P, Beavin-Bavelas J, Jackson D (1967) Some tentative axioms of communication. In *Pragmatics of Human Communication— A Study of Interactional Patterns, Pathologies and Paradoxes*, pp. 29–52. New York, W. W. Norton.)

level and to communicate downward to coworkers for whom the person is responsible.

LINEAR MODELS

The **linear model** is the simplest communication model, consisting of sender, message, receiver, and context. Linear models identify the process of communication focus only on the sending and receipt of messages, and do not necessarily consider communication as enabling the development of cocreated meanings between communicators.

- The **sender** is the source, or initiator of the message. The sender encodes the message (i.e., puts the message into verbal or nonverbal symbols that the receiver can understand). Encoding a message appropriately requires a clear understanding of the receiver's mental frame of reference (e.g., feelings, personal agendas, past experiences). Therapeutic communication requires that the helping person as sender has a health-related purpose.
- The **message** consists of the transmitted verbal or nonverbal expression of thoughts and feelings. Effective messages are relevant, authentic, and expressed in understandable language.
- The **receiver** is the recipient of the message. The receiver needs to be open to hearing what

the sender is saying. Once received, the receiver decodes the message and internally interprets its meaning to make personal sense of the message.) An open listening attitude and suspension of judgment strengthens the possibility of accurately decoding a sender's message.

The **context** of the interaction refers to all the factors that influence how a message is received. The most critical variable is the presence of **noise,** which is defined as anything that interferes with the effective transmission, reception, or understanding of a message. "Noise" is a concept found in both linear and transactional models. Linear models only consider external phenomena. *Physical* noise occurs in the form of environmental distractors such as people talking loudly, babies crying, children running around, music or TV playing, excessive room temperature, poor seating, and lack of privacy. In transactional models, noise also includes internal interference factors. *Physiological* noise includes internal distractors such as feeling tired, anxious, angry, worried, or being too sick to fully attend to the message. *Psychological* noise refers to a preconceived bias about the speaker or listener, differences in role status, ethnic or cultural differences that influence transmission of messages, and how they are received. *Semantic* noise is concerned with the use of uncommon abstract words, not easily understood by one of the communicators. Even one "noise" factor can compromise successful interpersonal communication.

TRANSACTIONAL MODELS OF COMMUNICATION

Transactional models expand the nature of linear models by including internal forms in the context of the communication, feedback loops, and validation. These models employ systems concepts in that the human system (client) receives information from the environment (input), internally processes the received data, and interprets its meaning (throughput). The result is new information or behavior (output). Feedback loops (from the receiver or the environment) validate the information or allow the human system to correct its original information. In doing so, transactional models draw attention to communication as having purpose, and meaning making attributes. Figure 1-1 shows the components of transactional models.

Transactional models conceptualize interpersonal communication as a reciprocal interaction in which sender and receiver influence each other as they converse. Each person constructs a mental picture of the other, including perceptions of the other person's attitude and possible reaction to the message. Individual perceptions influence the transmission of the message and its meaning to one or both of the communicators. Because the sender and receiver communicate at the same time, the conversation becomes a richer process and more than the sum of its parts.

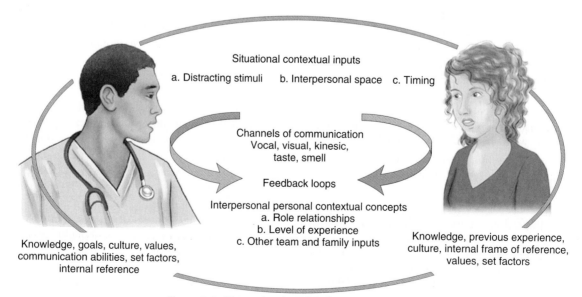

Figure 1-1   Transactional model of communication.

Transactional models capture the importance of interpersonal engagement in verbal and nonverbal communication. They reflect the development of collaborative meanings, which are cocreated from the symbolic exchanges between the communicators. Role relationships between communicators can influence communication. Often role relationships are unconsciously acted on, without taking their nature or implications for successful communication into account. Lack of awareness can compromise the effect of important messages. Exercise 1-4, Comparing Linear and Transactional Models of Communication, provides an opportunity to contrast the efficacy of linear versus transactional models.

People take either symmetric or complementary roles in communicating. **Symmetric role relationships** are equal, whereas **complementary role relationships** typically operate with one person holding a higher position than the other in the communication process. Nurses assume a *complementary* role of clinical expert available for information and consultation to achieve mutually determined health goals, and a *symmetric* role in working with the client as partner on developing mutually defined goals and the means to achieve them.

THERAPEUTIC COMMUNICATION

Therapeutic communication is a term originally coined by Ruesch (1961) to describe a goal-directed form of communication used in health care to achieve goals that promote client health and well-being. Doheny and colleagues (2007) observed that "when certain skills are used to facilitate communication between nurse and client in a goal directed manner, the therapeutic communication process occurs" (p. 5). Core dimensions of therapeutic communication—empathy, respect, helpful genuineness, and concreteness—are discussed in Chapters 5, 6 and 10.

FRAMEWORKS USED IN THERAPEUTIC RELATIONSHIPS

Commonly used frameworks used in professional nursing relationships include Erikson's psychosocial development theory, Maslow's basic human needs model, Peplau's psychosocial relationship nursing theory, general systems theory, and communication models.

Developmental Theory

Erik Erikson's theory of psychosocial development is considered an important conceptual framework for understanding human personal development (Erikson, 1950). Erikson's model represents one of the most solid theories of psychosocial development across the life span.

Nurses use this framework to assess developmental client needs and to design *developmentally* age-appropriate nursing interventions.

According to Erikson, human development occurs in universally defined sequential maturity stages. Each stage builds on the previous stage and requires a higher level of expected psychosocial competence. A person experiences each new set of expectations in the form of a psychosocial crisis. Confronting and successfully mastering tensions associated with each developmental psychosocial crisis, helps a person develop an associated ego strength. Failure to mature psychosocially results in a core weakness or pathology. Erikson identifies the first four stages of ego identity as building blocks for ego identity, which he considers the keystone of psychosocial development. The last three developmental stages help refine the ego identity in the adult segment of the life cycle.

EXERCISE 1-4	Comparing Linear and Transactional Models of Communication

Purpose: To help students see the difference between linear and circular models of communication.

Procedure
1. Role-play a scenario in which one person provides a scene that might occur in the clinical area using a linear model: sender, message, and receiver.
2. Role-play the same scenario using a circular model, framing questions that recognize the context of the message and its potential impact on the receiver, and provide feedback.

Discussion
1. Was there a difference in your level of comfort? If so, in what ways?
2. Was there any difference in the amount of information you had as a result of the communication? If so, in what ways?
3. What implications does this exercise have for your future nursing practice?

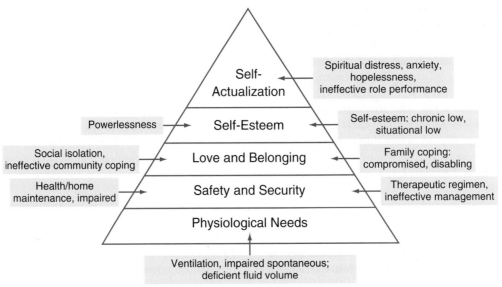

Figure 1-2   Nursing Diagnosis Categories corresponding with Maslow's hierarchy of needs.

Life circumstances, culture, and timing can affect age-related psychosocial ego development, such that it progresses at a faster or slower pace, and the behaviors indicating psychosocial competence may differ.

Peplau's Interpersonal Relationship Model

Hildegard Peplau (1952, 1997) offers the best-known nursing model for the study of interpersonal relationships in health care. Her model describes how the nurse-client relationship can facilitate the identification and accomplishment of therapeutic goals to enhance client and family well-being (see Chapter 10). In contemporary practice, Peplau's framework is more applicable today with long term relationships in rehabilitation centers, long-term care, and nursing homes. Despite the brevity of the alliances in acute care settings, basic principles of being a participant-observer in the relationship, building rapport, developing a working partnership, and terminating a relationship remain relevant.

Basic Needs Theory

The ICN declares, "human needs guide the work of nursing" (2010). Abraham Maslow's needs theory (1970) is a framework that nurses use to *prioritize* client needs, and develop relevant nursing approaches (see Chapters 2 and 10). Maslow's model proposes that people are motivated to meet their needs in an ascending order beginning with meeting basic survival needs.

As essential needs are satisfied, people move into higher psychosocial areas of development. Maslow defines basic (deficiency) needs as those required for human survival. First-level *basic physiological needs* include hunger, thirst, sexual appetites, and sensory stimulation. Maslow's second level, *safety and security needs*, includes both physical safety and emotional security, for example, financial safety, freedom from injury, safe neighborhood, and freedom from abuse.

Satisfaction of basic deficiency needs allows for attention to growth needs, which Maslow termed *love and belonging needs*, followed by self-esteem needs. Love and belonging needs relate to emotionally experiencing being a part of a family, and/or community. *Self-esteem needs* refer to a person's need for recognition and appreciation. A sense of dignity, respect, and approval by others for oneself is the hallmark of successfully meeting self-esteem needs.

Maslow's highest level of need satisfaction, self-actualization, refers to a person's need to achieve his or her maximum potential. Self-actualized individuals are not superhuman; they are subject to the same feelings of insecurity that all individuals experience, but they recognize and accept their vulnerability as part of the human condition. Not everyone reaches Maslow's self-actualization stage.

Figure 1-2 shows Maslow's model as a pyramid, with need requirements occurring in ascending fashion from basic survival needs through self-actualization.

EXERCISE 1-5	Maslow's Hierarchy of Needs

Purpose: To help students understand the usefulness of Maslow's theory in clinical practice.

Procedure
1. Divide the class into small groups, with each group assigned to a step of Maslow's hierarchy. Each group will then brainstorm examples of that need as it might present in clinical practice.
2. Identify potential responses from the nurse that might address each need.

3. Share examples with the larger group and discuss the concept of prioritization of needs using Maslow's hierarchy.

Discussion
1. In what ways is Maslow's hierarchy helpful to the nurse in prioritizing client needs?
2. What limitations do you see with the theory?

Nurses use Maslow's theory to prioritize nursing interventions. Exercise 1-5 provides practice with using Maslow's model in clinical practice.

APPLICATIONS

GENERAL SYSTEMS THEORY

A systems framework forms the contextual underpinning for the study of contemporary professional nursing in the United States. Beginning with the idea that each person is "different from and greater than the sum of his or her parts (Chinn and Kramer, 2011, p. 47), a systems framework provides a solid foundation for understanding the nature of communication and group dynamics. From a systems perspective, everything within the health care system is interrelated and interdependent (Porter O'Grady and Malloch, 2014). Collaboration and teamwork provider relationships, family relationships, continuity of care, and newly redefined system linkages between education, service, and research are best interpreted within a systems framework. The WHO has defined a health system as "all organizations, people and actions whose primary intent is to promote, restore or maintain health" (WHO, 2007, p. 2).

General systems theory (GST), initially described by Ludwig von Bertalanffy (1968), focuses on process and the interconnected relationships comprising the "whole." Over the years, systems thinking has been transformed into a "meta-language which can be used to talk about the subject matter of many different fields (Checkland, 1999). Even our bodily functions depend on an understanding of the interrelationships among body systems.

Adaptive system models help health professionals understand *how* the interrelationships among different

parts of the system contribute to its overall functioning at macro and micro levels. New skills and competencies introduced into nursing contemporary curriculums are based on systems approaches to help nurses collaborate effectively with other disciplines having different agendas and priorities to achieve common goals. Frenk and colleagues (2010) suggest that "the core space of every health system is occupied by the unique encounter between one set of people who need services and another who have been entrusted to deliver them" (p. 7). Note that patient/client is represented as the core of the health care system diagram in Figure 1-3.

A GST approach highlights the interdependence among all parts of a system and confirms how each part supports the system as a functional, ordered whole. Berkes and colleagues (2003) state that GST, "emphasizes connectedness, context and feedback, a key concept that refers to the result of any behavior that may reinforce (positive feedback) or modify (negative feedback) subsequent behavior" (p. 5).

In Figure 1-3, notice the outermost system ring relates to regulatory bodies. This relates to care delivered by integrated care facilities, which are subject to significant government regulation and joint commission oversight. Health care systems are viewed as integrated wholes whose properties cannot be effectively reduced to a single unit (Porter O'Grady and Malloch, 2014.) The interacting parts work together to achieve important goals. Only by looking at the whole picture can one fully appreciate its meaning of how its individual parts work together. How health providers use collaborative and networking skills to achieve clinical outcomes become the measure of competence from a systems perspective. There is a contemporary emphasis on interrelationships, and behavioral patterns within

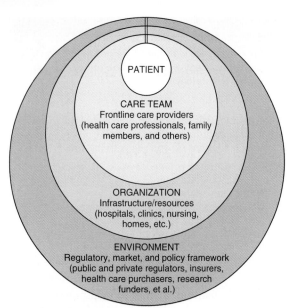

PATIENT

CARE TEAM
Frontline care providers
(health care professionals, family
members, and others)

ORGANIZATION
Infrastructure/resources
(hospitals, clinics, nursing,
homes, etc.)

ENVIRONMENT
Regulatory, market, and policy framework
(public and private regulators, insurers,
health care purchasers, research
funders, et al.)

Figure 1-3 Conceptual drawing of a four-level health care system, with the client (patient) as its core concept. *(From Reid PP, Compton WD, Grossman JH, et al., editors, for the Committee on Engineering and the Health Care System, National Academy of Engineering, Institute of Medicine. Building a better delivery system: a new engineering/health care partnership. Washington, DC, 2005, National Academies Press, p. 20. Available at* http://www.nap.edu/catalog/11378.html.)

the organizational system. Porter O'Grady and Malloch observe "to the extent that the balance and harmony are sustained, the organization's life is advanced." (p. 15).

System boundaries separate the system from the environment. Boundaries are arbitrary parameters, which distinguish what belongs with the system, and what lies outside of it. The environment consists of anything that affects system functioning, but it is not part of the system. Each system is separated by *boundaries,* which control the exchange of information, energy, and resources into and out of the system. Flexible boundaries allow new information to flow in and out of the system, whereas rigid boundaries do not. A system with flexible boundaries is termed an *open system.* A closed system has rigid boundaries; not much crosses its boundaries. *Outcomes* are referred to as *output.* Any changes in the system will influence the outcome or output. *Feedback loops* (what others from the environment say about the process) inform the system of changes needed for input so as to achieve more effective outcomes. For example, a client's response to a treatment offers feedback on whether to change a medication, or continue with it.

ISSUES RELATED TO HEALTH CARE REFORM

Creasia and Frieberg (2011) note that, historically significant changes in nursing and nursing education are linked to socioeconomic factors and nursing issues. Professional nursing is practiced today in an unprecedented era of shifting health care environments, momentous advances in health science, and unparalleled evolving technologies. Socioeconomic issues, such as the dramatic growth in health care options, population demographics, serious nursing, and physician shortages, the economics of health care, and documented concerns about safety and quality in health care, have prompted a fast-moving mandate to transform the current health care system. Most health care is delivered in community-based primary care settings with an emphasis on prevention and support for self-management of chronic health conditions. In 2000, the Pew Health Professions Report identified 21 competencies needed to reframe nursing practice for a new century (Bellack and O'Neil, 2000). These competencies are identified in Box 1-2.

Nurses are expected to have knowledge about and apply a variety of paradigms to real-life situations in clinical practice. Client roles have evolved from being passive recipients of health care into active autonomous partners with providers. Shared authority over decision making, and multiple perspectives in health care management across a continuum of care that extends into the community is the new norm.

In 2010, the Patient Protection and Affordable Care Act (PPACA) was signed into federal law. This law ushers in the most significant change to the U.S. health care system since the establishment of Medicare in 1965 (Kaiser Permanente, 2013). U.S. citizens and legal immigrants will be *required* to have a basic level of health care insurance.

Nurse practitioners (NPs), physicians, and physician assistants will continue to be the principal providers of primary care in the United States, and the need for continuity of care through collaborative team work will become even more important. To adequately dress increased expectations for skilled health care, special attention to the role of nurses, particularly advanced practice registered nurses (APRNs) becomes critical.

Managed care, the emergence of transdisciplinary professional roles as the preferred model of provider service delivery, public reporting of clinical outcomes, and inclusion of client quality of life and satisfaction with care are now expected clinical outcomes. Table 1-1 identifies seven conditions and their evolutionary correlates

BOX 1-2	Pew Commission's Recommendations to Nursing Programs: 21 Nursing Competencies Needed for the Twenty-First Century

1. Embrace a personal ethic of social responsibility and service.
2. Exhibit ethical behavior in all professional activities.
3. Provide evidence-based, clinically competent care.
4. Incorporate the multiple determinants of health in clinical care.
5. Apply knowledge of the new sciences.
6. Demonstrate critical thinking, reflection, and problem-solving skills.
7. Understand the role of primary care.
8. Rigorously practice preventive health care.
9. Integrate population-based care and services into practice.
10. Improve access to health care for those with unmet health needs.
11. Practice relationship-centered care with individuals and families.
12. Provide culturally sensitive care to a diverse society.
13. Partner with communities in health care decisions.
14. Use communication and information technology effectively and appropriately.
15. Work in interdisciplinary teams.
16. Ensure care that balances individual, professional, system, and societal needs.
17. Practice leadership.
18. Take responsibility for quality of care and health outcomes at all levels.
19. Contribute to continuous improvement of the health care system.
20. Advocate for public policy that promotes and protects the health of the public.
21. Continue to learn and help others learn.

From Bellack J, O'Neil E: Recreating nursing practice for a new century: recommendations and implications of the Pew Health Professions Commission's final report, *Nurs Health Care Perspect* 21(1):20, 2000.

TABLE 1-1	Criteria for Survival of the Nursing Profession Based on Evolutionary Principles
Criteria or Condition	**Evolutionary Principle**
Nursing needs to be relevant.	In nature, an organism will survive only if it occupies a niche, that is, performs a specific role that is needed in its environment.
Nursing must be accountable.	In every environment, there is a limited amount of resources. Organisms that are more efficient and use the available resources more effectively are much more likely to be selected by the environment.
Nursing needs to retain its uniqueness while functioning in a multidisciplinary setting.	In nature, an organism will survive only if it is unique. If it ceases to be so, it is in danger of losing its niche or role in the environment. In other words, it might lose out if the new species is slightly better adapted to the role, or if physically similar enough, it might even breed with that species and thus completely lose its identity. Successful organisms must also learn to coexist with many different species so that their role complements that of the other organisms.
Nursing needs to be visible.	In nature, organisms often are required to defend their niche and their territory usually by an outward display that allows other similar species to be aware of their presence. By being "visible," similar species can avoid direct conflict. In addition, visibility is also important for recognition by members of their own species, to allow for the formation of family and social units, based on cooperation and respect.
Nursing needs to have a global impact.	In nature, if a species is to survive, it must make its presence felt not just to its immediate neighbors but to all the members of its environment. Often, this results in a species adapting a unique presence, whether it is a color pattern, smell, or sound.
Nurses need to be innovators.	In evolution, the organisms that survive are, more often than not, innovators that have the flexibility to come up with new and different solutions to rapid changes in environmental conditions.
Nurses need to be both exceptionally competent and strive for excellence.	During evolution, when new niches open up, it is never possible for more than one species to occupy one niche. Only the best adapted and most competent among the competing organisms will survive; all others, even if only slightly less competent, will die.

From Bell (1997) as cited in Gottlieb L, Gottlieb B: Evolutionary principles can guide nursing's future development, *J Adv Nurs* 28(5):1099, 1998.

needed to secure a key player role for nurses in the new health care delivery system.

Porter O'Grady and Malloch (2014) refer to today's health care system as being radically transformed with new nonlinear and socially transformational realities. The context of professional interpersonal relationships in nursing and health care includes broader interconnections with other clinicians, health care decision makers, and other policy makers. Health care decision makers include the client as a key agent. The IOM recommendations described in the following section call for a systems-based team-care environment across clinical settings and collaborative teamwork across disciplines as the best means of reducing health disparities and promoting safe quality care. Communication skills and the development of stronger collaborative team-based professional interpersonal relationships will be key to integrating these competencies in health care delivery.

IMPACT OF INSTITUTE OF MEDICINE REPORT RECOMMENDATIONS

A series of IOM reports serve as a major force in driving and shaping the sweeping changes occurring in the health care delivery system nationally and globally. The overarching goals of these efforts relate to

1. Improving the patient's (client's) experience of care
2. Improving the health of individuals and populations
3. Reducing the per capita cost of health care

Over the past decade, a dramatic paradigm shift has emerged beginning with the publication of two IOM reports detailing serious quality and safety problems with health care delivery in the United States, and calling for radical change. Four priorities for national action were identified as depicted in Figure 1-4.

An initial IOM report, *To Err Is Human* (2000) drew attention to serious lapses in safety and quality in health care. A second report, *Crossing the Quality Chasm*, called for an innovative transformed health care system that is evidence-based, patient-centered, and systems oriented. It identified expected quality performance goals: effectiveness, timeliness, patient-centeredness, efficiency, and equity (IOM, 2001). The goals place clients at the center of the health care team. Subsequent IOM reports advocate an integrated inter-disciplinary team approach, with shared accountability for outcomes, as the preferred delivery system. Reports

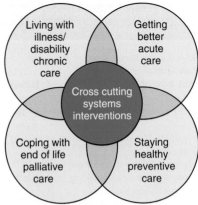

Figure 1-4 Priority Areas for National Action. Four stages of life and health are described in the four circles, connected by the need for coordination across time and health care. (*From Adams K, Corrigan JM, editors, for the Committee on Identifying Areas for Quality Improvement, Board on Health Care Services, Institute of Medicine.* Priority areas for national action: transforming health care quality. *Washington, DC, 2003, National Academies Press.*)

relevant to nursing and transformation in health care are presented in Table 1-2.

IOM recommendations have been endorsed by the American Association of Colleges of Nursing, National State Boards of Nursing, and the American Nurses Association. These reports serve as a dynamic foundation for aligning interprofessional competency domains with contextualized individual professional circumstances in professional education (Interprofessional Education Collaborative Expert Panel, 2011).

Expanded curriculum development is deemed essential to reforming the health care system. Frenk and colleagues (2010) describes the need to approach interdisciplinary education using "a global outlook, a multiprofessional perspective, and a systems approach" (p. 5).

The IOM report *Health Professions Education: A Bridge to Quality* (2003) calls for the restructuring of clinical education responsive to the twenty-first century health system transformation goals of providing the highest quality and safest medical care possible. This report identified five core areas of competency, required to cross the bridge to quality:

*   Delivering patient-centered care
*   Working as part of interdisciplinary teams
*   Practicing evidence-based medicine
*   Focusing on quality improvement
*   Using information technology (IOM, 2003)

TABLE 1-2	National Reports with Goals, Relevant to Nursing's Role in the Transformation of the Health Care System
Institute of Medicine Report	**Identified Goals**
2000: *To err is human: building a safer health system*	• Establish a national focus to enhance knowledge base of safety. • Develop a public mandatory reporting system to identify and learn from errors. • Implement safety systems to ensure safe practices at the delivery level. • Raise performance standards and expectations for safety improvement.
2003: *Health professions education: a bridge to quality*	Competency in: • Delivering patient-centered care, • Working as part of interdisciplinary teams, • Practicing evidence-based medicine, • Focusing on quality improvement and • Using information technology.
2009: *Redesigning continuing education in the health professions*	• Bring together health professionals from different disciplines in tailored learning environments. • Replace the current culture of continuing education (CE) with a new vision of professional development. • Establish a national interprofessional CE institute to foster improvements.
2010: *The future of nursing: leading change, advancing health*	• Practice at the full extent of their education and training • Achievement of higher levels of education and training through an improved education system that promotes seamless academic progression • Full partnership with physicians and other health professionals in redesigning health care in the United States • Better data collection and improved information infrastructure regarding workforce planning and policy making • Remove scope of practice barriers
2010: *Healthy People 2020* (www.healthypeople.gov)	1. Attain high-quality, longer lives free of preventable disease, disability, injury, and premature death. 2. Achieve health equity, eliminate disparities, and improve the health of all groups. 3. Create social and physical environments that promote good health for all. 4. Promote quality of life, healthy development, and healthy behaviors across all life stages.

Data from Institute of Medicine (IOM): *To err is human: building a safer health system*, Washington, DC, 2000, National Academies Press; IOM: *Health professions education: a bridge to quality*, Washington, DC, 2003, National Academies Press; IOM: *Redesigning continuing education in the health professions*, Washington, DC, 2009, National Academies Press; IOM: *The future of nursing: leading change, advancing health*, Washington, DC, 2010, National Academies Press; IOM: The future of nursing: accomplishments a year after the landmark report (editorial), *J Nurs Scholarsh* 44(1):1, 2012.

IOM competencies identified in Chapter 1 as conceptual underpinnings for communication and interpersonal relationships in professional nursing practice are discussed and integrated throughout the text. These are briefly described in the following sections.

Delivering Client-Centered Care

Whereas client-centered care is now *mandated* as an essential characteristic of contemporary health care delivery, it is a core value that nursing has always championed. The IOM defines **patient-centered care** as "care that is respectful of and responsive to individual patient preferences, needs, and values" (2001). Patient-centered approaches view the client as a primary source of influence and core decision maker on the health care team. Nurses are charged with understanding and anticipating client needs rather than simply interacting with presenting health care circumstances.

Carl Rogers' **person-centered relationship model** (1946) offers a conceptual basis for studying "client/patient-centered" care. Rogers believed that support for the individual integrity and self-responsibility of each client in an empathetic, accepting relationship empowered clients to become self-directed and develop new skills. He pointed to the primacy of the client as the most important source of knowledge, and a fundamental agent of healing. He described the client/health provider relationship as an equal partnership. Rogers believed that "the constructive forces in the individual can be trusted, and that the more deeply they are relied upon, the more deeply they are released" (Rogers, 1946, p. 418). Learning about the client's values, preferences, and perceptions related to the client's health care situation are critical dimensions of contemporary client-centered relationships (see Chapter 10).

Client-centered care requires that scientific guidelines be balanced with values-based nursing knowledge. Frist (2005) asserted that the focus of the twenty-first-century health care system must ensure that clients have access to the safest and highest-quality care, regardless of how much they earn, where they live, how sick they are, or the color of their skin (p. 468).

WORKING AS PART OF INTERDISCIPLINARY TEAMS

Health care reform calls for collaborative interdisciplinary teams of health care professionals, rather single practitioners assuming responsibility for the health care of clients (Batalden et al., 2006; IOM, 2003). The concept of collaboration is based on the premise that no single health care discipline can provide complete care for clients with multiple health and social care needs.

Interprofessional care teams are peopled by highly skilled professionals working together with a client for the common purpose of improving a client's health status. Professional team providers have complementary interdependent professional roles supported by mutual respect and power sharing. Collaborative health care efforts represent a non-hierarchal system of care delivery. Care coordination, and making connections between multiple care providers is viewed as an essential component of collaboration (Craig et al., 2011).

Recommendations from the IOM Report: *Health Professions Education: A Bridge to Quality* (2003) led to the Quality and Safety Education for Nurses (QSEN) initiative (Cronenwett et al., 2007) discussed in Chapter 2, and integrated throughout the text. QSEN competencies provide a solid conceptual framework for professional nursing education curriculums at all levels, and for clinical practice.

Bronstein's model is a frequently used conceptual framework (Kilgore and Langford, 2010) for the study of interdisciplinary collaboration. Each collaborative team takes collective ownership of treatment goals, determines the professional activities needed to achieve them, and has ongoing reflective communication about their process. Personal characteristics and the professional makeup of the team, the team's structural characteristics, and its level of experience with interdisciplinary collaborative approaches influence collaborative effectiveness (Bronstein, 2003). A multidimensional construct, defines "client," individually, or broadly as its core, and as an integral decision maker on the health care team.

Interprofessional collaboration requires communication and relationship skills that nurses can only be taught with interdisciplinary curriculum exposures involving more than one discipline (Bjorke and Haavie, 2006). Applications of interdisciplinary collaboration involve a socialization process that ideally begins early in the student's professional education. Students develop broader habits of inquiry and a comprehensive understanding of how to work with other professional disciplines productively. They learn firsthand about the value of a collective systems approach to diagnosis and treatment in a time of diminishing resources.

PRACTICING EVIDENCE-BASED NURSING

The scope of practice and nature of work for contemporary nurses has become multidimensional, multirelational, and highly complex. Practicing evidence based nursing (EBP) is every nurse's responsibility. What this means is that nurses should conscientiously keep up to date with the latest research and any published practice guidelines relevant to guiding their nursing practice (Rycroft-Malone et al., 2004). Applications for magnet status (Chapter 22) require proof of evidence-based practice. The strength of EBP lies in the blending of extensive clinical experience with sound clinical research and professional judgment in real-time client situations. EBP provides the foundational knowledge and facilitates the self-confidence new nurses need to interact effectively on interdisciplinary health care teams (Pfaff, et al., 2013). The collective wisdom of EBP is dynamically related to nursing theory through empirical ways of knowing. The concept of EBP consists of four elements:

1. *Best practices*, derived from consensus statements developed by expert clinicians and researchers
2. *Evidence from scientific findings* in research-based studies found in published journals

3. *Clinical nursing expertise* of professional nurses, including knowledge of pathophysiology, pharmacology, and psychology
4. *Preferences and values of clients* and family members (Sigma Theta Tau International, 2003)

Developing an Evidence-Based Practice

Stans S, Stevens A, Beurskens J. Interprofessional practice in primary care: development of a tailored process model. *J Multi Health Care.* 6:139-147, 2013.

Background: This qualitative study investigated interprofessional practice in a primary care setting, using the domains of the chronic care model as a framework. A target intervention consisting of three steps described targets for improvement for children with complex care needs, identified barriers and facilitators influencing interprofessional practice, and developed a tailored interprofessional process model.

Methodology: A qualitative methodology consisting of 13 semistructured interviews with the children's parents and professionals involved in the care of the children. Data were analyzed using direct content analysis. This step led to the development of a project group that formulated an interprofessional process through process mapping.

Findings: The most significant barrier to implementing the interprofessional practice related to the lack of structure in the care process and knowing what should be involved in the process in interprofessional practice. Study participants expressed the need to have structured communication through face-to-face meetings, and an electronic clinical information system.

Application to Your Clinical Practice: Regular multidisciplinary meetings, structured communication, and a defined system for division of tasks—"who does what" and "when" is *essential* for successful team process.

FOCUSING ON QUALITY IMPROVEMENT

Quality improvement in nursing historically began with Florence Nightingale's use of morbidity and mortality statistics to improve the quality of care during the Crimean War (Sousa and Corning-Davis, 2013). Batalden and Davidoff (2007) define **quality improvement** (QI) as "the combined and unceasing efforts of everyone—healthcare professionals, patients and their

families, researchers, payers, planners and educators—to make the changes that will lead to better patient outcomes (health), better system performance (care) and better professional development" (p. 2). Quality improvement (QI) is the responsibility of everyone in the organizational system, including clients. QI processes provide a measurable systematic way to ensure that the goals of care are

- *Appropriate:* for the client, and care requirements
- *Adequate:* to meet clinical requirements and client needs, including level of resources and skill mix of providers.
- *Effective:* care meets or exceed established standards of care
- *Efficient:* in terms of cost and time

Although the defining purpose of QI is health improvement, an essential component is identifying the resources to make care delivery an equitable reality for all (WHO, 2000). QI processes require that each organizational system, together with all of its stakeholders, develop a quality philosophy that matches the unique needs of the organization. Competency domains act as flexible practice guidelines, which are applicable across professions (Interprofessional Expert Panel, 2011).

USING INFORMATICS

The world from an interpersonal communication perspective is much different than it was even a decade ago—smaller and substantively better connected through technology. Smith and Wilson, (2010) note, "interpersonal relationships can be initiated, escalated, maintained, and dissolved either wholly, or in part, through mediated technology" (p. 14). Digital communication greatly expands interpersonal and professional communication, but a word of caution is needed. Texting, Instagrams, and e-mails do not allow the receiver to see facial expressions, hear the tonality of a message, or readily interpret an emotionally charged communication. Clarity and conciseness are essential, and all electronic messages are subject to HIPPA regulations.

Telehealth is fast becoming an integral part of the health care system, used both as a live interactive mechanism as presented earlier (particularly in remote areas, where there is a scarcity of health care providers), and as a way to track clinical data. Two important outcomes are reduction of health costs and access to care (Peck, 2005; Cipriano and Murphy, 2011).

The following case example represents a "virtual" application of communication through technology from the perspective of a Canadian nurse caring for a client in a remote area as it might occur in contemporary practice. The video system used in the case study has a monitoring device on both ends, with voice activation. The personalized contact allows clients and caregivers to communicate directly with each other from distant locations.

Case Example

The computer gently hums to life as community health nurse Rachel Muhammat logs into Nursenet. She asks a research partner, a cyberware specialist in London, England, for the results from a trial on neurologic side effects of ocular biochips. Rachel, as part of a 61-member team in 23 countries, is studying six clients with the chips. Then it is down to local business. Rachel e-mails information on air contaminant syndrome to a client down the street whose son is susceptible to the condition and tells her about a support group in Philadelphia. She contacts a qigong specialist to see if he can teach the boy breathing exercises and schedules an appointment with an environmental nurse specialist. Moments before her 9:45 appointment, Rachel gets into her El-van and programs it to an address 2 kilometers away. Her client, Mr. Chan, lost both legs in a subway accident and needs to be prepared for a bionic double-leg transplant. Together, they assess his needs and put together a team of health workers, including a surgeon, physical therapist, acupuncturist, and home care helpers. She talks to him about the transplant, and they hook up to his virtual reality computer to see and talk to another client who underwent the same procedure. Before leaving, Mr. Chan grasps her hand and thanks her for helping him. Rachel hugs him and urges him to e-mail her if he has any more questions (Sibbald, 1995, p. 33 [quoted in Clark, 2000]).

Technology advances provide nurses with new capabilities for transmission of data within and between care settings. Electronic records and communication technologies have revolutionized the way health information is processed (Cipriano and Murphy, 2011). Virtually every major health care system has switched to electronic medical record (EMR) keeping and bar code scanners for medications or identification. Web portals and other technological supports, which were not possible even a decade ago, assist clients at entry points to an increasingly complex health care system. Technology provides a powerful way to enhance access and coordination of health information across health care systems. Promoting greater availability of information transfer between client consumers and relevant health care providers can and improve patient/clinician

collaboration and decision-making. High quality technology can empower client self-management, and improve health outcomes (Wagner et al., 2010). Conversely, technology can contribute to dehumanization in health care delivery. It is only as useful as the ability of the people who control its use and the quality of information that is collected and shared. The client, not the information alone, should be the primary focus directing care.

The general public routinely uses computers and technical devices to access health-related information. Health care providers use the Internet to collaborate about research, and to seek consultation about the management of care delivery, referrals, and sharing of other health-related information and concerns. Secured Web portals that meet the Health Insurance Portability and Accountability Act (HIPAA) requirements are customized to meet the information needs of, or about, designated groups of people (Moody, 2005). Technology enhances the potential for global health care. Health experts in geographically distant areas throughout the world can share information and draw important conclusions about health care issues in real time.

Technology is routinely and extensively used in nursing education. Use of high-fidelity simulations help nurse educators and students develop critical thinking and collaborative management skills in a safe, realistic environment. Students receive feedback from the "simulated" patient. Simulations allow students from different health disciplines to share methods of reasoning, situational awareness, shared language, and behaviors in different clinical scenarios. As students communicate, and jointly explain their thinking processes about the clinical scenario, they develop a shared cognition that is more comprehensive than what could be attained by a single discipline focus.

THE FUTURE OF NURSING

The challenges and opportunities for professional nurses today are unparalleled. Currently, there is a major shortage of professional nurses. The rapid expansion of the populations requiring health care has caused the scope and complexity of nursing practice to expand exponentially particularly over the past decade.

Nursing is recognized as a critical professional body needed to transform the health care system in line with the IOM's (2001) vision of a "high performance, client centered health care system." A tidal wave of current and projected changes in the health care system creates the need for nurses to clearly "own" the essence of professional nursing and to redefine their professional role responsibilities within a collaborative interdisciplinary patient-centered health care system. IOM (2014) notes: Contemporary professionalism supports team based processes of multiple professions working together with cross-disciplinary responsibilities and accountability for achieving improved clinical outcomes IOM, 2014.

No longer labeled the "invisible profession" (Andrist et al., 2006), nurses are slated to become key players in a transformed health care system. In 2010, IOM and Robert Wood Johnson Foundation released its report on the future of nursing, entitled *The Future of Nursing: Leading Change, Advancing Health*. Four recommendations emphasize nursing's leadership role in facilitating the transformation of the health care system.

1. Nurses should practice to the full extent of their education and training.
2. Nurses should achieve higher levels of education and training through an improved education system that promotes seamless academic progression.
3. Nurses should be full partners, with physicians and other health professionals, in redesigning health care in the United States.
4. Effective workforce planning and policy making require better data collection and an improved information infrastructure (Litwack, 2013, IOM, 2010).

Changes in nursing education will be key to achieving these goals. Substantially more nurses will need to be educated at the graduate level; a baccalaureate degree in nursing will become essential (Aiken, 2011).

SUMMARY

Chapter 1 identifies various theory-based concepts important to the understanding of professional and nurse-client relationships in contemporary health care delivery. Concepts of nursing's metaparadigm, found across all nursing models include person, environment, health, and nursing. "Ways of knowing" help nurses to frame their interactions with clients and families based on forms of knowledge reflecting a different set of assumptions regarding client needs. These models bring order to nursing practice and provide a cognitive theoretical basis for nursing research. The process of communication is analyzed and the contributions of communication theory to the study of developmental theories used by nurses as presented in this chapter helps nurses integrate scientific understandings with a personalized approach to individual clients.

Hildegard Peplau's theory of interpersonal relationships forms a theoretical basis for understanding the nurse's role in the nurse-client relationship. Concepts from other developmental and psychological theories broaden the nurse's perspective and understanding of client behaviors. Nurses use Erikson's model of psychosocial development to provide nursing care in line with developmental needs of their clients and Maslow's need theory to prioritize care activities. Carl Rogers's emphasizes a client-centered approach and identifies conditions needed to facilitate personality change through increased insight and self understanding (Anderson, 2001). He offered basic concepts concerning characteristics the nurse needs for developing effective interpersonal relationships with clients. Therapeutic communication is used in the nurse-client relationship as a primary means of achieving treatment goals.

Dramatic transformational changes in the health care delivery system will require nurses to embrace new competencies consistent with advances in science, contemporary health care, and shifting demographic diversity of health care consumers. Highly skilled nurses are needed to provide complex care and leadership in a transdisciplinary health care system. IOM recommendations, and those of other nationally recognized health care experts, create a mandate for increased numbers of baccalaureate and advanced practice nurses to handle the complex demands of contemporary care delivery. Nurses have an unprecedented opportunity to make a difference and shape the future of nursing practice through communication at every level in health care delivery.

ETHICAL DILEMMA   What Would You Do?

Craig Montegue is a difficult client to care for. As his nurse, you find his constant arguments, poor hygiene, and the way he treats his family very upsetting. It is difficult for you to provide him with even the most basic care, and you just want to leave his room as quickly as possible. How could you use a patient-centered approach to understanding Craig? What are the ethical elements in this situation, and how would you address them in implementing care for Craig?

DISCUSSION QUESTIONS

1. In what ways does the discipline of nursing today reflect or refute the disciplines' original three themes identified in Donaldson and Crowley's seminal article of 1978?
2. How would you envision the nature of professional nursing practice in the future?
3. What do you consider to be the unique attributes of the nursing professionals today?

REFERENCES

Aiken L: Nurses for the future, *N Engl J Med* (364):196–198, 2011.

Alligood M: *Nursing Theory: Utilization and Application*, ed 4, Maryland Heights, MO, 2010, Mosby Elsevier.

Alligood M: *Nursing Theorists and Their Work 8th*, St. Louis MO, 2014, Mosby Elsevier.

Altmann T: An evaluation of the seminal work of Patricia Benner: theory or philosophy? *Contemp Nurs* 25:114–123, 2007.

American Nurses Association: *Scope and Standards of Nursing*, 2nd ed., Silver Spring, MD, 2010, American Nurses Association.

Anderson H: Postmodern collaborative and person-centered therapies: what would Carl Rogers say? *J Fam Ther* 23:339–360, 2001.

Andrist L, Nicholas P, Wolf K: *A history of nursing ideas*, Boston, 2006, Jones and Bartlett Publishers.

Arnold E: Caring from the graduate student perspective, *Int J Hum Caring* 1(3):32–42, 1997.

Batalden P, Ogrinc G, Batalden M: From one to many, *J Interprof Care* 20(5):549–551, 2006.

Baltaden P, Davidoff F: What is "quality improvement" and how can it transform health care, *Qual Saf Health Care* 16(1):2–3, 2007.

Bateson G: *Mind and nature*, New York, 1979, Dutton.

Bellack J, O'Neil E: Recreating nursing practice for a new century: recommendations and implications of the Pew Health Professions Commission's final report, *Nurs Health Care Perspect* 21(1):14–21, 2000.

Berkes F, Colding J, Folke C: *Navigating social-ecological systems: Building resilience for complexity and change*, New York, 2003, Cambridge University Press.

Bertalanffy LV: *General system theory: Foundations, development, applications*, New York, 1968, George Braziller.

Best A, Moor G, Holmes B, Clark PI, Bruce T, Leischow S, et al.: Health promotion dissemination and systems thinking: towards an integrative model, *Am. J. Health Behav.* 27(Suppl 3):S206–S216, 2003.

Bjorke G, Haavie N: Crossing boundaries: Implementing an interprofessional module into uniprofessional bachelor programmes, *J Interprof Care* 20(6):641–653, 2006.

Bronstein LR: A model for interdisciplinary collaboration, *Soc Work* 48:297–306, 2003.

Carper B: Fundamental patterns of knowing in nursing, *ANS Adv Nurs Sci* 1:13–23, 1978.

Chinn P, Kramer M: *Integrated theory and knowledge: Development in nursing*, 8th ed., St. Louis, MO, 2011, Mosby, Inc.

Checkland P: In Currie WL, Galliers. B, editors: Systems thinking in: *Rethinking management information systems*, Oxford NY, 1999, Oxford University Press, p 48.

Cipriano PF, Murphy J: Nursing informatics. The future of nursing and health IT: the quality elixir, *Nurs Econ* 29(5), 2011 286–282.

Clark DJ: Old wine in new bottles: delivering nursing in the 21st century, *J Nurs Scholarsh* 32(1):11–15, 2000.

Clark A: Empathy: An integral model in the counseling program, *J. Couns Dev.* 88(3):348–356, 2010.

Creasia J, Friberg E: *Conceptual Foundations: The Bridge to Professional Nursing Practice*, St. Louis, Missouri, 2011, Elsevier Mosby.

Cronenwett L, Sherwood G, Barnsteiner J, Disch J, Johnson J, Mitchell P, Warren J: Quality and safety education for nurses, *Nurs Outlook* 55:122–131, 2007.

Craig C, Eby D, Whittington J: Care coordination model: Better care at lower cost for people with multiple health and social needs. IHI innovation series white paper, Cambridge Massachusetts , *Institute for Healthcare Improvement*, 2011. Available on www.IHI.org.

Crowe M: The nurse-client relationship: a consideration of its discursive content, *J Adv Nurs* 31(4):962–967, 2000.

D'Antonio P: *American nursing: A history of knowledge*, Baltimore MD, 2010, Johns Hopkins University Press.

Doheny M, Cook C, Stopper M: *The discipline of nursing*, Stamford, CT, 2007, Appleton & Lange.

Donaldson SK, Crowley DM: The discipline of nursing, *Nurs Outlook* 26:113–120, 1978.

Egenes K: History of nursing. In Roux G, Halstead J, editors: *Issues and Trends in Nursing: Essential Knowledge for Today and Tomorrow*, Sudbury, MA, 2009, Jones and Bartlett.

Erikson E: *Childhood and society*, New York, 1950, WW Norton.

Finkelman AW, Kenner C: *Teaching the IOM: implications of the IOM reports for nursing education*, Silver Spring, MD, 2009, American Nurses Association.

Frenk J, Chen L, Bhuta Z, et al.: Health professionals for a new century: Transforming education to strengthen health care systems, *Lancet* 376:1923–1958, 2010.

Frist W: Health care in the 21st century, *N Engl J Med* 352:267–272, 2005.

Gottlieb L, Gottlieb B: Evolutionary principles can guide nursing's future development, *J Adv Nurs* 28(5):1099, 1998.

Gramling K: A narrative study of nursing art in critical care, *J Holist Nurs* 22(4):379–398, 2004.

Greene S, Tuzzio l, Cherkin D: A framework for making patient-centered care front and center, *Perm. J* 16(3):49–53, 2012.

Hargie O: *Skilled Interpersonal Communication: Research, Theory and Practice*, 5th ed., New York: NY, 2011, Routledge.

Henly S, Wyman J, Findorff M: Health and illness over time: The trajectory perspective in nursing science, *Nurs Res* 60(3 suppl):S5–14, 2011.

Holtslander L: Patterns of knowing hope: Carper's fundamental patterns as a guide for hope research with bereaved palliative care givers, *Nurs Outlook* 56(4):25–30, 2008.

Institute of Medicine (IOM): *Crossing the quality chasm: a new health system for the 21st century*, Washington, D.C, 2001, National Academies Press.

Institute of Medicine (IOM): *To err is human: building a safer health system*, Washington, DC, 2000, National Academies Press.

Institute of Medicine (IOM): *Health professions education: a bridge to quality*, Washington, DC, 2003, National Academies Press.

Institute of Medicine (IOM): *Redesigning continuing education in the health professions*, Washington, DC, 2009, National Academies Press.

Institute of Medicine (IOM): *The future of Nursing: Leading change, advancing health*, Washington, DC, 2010, National Academies Press.

Institute of Medicine (IOM): The future of nursing: accomplishments a year after the landmark report (Editorial), *J Nurs Scholar* 44(1):1, 2012.

Institute of Medicine (IOM): *Establishing transdisciplinary professionalism for improving health outcomes: Workshop summary*, Washington DC, 2014, The National Academies Press.

International Council of Nurses (ICN): *Definition of nursing*. Retrieved from http://www.icn.ch/about-icn/icn-definition-of-nursing/, 2014. retrieved June 30, 2014.

Interprofessional Education Collaborative Expert Panel: *Core competencies for interprofessional collaborative practice: Report of an expert panel*, Washington, D.C., 2011, Interprofessional Education Collaborative.

Jarrin O: The integrality of situated caring, *Adv Nurs Sci* 35(1):14–24, 2012.

Karnick P: The importance of defining theory in nursing: Is there a common denominator? *Nurs Science Quarterly* 26(1):29–30, 2013.

Kaiser Permanente: Understanding the affordable care act, *Affordable Care Act: Obamacare and health reform facts*, 2013. Accessed June 5, 2013 http://healthreform.kaiserpermanente.org.

Kilgore R, Langford R: Defragmenting care: Testing an intervention to increase the effectiveness of interdisciplinary health care teams, *Crit Care Nurs Clin North Am* 22:271–278, 2010.

Kim I: *The Nature of Theoretical Thinking in Nursing*, 3rd ed., New York, NY, 2010, Springer Publishing Co LLC.

Leight S: Starry night: using story to inform aesthetic knowing in women's health nursing, *J Adv Nurs* 37(1):108–114, 2002.

Litchfield M, Jonsdottir H: A practice discipline that is here and now, *Adv Nurs Sci.* 31(1):79–91, 2008.

Litwack K: The future of nursing: You can't have knowledge you don't have, *J Perianesth Nurs* 28(3):192–193, 2013.

Malloch K: Beyond transformational leadership to greater engagement: Inspiring innovation in complex organizations, *Nurs Leader* 12(2):60–63, 2014.

Marrs J, Lowry L: Nursing theory and practice: connecting the dots, *Nurs Sci Q* 19(1):44–50, 2006.

Maslow A: *Motivation and personality*, ed 2, New York, 1970, Harper & Row.

McGibbon E, Etowa A, McPherson C: Health access as a social determinant of health, *Can Nurs* 104(7):23–27, 2008.

Moody L: E-health web portals: Delivering holistic healthcare and making home the point of care, *Holist Nurs Pract* 19(4):156–160, 2005.

Nordstrom K, Coff C, Jonson H, et al.: Food and health: Individual, cultural, or scientific, *Genes Nutr* 8:857–863, 2013.

Peck A: Changing the face of standard nursing practice through telehealth and telenursing, *Nurs Adm Q* 29(4):339–343, 2005.

Nightingale F: In Skretkowicz. Victor, editor: *Commemorative edition Notes on Nursing, with historical commentary*, New York, 2010, Springer Publishing Company.

Pelletier L, Stichler J: Action brief: Client engagement and activation: A health reform imperative and improvement opportunity for nursing, *Nurs Outlook* 51–54, 2013.

Peplau H: *Interpersonal relations in nursing*, New York, 1952, Putnam.

Peplau H: Peplau's theory of interpersonal relations, *Nurs Sci Q* 10(4):162–167, 1997.

Pfaff K, Baxter P, Jack S, Ploeg J: An integrative review of the factors influencing new graduate nurse engagement in interprofessional collaboration, *J Adv Nurs* 7(1):4–20, 2013.

Porter S, O'Halloran P, Morrow E: Bringing values back into evidenced based nursing: Role of clients in resisting empiricism, *Nurs Sci Q* 34(2):106–118, 2011.

Porter-O'Grady T, Malloch K: *Q Quantum Leadership Building Better Partnerships for Sustainable Health*, 4th ed., Burlington MA, 2014, Jones & Bartlett Learning.

Reed P, Shearer N, 2007 Perspectives on nursing theory Lippincott: Philadelphia

Ritter-Teitel J: The impact of restructuring on professional nursing practice, *J Nurs Admin* 31(1):31–41, 2002.

Rogers C: Significant aspects of patient-centered therapy, *Am Psychol* 1:415–422, 1946.

Ruesch J: *Therapeutic communication*, New York, 1961, Norton.

Rycroft-Malone J, Seers K, Titchen A, McCormack B: What counts as evidence in evidence-based practice, *J Adv Nurs* 47(1):81–90, 2004.

Shaller D, 2007 October, *Patient-centered care: what does it take?* The Commonwealth Fund. Available online http://www.commonwealth fund.org/publications/fund-reports/2007/oct/patient-centered-care–what-does-it-take. Accessed December 18, 2009.

Sibbald B: 2020-Vision of the Future, *Can Nurse, March* 91:33–36, 1995.

Sigma Theta Tau International: *position statement on evidence-based nursing* 2003. Available online http://www.nursingsociety.org.

Smith M, McCarthy MP: Disciplinary knowledge in nursing education: Going beyond the blueprints, *Nurs Outlook* 58:44–51, 2010.

Smith S, Wilson S: *New directions in interpersonal communication*, Thousand Oaks, CA, 2010, Sage Publications.

Sousa M, Corning-Davis B: Management and leadership: Quality improvement: friend or foe, *Journal of Radiology Nursing* 32(3):141–143, 2013.

U.S. Department of Health and Human Services (DHHS): *Healthy people 2020*. Accessed March 15, 2013 www.healthypeople.gov

Wagner DJ, Whaite B: An exploration of the nature of caring relationships in the writings of Florence Nightingale, *J Holist Nurs* 4:225–234, 2010.

Watzlawick P, Beavin-Bavelas J, Jackson D: Some tentative axioms of communication. *Pragmatics of Human Communication—A Study of Interactional Patterns, Pathologies and Paradoxes*, New York, W. W, 1967, Norton, pp 29–52.

Watson J: *Caring Science as Sacred Science*, Philadelphia, PA, 2005, FA Davis Company.

World Health Organization (WHO), 2001 International classification of functioning, disability and health WHO: Geneva

World Health Organization (WHO). Preamble to the Constitution of the World Health Organization as adopted by the International Health Conference, New York, 19–22 June, 1946 www.who.int/abou t/definition/en/print.html. Accessed, Aug. 2, 2013.

World Health Organization (WHO): *World Health Report 2000*, Geneva, 2000, World Health Organization.

Zander P: Ways of knowing in nursing: the historical evolution of a concept, *J Theor Construct Test* 11(1):7–11, 2007.

Zolnierek C: An integrative review of knowing the patient, *J Nurs Scholarsh* 46(1):3–10, 2014.

CHAPTER 2

Professional Guides for Nursing Communication

Kathleen Underman Boggs

OBJECTIVES

At the end of the chapter, the reader will be able to:

1. Describe the impact on nursing communication of standards and guidelines for care and communication issued by multiple organizations.
2. Discuss competencies expected of the newly graduated nurse as listed by Quality and Safety Education for Nurses (QSEN) and other organizations, specifically as they affect communication.
3. Discuss legal and ethical standards in nursing practice relevant to communication.
4. Discuss client privacy in light of the Health Insurance Portability and Accountability Act (HIPAA) of 1996—regulations, confidentiality, and informed consent—as guides to action in nurse-client relationships.

This chapter introduces the student to standards and guidelines that directly or indirectly influence nursing communication. Included in this chapter is a brief overview of the nursing process.

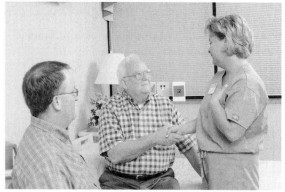

The nurse in all professional relationships, practices with compassion and respect for the inherent dignity, worth, and uniqueness of every individual.

BASIC CONCEPTS

STANDARDS AS GUIDES TO COMMUNICATION IN CLINICAL NURSING

As nurses we are guided by standards, policies, ethical codes, and laws. Factors external to the nursing profession, such as technology innovations, research reports, and government mandates, are driving major changes in the way nurses communicate. As described in Chapter 1, American laws such as Patient Protection and Affordable Care Act (2010), as well as guidelines from professional organizations, affect our practice and communications.

In an ideal work environment, we nurses demonstrate professional conduct by using established evidence-based "best practices" to provide safe, high-quality care for our clients. In an ideal work environment, we have excellent communication with our client and their families. In an ideal work environment, we have excellent, effective communication with all members of the interdisciplinary health care team, while maintaining confidentiality (Amer, 2013).

Nursing is working toward these goals by implementing new clear, complete communication practices. This is essential to workplace efficiency and delivery of high-quality, safe care to clients. A number of international, national, and professional organizations have issued standards, guidelines, and recommendations impacting the way nurses communicate.

EFFECTIVE COMMUNICATION

Effective communication is defined as *a two-way exchange of information* among clients and health providers ensuring that the expectations and responsibilities of all are clearly understood. It is an active process for all involved. Two-way communication provides feedback, which enables understanding by both senders and receivers. It is *timely, accurate, and usable*. Messages are processed by all parties until the information is clearly understood by all and integrated into care (adapted from The Joint Commission [TJC, 2011]. Effective and correct communication is clear, concise, concrete, complete, and courteous.

Communication problems occur when there are failures in one or more categories: the system, the transmission, or in the reception. **System failures** occur when the necessary channels of communication are absent or not functioning. **Transmission failures** occur when the channels exist but the message is never sent or is not clearly sent. **Reception failures** occur when channels exist and necessary information is sent, but the recipient misinterprets the message.

Why are nurses interested in using communication standards to modify and clarify their own communication? Ideally because we are motivated to provide the best, safest possible care. Failure to adhere to established nursing practice and professional performance standards could result in a negative civil judgment against a professional nurse. Consider the unfortunate but true case of a new graduate nurse as shown in the following case example.

Case Example: Graduate Nurse Kay

Immediately following graduation from her nursing program, Kay Smite, GN, takes an entry position on a busy surgical unit in a small-size general hospital. With no orientation she was assigned to work evening shift, with one registered nurse and two aides. During her second week when the registered nurse calls in ill, Kay is told by the evening supervisor that she is "charge nurse" this evening, and a float nurse will be sent as soon as possible to help with the workload. A surgeon arrives and rapidly gives verbal instructions to limit his pre-op craniotomy patient's head hair shaving to the incision site only tomorrow when the preparation procedure is done in the operating suite. As a student, Kay never spoke to a physician. He writes an order stating "client will be shaved according to head nurse's instructions." He asks Kay to call the operating room to relay these instructions, which she does. Nothing is in the record describing the area to be shaved. When the day shift arrives in the surgical suite, the telephone message from Kay is not passed on. The client's head is completely shaved, and a lawsuit is threatened.

1. What standards of communication were violated?
2. What do you think is wrong with this entire work environment?
3. What would you change in this unfortunate but true situation?

ORGANIZATIONS OR AGENCIES ISSUING HEALTH CARE COMMUNICATION GUIDELINES

The **World Health Organization (WHO)**, a part of the United Nations, has actively sought to improve worldwide client safety and this has affected expectations for nursing communication. In 2005 WHO designated The Joint Commission International as the WHO Collaborating Center for patient safety solutions. In 2007, WHO (TJC International, n.d.) published nine solutions for increasing health care safety. Number two is "correctly identifying the patient," and number three is "better communication during patient hand-over" (from one caregiver to another).

The Code of Ethics of the **International Council of Nurses (ICN)** describes nurse activities in relation to people, practice, profession, and coworkers (ICN, 2012). Description of elements set expectations for communication. One example would be "ensures confidentiality."

As highlighted in the **Institute of Medicine (IOM)** report "Crossing the Quality Chasm" described in Chapter 1, health care providers are refocusing on patient-centered care as the core concept in improving our health care system. Since the IOM implicated poor communication as a causative factor in 70% of health care errors, many other organizations have issued standards and guidelines that affect the way nurses communicate. The IOM specifically included "accurate, complete communication" as one of eight goals they established to improve safe care outcomes for clients. IOM specifically advocates use of **standardized communication tools.** Standardized formats and tools for communication are described in Chapter 4. One example of standardized communication is the situation, background, assessment, recommendation (SBAR) format.

Situation (What is going on with the client?)
Background (What is key information/context?)
Assessment (What do I think the problem is?)
Recommendation (What do I want to be done?)

Since every member of the health team uses this same standard format for communicating problems, they easily understand each other.

The **Agency for Healthcare Research and Quality (AHRQ)** in the U.S. Department of Health and Human Services has taken a leading role in health care in the United States to improve client safety. AHRQ's role, as mandated by Congress, is to prevent medical errors and promote client safety. They fund research and compile evidence to develop and publish "best practices" evidenced-based care protocols. An amazing number of resources can easily be accessed on the Internet such as (www.ahrq.gov/).

PROFESSIONAL NURSING ORGANIZATIONS ISSUING HEALTH CARE COMMUNICATION GUIDELINES

Professional nursing organizations all over the world have established standards for nursing care that specify clear, comprehensive communication as a requirement. Nurses are expected to demonstrate communication skills to effectively implement care and client safety within the context of the interprofessional health care team (American Association of Colleges of Nursing [AACN], 2008). Internationally, examples include guidelines from the College of Nurses of Ontario, Canada, who advocate that among other behaviors, nurses develop clear goal-directed communication processes, sharing information frequently with clients, families, and colleagues (www.cno.org/Global/docs/prac/41070_refusing.pdf). Other countries such as Great Britain also address the need for effective nurse communication.

The **American Nurses Association (ANA)** is a national professional organization for registered nurses. The ANA publishes standards of performance such as ANA's *Scope and Standards of Nursing Practice.* These help ensure professional nursing competence

and safe ethical clinical practice. Professional standards of practice serve the dual purpose of providing a standardized benchmark for evaluating the quality of their nursing care and offering the consumer a common means of understanding nursing as a professional service relationship. In this way, they communicate with the public as to what can be expected from professional nurses. In support of recommendations from a IOM and a Robert Wood Johnson (RWJ)–funded initiative to transform the practice of nursing (IOM, 2010), ANA is encouraging nurses to act as full partners in redesigning the health care system, especially by taking an active part in collecting and communicating information.

The **American Association of Colleges of Nursing (AACN)** makes recommendations for nursing curricula. For example, they suggest nursing students learn application of evidence-based clinical practices. An example of a specific communication recommendation is learning standard protocol for "handing off" communication when one nurse turns over care of the client to another. Another is mastering open communication and interdisciplinary cooperation techniques especially for working in health care teams (AACN, 2006).

QUALITY AND SAFETY IN NURSING EDUCATION

More than a decade ago, nursing leaders established a national initiative, **Quality and Safety Education for Nurses (QSEN),** to transform nursing education by building on IOM's recommendations to identify essential competencies for nurses, to be taught within nursing curricula (Cronenwett et al., 2007). QSEN identifies six areas of nursing competency as well as the knowledge, skills, and attitudes (KSA) associated with each competency as needed by all nurses (Barnsteiner et al., 2013; Disch, 2012). With significant funding from the Robert Wood Johnson Foundation, a national advisory board at QSEN continues to help educational institutions pursue quality and safety goals by providing training, resources, and consultants to translate QSEN competencies into teaching strategies. In each of the six competencies, QSEN specifies the *knowledge*, *skills*, and *attitudes* that are the learning objectives for each competency (see Table 2-1 for examples).

Patient-centered care is the first competency. Defined as empowering the client/family to be a full partner in providing compassionate, coordinated care. In terms of "knowledge," you are expected to integrate

TABLE 2-1	QSEN's Six Prelicensure Competencies, Definitions, and Selected Communication Examples	
Competency	**Definition**	**Partial Examples:** **K = knowledge; S = skill; A = attitude**
1. Patient-centered care (Arnold and Boggs discussed in every chapter)	Focus on fully partnering with client to provide care that incorporates his or her values and preferences to give safe, caring, compassionate effective care. To do so requires us to communicate client preferences to other health team members.	(K) Integrate understanding of arts, sciences, including communication, to apply nursing process. (S) Use communication skills in intake clinical interview to ask about client preferences, to develop care plan, to communicate these to others. Use communication tools. (A) Value client expertise and input.
2. Teamwork and collaboration (Arnold and Boggs discussed in Chapters 2, 4, 6, and 22-24)	For teamwork we need mutual respect, open communication, and shared decision making with all team members.	(K) Know scope of practice. Analyze differences in communication styles. (S) Adapt own style to the needs of the team in the current situation. Communicate openly, share in decision making, resolve potential conflicts. (A) Respect contributions of every team member.
3. Evidence-based practice (EBP) (Arnold and Boggs discussed in Chapters 1, 2, 4, and 23, with examples and application to practice in every chapter)	Incorporate the best practices based on newest evidence with our clinical expertise to deliver optimal care.	(K) Identify sources of EBP. Differentiate quality of evidence. (S) Use EBPs, after analyzing research findings and care protocols relevant to our client's diagnosis; communicate these to others. (A) Value research, appreciate need to seek EBP information.
4. Quality improvement (Arnold and Boggs discussed in Chapters 4 and 25)	Collect data on common outcome measures of our care to compare with accepted outcomes (benchmarks).	(K) Identify differences between our agency practices and "best practices." (S) Use communication tools to make client care explicit. (A) Value own and others contributions.
5. Safety (Arnold and Boggs incorporated throughout with focused discussion in Chapters 4 and 25)	Minimize risk of harm…, analyzing root causes of error, moving from a blame culture to a just culture should increase communication, prevent future problems, result is safer care.	(K) Analyze safety processes in own workplace. (S) Speak up proactively (about potential safety violations) and report near misses. (A) Appreciate how variation from established protocols creates risk.
6. Informatics (Arnold and Boggs discussed in Chapters 4, 25, and 26)	Use technology to effectively communicate and manage client care…, make decisions, and access evidence-based treatment information.	(K) Contrast benefits and limitations of different communication technologies. (S) Use electronic skills to access available databases to design an effective, evidence-based care plan. (A) Protect confidentiality.

QSEN, Quality and Safety Education for Nurses.

multiple dimensions of care, including communication, to involve the client and family. In terms of "skills," you are expected to elicit client values and preferences during your initial interview and care plan development and to communicate client preferences to other members of the health care team. In terms of "attitudes," you are to value expressions of client values, as well as their expertise regarding their own health status. In meeting the QSEN competency of providing patient-centered care, do you communicate with client and family members to engage them in planning care?

Teamwork and collaboration is another expected nurse competency. You are expected to be able to function effectively within nursing and an interprofessional team, to foster open communication, mutual respect, and shared decision making to achieve quality care. A partial example of expected knowledge objectives for this competency are that you know the various roles and scope of practice for team members and are able to analyze differences in communication style preferences for client, family, and for other members of the health care team. In terms of "skill," you are expected to be able to adapt your own style of communicating and able to initiate actions to resolve any conflicts. In terms of "attitudes," your behavior shows that you value teamwork and different styles of communication (www.QSEN.org/). As a student, are you having experiences in which you directly communicate with physicians?

As you can see in Table 2-1, *communication is a major component* of most of these six competencies. The QSEN web site gives you access to the case study of Lewis Blackman, a healthy, active 15-year-old, who died unnecessarily following elective surgery (www.qsen.org/videos/the-lewis-blackman-story). This case details a series of miscommunications and lack of intervention by staff nurses and physicians. In addition to the inaction on the part of nurses, fragmentation of the care system and the barrier of the physician-nurse power hierarchy are implicated. When members of the health care team are not empowered to speak up and participate, a major threat to client safety occurs. Just as it does when members of family are not empowered (Acquaviva, 2013). Blackman's mother, Helen Haskell, states that it is her belief that "Lewis' death could have been averted by a knowledgeable, assertive nurse." Effectively working as part of a health care team requires open communication, mutual respect, and shared decision making with client and family included.

Additional QSEN competencies are defined for graduate nursing education (Disch and Barnsteiner, 2012).

These and other QSEN competencies will be discussed throughout this book, as related to communication. For more information and descriptions of the knowledge, skills, and attitudes attached to each competency, refer to www.QSEN.com. Other models are also available that identify core competencies expected of nurses. All of them stress excellent communication, coordination, and collaborative skills. For example, Lenburg's Competency Outcomes Performance Assessment Model (COPA) includes oral skills, writing skills, and electronic skills (Amer, 2013).

OTHER PROFESSIONAL ORGANIZATIONS AND ACCREDITING AGENCIES ISSUING COMMUNICATION GUIDELINES AFFECTING NURSING

The **Joint Commission (TJC)** is the organization that regulates hospitals in the United States. To obtain reimbursement from insurance, a health care organization must have TJC accreditation. TJC attributes more than 60% of sentinel events to miscommunication. So they specifically have some regulations focused on improving communication, such as requirements to use checklists. TJC mandates that hospitals effectively communicate with patients when providing services, identifying client oral and written communication needs to facilitate the exchange of information during the care process (TJC, *R3 Report*, n.d., PC.02.01.21). TJC's Accreditation Manual for Hospitals says that staff must be aware of relevant policies for meeting patient communication needs (TJC, 2011a).

TJC defines **effective communication** as that which is timely, accurate, complete, unambiguous, and understood by the recipient. Goal number 2 of their National Patient Safety Goals (TJC, 2011b) aims at structuring and improving communication to improve effectiveness among caregivers. Section 2E of the goals specifically addresses communication guidelines needed to manage handoff communication. When your client is handed off or transferred into the care of another caregiver on your unit or to another location, TJC encourages staff to follow a standard communication protocol. These **standardized communication tools** are described in detail in Chapter 4.

TJC also mandates that written nursing policies with specific standards of care be available on all nursing units. TJC has 15 standards-based performance areas. Professional standards of practice provide definitions of the minimum competencies needed for quality professional nursing practice. Presented as principled statements, they designate the knowledge and clinical skills required of nurses to practice competently and safely.

ETHICAL STANDARDS AND ISSUES

Nurses are subjected to numerous ethical and legal duties in their professional role (McGowan, 2012). Nurses have an ethical accountability to the clients they serve that extends beyond their legal responsibility in everyday nursing situations. Ethical issues of particular relevance to the nurse-client relationship relate to caring for clients in ambulatory managed care settings, the rights of clients participating in research, caring for mature minors, client education, right to die issues, transfer to long-term care of elderly clients, and telehealth nursing. The process for applying ethical decision making will be described in Chapter 3.

ETHICAL CODES

All legitimate professions have standards of conduct. Nurses of every nation are guided by written professional ethical codes. An International Code of Ethics was adopted by ICN in 1953 and revised in 2012. This code identifies four fundamental nursing responsibilities as being to promote health, prevent illness, restore health, and alleviate suffering. Moreover the code says each nurse has the responsibility to maintain a clinical practice that promotes ethical behavior, while sustaining collaborative, respectful relationships with coworkers. Among many elements of the code, those addressing communication state we need to ensure that each client receives accurate, sufficient communication in a timely manner and to maintain confidentiality.

Professional nurses, regardless of setting, are expected to follow ethical guidelines in their practice. As listed in Box 2-1, American Nurses Association Code of Ethics for Nurses (with interpretive statements) (ANA, 2001) establishes principled guidelines designed to protect the integrity of clients related to their care, health, safety, and rights. It provides ethical guidelines for nurses designed to protect client

| BOX 2-1 | American Nurses Association Code of Ethics for Nurses |

1. The nurse, in all professional relationships, practices with compassion and respect for the inherent dignity, worth, and uniqueness of every individual, unrestricted by considerations of social or economic status, personal attributes, or the nature of health problems.
2. The nurse's primary commitment is to the patient, whether an individual, family, group, or community.
3. The nurse promotes, advocates for, and strives to protect the health, safety, and rights of the patient.
4. The nurse is responsible and accountable for individual nursing practice and determines the appropriate delegation of tasks consistent with the nurse's obligation to provide optimum patient care.
5. The nurse owes the same duties to self as to others, including the responsibility to preserve integrity and safety, to maintain competence, and to continue personal and professional growth.
6. The nurse participates in establishing, maintaining, and improving health care environments and conditions of employment conducive to the provision of quality health care and consistent with the values of the profession through individual and collective action.
7. The nurse participates in the advancement of the profession through contributions to practice, education, administration, and knowledge development.
8. The nurse collaborates with other health professionals and the public in promoting community, national, and international efforts to meet health needs.
9. The profession of nursing, as represented by associations and their members, is responsible for articulating nursing values, for maintaining the integrity of the profession and its practice, and for shaping social policy.

Reprinted from the American Nurses Association (ANA, 2001) by permission.

rights, provide a mechanism for professional accountability, and educate professionals about sound ethical conduct. Codes of ethics for nurses are found in most other nations. For example, there is the Canadian Nurses Association Code of Ethics for Registered Nurses (1997).

A Code of Ethics for Nurses provides a broad conceptual framework outlining the principled behaviors and value beliefs expected of professional nurses

EXERCISE 2-1	Applying the Code of Ethics for Nurses to Professional and Clinical Situations

Purpose: To help students identify applications of the Code of Ethics for Nurses.

Procedure

Break into small groups of four or five students to consider the following clinical scenarios:

1. Barbara Kohn is a 75-year-old woman who lives with her son and daughter-in-law. She reveals to you that her daughter-in-law keeps her locked in her room when she has to go out because she does not want her to get in trouble. She asks you not to say anything as that will only get her into trouble.

2. The nursing supervisor asks you to "float" to another unit that will require some types of skills that you believe you do not have the knowledge or skills to perform. When you explain your problem, she tells you that she understands, but the unit is short staffed and she really needs you to do this.

3. Bill Jackson is an elderly client who suffered a stroke and is uncommunicative. He is not expected to live. The health care team is considering placement of a feeding tube based on his wife's wishes. His wife agrees that he probably will not survive, but wants the feeding tube just in case the doctors are wrong.

4. Dr. Holle criticizes a nurse in front of a client and the client's family.

Share each ethical dilemma with the group and collaboratively come up with a resolution that the group agrees on, using the nurse's code of ethics to work through the situation.

Discussion

1. What types of difficulty did your group encounter in resolving different scenarios?
2. What type of situation offers the most challenge ethically?
3. Were there any problems in which the code of ethics was not helpful?
4. How can you use what you learned in this exercise in your nursing practice?

in delivering health care to individuals, families, and communities. Ethical standards of behavior require a clear understanding of the multidimensional aspects of an ethical dilemma, including intangible human factors that make each situation unique (e.g., personal and cultural values or resources).

When an ethical dilemma cannot be resolved through interpersonal negotiation, an ethics committee composed of biomedical experts reviews the case and makes recommendations. Of particular importance to the nurse-client relationship are ethical directives related to the nurse's primary commitment to

- The client's welfare
- Respect for client autonomy
- Recognition of each individual as unique and worthy of respect and advocacy
- Truth telling

Exercise 2-1 provides an opportunity to consider the many elements in an ethical nursing dilemma.

LEGAL STANDARDS

As stressed in the IOM/RWJ report, nurses must be accountable for their own contributions to delivery of high-quality care (2010). As professional nurses, we are held legally accountable for all aspects of the nursing care we provide to clients and families, including documentation and referral. Of special relevance to communication within the nurse-client relationship are issues of professional liability, informed consent, and confidentiality.

CLASSIFICATIONS OF LAWS IN HEALTH CARE

As nurses, we need to take into consideration two types of law related to our care. *Statutory laws* are legislated laws, drafted and enacted at federal or state levels. Medicare and Medicaid amendments to the Social Security Act are examples of federal statutory laws. Each state's Nurse Practice Act is an example of statutory law.

Civil laws are developed through court decisions, which are created through precedents, rather than written statutes. Most infractions for malpractice and negligence are covered by civil law and are referred to as *torts*. A tort is defined as a private civil action that causes personal injuries to a private party. Deliberate intent is not present. Four elements are necessary to qualify for a claim of malpractice or negligence.

- The professional duty was owed to client (professional relationship).

- A breach of duty occurred in which the nurse failed to conform to an accepted standard of care.
- Causality in which a failure to act by professional standards was a proximate cause of the resulting injury.
- Actual damage or injuries resulted from breach of duty.

As nurses, we are legally bound by the principles of civil tort law to provide the care that any reasonably prudent nurse would provide in a similar situation. If taken to court, this standard would be the benchmark against which our actions would be judged.

Criminal law is reserved for cases in which there is intentional misconduct or a serious violation of professional standards of care. The most common nurse violation of criminal law is failure to renew a professional nursing license, which means that a nurse is practicing nursing without a license.

LEGAL LIABILITY IN NURSE-CLIENT RELATIONSHIPS

In the nurse-client relationship, the nurse is responsible for maintaining the professional conduct of the relationship. Examples of unprofessional conduct in the nurse-client relationship include:

- Breaching client confidentiality
- Verbally or physically abusing a client
- Assuming nursing responsibility for actions without having sufficient preparation
- Delegating care to unlicensed personnel, which could result in client injury
- Following a doctor's order that would result in client harm
- Failing to assess, report, or document changes in client health status
- Falsifying records
- Failing to obtain informed consent
- Failure to question a physician's orders, if they are not clear
- Failure to provide required health teaching
- Failure to provide for client safety (e.g., not putting the side rails up on a client with a stroke)

Effective and frequent communication with clients and other providers is one of the best ways to avoid or minimize the possibility of harm leading to legal liability.

DOCUMENTATION AS A LEGAL RECORD

As described in Chapter 25, nurses are responsible for accurate and timely documentation of nursing assessments, care given, and the responses of the client. This documentation represents a permanent record of the client's health care experience. In the eyes of the law, failure to document in written form any of these elements means the actions were not taken.

APPLICATIONS

As illustrated in Figure 2-1, Communication in the Nursing Process, communication standards and skills are an integral component of the knowledge, experience and skills, and attitudes encompassed in using the nursing process to deliver care. Standards for nurse behaviors are specified in professional codes and guidelines, including clarity and completeness of communication. Nursing students need opportunities to practice effectively communicating before entering the workforce. Throughout this book, emphasis is placed on the importance of guiding your practice through application of both professional standards and evidence-based practices in your nursing care. Discussing case studies and exercises offers opportunities to hone communication skills.

EVIDENCE-BASED PRACTICE

As discussed in Chapter 1, **evidenced-based practice (EBP)** guidelines are clinical behaviors compiled from the best current research evidence available and the expertise of clinicians. IOM's *The Future of Nursing* report specifies that nursing education provide opportunities for students to develop competency in the use of EBP and collaborative teamwork to ensure the delivery of safe, patient-centered care across settings (IOM, 2010). Use of EBPs are also a QSEN competency. Each nurse is expected to be able to integrate "best current evidence" with clinical expertise and client/family preferences and values to deliver optimum care (Barnsteiner et al., 2013). In developing this skill, you learn to determine which data are scientifically valid and useful in guiding your practice. By consulting EBP guidelines, your ability to make specific clinical decisions about care for your client is enhanced, so you can give the highest quality care. Do you have a clinical question? Many sources are available to you, such as guidelines from agencies such as AHRQ or speciality nursing organizations (www.guideline.gov/index.aspx).

Much of nursing and medicine is not yet based on evidence. When a guideline is not yet available, you

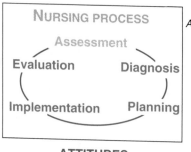

Figure 2-1   Communication in the nursing process. *(Modified from Potter PA, Perry AG, Stockert PA, et al. Fundamentals of nursing, ed 8, St. Louis, 2013, Mosby.)*

can access specific journal research articles using any of several databases such as CINAHL (QSEN module on EBP). Careful critical thinking is needed when relying on just one study's findings. As Disch (2012,b) points out, even when we have available best evidence, sometimes we choose to not apply it. Her example is that oral care is often not done, even though strong evidence exists that oral care reduces ventilator-associated pneumonia. Use the EBP samples provided in this book to stimulate discussion and to encourage you to seek out those you can apply in your clinical practice.

STANDARDS

Application of standards of professional communication necessitates use of critical thinking and problem-solving skills in all aspects of care (described in Chapter 3). Clarity of communication is crucial. Many of the organizations cited earlier recommend use of standardized communication formats. Failure to follow accepted codes and standards of behavior can result in potential harm to clients, termination of employment, state licensure disciplinary action, or litigation.

USING THE NURSING PROCESS IN NURSE-CLIENT RELATIONSHIPS

The nurses' primary duty is to provide the client with competent, safe, consistent, and ethical care. The most common configuration for collecting, organizing, and analyzing client data remains the nursing process. The purpose of the nursing process is to diagnose and treat human responses to actual or potential health problems (ANA, 2010). Since the nursing process is an interpersonal, client-centered process involving many team members, communication is a major component. Assessment data, nursing diagnosis, and goals for treatment are systematically documented and shared with nurses and other health professionals. Figure 2-1 illustrates how the nursing process is central to our care of clients. Input from your knowledge, skills/experience, and your attitudes contribute to your use of the nursing process, just as do the standards we discuss in this chapter. While standards include standards for nursing practice and evidence-based practice guidelines, we focus chapter discussion on *communication standards.*

Developing an Evidence-Based Practice

This is an example of one of several research studies reviewed by experts to compile the *Mosby's Nursing Consult Evidence-Based Nursing Recommendations* for the category **Pressure Ulcers** (http://www.nursingconsult.com/nursing/login?env=PROD&URI=/nursing/evidence-based-nursing/monograph%3Fmonograph_id%3D189626).

Moore Z, Cowman S, Conroy RM. A randomized controlled clinical trial of repositioning, using the 30-degree tilt for the prevention of pressure ulcers, *J Clin Nurs* 20(17/18): 2633-2644, 2011.

This was a prospective, randomized study that compared two methods of positioning 213 geriatric clients to prevent development of pressure ulcers (bed sores). The treatment group had their positions changed using a tilt every 2 hours during the night, while control group members were repositioned the standard position change schedule of every 6 hours during the night.

Results: Thirteen of the control group developed pressure ulcers as compared to only three in the group whose positions were changed more frequently. The authors concluded that more frequent repositioning especially using the 30-degree tilt is more effective.

Application to your clinical practice: The Mosby evidence-based practice (EBP) site reviewed additional studies and summarized the data to make EBP recommendations for nursing care. Among many guidelines they listed these nursing actions:

- Nurses need to access skin condition and risk for ulcers on admission and at least daily.
- Nurses should reposition immobile clients at least every 2 hours using a 30-degree tilt during the night.
- Nurses should reposition chair-bound clients every hour if they cannot change their position themselves.
- Nurses need to keep client skin clean and dry and avoid vigorous massage of skin over bony prominences.

This site also provides you with information for discharge planning and evaluation. It goes on to list the Nursing Outcomes Classification (NOC) and Nursing Interventions Classification (NIC) categories and codes.

Explore this web site for other specific EBP guidelines. Then for fun, check out the sites available to you from the Agency for Healthcare Research and Quality (AHRQ.gov), including their hyperlinks to YouTube, for videos that you can use in teaching young clients (www.youtube.com/user/AHRQHealthTV/).

Just click on "prevention is the key to a healthy life" or other topics.

The nursing process consists of five progressive phases: assessment, problem identification and diagnosis, outcome identification and planning, implementation, and evaluation. As a dynamic, systematic clinical management tool, it functions as a primary means of directing the sequence, planning, implementation, and evaluation of nursing care to achieve specific health goals. Continual and timely communication is a component of each step in the nursing process. Specifically the role communication plays is

- Establishing and maintaining a therapeutic relationship
- Helping client to promote, maintain, or restore health, or to achieve a peaceful death
- Facilitating client management of difficult health care issues through communication
- Providing quality nursing care in a safe and efficient manner

The nursing process is closely aligned with meeting professional nursing standards in the total care of the client. Table 2-2 illustrates the relationship.

The nursing process begins with your first encounter with a client and family, and ends with discharge or referral. Although there is an ordered sequence of nursing activities, each phase is flexible, flowing into and overlapping with other phases of the nursing process. For example, in providing a designated nursing intervention, you might discover a more complex need than what was originally assessed. This could require a modification in the nursing diagnosis, identified outcome, intervention, or the need for a referral.

ASSESSMENT

You employ communication skills in beginning the initial step in your client-centered approach to assessment. You systematically gather data about the client seeking service. The assessment process begins when you first meet the client and family. Introducing yourself and explaining the purpose of the assessment interview helps put the client at ease.

Next in this assessment process is the intake assessment, done to obtain information about the client's problem history. Using your verbal interviewing skills as well as observations about nonverbal cues, you use open-ended and focused questions to collect data about

TABLE 2-2	Relationship of the Nursing Process to Professional Nursing Standards in the Nurse-Client Relationship
Nursing Process: Assessment	**Related Nursing Standard**
Collects data/information from: • Client history/interview • Own observations; physical examination • The family • Past records/tests • Other members of health team	The nurse collects data throughout the nursing process related to client strengths, limitations, available resources, and changes in the client's condition.
Analyzes data	The nurse organizes cluster behaviors and makes inferences based on subjective and objective client data, combined with personal and scientific nursing knowledge.
Verifies data	The nurse verifies data and inferences with client to ensure validity.
Nursing Process: Diagnosis	
Identifies health care needs/problems and formulates biopsychosocial statements	The nurse develops a comprehensive biopsychosocial statement that captures the essence of the client's health care needs/problems (see Box 2-2, Gordon's Functional Health Patterns)
	Nurse validates the accuracy of the statement with the client and family; this statement becomes the basis for nursing diagnoses.
Establishes nursing diagnosis Nurse uses NANDA approved diagnoses and codes	The nurse develops relevant nursing diagnoses. Prioritizes them based on the client's most immediate needs in the current health care situation (see Table 2-3, Identifying Nursing Problems Associated with Maslow's Hierarchy of Needs).
Nursing Process: Outcome Identification and Planning	
Identifies expected outcomes (for each NANDA diagnosis, there are several NOC suggested outcomes)	The nurse and client mutually and realistically develop expected outcomes based on client needs, strengths, and resources.
Specifies short-term goals	The nurse and client mutually and realistically develop expected outcomes based on client needs, strengths, and resources.
Nursing Process: Implementation	
Takes appropriate nursing action interventions. Nursing interventions alter client's status/symptoms.	The nurse encourages, supports, and validates the client in taking agreed-on action to achieve goals and expected outcomes through integrated, therapeutic nursing interventions and communication strategies.
Nursing Process: Evaluation	
Evaluates goal achievement. Expected outcome is stated and nurse is quickly able to identify client's current status.	The nurse and client mutually evaluate attainment of expected outcomes and survey each step of the nursing process for appropriateness, effectiveness, adequacy, and time efficiency.
	Modifies the plan if evaluation shows expected outcome not achieved.

NANDA, North American Nursing Diagnosis Association; *NOC,* Nursing Outcomes Classification.

- The current problem for which the client seeks treatment
- The client's perception of his or her health patterns
- Presence of other health risk and protective factors
- Relevant social, occupational, and family history
- The client's medical and psychiatric history (e.g., previous hospitalizations, family history, medical and psychiatric treatment, and medications)
- The client's coping patterns
- Level and availability of the client's support system

BOX 2-2	Gordon's Functional Health Patterns

1. Health perception-health management pattern
2. Nutritional-metabolic pattern
3. Elimination pattern
4. Activity-exercise pattern
5. Sleep-rest pattern
6. Cognitive-perceptual pattern
7. Self-perception-self-concept pattern
8. Role-relationship pattern
9. Sexuality-reproductive pattern
10. Coping-stress tolerance pattern
11. Value-belief pattern

Assessment of client needs should take the client's entire experience of an illness, rather than simply focusing on clinical data related to the diagnosis. In addition to your interview, assessment includes information you obtain from existing records, past diagnostic testing, information from family, and in some instances, contact with previous health care providers, schools, or other referral sources. As new information becomes available, you are expected to refine and update the original assessment.

Two types of data are collected during an assessment interview. **Subjective data** refers to the client's perception of data and what the client or family says about the data (e.g., "I have a severe pain in my chest"). Client data about alternative forms of treatment, medications, and previously used care systems are relevant pieces of information. **Objective data** refers to data that are directly observable or verifiable through physical examination or tests (e.g., an abnormal electrocardiogram). Combined, these data will present a complete picture of the client's health problem.

Observations of the client's appearance and nonverbal behaviors can help you make inferences. Throughout the assessment phase, you will need to validate the information you receive from the client and significant others to make sure that the data are complete and accurate. Ask the client for confirmation that your perceptions and problem analysis are correct periodically throughout the assessment interview, and summarize your impressions at the end.

NURSING DIAGNOSES

Once the assessment is complete and you have baseline data, the next step is to analyze the information and identify gaps in the data collection or content. One way to do this is to compare individual client data

with normal health standards, behavior patterns, and developmental norms. Gordon's Functional Health Patterns (Box 2-2) provide a useful structure for clustering assessment data and help direct the choice of nursing diagnoses. The determination of whether a pattern is functional or dysfunctional is based on established norms for age and sociocultural standards (Gordon, 2007).

A nursing diagnoses describes the client's human responses to health issues and medical diagnoses. They provide a platform for independent and dependent nursing actions and should complement, not compete, with the actual medical diagnosis of a health problem.

The nursing diagnosis consists of three parts: problem, cause, and evidence (North American Nursing Diagnosis Association [NANDA], 2011).

- *Problem:* A statement identifying a health problem or alteration in a client's health status, requiring nursing intervention. Using a list of the most recent NANDA diagnoses, you would pick a NANDA diagnosis that best represents the identified problem or potential problem.
- *Cause:* A statement specifying the probable causative or risk factors contributing to the existence or maintenance of the health care problem. The cause of a problem can be psychosocial, physiologic, situational, cultural, or environmental in nature. The phrase "related to" (R/T) serves to connect the problem and causative statements. Example: "Impaired communication related to a cerebrovascular accident."
- *Evidence:* A statement identifying the clinical evidence (behaviors, signs, symptoms) that support the diagnosis. An example of a nursing diagnosis statement would be "Impaired verbal

communication related to a cerebrovascular accident, as manifested by incomplete sentences and slurred words."

Prioritize. Traditionally nurses have used Maslow's Hierarchy of Needs (see Chapter 1) to prioritize goals and objectives. Examples of nursing problems associated with each level of Maslow's hierarchy are included in Table 2-3. Priority attention should be given to the most immediate, life-threatening problems. Use communication skills to validate these priorities with your client and health team. Try Exercise 2-2 to practice considering cultural, age, and gender-related themes when using the nursing process with different types of clients.

Identify Outcomes. Outcomes should be client-centered (e.g., "The client will...") and described in specific, measurable terms. An appropriate treatment outcome for a client after surgery might be: "The client will show no signs of infection as evidenced by the incision being well-approximated and free of redness and swelling, normal temperature, and white blood cell count within normal limits by 3/21/14." Nursing outcomes should be

- Based on diagnoses
- Documented in measurable terms
- Developed collaboratively with the client and other health providers
- Realistic and achievable

Each treatment outcome specifies the action or behavior that the client will demonstrate once the health problem is resolved. Outcome criteria are stated as long- and short-term treatment goals. Using measurable action verbs to describe what the client will be doing to achieve a short-term goal is key to effective identification of treatment outcomes; for example, "The client will take his medicine, as prescribed" is measurable: He either takes his medicine or he does not. Other measurable verbs include "perform," "identify," "discuss," and "demonstrate." Broad-spectrum verbs

TABLE 2-3	Identifying Nursing Problems Associated with Maslow's Hierarchy of Needs
Physiologic survival needs	Circulation, food, intake/output, physical comfort, rest
Safety and security needs	Domestic abuse, fear, anxiety, environmental hazards, housing
Love and belonging	Lack of social support, loss of significant person or pet, grief
Self-esteem needs	Loss of a job, inability to perform normal activities, change in position or expectations
Self-actualization	Inability to achieve personal goals

EXERCISE 2-2   **Using the Nursing Process as a Framework in Clinical Situations**

Purpose: To help students develop skills in considering cultural, age, and gender role issues in assessing each client's situation and developing relevant nursing diagnoses.

Procedure

1. In small groups of three to four students, discuss how you might assess and incorporate differences in client/family values, knowledge, beliefs, and cultural background in delivery of care for each of the following clients. Indicate what other types of information you would need to make a complete assessment.
2. Identify and prioritize nursing diagnoses for each client to ensure client-centered care.
   - Michael Sterns was in a skiing accident. He is suffering from multiple internal injuries, including head injury. His parents have been notified and are flying in to be with him.
   - Lo Sun Chen is a young Chinese woman admitted for abdominal surgery. She has been in this country for only 8 weeks and speaks very little English.
   - Maris LaFonte is a 17-year-old unmarried woman admitted for the delivery of her first child. She has had no prenatal care.
   - Stella Watkins is an 85-year-old woman admitted to a nursing home after suffering a broken hip.

Discussion

1. In what ways might the needs of each client be different based on age, gender role, or cultural background? How would you account for the differences?
2. Were there any common themes in the types of information each group decided it needed to make a complete assessment?
3. How could you use what you learned from this exercise in your clinical practice?

such as "understand," "know," and "learn" are not easily measurable and should not be used. Note the conditions or circumstances for outcome achievement "as prescribed" is specifically identified. Documentation of clinical outcomes should include client response.

PLANNING

Use communication skills to collaborate with health team members and with client and family members to identify expected outcomes for your nursing care. Based on the assessment data, you collaborate with the client to develop a mutually agreed-on plan of care and anticipated outcomes. The plan of care plan serves as the structural framework for providing safe quality care. Its purpose is to provide continuity and supply a basis for interventions and documentation of client progress. Each plan of care should be individualized to reflect client values, clinical needs, and preferences.

IMPLEMENTATION

During the implementation phase, you and others make interventions and evaluate corresponding client responses. This includes giving direct physical care and using your communication skills to delegate some care (indirect care). You also use communication skills to provide support to clients and families, provide needed teaching, and document progress.

EVALUATION

In the evaluation phase, the nurse and client mutually examine the client's progress or lack of progress toward achievement of treatment outcomes, mutually determined during the planning phase. Use your communication skills to obtain feedback from your client, contrasting actual progress with expected outcomes. Analyze factors that might have effected goal achievement. Communicate with team members to modify interventions as needed.

APPLICATION OF ETHICAL AND LEGAL GUIDELINES

MORAL DISTRESS

Moral distress occurs when an agency attempts to require you to act contrary to your personal values or in a way you know is ethically inappropriate (American Association of Critical Care Nurses [AACCN], 2008). The process of moral decision making is discussed in Chapter 3. ANA (2013) describes their Code of Ethics

as "nonnegotiable, encompassing all nursing activities and may supersede specific policies of institutions." If you are unable to provide care, you are obligated to ensure that the client will have care from another well-qualified nurse.

ANA supports the rights of clients to self-determination. As a nurse you have an ethical obligation to support clients in their choices.

PROTECTING THE CLIENT'S PRIVACY

ANA supports a client's right to privacy, which is to have control over personal identifiable health information, whereas confidentiality refers to your obligation not to divulge anything said in a nurse-client relationship. Institutional policies and federal law provide specific guidelines that all health care providers are required to follow. The client's right to have personal control over personal information is upheld through federal regulations. The ANA Code of Ethics (2001) specifically addresses the nurse's responsibility to safeguard the client's right to privacy.

Health Insurance Portability and Accountability Act Regulatory Compliance

In the United States, federal legislation known as the Health Insurance Portability and Accountability Act (HIPAA) of 1996 went into effect in 2003 to protect client privacy.

The goals of HIPAA regulations are to assure that individual's information is protected while allowing the flow of information needed to provide quality care. A nurse is obligated to protect confidential information, unless required by law to disclose that information. Health care providers must provide clients with a written notice of their privacy practices and procedures. Agencies are audited for compliance. The key elements of the HIPAA privacy regulations are presented in Box 2-3.

HIPAA privacy rules govern the use and disbursement of individually identifiable health information, and give individuals the right to determine and restrict access to their health information. Clients have the right to access their medical records, request copies, and/or request amendments to health information contained in the record. The Fair Health Information Practices Act of 1997 stipulates civil and criminal penalties for not allowing clients to review their medical records. The Affordable Care Act of 2010 further strengthened privacy regulations.

| BOX 2-3 | Overview of Federal HIPAA Guidelines Protecting Client Confidentiality |

- All medical records and other individually identifiable health information used or disclosed in any form, whether electronically, on paper, or orally, are covered by HIPAA regulations.
- Providers and health plans are required to give clients a clear written explanation of how their health information may be used and disclosed.
- Clients are able to see and get copies of their own records and request amendments.
- Health care providers are required to obtain client consent before sharing their information for treatment, payment, and health care operations. Clients have the right to request restrictions on the uses and disclosures of their information.
- People have the right to file a formal complaint with a covered provider or health plan, or with the U.S. Department of Health and Human Services (DHHS), about violations of Health Insurance Portability and Accountability Act (HIPAA) regulations.
- Health information may not be used for purposes not related to health care (e.g., disclosures to employers to make personnel decisions) without explicit authorization.
- Disclosure of information is limited to the minimum necessary for the purpose of the disclosure.
- Written privacy procedures must be in place to cover anyone who has access to protected information related to how information will be used and disclosed.
- Training must be provided to employees about the use of HIPAA privacy procedures.
- Health plans, providers, and clearinghouses that violate these standards will be subject to civil liability, and if knowingly violating client privacy for personal advantage, can be subject to criminal liability.
- Use and disclosure is permitted for treatment, payment and health care operations activities; for notification; for public health for preventing or controlling disease to lessen an imminent threat; or in cases of abuse, disclosure is permitted to government authorities.

Adapted from Health Insurance Portability and Accountability Act (HIPAA) Guidelines: www.hss.gov/ocr/privacy.

HIPAA regulations protect the confidentiality, accuracy, and availability of all electronic protected information, whether created, received, or transmitted. Strict maintenance of written records in a protected, private environment is required. Other potential issues of concern about privacy involve cell phones, picture taking, use of handheld devices, use of fax machines, Internet user ID and passwords, and use of electronic monitoring devices (Kerr, 2009).

Health care providers must get written authorization from clients before disclosing or sharing any personal medical information. Client authorization is not required in situations concerning the public's health, criminal and legal matters, quality assurance, and aggregate record reviews for accreditation. Information can be shared among health care providers. The Office of Civil Rights enforces HIPAA regulations. Agencies and providers face severe penalties for violations, with improper disclosure of medical information punishable by fines or imprisonment. Study your agency's policies to determine to whom and under what conditions personal health information can be released. More information can be obtained through their web site (www.cms.gov/Regulations-and-Guidance/HIPPA).

The Joint Commission Privacy Regulations

TJC requires agencies to have written privacy policies, to orient the staff to these policies, and to demonstrate staff awareness of their privacy policy (TJC, 2011a).

Ethical Responsibility to Protect Client Privacy in Clinical Situations

In addition to legally mandated informational privacy, informal protection of the client's right to control the access of others to one's person in clinical situations is an ethical responsibility. The client and family usually view protecting the client's privacy in the clinical setting as a measure of respect. Simple strategies that nurses can use to protect the client's right to privacy in clinical situations include:

- Providing privacy for the client and family when disturbing matters are to be discussed
- Explaining procedures to clients before implementing them
- Entering another person's personal space with warning (e.g., knocking or calling the client's name) and, preferably, waiting for permission to enter
- Providing an identified space for the client's personal belongings

- Encouraging the inclusion of personal and familiar objects on the client's nightstand
- Decreasing direct eye contact during hands-on care
- Minimizing body exposure to what is absolutely necessary for care
- Using only the necessary number of people during any procedure
- Using touch appropriately

Confidentiality

Protecting the privacy of client information and confidentiality are related, but separate concepts. **Confidentiality** is defined as providing *only* the information needed to provide care for the client to other health professionals who are directly involved in the care of the client. The need to share information with other health professionals directly involved in care on a "need to know" basis should be made clear to the client as they enter the clinical setting. Other than these individuals, the nurse must have the client's written permission to share his or her private communication, unless the withholding of information would result in harm to the client or someone else, or in cases where abuse is suspected. Confidential information about the client cannot be shared with the family or other interested parties without the client or designated legal surrogate's written permission. Shared confidential information, unrelated to identified health care needs, should not be communicated or charted in the client's medical record.

Confidentiality within the nurse-client relationship involves the nurse's legal responsibility to guard against invasion of the client's privacy related to the following:
- Releasing information about the client to unauthorized parties
- Unwanted visitations in the hospital
- Discussing client problems in public places or with people not directly involved in the client's care
- Taking pictures of the client without consent or using the photographs without the client's permission
- Performing procedures such as testing for human immunodeficiency virus (HIV) without the client's permission
- Publishing data about a client in any way that makes the client identifiable without the client's permission

Professional Sharing of Confidential Information. Nursing reports and interdisciplinary team case conferences are acceptable forums for the discussion of health-related communications shared by clients or families. Other venues include change-of-shift reports, one-on-one conversations with other health professionals about specific client care issues, and client-approved consultations with client families. Discussion of client care should take place in a private room with the door closed. Only relevant information specifically related to client assessment or treatment should be shared. Discussing private information casually with other health professionals, such as in the lunch room or on social media, without the client's permission is an abuse of confidentiality. The ethical responsibility to maintain client confidentiality continues even after the client is discharged from care.

Mandatory Reporting

Disclosure should be limited (ANA, 2001). But under certain circumstances you are required to report client personal health information. Certain communicable or sexually transmitted diseases, child and elder abuse, and the potential for serious harm to another individual are considered exceptions to sharing of confidential information. Legally required mandatory disclosures may differ slightly from state to state. In general, nurses are required to report all notifiable infectious diseases and abuse to appropriate state and local reporting agencies. This duty to report supersedes the client's right to confidentiality or privileged communication with a health provider. Relevant client data should be released only to the appropriate agency and handled as confidential information. The information provided must be the minimum amount needed to accomplish the purposes of disclosure, and the client needs to be informed about what information will be disclosed, to whom, and for what reason(s).

Informed Consent

Client rights such as autonomy and self-determination as well as ethical principles, such as beneficence, are the basis for **informed consent.** In today's health care market, legal decision making requires that you educate clients about their care. Informed consent is a legal right protected by common law and case law. It is defined as a client-focused acquiescence or voluntary yielding of will to the proposition of

BOX 2-4	Elements of a Legally Valid Informed Consent

- Is a client-based decision
- Is signed voluntarily, without coercion
- Client has full knowledge of purpose, risks, benefits
- Nurse has verified client is competent to make decision
- Client has knowledge of possible alternative procedures
- Client knows he or she has the right to refuse or discontinue care
- If risk is involved, a written consent form is signed (and witnessed) except in emergencies

another, requiring full knowledge of the purpose, risks and possible benefits of submitting to treatment (Philipsen, 2013). It is a focused communication process in which you provide all relevant information related to a procedure or treatment, offering full opportunity for discussion, questions, and expressions of concern, before asking the client or health care agent for the client to sign a legal consent form. EBP indicates that you use more than one method for educating the client about the procedure (Mahjoub and Rutledge, 2011). Unless there is a life-threatening emergency, all clients have the right to decide about whether to consent. Part of the ICN Code of Ethics says the nurse ensures that the individual receives accurate, sufficient, and timely information in a culturally appropriate manner on which to base consent for care and related treatment, maintaining the client's right to choose or refuse treatments (ICN, 2012). Box 2-4 lists elements that must be a part of an informed consent for it to be legal.

Allowing a client to sign a consent form without fully understanding the meaning invalidates the legality of consent. Ending the conversation leading to the actual signing of the consent form should always include the question, "Is there anything else that you think might be helpful in making your decision?" This type of dialogue gives the client permission to ask a question or address a concern that the nurse may not have given thought to in the informed consent discussion.

Nurses are accountable for verifying the competency of a client to give consent. Only legally competent adults can give legal consent; adults who are mentally retarded, developmentally disabled, or cognitively impaired cannot give legal consent. Evaluation of competency is made on an individual basis (e.g., in the case of emancipated adolescents no longer under their parent's control, brain-injured clients, or clients with early dementia) to determine the extent to which they understand what they are signing.

Legislation exists in all states stipulating that a legal guardian or personal health care agent can provide consent for the medical treatment of adults who lack the capacity to consent on their own behalf. In most cases, legal guardians or parents must give legal consent for minor children, defined as those younger than 18, unless the youth is legally considered an emancipated minor. Minors can also give consent in cases of immediate emergencies. Emancipated minors are mentally competent adolescents younger than 18 who petition the courts for adult status. To be considered, adolescents must be financially responsible for themselves, and no longer living with their parents. Other criteria include being married, having a child, and/or being in military service.

There is no recommended duration of consent unless it is stipulated in the document, so a form could address repeated procedures. But a new consent form should be signed if the client's condition changes (Woods, 2012). Many agencies require that the signature on a consent form be witnessed.

SUMMARY

This chapter addresses major factors effecting current nursing communication. Standards issued by various agencies and organizations guide nurses in their communications with and about clients. Standards provide a measurement benchmark, used to assess nursing competency as they apply EBP and clinical guidelines. Ethical and legal aspects of nursing communication, especially HIPAA privacy regulations, were described. The ANA Code of Ethics for Nurses provides an important guide to choice of communication in nurse-client relationships. The nursing process serves as a clinical management framework. Communication is woven into each of the sequential, overlapping phases: assessment, planning, diagnosis, planning, care implementation, and evaluation of client outcomes. All phases are client-centered, where the client is an active participant and decision maker.

ETHICAL DILEMMA   What Would You Do?

As a student nurse, you observe a fellow nursing student making a medication error. She is a good friend of yours and is visibly upset by her error. She also is afraid that if she tells the instructor, she could get a poor grade for clinical, and she needs to have a good average to keep her scholarship. The client was not actually harmed by the medication error, and your friend seems sufficiently upset by the incident to convince you that she would not make a similar error again. What would you do?

DISCUSSION QUESTIONS

1. Identify three ways to communicate effectively with each member of your client's health care team.
2. Can you give some examples of nurses choosing to not follow written standards for communication? Why didn't they?

REFERENCES

Acquaviva K: Human cognition and the dynamics of failure to rescue: The Lewis Blackman Case, *J Prof Nurs* 29(2):95–101, 2013.

Agency for Healthcare and Quality (AHRQ).

Amer KS: *Quality and Safety for Transformational Nursing: Core Competencies*, Boston, 2013, Pearson Inc.

American Nurses Association (ANA)
- ANA. 2001. Code of ethics for nurses with interpretive statements. Author: Washington, DC. www.nursingworld.org/MainMenuCategories/ThePracticeofProfessionalNursing/EthicsStandards/CodeofEthics.aspx. Accessed 10/20/13.
- ANA. 2010. Nursing: scope and standards of practice Author: Washington, DC.
- ANA. 2013. The nonnegotiable nature of ANA Code for Nurses with Interpretive Statements. 2013. www.nursingworld.org/MainMenuCategories/Policy-Advocacy/Positions-and-Resolutions/ [choose Positionstatements/

American Association of Colleges of Nursing (AACN).
- AACN. 2008. Essentials of Baccalaureate Education for Professional Nursing Practice. 2008. Author. www.aacn.org/. Accessed 10/15/13.
- AACN. 2006. Hallmarks of quality and safety: Recommended baccalaureate competencies and curricular guidelines to ensure high-quality and safe patient care. *J Prof Nurs* 22(6), 329-330.

American Association of Critical Care Nurses (AACCN): Public policy statement: Moral Distress, http://www.aacn.org/wd/practice/docs/moral_distress.pdf, 2008.

Barnsteiner J, Disch J, Johnson J, McGuinn K, et al.: Diffusing QSEN competencies across Schools of Nursing: The AACN/RWJF faculty development institutes, *J Prof Nurs* 29(2):1–8, 2013.

Canadian Nurses Association: *The code of ethics for registered nurses.* Available online Canada, 1997, Author: Alberta. [search code of ethics] http://www.cna-aiic.ca/en.

College of Nurses, Ontario. Entry into Practice: Competencies for Ontario Registered Nurses. www.cno.org/Global/docs/prac/41070_refusing.pdf (practice guidelines: communication).

Cronenwett L, Sherwood G, Barnsteiner J, et al.: Quality and Safety education for nurses, *Nurs Outlook* 55(6):122–131, 2007.

Disch J: Are we evidence-based when we like the evidence? *Nurs Outlook* 60(1):1–3, 2012a.

Disch J: QSEN? What is QSEN? *Nurs Outlook* 60(2):58–59, 2012b.

Disch J, Barnsteiner J: Second Generation QSEN, *Nurs Clin North Am* 47(3):323–416, 2012.

Gordon M: *Manual of nursing diagnoses*, Sudbury, MA, 2007, Ed 11 Jones and Bartlett Publishers.

Health Insurance Portability and Accountability Act (HIPAA): U.S. Department of Health and Human Services (DHHS), *Summary of the HIPAA privacy rule*, 1996. Accessed 10/17/13. http://www.hhs.gov/ocr/privacy/.

International Council of Nurses (ICN): *The ICN Code of Ethics for Nurses, revised.* Author, 2012. Accessed 10/4/13. www.ICN.ch/about-ICN/code-of-ethics-for-nurses/.

Institute of Medicine (IOM)
- IOM. 2010. The Future of Nursing: Leading change, advancing health. Institute of Medicine. Author.
- IOM. 2001. Crossing the quality chasm: A new health system for the 21st century. Washington, DC: National Academy Press.

Joint Commission, The (TJC)
- TJC. 2011a. Comprehensive Accreditation Manual for Hospitals Author: Chicago.
- TJC. 2011b. National Patient Safety Goals www.patientsafety.gov/
- TJC. R3 Report. www.jointcommssion.org/ [search r3 report].

Kerr P: Protecting patient education in an electronic age: A sacred trust, *Urol Nurs* 29(5):315–319, 2009.

Quality and Safety Education for Nurses (QSEN) Institute. *Lewis Blackman Story.* www.qsen.org/videos/the-lewis-blackman-story/. Accessed 11/1/13.

Mahjoub R, Rutledge DN: Perceptions of informed consent for care practices: Hospitalized patients and nurses, *Appl Nurs Res* 24(4):1–6, 2011.

McGowan C: Patients' confidentiality, *Crit Care Nurse* 32(5):61–64, 2012.

NANDA: *Nursing diagnoses: definitions & classification 2012-2014*, Philadelphia, 2011, NANDA International.

Philipsen N, Murray T, Wood C, Bell-Hawkins A, et al.: Surrogate decision-making: How to promote best outcomes in difficult times, *J Nurs Pract* 9(9):1–7, 2013.

Quality and Safety Education for Nurses (QSEN). www.qsen.org/

World Health Organization, Woods KD: Reply to question on Informed Consent for repeated procedures, *AORN J* 96(6):1–7, 2012. Clinical issues-December 2012. www.WHO.int.

CHAPTER 3

Clinical Judgment and Ethical Decision Making

Kathleen Underman Boggs

OBJECTIVES

At the end of the chapter, the reader will be able to:

1. Define client-centered care communication terms related to thinking, ethical reasoning, and critical thinking.
2. Identify and discuss three principles of ethics underlying bioethical reasoning.
3. Describe the 10 steps of critical thinking.
4. Discuss the application of ethics in nurse-client relationships.
5. Analyze and apply the critical thinking process used in making clinical decisions with clients.
6. Demonstrate ability to analyze, synthesize, and evaluate a complex simulated case situation to make a clinical judgment.
7. Utilize evidenced-based practice competency by discussing application of findings from a research study to clinical practice.

This chapter examines the principles of ethical decision making and the process for critical thinking. Both are essential foundational knowledge for you to make effective nursing clinical judgments. Your ability to use critical thinking and ethical reasoning skills and communicate these will be a determining factor in your competency as a nurse. Successfully developing these abilities contributes to success on the NCLEX-RN licensure examination (Chang et al., 2011). Ethical responsibility is a big aspect of nursing care. It is a much wider concept than legal responsibility, engaging not only your clients but your entire community (Tschudin, 2013). Making ethical decisions requires that you understand the process. In this book, the focus is on the current literature in bioethics as held in Western society. In addition to basic content presented in this chapter, an ethical dilemma is included in subsequent chapters to help you begin applying your reasoning process.

Critical thinking is a learned skill that teaches you how to use a systematic process to make your clinical decisions. In the past, expert nurses accumulated this skill with on-the-job experience, through trial and error. But this essential nursing skill can be learned with continual practice and conscientious applications while in school. The Applications section of this chapter specifically walks you through the reasoning process in applying the 10 steps of critical thinking.

BASIC CONCEPTS
TYPES OF THINKING

There are many ways of thinking (Figure 3-1). Students often attempt to use total recall by simply memorizing a bunch of facts (e.g., memorizing the cranial nerves by using a **mnemonic** such as "On Old Olympus' Towering Tops. . ."). At other times, we rely on developing habits by repetition, such as practicing cardiopulmonary resuscitation (CPR) techniques. More structured methods of thinking, such as **inquiry**, have been developed in disciplines related to nursing. For example, you are probably familiar with **the scientific method**. As used in research, this is a logical, linear method of systematically gaining new information, often by setting up an experiment to test an idea. The nursing process uses a method of systematic steps: assessment before planning, planning before intervention, and evaluation.

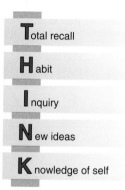

Total recall

Habit

Inquiry

New ideas

Knowledge of self

Figure 3-1 Mnemonics can be useful tools.

This chapter focuses on the most important concepts that help you develop your clinical judgment abilities.

ETHICAL REASONING

As nurses, we often face ethical dilemmas that may leave us in moral distress (Pavlish et al., 2011). Most nurses report facing ethical dilemmas in their work at least on a weekly basis. The most commonly reported issues involve client choice, quality of life, and end-of-life decisions. As a nurse you will frequently have to act in value-laden situations. For example, you may have clients who request abortions or who want "do not resuscitate" (DNR; "no code") orders. Your decisions affect your client's rights and quality of life. Remember, your willingness to comply with ethical and professional standards is a hallmark of a professional.

Members of many professions have difficulty applying ethical principles to clinical care situations. Fero's study (2010) showed that nursing students have difficulty even recognizing the problem. Professionals, including physicians and nurses, when tested respond correctly to ethical dilemma questions less than half of the time. Is being ethically correct less than half the time acceptable? Student practice in applying ethical principles is important. Although it is true that most health care agencies now have ethics committees that often are the primary party involved in resolving difficult ethical dilemmas, you, the nurse, will be called on to make ethical decisions.

As nurses, we need to have a clear understanding of the ethics of the nursing profession. Nursing organizations have formally published ethical codes, such as those from the Federation of European Countries or from the American Nurses Association (ANA). Refer to ANA's Code of Ethics listed in Chapter 2.

Case Example

During an influenza pandemic, Ada Kelly, RN, is reassigned to work on an unfamiliar pulmonary intensive care unit. Clients there have a severe form of infectious flu with respiratory complications and are receiving mechanical ventilation. She worries that if she refuses to care for these assigned clients, she could lose her job or even her license. But she also fears carrying this infection home to her two preschool children.

This case highlights conflicting duties: employer/client versus self/family. According to the American Nurses Association (ANA), nurses are obligated to care for all clients, but there are limits to the personal risk of harm a nurse can be expected to accept. It is her *moral duty* if clients are at significant risk for harm that her care can prevent. This situation becomes a *moral option* only if there are alternative sources of care (i.e., other nurses available).

ETHICAL THEORIES AND DECISION-MAKING MODELS

Ethical theories provide the bedrock from which we derive the principles that guide our decision making. There is no one "right" answer to an ethical dilemma: The decision may vary depending on which theory the involved people subscribe to. The following section briefly describes the most common models currently used in bioethics. They are, for the most part, representative of a Western European and Judeo-Christian viewpoint. As we become a more culturally diverse society, other equally viable viewpoints may become acculturated. This discussion focuses on three decision-making models: utilitarian/goal-based, duty-based, and rights-based models.

The **utilitarian/goal-based model** says that the "rightness" or "wrongness" of an action is always a function of its consequences. Rightness is the extent to which performing or omitting an action will contribute to the overall good of the client. Good is defined as maximum welfare or happiness. The rights of clients and the duties of a nurse are determined by what will achieve maximum welfare. When a conflict in outcome occurs, the correct action is the one that will result in the greatest good for the majority. An example of a decision made according to the goal-based model is forced mandatory institutionalization of a client with tuberculosis who refuses to take medicine to protect other members of the community. The client's hospitalization produces the greatest balance of good over harm for the majority. Thus, "goodness" of an action is determined solely by its outcome.

The **deontologic** or **duty-based model** is person centered. It incorporates Immanuel Kant's deontologic philosophy, which holds that the "rightness" of an action is determined by other factors in addition to its outcome. Respect for every person's inherent dignity is a consideration. For example, a straightforward implication would be that a physician (or nurse) may never lie to a client. Do you agree? Decisions based on this duty-based model have a religious-social foundation. Rightness is determined by moral worth, regardless of the circumstances or the individual involved. In making decisions or implementing actions, the nurse cannot violate the basic duties and rights of individuals. Decisions about what is in the best interests of the client require consensus among all parties involved. Examples are the medical code "do no harm" and the nursing duty to "help save lives."

The **human rights–based model** is based on the belief that each client has basic rights. Our duties as health care providers arise from these basic rights. For example, a client has the right to refuse care. Conflict occurs when the provider's duty is not in the best interests of the client. The client has the right to life and the nurse has the duty to save lives, but what if the quality of life is intolerable and there is no hope for a positive outcome? Such a case might occur when a neonatal nurse cares for an infant with anencephaly (born without brain tissue in the cerebrum) in whom even the least invasive treatment would be extremely painful and would never provide any quality of life.

Ethical dilemmas arise when an actual or potential conflict occurs regarding principles, duties, or rights. Of course, many ethical or moral concepts held by Western society have been codified into law. Laws may vary from state to state, but a moral principle should be universally applied. Moral principles are shared by most members of a group, such as physicians or nurses, and represent the professional values of the group. Conflict arises when a nurse's professional values differ from the law in her state of residence. Conflict may also arise when you have not come to terms with situations in which your personal values differ from the profession's values. One example is doctor-assisted suicide (euthanasia). *Legally*, at the turn of the twenty-first century, such an act was legal in Oregon but illegal in Michigan. *Professionally*, the ANA Code of Ethics

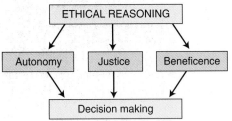

Figure 3-2 Guiding ethical principles that assist in decision making.

guides you to do no harm. *Personally*, your belief about whether euthanasia is right or wrong may be at variance with either of the above.

Bioethical Principles

To practice nursing in an ethical manner, you must be able to recognize the existence of a **moral problem**. Once you recognize a situation that puts your client in jeopardy, you must be able to take action. Three essential, guiding ethical principles have been developed from the theories cited earlier. The three principles that can assist us in decision making are autonomy, beneficence (nonmaleficence), and justice (Figure 3-2).

Autonomy Versus Medical Paternalism. Autonomy is the client's right to self-determination. In the medical context, respect for a client's autonomy is a fundamental ethical principle. It is the basis for the concept of informed consent, which means your client makes a rational, informed decision without coercion. In the past, nurses and physicians often made decisions for clients based on what they thought was best for the client. This *paternalism* sometimes discounted the wishes of clients and their families. The ethical concept of client autonomy has emerged strongly as a client right in Western countries. Aspects involving the individual's right to participate in medical decisions about his own care have become law.

This moral principle of autonomy means that each client has the right to decide about his or her health care. Clients who are empowered to make such decisions are more likely to comply with your treatment plan. Internal factors such as pain may interfere with a client's ability to choose. External factors such as coercion by a care provider may also interfere. As a nurse, you and your employer must legally obtain the client's permission for all treatment procedures. In the United States, under the Patient Self-Determination Act of 1991, all clients of agencies receiving Medicaid funds must receive written information about their rights to make decisions about their medical care. Nurses, as well as physicians, must provide clients with all the relevant and accurate information they need to make an "informed" decision whether they agree to treatments. The ANA states that it is the nurse's responsibility to assist clients to make these decisions, as discussed in Chapter 2 (see Informed Consent section).

Many of the nursing theories incorporate concepts about autonomy and empowering the client to be responsible for self-care, so you may find this easy to accept as part of your nursing role. However, what happens if the client's right to autonomy puts others at risk? Whose rights take precedence?

The concept of autonomy has also been applied to the way we practice nursing, but our professional autonomy has some limitations. For example, the American Medical Association's Principles of Medical Ethics says a physician can choose whom to serve, except in an emergency; however, the picture is a little different in nursing practice. According to the ANA Committee on Ethics, nurses are ethically obligated to treat clients seeking their care. For example, you could not refuse to care for a client with acquired immunodeficiency syndrome (AIDS) who is assigned to you.

A nurse has autonomy in caring for a client, but this is somewhat limited because legally she must also follow physician orders and be subject to physician authority. Before the nurse or physician can override a client's right to autonomy, he or she must be able to present a strong case for their point of view based on either or both of the following principles: beneficence and justice.

Autonomy Case Example

Ms. Dorothy Newt, 72 years of age, refuses physician-assisted suicide after being diagnosed with Alzheimer disease. She also refuses entry into a long-term care facility, deciding instead to rely on her aged, disabled spouse to provide her total care as she deteriorates physically and mentally. As her home health nurse, you find he is unable to provide needed care, and ask her physician to transfer her to an extended-care facility.

Beneficence and Nonmaleficence

Beneficence implies that a decision results in the greatest good or produces the least harm to the client. This is based on the Hippocratic Oath and its concept of "do no harm." Avoiding actions that bring harm to another person is known as *nonmaleficence.* An example is the Christian belief of "do not kill,"

which has been codified into law but has many exceptions (e.g., soldiers sent to war are expected to kill the enemy).

In health care, beneficence is the underlying principle for the ANA Code of Ethics, saying that the good of your client is your primary responsibility. Nursing theorists have incorporated this into the nursing role, so you may find this easy to accept. Helping others may be why you chose to become a nurse. In nursing, you not only have the obligation to avoid harming your clients, but you also are expected to advocate for your clients' best interests.

Beneficence is challenged in many clinical situations (e.g., requests for abortion or euthanasia). Currently, some of the most difficult ethical dilemmas involve situations where decisions may be made to withhold treatment. For example, decisions are made to justify such violations of beneficence in the guise of permitting merciful death. Is there a moral difference between actively causing death or in withholding treatment, when the outcome for the client is the same death? There are clear legal differences. In most states, a health care worker who intentionally acts to cause a client's death is legally liable.

Other challenges to beneficence occur when the involved parties hold different viewpoints about what is best for the client. Consider a case in which the family of an elderly, post stroke, comatose, ventilator-dependent client wants all forms of treatment continued, but the health care team does not believe it will benefit the client. The initial step toward resolution may be holding a family conference and really listening to the viewpoints of family members, asking them whether the client ever expressed wishes verbally or in writing in the form of an advance directive. Maintaining a trusting, open, mutually respectful communication may help avoid an adversarial situation.

Beneficence Case Example

Mr. Harper, 62 years of age, is admitted with end-organ failure. You are expected to assess for pain that he has and treat it. Do you seek a palliative order even though his liver cannot process drugs? It is estimated that more than 50% of conscious clients spend their last week of life in moderate to severe pain. Who is advocating for them?

Justice

Justice is actually a legal term; however, in ethics, it refers to being fair or impartial. A related concept is equality (e.g., the just distribution of goods or resources, sometimes called *social justice* or *distributive justice*). Within the health care arena, this distributive justice concept might be applied to scarce treatment resources. As new and more expensive technologies that can prolong life become available, who has a right to them? Who should pay for them? If resources are scarce, how do we decide who gets them? Should a limited resource be spread out equally to everyone? Or should it be allocated based on who has the greatest need?

Unnecessary Treatment. Decisions made based on the principle of justice may also involve the concept of unnecessary treatment. Are all operations that are performed truly necessary? Why do some clients receive antibiotics for viral infections, when we know they do not kill viruses? Are unnecessary diagnostic tests ever ordered solely to document that a client does not have Condition X, just in case there is a malpractice lawsuit?

Social Worth. Another justice concept to consider in making decisions is that of social worth. Are all people equal? Are some more deserving than others? If a client, Dan, is 7 years old instead of 77 years old, and the expensive medicine would cure his condition, should these factors affect the decision to give him the medicine? If there is only one liver available for transplant today, and there are two equally viable potential recipients—Larry, age 54 years, whose alcoholism destroyed his own liver; or Kay, age 32 years, whose liver was destroyed by hepatitis she got while on a life-saving mission abroad—who should get the liver?

Veracity. Truthfulness is the bedrock of trust. And trust is an essential component of the professional nurse-client relationship. Not only is there a moral injunction against lying, but it is also destructive to any professional relationship. Generally, nurses would agree that a nurse should never lie to a client. However, there is controversy about withholding information from a client. We need clarity about truth telling. There will be times when we need to exercise some judgment about to whom to disclose information. We have an obligation to protect potentially vulnerable clients from information that would cause emotional distress. Although it is never acceptable to lie, nurses have evaded answering questions by saying, "You need to ask your physician about that." Can you suggest another response?

Justice Case Example

Lee, age 18 years, is admitted to the emergency department (ED) bleeding from a chest wound. His blood pressure is falling, shock is imminent. Tomas, Sue, and Mary were registered ahead of Lee, but do not have life-threatening complaints. ED's triage protocol says care for the least stable client is a priority. Is this a "just distribution" of ED resources?

STEPS IN ETHICAL DECISION MAKING

The process of moral reasoning and making ethical decisions has been broken down into steps. These steps are only a part of the larger model for critical thinking. If you are the moral agent making this decision, you must be skillful enough to implement the actions in a morally correct way.

In deciding how to spend your limited time with these clients, do you base your decision entirely on how much good you can do for each client? Under distributive justice, what should happen when the needs of these four conflict? You could base your decision on the principle of beneficence and do the greatest good for the most clients, but this is a very subjective judgment. Would one of these clients benefit more from nursing care than the others?

In using ethical decision-making processes, nurses must be able to tolerate ambiguity and uncertainty. One of the most difficult aspects for the novice nurse to accept is that there often is no one "right" answer; rather, usually several options may be selected, depending on the person or situation.

Ethical Decision-Making Case Example

You are assigned to four critical clients on your unit. Mrs. Rae, 83 years of age, is unconscious, dying, and needs suctioning every 10 minutes. Mr. Jones, 47 years of age, has been admitted for observation for severe bloody stools. Mr. Hernandez, 52 years of age, has newly diagnosed diabetes and is receiving intravenous (IV) drip insulin; he requires monitoring of vital signs every 15 minutes. Mr. Martin, 35 years of age, is suicidal and has been told today he has inoperable cancer.

CRITICAL THINKING

Critical thinking is a tool of inquiry (Facione, 2007). It is an analytical process in which you purposefully use specific thinking skills to make complex clinical decisions. You are able to reflect on your own thinking process to make effective decisions that improve your client's outcome (Ryan and Tatum, 2013). Although no consensus has been reached on a critical thinking definition in the nursing arena, we generally define critical thinking as the purposeful use of a specific cognitive framework to identify and analyze problems. Critical thinking enables us to recognize emergent client situations, make clear, objective clinical decisions, and intervene appropriately to give safe, effective care. It encompasses the steps of the nursing process, but possibly in a more circular loop than we usually envision the nursing process. By thinking critically, we can modify our client's care plan based on responses to our nursing interventions.

Critical thinking is more than just a *cognitive process* of following steps. It also has an *affective component*—the willingness to engage in self-reflective inquiry. As you learn to be a critical thinker, you improve and clarify your thinking process skills, so that you are more accurately able to solve problems based on available evidence. Although cognitive thinking skills can be taught, you also need to be willing to consciously choose to apply this process.

CHARACTERISTICS OF A CRITICAL THINKER

Critical thinkers are skilled at using inquiry methods. They approach problem solutions in a systematic, organized, and goal-directed way when making clinical decisions. They continually use past knowledge, communication skills, new information, and observations to make these clinical judgments. Table 3-1 summarizes the characteristics of a critical thinker.

Expert nurses recognize that priorities change continually, requiring constant assessment and alternative interventions. When the authors analyzed the decision-making process of expert nurses, they all used the critical thinking steps described in this chapter when they made their clinical judgments, even though they were not always able to verbally state the components of their thinking processes. Expert nurses organized each input of client information and quickly distinguished relevant from irrelevant information. They seemed to categorize each new fact into a problem format, obtaining supplementary data and arriving at a decision about diagnosis and intervention. Often, they commented about comparing this new information with prior knowledge, sometimes

TABLE 3-1	Characteristics of a Critical Thinker
Attitude	• Be inquisitive and desire to seek the truth • Develop an analytical thinking ability • Maintain an inquisitive mind set, systematically seeking solutions • Display open-minded and flexible thinking process
Thought Processes	• Think in an orderly way, using logical reasoning in complex problem situations • Be reflective and anticipate consequences • Combine existing knowledge and standards with new information (transformation) • Incorporate creative thinking • Diligently persevere in seeking relevant information • Discard irrelevant information (discrimination) • Consider alternative solutions
Actions	• Recognize when information is missing and seeks new input • Revise actions based on new input • Evaluate solutions and outcomes

from academic sources and "best practice protocols" but most often from information gained from other nurses. They constantly scan for new information, and constantly reassess their client's situation. This is not linear. New input is always being added. This contrasts with novice nurses who tend to think in a linear way, collect lots of facts but not logically organize them, and fail to make as many connections with past knowledge. Novice nurses' assessments are more generalized and less focused, and they tend to jump too quickly to a diagnosis without recognizing the need to obtain more facts.

Because nurses are responsible for a significant proportion of decisions that affect client care, and are key gatekeepers in preventing harm, employing agencies periodically retest staff nurses for competencies. This procedure was initially done just to retest or recertify technical skills, such as CPR. Now many agencies routinely add other competency testing, including evaluation of critical thinking and clinical judgment skills.

BARRIERS TO THINKING CRITICALLY AND REASONING ETHICALLY

Attitudes and Habits

Barriers that decrease a nurse's ability to think critically, including attitudes such as "my way is better," interfere with our ability to empower clients to make their own decisions. Our thinking habits can also impede communication with clients or families making complex bioethical choices. Examples include becoming accustomed to acknowledging "only one right answer" or selecting only one option. Behaviors that act as barriers include automatically responding defensively when challenged, resisting changes, and desiring to conform to expectations. Cognitive barriers, such as thinking in stereotypes, also interfere with our ability to treat a client as an individual.

Cognitive Dissonance

Cognitive dissonance refers to the mental discomfort you feel when there is a discrepancy between what you already believe and some new information that does not go along with your view. In this book, we use the term to refer to the holding of two or more conflicting values at the same time.

Personal Values Versus Professional Values

We all have a *personal value system* developed over a lifetime that has been extensively shaped by our family, our religious beliefs, and our years of life experiences. Our values change as we mature in our ability to think critically, logically, and morally. Strongly held values become a part of self-concept. Our education as nurses helps us acquire a *professional value system*. In nursing school, as you advance through your clinical experiences, you begin to take on some of the values of the nursing profession (Box 3-1). You are acquiring these values as you learn the nursing role. The process of this role socialization is discussed in Chapter 22. For example, maintaining client confidentiality is a professional value, with both a legal and a moral requirement. We must take care that we do not allow our personal values to obstruct care for a client who holds differing values.

VALUES CLARIFICATION AND THE NURSING PROCESS

The nursing process offers many opportunities to incorporate *values clarification* into your care. During the assessment phase, you can obtain an assessment of the *client's values* with regard to the health system. For

BOX 3-1	Five Core Values of Professional Nursing

Five *core values of professional nursing* have been identified by the American Association of Colleges of Nursing (AACN):
- Human dignity
- Integrity
- Autonomy
- Altruism
- Social justice

example, you interview a client for the first time and learn that he has obstructive pulmonary disease and is having difficulty breathing, but he insists on smoking. Is it appropriate to intervene? In this example, you know that smoking is detrimental to a person's health and you, as a nurse, find the value of health in conflict with your client's value of smoking. It is important to understand your client's values. When your values differ, you attempt to care for this client within his or her reality. Your client has the right to make decisions that are not always congruent with those of his health care providers.

When identifying specific nursing diagnoses, it is important that your diagnoses are not biased. Examples of value conflicts might be spiritual distress related to a conflict between spiritual beliefs and prescribed health treatments, or ineffective family coping related to restricted visiting hours for a family in which full family participation is a cultural value. In the planning phase, it is important to identify and understand the client's value system as the foundation for developing the most appropriate interventions. Plans of care that support rather than discount the client's health care beliefs are more likely to be received favorably. Your interventions include values clarification as a guideline for care. You help clients examine alternatives. During the evaluation phase, examine how well the nursing and client goals were met while keeping within the guidelines of the client's value system.

To summarize, in case of conflict (with own personal ethical convictions), nurses must put aside their own moral convictions to provide necessary assistance in a case of emergency when there is imminent risk to a patient's life (Sasso et al., 2008). Ethical reasoning and critical thinking skills are essential competencies for making clinical judgments, in an increasingly complex health care system. To apply critical thinking to a

Developing an Evidence-Based Practice

Lancaster R. Analysis of work-arounds. Research paper presented at the 2013 QSEN National Forum, May 30-31, 2013, Atlanta, Georgia.

Fourth-year baccalaureate student nurses used Quality and Safety Education for Nurses (QSEN)'s Staff Work-Around Assignment (www.qsen.org) to describe their observations of their staff nurse preceptors engaging in work-arounds over a 1-year period. (A work-around is defined as an improvised response, a break in the established work policies.) Using a quantitative design, a content analysis of data was utilized to identify themes.

Results: The following themes emerged as possible influences or reasons for nurses to engage in work-arounds: workload, patient needs, equipment/technology, nursing knowledge, or judgment.

Application to your Practice: Lancaster suggests a need to address the cognitive dissonance that occurs when students observe the occurrence of risky behaviors contrary to what has been taught. Consider the following issues:
1. What rationale (ethical principle) does a nurse use when "borrowing" a similar pain medication from another client's drawer, instead of waiting for the newly ordered med to arrive from pharmacy for a client in severe discomfort? Are there risks to her client's safety if the nurse mistakes the ordered dosage?
2. What rationale does a staff member use when he rips off the finger of his latex glove to palpate for a pulse when performing a venipuncture (blood draw)? Is there risk of harm to self or other clients?
3. What workload factors might induce a nurse to scan all bar codes at once in the medication room rather than carrying the scanner into each client's separate room to scan?

clinical decision, we need to base our intervention on *the best evidence* available. These skills can be learned by participating in simulated patient case situations. Acquiring these skills will enable you to provide higher quality nursing care (Fero et al., 2009).

APPLICATIONS

Accrediting agencies for nursing curriculums require inclusion of critical thinking curriculum. Accepted teaching-learning methods for assessing critical thinking include case studies, questioning, reflective journalism, client simulations, portfolios, concept maps, and problem-based learning. As a nurse, you are faced with processing copious amounts of information to be considered before making a decision about your client's situation. Often, you must consider more than one possibility but make your decision quickly. To provide safe care, you must be able to apply critical thinking skills to clinical situations (Fero et al., 2009).

PARTICIPATION IN CLINICAL RESEARCH

You or your clients may be called on at some time to participate in clinical research trials. The focus of this book is to examine ethical dilemmas faced in nursing practice, and this does not encompass the ethical aspect of conducting or participating in research studies. To examine what makes clinical research ethical, consult a nursing research book.

SOLVING ETHICAL DILEMMAS IN NURSING

Nurses indicate a need for more information about dealing with the ethical dilemmas they encounter, yet most say they receive little education in doing so. Exercises 3-1 (autonomy), 3-2 (beneficence), and 3-3 (justice) give you this opportunity.

The ethical issues that nurses commonly face today can be placed in three general categories: moral uncertainty, moral or ethical dilemmas, and moral distress. *Moral uncertainty* occurs when a nurse is uncertain as to which moral rules (i.e., values, beliefs, or ethical principles) apply to a given situation. For example, should a terminally ill client who is in and out of a coma and chooses not to eat or drink anything be required to have intravenous (IV) therapy for hydration purposes? Does

EXERCISE 3-1   Autonomy

Purpose: To stimulate class discussion about the moral principle of autonomy.

Procedure
In small groups, read the three case examples on page *** and discuss whether the client has the autonomous right to refuse treatment if it affects the life of another person.

Discussion
Prepare your argument for an in-class discussion.

EXERCISE 3-2	Beneficence

Purpose: To stimulate discussion about the moral principle of beneficence.

Procedure

Read the following case example and prepare for discussion:

Dawn, a staff nurse, answers the telephone and receives a verbal order from Dr. Smith. Ms. Patton was admitted this morning with ventricular arrhythmia. Dr. Smith orders Dawn to administer a potent diuretic, furosemide (Lasix) 80 mg, IV, STAT. This is such a large dose that she has to order it up from pharmacy.

As described in the text, you are legally obliged to carry out a doctor's orders unless they threaten the welfare of your client. How often do nurses question orders? What would happen to a nurse who questioned orders too often? In a research study using this case simulation, nearly 95% of the time the nurses participating in the study attempted to implement this potentially lethal medication order before being stopped by the researcher!

Discussion
1. What principles are involved?
2. What would you do if you were this staff nurse?

EXERCISE 3-3	Justice

Purpose: To encourage discussion about the concept of justice.

Procedure

Consider that in Oregon several years ago, attempts were made to legislate some restrictions on what Medicaid would pay for. A young boy needed a standard treatment of bone marrow transplant for his childhood leukemia. He died when the state refused to pay for his treatment.

Read the following case example and answer the discussion questions:

Mr. Diaz, age 74 years, has led an active life and continues to be the sole support for his wife and disabled daughter. He pays for health care with Medicare government insurance. The doctors think his cancer may respond to a very expensive new drug, which is not paid for under his coverage.

Discussion
1. Does everyone have a basic right to health care, as well as to life and liberty?
2. Does an insurance company have a right to restrict access to care?

---

giving IV therapy constitute giving the client extraordinary measures to prolong life? Is it more comfortable or less comfortable for the dying client to maintain a high hydration level? When there is no clear definition of the problem, moral uncertainty develops, because the nurse is unable to identify the situation as a moral problem or to define specific moral rules that apply. Strategies that might be useful in dealing with moral uncertainty include using the values clarification process, developing a specific philosophy of nursing, and acquiring knowledge about ethical principles.

Ethical or moral dilemmas arise when two or more moral issues are in conflict. An ethical dilemma is a problem in which there are two or more conflicting but equally right answers. Organ harvesting of a severely brain-damaged infant is an example of an ethical dilemma. Removal of organs from one infant may save the lives of several other infants. However, even though the brain-damaged child is definitely going to die, is it right to remove organs before the child's death? It is important for the nurse to understand that, in many ethical dilemmas, there is often no single "right" solution. Some decisions may be "more right" than others, but often what one nurse decides is best differs significantly from what another nurse would decide.

The third common kind of ethical problem seen in nursing today is *moral distress*. Moral distress results when the nurse knows what is "right" but is bound to do otherwise because of legal or institutional constraints. When such a situation arises (e.g., a terminally ill client who does not have a "do not resuscitate" medical order and for whom, therefore, resuscitation attempts must be made), the nurse may experience inner turmoil.

Nurses have reported that three of their most commonly encountered ethics problems have to do with resuscitation decisions for dying clients with unclear, confusing, or no code orders; patients and families who wanted more aggressive treatment; and colleagues who discussed clients inappropriately.

Because values underlie all ethical decision making, nurses must understand their own values thoroughly before making an ethical decision. Instead of responding in an emotional manner on the spur of the moment (as people often do when faced with an ethical dilemma), the nurse who uses the values clarification process can respond rationally. It is not an easy task to have sufficient knowledge of oneself, of the situation, and of legal and moral constraints to be able to implement ethical decision making quickly. Expert nurses still struggle. Taking time to examine situations can help you develop skill in dealing with ethical dilemmas in nursing, and the exercises in this book will give you a chance to practice. Each chapter in this book has included at least one ethical dilemma, so you can discuss what you would do.

As nurses, we advocate for our client's best interests. To do so, we avoid a "paternalistic" imposing of what we think is in their best interests, instead listening and eliciting their preferences, to work collaboratively with the health care team in developing an ethical patient-centered plan of care (Pavlish et al., 2011). Issues most frequently necessitating ethical decisions occur at the beginning of life and at the close of life.

Finally, reflect on your own ethical practice. How important it is for your client to be able to always count on you? Consider the following client journal entry (Milton, 2002):

I ask for information, share my needs, to no avail.
You come and go. . .
"Could you find out for me?" "Sure, I'll check on it."
[But] check on it never comes. . .
Who can I trust? I thought you'd be here for me. . .
You weren't. What can I do?
Betrayal permeates. . .

PROFESSIONAL VALUES ACQUISITION

Professional values or ethics consist of the values held in common by the members of a profession. Professional values are formally stated in professional codes. One example is the ANA Code of Ethics for Nurses. Often, professional values are transmitted by tradition in nursing classes and clinical experiences. They are modeled by expert nurses and assimilated as part of the role socialization process during your years as a student and new graduate. Professional values acquisition should perhaps be the result of conscious choice by a nursing student. This is the first step in values

acquisition. Can you apply it to your own life? It may also help you understand the value system of your clients.

Values are a strong determinant in making selections between competing alternatives. Consider whether the nursing profession holds values regarding the following situation: What if you observed a nurse charting that a medicine was given to a client when you know it was not? What professional value should guide your response?

APPLYING CRITICAL THINKING TO THE CLINICAL DECISION-MAKING PROCESS

This section discusses a procedure for developing critical thinking skills as applied to solving clinical problems. Different examples illustrate the reasoning process developed by several disciplines. Unfortunately, each discipline has its own vocabulary. Table 3-2 shows that we are talking about concepts with which you are already familiar. It also contrasts terms used in education, nursing, and philosophy to specify 10 steps to help you develop your critical thinking skills. For example, the nurse performs a "client assessment," which in education is referred to as "collecting information" or in philosophy may be called "identifying claims."

The process of critical thinking is systematic, organized, and goal directed. As critical thinkers, nurses are able to explore all aspects of a complex clinical situation. This is a learned process. Among many teaching-learning techniques helping you develop critical thinking skills, most are included in this book: reflective journaling, concept maps, role-playing, guided small group discussion, and case study discussion. An extensive case application follows. During your learning phase, the critical thinking skills are divided into 10 specific steps. Each step includes a discussion of application to the clinical case example provided.

To help you understand how to apply critical thinking steps, read the following case and then see how each of the steps can be used in making clinical decisions. Components of this case are applied to illustrate the steps and stimulate discussion in the critical thinking process; many more points may be raised. From the outset, understand that, although these are listed as steps, they do not occur in a rigid, linear way in real life. The model is best thought of as a circular model. New data are constantly being sought and added to the process.

TABLE 3-2	Reasoning Process		
Generic Reasoning Process	Diagnostic Reasoning in the Nursing Process	Ethical Reasoning	Critical Thinking Skill
Collect and interpret information	Gordon's functional patterns of health assessment	Identify ethical problem (parties, claim, basis)	1. Clarify concepts 2. Identify own, client, and professional values and differentiate
Identify problem	Statement of nursing diagnosis	Consider ethical dilemma: • State the problem • Collect additional information • Develop alternatives for analysis	3. Integrate data and identify missing data 4. Collect new data 5. Identify problem 6. Apply criteria 7. Look at alternatives 8. Examine skeptically 9. Check for change in context
Plan for problem solving	Prioritization of problems/ interventions	Prioritized claims	10. Make decision, select best action plan, and act to implement
Implement plan	Nursing action	Take moral action	
Evaluate	Outcome evaluation	Moral evaluation of outcome and reflect on the process used	Evaluate the outcome and reflect on the process

Case Example

Day 1—Mrs. Vlios, a 72-year-old widowed teacher, has been admitted to your unit. Her daughter, Sara, lives 2 hours away from her mother, but she arrives soon after admission. According to Sara, her mother lived an active life before admission, taking care of herself in an apartment in a senior citizens' housing development. Sara noticed that for about 3 weeks now, telephone conversations with her mother did not make sense or she seemed to have a hard time concentrating, although her pronunciation was clear. The admitting diagnosis is dehydration and dementia, rule out Alzheimer disease, organic brain syndrome, and depression. An intravenous (IV) drip of 1000 mL dextrose/0.45 normal saline is ordered at 50 drops/hour. Mrs. Vlios's history is unremarkable except for a recent 10-pound weight loss. She has no allergies and is known to take acetaminophen regularly for minor pain.

Day 2—When Sara visits her mom's apartment to bring grooming items to the hospital, she finds the refrigerator and food pantry empty. A neighbor tells her that Mrs. Vlios was seen roaming the halls aimlessly 2 days ago and could not remember whether she had eaten. As Mrs. Vlios's nurse, you notice that she is oriented today (to time and person). A soft diet is ordered, and her urinary output is now normal.

Day 5—In morning report, the night nurse states that Mrs. Vlios was hallucinating and restraints were applied. A nasogastric tube was ordered to suction out stomach contents because of repeated vomiting. Dr. Green tells Sara and her brother, Todos, that their mother's prognosis is guarded; she has acquired a serious systemic infection, is semicomatose, is not taking nourishment, and needs antibiotics and hyperalimentation. Sara reminds the doctor that her mother signed a living will in which she stated she refuses all treatment except IVs to keep her alive. Todos is upset, yelling at Sara that he wants the doctor to do everything possible to keep their mother alive.

STEP 1: CLARIFY CONCEPTS

The first step in making a clinical judgment is to identify whether a problem actually exists. Poor decision makers often skip this step. To figure out whether there is a problem, you need to think about what to observe and what basic information to gather. If it is an ethical dilemma, you not only need to identify the existence of the moral problem, but you need to also identify all the interested parties who have a stake in the decision. Figuring out exactly what the problem or issue is may not be as easy as it sounds.

Look for Clues

Are there hidden meanings to the words being spoken? Are there nonverbal clues?

Identify Assumptions

What assumptions are being made?

Case Discussion

This case is designed to present both physiologic and ethical dilemmas. In clarifying the problem, address both domains.

- Physiological concerns: Based on the diagnosis, the initial treatment goal was to restore homeostasis. By day 5, is it clear whether Mrs. Vlios's condition is reversible?
- Ethical concerns: When is a decision made to initiate treatment or to abide by the advance directive and respect the client's wishes regarding no treatment?
- What are the wishes of the family? What happens when there is no consensus?
- Assumptions: Is the diagnosis correct? Does the client have dementia? Or was her confusion a result of dehydration and a strange hospital environment?

STEP 2: IDENTIFY YOUR OWN VALUES

Values clarification helps you identify and prioritize your values. It also serves as a base for helping clients identify the values they hold as important. Unless you are able to identify your client's values and can appreciate the validity of those values, you run the risk for imposing your own values. It is not necessary for your values and your client's values to coincide; this is an unrealistic expectation. However, whenever possible, the client's values should be taken into consideration during every aspect of nursing care. Discussion of the case of Mrs. Vlios presented in this section may help you with the clarification process.

Having just completed the exercises given earlier should help your understanding of your own personal values and the professional values of nursing. Now apply this information to this case.

Case Discussion

Identify the values of each person involved:

- Family: Mrs. Vlios signed an advance directive. Sara wants it adhered to; Todos wants it ignored. Why? (Missing information: Are there religious beliefs? Is there unclear communication? Is there guilt about previous troubles in the relationship?)
- Personal values: What are yours?
- Professional values: The ANA says nurses are advocates for their clients; beneficence implies nonmaleficence

("do no harm"), but autonomy means the client has the right to refuse treatment. What is the agency's policy? What are the legal considerations? Practice refining your professional values acquisition by completing the values exercises in this chapter.

In summary, you need to identify which values are involved in a situation or which moral principles can be cited to support each of the positions advocated by the involved individuals.

STEP 3: INTEGRATE DATA AND IDENTIFY MISSING DATA

Think about knowledge gained in prior courses and during clinical experiences. Try to make connections between different subject areas and clinical nursing practice.

- Identify what data are needed. Obtain all possible information and gather facts or evidence (evaluate whether data are true, relevant, and sufficient). Situations are often complicated. It is important to figure out what information is significant to this situation. Synthesize prior information you already have with similarities in the current situation. Conflicting data may indicate a need to search for more information.
- Compare existing information with past knowledge. Has this client complained of difficulty thinking before? Does she have a history of dementia?
- Look for gaps in the information. Actively work to recognize whether there is missing information. Was Mrs. Vlios previously taking medications to prevent depression? For a nurse, this is an important part of critical thinking.
- Collect information systematically. Use an organized framework to obtain information. Nurses often obtain a client's history by asking questions about each body system. They could just as systematically ask about basic needs.
- Organize your information. Clustering information into relevant categories is helpful. For example, gathering all the facts about a client's breathing may help focus your attention on whether the client is having a respiratory problem. In your assessment, you note rate and character of respirations, color of nails and lips, use of accessory muscles, and grunting noises. At the same time, you exclude information about bowel sounds or deep tendon reflexes as not

being immediately relevant to his respiratory status. Categorizing information also helps you notice whether there are missing data. A second strategy that will help you organize information is to look for patterns. It has been indicated that experienced nurses intuitively note recurrent meaningful aspects of a clinical situation.

Case Discussion

Rely on prior didactic knowledge or clinical experience. Cluster the data. What was Mrs. Vlios's status immediately before hospitalization? What was her status at the time of hospitalization? What information is missing? What additional data do you need?

- Physiology: Consider pathophysiologic knowledge about the effects of hypovolemia and electrolyte imbalances on the systems such as the brain, kidneys, and vascular system. What is her temperature? What are her laboratory values? What is her 24-hour intake and output? Is she still dehydrated?
- Psychological/cognitive: How does hospitalization affect older adults? How do restraints affect them?
- Social/economic: Was weight loss a result of dehydration? Why was she without food? Could it be due to economic factors or mental problems?
- Legal: What constitutes a binding advance directive in the state in which Mrs. Vlios lives? Is a living will valid in her state, or does the law require a health power of attorney? Are these documents on file at the hospital?

STEP 4: OBTAIN NEW DATA

Critical thinking is not a linear process. Expert nurses often modify interventions based on the response to the event, or change in the client's physical condition (Fero et al., 2009). Constantly consider whether you need more information. Establish an attitude of inquiry and obtain more information as needed. Ask questions; search for evidence; and check reference books, journals, the ethics sources on the Internet, or written professional or agency protocols.

Evaluate conflicting information. There may be time constraints. If a client has suspected "respiratory problems," you may need to set priorities. Obtain data that are most useful or are easily available. It would be useful to know oxygenation levels, but you may not have time to order laboratory tests. But perhaps there is a device on the unit or in the room that can measure oxygen saturation.

Sometimes you may need to change your approach to improve your chances of obtaining information. For example, when the charge nurse caring for Mrs. Vlios used an authoritarian tone to try to get the sister and brother to provide more information about possible drug overdose, they did not respond. However, when the charge nurse changed his approach, exhibiting empathy, the daughter volunteered that on several occasions her mother had forgotten what pills she had taken.

Case Discussion

List sources from which you can obtain missing information. Physiologic data such as temperature or laboratory test results can be obtained quickly; some of the ethical information, however, may take longer to consider.

STEP 5: IDENTIFY THE SIGNIFICANT PROBLEM

- Analyze existing information: Examine all the information you have. Identify all the possible positions.
- Make inferences: What might be going on? What are the possible diagnoses? Develop a working diagnosis.
- Prioritize: Which client problem is most urgently in need of your intervention? What are the appropriate interventions?

Case Discussion

A significant physiologic concern is sepsis, regardless of whether it is an iatrogenic (hospital-acquired) infection or one resulting from immobility and debilitation. A significant ethical concern is the conflict among family members and client (as expressed through her living will). At what point do spiritual concerns take priority over a worsening physical concern?

STEP 6: EXAMINE SKEPTICALLY

Thinking about a situation may involve weighing positive and negative factors, and differentiating facts that are credible from opinions that are biased or not grounded in true facts.

- Keep an open mind.
- Challenge your own assumptions.
- Consider whether any of your assumptions are unwarranted. Does the available evidence really support your assumption?

- Discriminate between facts and inferences. Your inferences need to be logical and plausible, based on the available facts.
- Are there any problems that you have not considered?

In trying to evaluate a situation, consciously raising questions becomes an important part of thinking critically. At times there will be alternative explanations or different lines of reasoning that are equally valid. The challenge is to examine your own and others' perspectives for important ideas, complicating factors, other plausible interpretations, and new insights. Some nurses believe that examining information skeptically is part of each step in the critical thinking process rather than a step by itself.

Case Discussion

Challenge assumptions about the cause of Mrs. Vlios's condition. For example, did you eliminate the possibility that she had a head injury caused by a fall? Could she have liver failure as a result of acetaminophen overdosing? Have all the possibilities been explored? Challenge your assumptions about outcome: Are they influenced by expected probable versus possible outcomes for this client? If she, indeed, has irreversible dementia, what will the quality of her life be if she recovers from her physical problems?

STEP 7: APPLY CRITERIA

In evaluating a situation, think about appropriate responses.

- Access standards for "best practices" related to your client's situation.
- Laws: There may be a law that can be applied to guide your actions and decisions. For example, by law, certain diseases must be reported to the state. If you suspect physical abuse, there is a state statute that requires professionals to report abuse to the Department of Social Services.
- Legal precedents: There may have been similar cases or situations that were dealt with in a court of law. Legal decisions do guide health care practices. In end-of-life decisions, when there is no legally binding health care power of attorney, the most frequent hierarchy is the spouse, then the adult children, then the parents.
- Protocols: There may be standard protocols for managing certain situations. Your agency may have standing orders for caring for Mrs. Vlios if

she develops respiratory distress, such as administering oxygen per face mask at 5 L/min.

Case Discussion

Many criteria could be used to examine this case, including the Nurse Practice Act in the area of jurisdiction, the professional organization code of ethics or general ethical principles of beneficence and autonomy, the hospital's written protocols and policies, state laws regarding living wills, and prior court decisions about living wills. Remember that advance directives are designed to take effect only when clients become unable to make their own wishes known.

STEP 8: GENERATE OPTIONS AND LOOK AT ALTERNATIVES

- Evaluate the major alternative points of view.
- Involve experienced peers as soon as you can to assist you in making your decision.
- Use clues from others to help you "put the picture together."
- Can you identify all the arguments—pro and con—to explain this situation? Almost all situations will have strong counterarguments or competing hypotheses.

Case Discussion

The important concept is that neither the physician nor the nurse should handle this alone; rather, others should be involved (e.g., the hospital bioethics committee, the ombudsman client representative, the family's spiritual counselor, and other medical experts such as a gerontologist, psychologist, and nursing clinical specialist).

STEP 9: CONSIDER WHETHER FACTORS CHANGE IF THE CONTEXT CHANGES

Consider whether your decision would be different if there were a change in circumstances. For example, a change in the age of the client, in the site of the situation, or in the client's culture may affect your decision. A competent nurse prioritizes which aspects of the situation are most relevant and can modify her actions based on the client's responses. A competent nurse anticipates consequences.

Case Discussion

If you knew the outcome from the beginning, would your decisions be the same? What if you knew Mrs.

Vlios had a terminal cancer? What if Mrs. Vlios had remained in her senior housing project and you were the home health nurse? What if Mrs. Vlios had remained alert during her hospitalization and refused IVs, hyperalimentation, nasogastric tubes, and so on? What if the family and Mrs. Vlios were in agreement about no treatment? Would you make more assertive interventions to save her life if she were 7 years old, or a 35-year-old mother of five young children?

STEP 10: EVALUATE AND MAKE THE INTERVENTION

After analyzing available information in this systematic way, you need to make a judgment or decision. An important part of your decision is your ability to communicate it coherently to others and to reflect on the outcome of your decision for your client.

- Justify your conclusion.
- Evaluate outcomes.
- Test out your decision or conclusion by implementing appropriate actions.

As a critical thinker, you need to be able to accept that there may be multiple solutions that can be equally acceptable. In other situations, you may need to make a decision even when there is incomplete knowledge. Be able to cite your rationale or present your arguments to others for your decision choice and interventions.

Revise interventions as necessary. After you implement your interventions, examine the client outcomes. Was your assessment correct? Did you obtain enough information? Did the benefits to the client and family outweigh the harm that may have occurred? In retrospect, do you know you made the correct decision? Did you anticipate possibilities and complications correctly? This kind of self-examination can foster self-correction. It is this process of reflecting on one's own thinking that is the hallmark of a critical thinker.

USE OF CASE STUDIES AND CLINICAL SIMULATIONS

A number of techniques provide you with opportunities to master the skills described in this chapter. Analyze and apply these new ways of making clinical decisions before facing actual clinical crises. In addition to using peer discussions of the case studies provided in this chapter, students use videotaped or live client simulated problems, or computer generated animated pedagogical agents (APAs), which give opportunity for practice (Fero, 2010).

SUMMARIZING THE CRITICAL THINKING LEARNING PROCESS

The most effective method of learning these steps in critical thinking results from repeatedly applying them to clinical situations. This can occur in your own clinical care. A new graduate nurse must, at a minimum, be able to identify essential clinical data, know when to initiate interventions, know why a particular intervention is relevant, and differentiate between problems that need immediate intervention versus problems that can wait for action. Repeated practice in applying critical thinking can help a new graduate fit into the expectations of employers.

Students have demonstrated that critical thinking can be learned in the classroom, as well as through clinical experience. Effective learning can occur when opportunities are structured that allow for repeated in-class applications to client case situations. This includes using real-life case interviews with experienced nurses, which allow you to analyze their decision-making process. The interview and analysis of an expert nurse's critical thinking described in Exercise 3-4 explains how this is done using a 10-minute recording.

You may also help increase your critical thinking and clinical problem-solving skills by discussing the following additional case example. Remember that most clinical situations requiring decision making will not involve the types of ethical dilemmas discussed earlier in this chapter.

Case Example

Mr. Gonzales has terminal cancer. His family defers to the attending physician, who prescribes aggressive rescue treatment. The hospice nurse is an expert in the expressed and unexpressed needs of terminal clients. She advocates for a conservative and supportive plan of care. A logical case could be built for each position.

SUMMARY

Ethical reasoning and critical thinking are systematic, comprehensive processes to aide you in making clinical decisions. An important concept is to forget the idea that there is only one right answer in discussing ethical dilemmas. Accept that there may be several equally correct solutions depending on each individual's point of view.

Critical thinking is not a linear process. Analysis of the thinking processes of expert nurses reveals that they

EXERCISE 3-4	Your Analysis of an Expert's Critical Thinking: Interview of Expert Nurse's Case

Purpose: To develop awareness of critical thinking in the clinical judgment process.

Procedure

Find an experienced nurse in your community and record him or her describing a real client case. You can use a computer or cell phone with recording capability, videotape, or audiotape to record an interview that takes less than 10 minutes. During the interview, have the expert describe an actual client case in which there was a significant change in the client's health status. Have the expert describe the interventions and thinking process that took place during this situation. Ask what nursing knowledge, laboratory data, or experience helped the nurse make his or her decision. You can work with a partner. Remember to protect confidentiality by omitting names and other identifiers.

Discussion

Analyze the recording using an outline of the 10 steps in critical thinking. Discussion should first include citation examples of each step noted during their review of the taped interview, followed by application to the broad principles. Discussion of steps missed by the interviewed expert can be enlightening, as long as care is taken to avoid any criticism of the guest "expert."

continually scan new data and simultaneously apply these steps in clinical decision making. They monitor the effectiveness of their interventions in achieving desired outcomes for their client. A nurse's moral reasoning and critical thinking abilities often have a profound effect on the quality of care given to a client, even affecting client mortality outcomes. Functioning as a competent nurse requires that you have knowledge of medical and nursing content, "best practice" guidelines, an accumulation of clinical experiences, and an ability to think critically.

Almost daily, we confront ethical dilemmas and complicated clinical situations that require expertise as a decision maker. We can follow the 10 steps of the thinking process described in this chapter to help us respond to such situations. Developing skill as a critical thinker is a learned process, one which requires repeated application.

ETHICAL DILEMMA	What Would You Do?

The Moyers family has power of attorney over hospitalized, terminally ill Gail Midge, age 42 years. They are consistently at her bedside and refuse to allow you and other nurses to administer pain medication ordered by Mrs. M's physician, since they fear it will overdose her, causing her death. Gail often moans, cries with pain, and begs you for pain meds. The family threatens a lawsuit if she is given anything and then dies. What would you do?

[Based on a case reported by Pavlish et al., 2011, p. 390. The nurse in this case considered conflicting variables from each point of view and assumed responsibility for initiating action, calling the palliative care team and the ethics consultation team.]

DISCUSSION QUESTIONS

1. Reflect on the characteristics of a **critical thinker** listed in Table 3-1. Which did you develop prior to entering nursing? Were they innate or when did you acquire them?
2. Consider the Quality and Safety Education for Nurses (QSEN) competency of patient-centered care and the concept of autonomy: When does a client have the right to refuse treatment?
3. By choosing to become a nurse, do you assume an **ethical** obligation to treat any client assigned to you? When are there exceptions?

REFERENCES

American Association of Colleges of Nursing (AACN): Moral distress statement. www.aacn.org/WD/practice/DOCS/moral_distress.pdf 2008.

Chang MJ, Chang Y, Kuo S, Yang Y, Chou F: Relationship between CT and nursing competence in clinical nurses, *J Clin Nurs* 20:3224–3232, 2011.

Facione PA: *Critical thinking: what is it and why it counts*, Milbrae, CA, 2007, California Academic Press.

Fero LJ: Critical thinking skills in nursing students: Comparison of simulation-based performance with metrics, *J Adv Nurs* 66(10):2182–2193, 2010.

Fero LJ, Witsberger CM, Wesmiller SW, et al.: Critical thinking ability of new graduate and experienced nurses, *J Adv Nurs* 65(1):139–148, 2009.

Milton C: Ethical implications for acting faithfully in nurse-person relationships, *Nurs Sci Q* 15:21–24, 2002.

Pavlish C, Brown-Sullivan K, Herish M, Shirk M, Rounkle A: Nursing priorities, actions, and regrets for ethical situations in clinical practice, *J Nurs Scholarsh* 43(4):385–395, 2011.

Quality and Safety Education for Nurses (QSEN) Competencies. (n.d.) www.qsen.org/competencies.

Romeo EM: Quantitative research on CT and predicting nursing students' NCLEX-RN performance, *J Nurs Educ* 49(7):378–386, 2010.

Ryan C, Tatum K: Customizing orientation to improve the CT ability of newly hired pediatric nurses, *J Nurs Admin* 43(4):208–214, 2013.

Sasso L, Stievano A, Jurado MG, et al.: Code of ethics and conduct for European nursing, *Nurs Ethics* 15(6):821–836, 2008.

Tschudin V: Two decades of nursing ethics: Some thoughts on changes, *Nurs Ethics* 20(2):123–125, 2013.

CHAPTER 4

Clarity and Safety in Communication

Kathleen Underman Boggs

OBJECTIVES

At the end of the chapter, the reader will be able to:

1. Identify client communication safety goals.
2. Define the role of communication in a "culture of safety."
3. Describe why client safety is a complex system issue, as well as an individual function.
4. Describe how open communication and organizational error reporting contribute to a culture of safety.
5. Discuss how to advocate for safe, high-quality care as a team member.
6. Use simulations to demonstrate use of standardized tools for clear communication affecting client care, such as using situation, background, assessment, recommendation (SBAR) in a simulated conversation with a physician.

This chapter focuses on communication concepts designed to assist nurses and their health team colleagues in creating a safe environment for their clients. Health care regulators, legislation, and standards of practice for all health disciplines all address safety. Client safety is and has always been a priority in nursing care, as part of our mission to give the highest quality of care. The ability to give safe and effective care is identified by Quality and Safety Education for Nurses (QSEN) as an essential competency (QSEN, www.qsen.org/).

Clear, accurate communication is the bedrock of safe care. Accurate, clear communication and best practice are indicators of quality of care and serve to maintain a safe environment (Agency for Healthcare Research and Quality [AHRQ n.d.{a}; 2009]). Threats to safe care occur at multiple levels in the care system. Some examples are wrong site surgery, equipment failure, incorrect labeling of specimens, and medication errors. However, miscommunication is the dominant factor in harmful errors, cited by The Joint Commission (TJC) in 60% to 70% of reported cases (TJC, 2008).

GOAL

A major international effort is underway to prioritize safety goals by improving communication about clients among their various providers. The aim is to reduce client mortality, decrease medical errors, and promote effective health care teamwork. These goals need to be mutually established by organizations and by individuals in the health team in a climate of respect to assure maximum clarity.

A number of agencies and professional organizations are issuing guidelines for promoting levels of communication that act to prevent errors and prevent adverse client outcomes. The goal is to increase the quality of care and safety of our clients by embedding a "culture of safety" within all levels of health care. Since nurses play a critical role in client safety, holding all nurses accountable for making safety a priority is one component (Brickell and McLeane, 2011). This chapter discusses communication strategies designed to promote a safe environment and focuses on commonly used **standardized tools** for clear communication.

BASIC CONCEPTS

SAFETY DEFINITION

Multiple health care organizations have issued definitions of safety. Safety is defined by the Institute of

Medicine (IOM) as freedom from accidental injury (IOM, 2000). The nursing profession has always had safe practice as a major goal, as identified in the American Nurses Association (ANA) Code of Ethics for Nurses. The National Patient Safety Foundation (NPSF) has a more specific definition: "avoidance, prevention, amelioration of adverse outcomes or injuries stemming from the process of health care itself" (NPSF, online, n.d.).

QSEN and the American Association of Colleges of Nursing (AACN, 2006, b) offer a broader definition: safety is "the minimization of risk for harm to patients and to providers through both system effectiveness and individual performance" (Cronenwett et al., 2007).

SAFETY INCIDENCES

In the United States, one in four hospitalized clients suffers some level of harm. Hospitals with higher satisfaction scores for physician-nurse communication on average have fewer safety events (Hospital Safety Score, 2013). And almost as many errors are likely to occur in physician offices. When asked to identify which profession was responsible for client safety, 90% to 96% of all professional disciplines surveyed said the nurse was responsible (Abrahamson et al., 2012).

Case Example: Adele Kelly

Dr. Kelly, RN, is principle investigator on an outcome review study of catheter infections in California hospitals and nursing homes. When analyzing data for 2013, she finds that catheter-related infections are 56% more common in agencies reporting poor physician-nurse communication than those with better communication.

PRINCIPLES RELATED TO OCCURRENCE OF UNSAFE EVENTS

Miscommunication. Much has changed in health care practice since the landmark 1999 IOM study that found that preventable health care errors were responsible for almost 98,000 deaths each year in the United States. The series of IOM reports, described in Chapter 1, instigated a major effort to make client safety a national American priority. Yet, hospitalized clients still suffer harm. Failure to communicate or communicating inaccurately results in an inability to detect and correct error (Hospital Safety Score, 2013).

Multiple studies have pinpointed miscommunication as a major causative agent in sentinel events, that is, errors resulting in unnecessary death and serious injury. According to The Joint Commission International, miscommunication is the root cause in nearly 70% of reported sentinel events.

Professional Silos. In the past decades health care professionals were educated in separate areas, each with a different professional language, leading to miscommunication and misunderstandings or lack of appreciation for the other's point of view.

Case Example: Student Nurse Mary

Student nurse Mary [to staff RN]: "I am assigned to give the meds today." However, she meant all the oral meds for the team, since her instructor assigned these to her, but not the intravenous medications. Fortunately her instructor was there to clarify the message. When policy says to report near misses as well as errors, does your agency track near misses by students?

Errors are Usually System Problems. While health care traditionally viewed errors as failings on the part of individuals, use of systems theory shows us that adverse events are usually the result of an accumulation of multiple, smaller errors that slip through because of flaws in the overall system. This newer approach is termed "the Swiss cheese model of medical errors," in which holes appear when you line up the slices. Efforts to improve safety focus on analysis of the steps that lead to the breakdown of safety (PSNet, Systems Approach, PrimerID=21). Often these are communication errors. The problem is complex; therefore, solutions also will be complex.

Most Errors are Preventable. It is estimated that 70% of reported errors are preventable. "Preventable" means the error occurs through a medical intervention, not because of the client's illness. Fatigue is repeatedly cited as a factor contributing to errors. The most common cause of error is incomplete communication during the very many "handoffs" transferring responsibility for client care to another care provider, another unit, or agency. It is estimated that in 1 day, a client may experience up to eight handoffs. Errors have a high financial cost in addition to the human cost, exceeding $29 billion per year just in the United States (AHRQ, n.d.[b]).

GENERAL SAFETY COMMUNICATION GUIDELINES FOR ORGANIZATIONS

Safe client care is always a priority. General standards for communication issued by organizations and agencies are discussed in Chapter 2. These include specific guidelines designed to promote safe communication. Unlike other countries such as Great Britain, in the United States there is no one national database for reporting unsafe care, making data less readily accessible. The Centers for Medicare and Medicaid Services (CMS) does require reporting for clients who have Medicare. Other U.S. government agencies (e.g., AHRQ, IOM) and professional nursing groups (e.g., AACN, ANA, QSEN) have made recommendations for clear communication strategies to provide safer care that affect both your communication with other nurses and with other health team members. AACN recommends using safety communication strategies from research-based and evidence-based knowledge as a basis for your clinical practice (2006a).

BARRIERS TO SAFE, EFFECTIVE COMMUNICATION IN THE HEALTH CARE SYSTEM

Fragmentation. Health care organizations are complex systems, often a result of an amalgamations of a number of previously unaffiliated agencies and practices. This organizational hodge-podge impedes communications. Fragmentation is a barrier to safer care. Evidenced-based practices have to be reinforced and implemented at a system-wide level. Although most hospitals and agencies have some form of error reporting, they lack a system-wide department for processing safety information. One model to be emulated is that of Kaiser Permanente, which implemented a national patient safety plan in 2000.

Handoffs or transfers of client care. Miscommunication errors most often occur during a handoff procedure, when one staff member transfers responsibility for care to another staff member. More than half of incidences, perhaps 80%, of reported serious miscommunications occurred during *client handoff and transfer,* when those assuming responsibility for the client (coming on duty) are given a verbal, face-to-face synopsis of the client's current condition by those who had been caring for the patient and are now going off duty (Henkind and Sinnett, 2008).

Client care is constantly being handed off to the next shift of nurses, or when the client is transferred to another unit. Transition times are high risk for incomplete communication. This has been attributed to frequent interruptions, inconsistent report format, and omission of key information (Cornell and Gervis, 2013). Some agencies have adopted standardized handoff communication tools, including those used on handheld devices (Yee et al., 2013).

Underreporting of Errors in a Punitive Climate. Providers are concerned about negative consequences of disclosing errors, such as malpractice litigation, reputation damage, job security, and personal feelings such as loss of self-esteem, among others. This has led to serious underreporting. In the United States, according to IOM, only a tiny fraction of unsafe care incidents are reported (IOM, 2000). Some estimate that more than 90% of errors go unreported (Haw and Cahill, 2013). Adequate error and near-miss event reporting are necessary to designing better, safer systems. Failure to repost and track errors and near misses actually increases the likelihood of other errors (Barnsteiner and Disch, 2012). A redesign is needed if we are to create a culture of safety. A culture of safety is characterized by installing a strong, nonpunitive reporting system; supporting care providers after adverse events; and developing a method to inform and compensate clients who were harmed. The health care industry is looking at models created by other industries such as aviation or nuclear power, which have excellent safety records. Aviation's successful crew resource management practice model has been used as a template. One needed step is to require the reporting of "near misses" so new, safer protocols can be created. Another is to create a database so errors and near misses can be analyzed in order to design a safer system. A study by Elder and colleagues (2008) reported that nurses remain strongly conflicted about disclosing their errors to peers and physicians. In their survey, less than half of the intensive care unit nurses witnessing a near-miss error were likely to report it. Creating a new safety climate would require retraining nurses in error disclosure to help prevent future errors. Meanwhile providers struggle with the current systems for reporting errors. *We need* *to establish a nonpunative climate. We need to create this new climate of safety in which agencies, policies, and employees maintain a vigilant, proactive attitude toward adverse events.* Recognizing that human error occurs, everyone's focus needs to be on correcting system flaws to avoid future adverse events, rather than finding the one to blame.

FATIGUE

Risk of error nearly doubles when nurses worked more than 12 consecutive hours in a study by Scott and associates (PSNet, Medication Errors, PrimerID=23). Graduate medical education guidelines require resident's work hours per week to be 80 or less rather than the formerly common 100 hours per week, although impact on client's safety is less clear-cut.

INNOVATIONS THAT FOSTER SAFETY

Communication problems and communication solution strategies identified as "best practice" for creating a culture of safety are summarized in Table 4-1. Beyond individual changes to create safer climates for our clients, we need to advocate for organizational system changes. Leadership is needed to incorporate the three C's that promote safer clinical practice:

1. Communication clarity
2. Collaboration
3. Cooperation

TABLE 4-1	Safe Communication: Problems and Recommended Best Practices
Communication Problem	**Best Practice Communication Solution**
Health care system complexity	Agency establishes safety as a priority.
	Agency policies adopt procedures to promote transparency and accountability.
Hierarchical status difference with decreased willingness to communicate	Team training such as TeamSTEPPS.
	Clarify duties of each team member.
Distracted or preoccupied	Policy that isolates you from interruptions (signal to others not to interrupt, such as wearing vest when administering meds).
	Team members maintain safety awareness as a priority.
	Control high levels of ambient noise/alarm fatigue.
	Establish policy to limit interruptions during crucial times.
Heavy workload	Held accountable for evidence-based practice (EBP).
	Support from administration and colleagues.
	Team members share common goal of safety, which each see as their responsibility.
Stress and practice pressures due to lack of time leading to use of shortcuts and poor communication	Adherence to safety protocols, especially in med administration.
	Team huddles, meetings, bedside rounds.
Staff fail to say what they mean; fail to speak up about safety concerns (lack of assertiveness)	All staff receive continual educational programs that emphasize safety promotion. Communication and assertiveness training.
	Use of time-outs.
Attitude of not believing in usefulness of practice guidelines	Ease of access and increased availability of EBP guidelines specifically relevant to your client.
	Value electronic decision-support apps.
	Participate in team meetings, conference calls and opportunities to share successes.
Education silos in which each discipline has own jargon and assumptions	Use of standardized communication tools.
	Team training.
	Each team member is encouraged to give input.
Cultural differences or language issues	Cultural sensitivity education, especially relevant to adapting communication strategies.

TABLE 4-1	Safe Communication: Problems and Recommended Best Practices—cont'd	
Communication Problem	**Best Practice Communication Solution**	
Miscommunication	Adapt communication and verify receipt of message.	
	Use standardized communication.	
	Participate in simulations, critical event training scenarios, to foster clear, efficient communication.	
	Read back and record verbal orders immediately.	
	With clients, use teach-backs or "show me" techniques.	
	Solicit questions.	
Avoidance of confrontation and communication with the conflict person	Use conflict resolution skills.	
	Practices open communication.	
	Be assertive in confronting the problem.	
Cognitive difficulty obtaining, processing, or understanding	Continuing education units (CEUs) about effective communication skills.	
	Avoidance of factors interfering with decision-making such as fatigue.	
Lack of training	Seek CEUs, in-service.	
Resistance from client or family to following guidelines for safe, effective care	Team recognizes that safe outcomes require work and communicates that this must involve client and family.	
	Bedside rounds, briefings, and involving client in daily care plan goal setting.	

TeamSTEPPS, Team Strategies and Tools to Enhance Performance and Patient Safety.

CREATE A CULTURE OF SAFETY

Agencies are working toward promoting a culture of safety in many ways (PSNet, Safety Culture, PrimerID=5). A major focus is to improve **clarity of communication**. This occurs through use of standardized communication tools and team training. This is evidenced by more than 6000 recent articles and the assessment and intervention tools available from AHRQ's PSNet (http://psnet.ahrq.gov/).

Leadership is essential to change to a just culture model, in which the organization creates a balance between accountability between individuals and the institutional system (Ring and Fairchild, 2013). Establishment of an organizational culture of safety requires us to acknowledge the complexity of any health care system. Strong leaders can change the focus to safety practices as a shared value. Creating a safe environment requires us to communicate openly, to be vigilant, to be willing to speak up, and to be held accountable.

Create a Team Culture of Collaboration and Cooperation

Team culture includes shared norms, values, beliefs, and staff expectations. Creating effective health teams means getting all team members to value teamwork more than individual autonomy. Team *collaborative communication strategies* involve shared responsibility for maintaining open communication, mutual problem solving and decision making, as well as coordination of care. Teamwork failures, including poor communication and failures in physician supervision, have been implicated in two-thirds of harmful errors to clients (Singh et al., 2007). Creating a safe environment requires all team members to communicate openly, to be vigilant and accountable, and to express concerns and alert team members to unsafe situations.

Create a Nonpunative Culture

Establishing a **just culture** system creates expectations of a work environment in which staff can speak up and express concerns and alert team members to unsafe situations. Just culture does not mean eliminating individual accountability but rather puts greater emphasis on analysis of problems that contribute to adverse events in a system (Rideout, 2013).

Establishing open communication about errors is an important aspect of just culture. Most state boards of nursing require nurses to report unsafe practice by coworkers, but many nurses have mixed feelings about reporting a colleague, especially to a state agency. Physicians also have reservations about reporting problems (Zbar et al., 2009). Barriers to reporting include fear, threat to self-esteem, threat to professional livelihood, and lack of timely feedback and support. Ethical incentives to reporting are protection of the client and professional protection (Hartnell et al., 2012).

One focus of team training can be creating an in-house agency system climate in which team members feel comfortable speaking out about their safety concerns. In a nonpunitive reporting environment, staff are encouraged to report errors, mistakes, and near misses. They work in a climate in which they feel comfortable making such reports. In safety literature, compiling a database that includes near-miss situations that could have resulted in injury is important information in preventing future errors. A complete error reporting process should include timely feedback to the person reporting. Administrators should assume errors will occur and put in place a plan for "recovery" that has well-rehearsed procedures for responding to adverse events.

BEST PRACTICE: COMMUNICATING CLEARLY FOR QUALITY CARE

AHRQ and medical and nursing organizations, as well as health care delivery organizations, have undertaken initiatives designed to foster "**best practice**" safer client care by designing protocols for care that are evidence-based. *Use "best practices" by increasing use of evidence-based "best practice" versus "usual practice."* AHRQ funds research to identify the most effective methods of promoting clear communication among health team members and agencies, as well as the most effective treatments. This information is used to develop and distribute protocols for best practice, including formats of standard communication techniques. We need more studies of interventions to promote best communication between nurse and physician with documented outcomes for clients.

Developing an evidence-based best practice requires closing the gap between best evidence and the way communication occurs in your current practice (Figure 4-1). Apply information from evidence-based best practice databanks for safe practice. The process for development of practice guidelines, protocols, situation checklists, and so on is not transparent or easy. Solutions include gathering more evidence

on which to base our practice. When is the "evidence" sufficiently strong to warrant adoption of a standardized form of communication about care? Many best practice protocols are available on free web sites such as AHRQ's (www.ahrq.gov), proprietary sites such as Mosby's Nursing Consult, or in books such as *Patient Safety and Quality: An Evidence-Based Handbook for Nurses* (Hughes, 2008).

Computerized Order Entry. Computerized order provider entry (COPE) associated with electronic health records (EHRs) are replacing written paper orders. This should greatly improve safety, for example, eliminating confusion due to illegible handwriting. But the COPE system offers many more aides such as alerts for incompatible meds, alerts for client allergies, and so on. COPE will be discussed in Chapter 25.

EHRs improve safety of care and empower providers to have better quality care delivery as well as better accountability for preventive care and compliance with standard care protocols. They aide in decision support. For example, providing data for the physician about the number of clients who need mammograms (Parsons, 2013). EHRs are discussed in Chapter 25.

STANDARDIZED COMMUNICATION AS AN INITIATIVE FOR SAFER CARE

We are redeveloping our health care system to make client care safer. There is consensus that this reuires improving communication. Best nurse-physician collaborative communication has empirically been associated with lower risk for negative client outcomes and greater satisfaction. Renewed focus on improving patient safety is causing standardization of many health care practices. **Standardization of communication** is an effective tool to avoid incomplete or misleading messages. Standardization needs to be institutionalized at the system level and implemented consistently at the staff level. Safe communication about client care matters needs to be clear, unambiguous, timely, accurate, complete, open, and understood by the recipient to reduce errors.

Client Safety Outcomes

Evidence that use of standardized tools for clear communication is beginning to reveal that use of these tools prevents harm to clients. Standardization is becoming best practice. Regulatory agencies have begun mandating use of standardized communication tools in certain areas of practice.

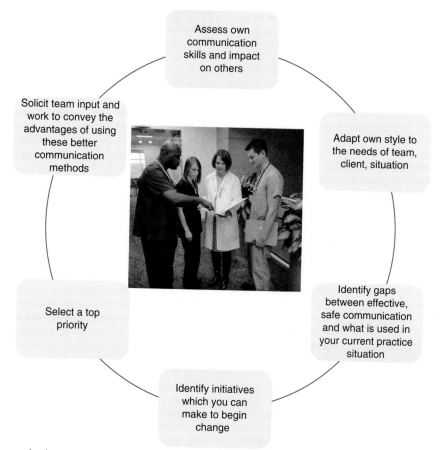

Figure 4-1   Communication competencies for creating safer care. *(Adapted from Carey M, Buchan H, Sanson-Fisher R: The cycle of change: implementing best-evidence clinical practice, Int J Qual Healthc 21(1):37-43, 2009; Cronenwett L, Sherwood G, Barnsteiner J, et al: Quality and safety education for nurses, Nurs Outlook 55(3):122-131, 2007.)*

Nurse-Specific Initiatives

Nurses are often the "last line of defense" against error. As staff nurses, we are in a position to prevent, intercept, or correct errors. In order to prevent error, we need to be communicating clearly to others in the health team. Your clarity of communication can prevent safety risks such as medication errors, client injuries from falls, clinical outcomes related to client nonadherence to the treatment plan, and rehospitalization rates. With poor communication, you can compromise client safety. One sample case might be that of Nurse Kay in the following case example.

Case Example: Kay

Ms. Kay, RN, newly hired staff nurse, has eight clients assigned to her on a surgical unit. She calls the resident for additional pain medication for a client. Dr. Andrews, first-year resident, on a thoracic surgery 3-month rotation, has responsibility for more than 80 patients this weekend when he is on call. Many of these he has never seen. In the phone call, Ms. Kay uses nursing diagnoses to describe the client and is irritated when Dr. Andrews does not seem to recognize the client, nor understand her.

Interruptions interfere with a nurse's ability to perform a task safely, yet interruptions have become an almost continual occurrence. These interruptions are tied to an increased risk of errors (PSNet, Nursing and Patient Safety, PrimerID=22). Nonverbal strategies to signal others to avoid distracting communication have been suggested, such as wearing an orange vest when preparing and administering medications.

Medication Process. Particular focus for error reduction is the entire medication process, ranging from ordering to administration. The definition of an adverse medication event is harm to a client as a result of exposure to a drug, occurring in at least 5% of all hospitalized clients (PSNet, Handoffs and Signouts, PrimerID=9). We have expanded the definition to include near misses. For example, a nurse prepares an ordered med but recognizes that the ordered dose far exceeds safe parameters. While some medication errors stem from lack of knowledge about the drug, side effects, incompatibility, and other factors involved in ordering or compounding, the majority occur during the nurse's actions in administering the medication. TJC (2007) concluded that drug errors occur when communication is unclear or when a nurse fails to follow the rules for verification: right med, right client, right dose, and right time.

Developing an Evidence-Based Practice

Abrahamson KA, Fox RL, Doebbeling BN: Facilitators and barriers to clinical practice guidelines use among nurses, Am J Nurs 112(7), 26-35, 2012. Nurses working in 134 Veterans Association hospitals were surveyed to learn their perceptions of factors that facilitate or act as barriers to their use of clinical practice guidelines. Clinical practice guidelines are designed to foster evidence-based practice by applying research findings to actual clinical practice. An open-ended survey questionnaire was used.

Results: The 575 registered nurse respondents identified system issues and social factors, such as the support given them by their organization, as key in their choice to use clinical practice guidelines. Interestingly, many of the participants provided additional information by texting the researchers, suggesting a high level of interest in the study. Barriers to use included workload (44%), and communication difficulties (22%). Factors outside the individual nurse's control were cited by 94% and included lack of training, staffing, and workload problems, lack of knowledge that a guideline exists for a client's specific diagnosis, and lack of administrative support.

Application to Your Practice: Use of clinical practice guidelines is based on your knowledge, attitude, motivation, and ease of access. Guidelines can help you make a decision about your specific care of your client today. How can you increase your knowledge of specific guidelines? What web sites can you access?

APPLICATIONS

Communication interventions shown to improve safe communication are listed in Table 4-1. These are best practices. For example, when there is conflicting information or a concern about a potential safety breech, nurses use the "two challenge rule." The nurse states his or her concern twice. This is theoretically enough cause to stop the action for a reassessment.

A discussion of **standardized tools** used to promote safe interdisciplinary and nursing communication will be the main focus of our application section. Quality and safety education competencies have been developed for all nurses by national nurse leaders, which emphasize safety (QSEN, 2013, online). The mantra for safe communication should be "simplify, clarify, verify" (Fleischmann, 2008).

Attitude

The IOM has urged organizations to create an environment in which safety is a top priority. Strive to develop an attitude in which safety is always a priority. Our prime goal is to improve communication about client condition among all the people providing care to that client. Errors occur when we assume someone else has addressed a situation.

Client Safety Outcome

Once nurses understand the use of clinical guidelines and evidence-based practice procedures and become comfortable accessing this information, they see that they are giving higher quality care, improving their decision-making skills, and avoiding errors, resulting in safer care for their clients. They have fewer error incident reports, fewer client falls, fewer medication events, less delay in treatment for clients, and fewer wound infections, among other outcomes (Saintsing et al., 2011).

TOOLS FOR SAFER CARE

USE OPPORTUNITIES FOR CLINICAL PRACTICE SIMULATIONS

Opportunities to practice honing communication and practice skills are provided with clinical situation simulations. Ideally, these are interdisciplinary. Virtual client-nurse scenarios, whether using technologically enhanced dummies or active learning situations, such as the case studies provided in this textbook, allow practice without risk for potentially devastating outcomes with an actual client care situation. Practice scenarios can be viewed on the Internet (even on sites such as YouTube). Nursing education programs use "live models" to simulate clients. Actors are trained to portray clients with specific illnesses. Student nurses practice communicating with them to elicit histories, as well as practicing skills such as physical examinations. Hospital continuing education departments are engaging staff in interdisciplinary simulations for continuous refreshers.

Simulations are designed to increase cognitive decision-making skills, increase technical proficiency, and enhance teamwork, including efficient communication skills.

Client Safety Outcome

More research is needed about the impact of practice simulations on nursing communications that affect actual client safe care. Certainly strong evidence shows increased skill proficiency, for example, in cardiopulmonary resuscitation.

INTRODUCTION TO USE OF STANDARDIZED COMMUNICATION TOOLS, INCLUDING SBAR AND CREW RESOURCE MANAGEMENT

While a nurse's clinical judgment remains a valid, essential aspect of communication, other safety communication improvement solutions include using standardized verbal and electronic communications tools, participating in team-training communication seminars, adopting technology-oriented tools, and empowering clients to be partners in safer care. Communication that promotes client safety needs to include both communication of concise critical information and active listening. Educational programs impart very different communication expectations for nurses than those taught to medical students, pharmacists, and other health team members. Nurses are taught to communicate in detailed narrative form, to describe the broad picture when discussing a client with his physician. Physicians are taught to speak concisely, to diagnose and summarize. As Leonard and Bonacum (2008) said, "Physicians want bullet points," or just the headlines. Each group holds slightly different expectations about communication content and may have separate vocabularies.

Nurses want their observations or assessments taken seriously. Solutions include team training and use of standardized communication tools. Although currently there is no one universally accepted process, use of a shared format across disciplines can promote effective communication and client safety.

USE OF CHECKLISTS

A checklist is defined as a specific, structured list of actions to be performed in a specific clinical setting whose contents are based on evidence (PSNet, Checklists, PrimerID=14). The user's goal is that no step in the process will be forgotten. Following a checklist ensures that key steps will not be omitted and important information missed due to *fatigue, pressure, distraction* or other factors. They are a cognitive guide to accurate task completion or to complete communication of information. If every step on the list is completed, the possibility of miscommunication or slips leading to error are greatly reduced. Some examples include the *World Health Organization (WHO) surgical safety list.* Since it was introduced in 2008, use of the WHO list has nearly doubled the adherence to surgical standards of care. Another example is the *Association of Perioperative Registered Nurses (AORN) competency checklist* (Denholm, 2013). This list combines WHO suggestions and TJC guidelines to produce a color-coded list.

Surgical suites and emergent care sites are places that use time-out checklists; these stop everyone in their tasks to verify correctness. Staff verbally run down completion of the list to avoid wrong client, wrong procedure/surgery, and wrong site. TJC, with its universal protocol, does not mandate a specific checklist, just requires that one be used. In 2012, CMS issued requirements to use checklists. AORN has advocated use of a preoperative checklist for years.

Unit checklists are used when, for example, the floor nurse uses a preoperative checklist to verify that everything has been completed before sending the client to the surgical suite, but then this list is again checked when the client arrives but before the actual surgery. Such system redundancies are used to prevent errors. But they have limited and specific uses, and do not address underlying communication problems. No standardized protocol exists for checklist development, but use of expert panels with multiple pilot testing is recommended. One example found in most agency preoperative areas is a checklist where standard items are marked as having been done and available in the client's record or chart. For example, laboratory results are documented regarding blood type, clotting time, and so forth. Adoption of assertion checklists empowers any team member to speak up when they become aware of missing information.

Client Safety Outcomes

Evidence shows use of checklists improves communication and client safety, especially in areas managing rapid change, such as preoperative areas, emergency departments, and anesthesiology. According to Amer (2013) use of a simple checklist saved more than 1500 lives in a recent 18-month test period. A study by Semel and colleagues (2010) found that if a hospital has a baseline major complication rate following surgery of more than 3%, the use of a checklist would generate cost savings once it prevented five major complications. Some nurses in surgical areas have complained that lists are redundant, take too much time, or are not used by all surgeons.

USE OF SBAR

The situation, background, assessment, recommendation **(SBAR)** uses a standardized verbal communication tool with a structured format to create a common language between nurses and physicians and others on the health team. It is especially useful when brief clear communication is needed in acute situations such as emergent declines in client status or during handoffs. See Table 4-2 for the SBAR format.

SBAR is designed to convey only the most critical information by eliminating excessive language. It eliminates the authority gradient, flattening the traditional physician-to-nurse hierarchy, making it possible for staff to say what they think is going on. This improves communication and creates collaboration. This concise format has gained wide adoption in the United States and Great Britain (Fleishman and Rabatin, 2008; Leonard and Bonacum, 2008; Schroeder, 2011).

SBAR is used as a situational briefing, so the team is "on the same page" (Bonacum, 2009). It is used across all types of agencies, groups, and even in e-mails. SBAR simplifies verbal communication between nurses and physicians because content is presented in an expected format. Some hospitals use laminated SBAR guidelines at the telephones for nurses to use when calling physicians about changes in client status and requests for new orders. Documenting the new order is the only part of SBAR that gets recorded. Refer to Box 4-1 for an example. Then practice your use of SBAR format in Exercises 4-1, 4-2, and 4-3.

Client Safety Outcomes

Evidence-based reports show that client adverse events have decreased through use of SBAR, including decreases in unexpected deaths (De Meester et al., 2013). Practicing use of standardized communication formats by student nurses has been found to improve their ability to effectively communicate with

	TABLE 4-2	SBAR Structured Communication Format
S	Situation	Identify yourself; identify the client and the problem. In 10 seconds, state what is going on. This may include client's date of birth, hospital ID number, verification that consent forms are present, etc.
B	Background	State relevant context and brief history. Review the chart if possible before speaking or telephoning to the physician. Relate the client's background, including client's diagnosis, problem list, allergies, as well as relevant vital signs, medications that have been administered, laboratory results, etc.
A	Assessment	State your conclusion, what you think is wrong. List your opinion about the client's current status. Examples would be client's level of pain, medical complications, level of consciousness, problem with intake and output, or your estimate of blood loss, etc.
R	Recommendation or request	State your informed suggestion for the continued care of this client. Propose an action. What do you need? In what time frame does it need to be completed? Always should include an opportunity for questions. Some sources recommend that any new verbal orders now be repeated for feedback clarity. If no decision is forthcoming, reassert your request.

Adapted from personal interviews: Bonacum D: CSP, CPHQ, CPHRM, Vice President, Safety Management, Kaiser Foundation Health Plan, Inc., February 25, 2009; Fleischmann JA: Medical Vice President of Franciscan Skemp, Mayo HealthCare System, LaCrosse, WS, May 29, 2008.

BOX 4-1	SBAR Example

Clinical Example of Use of SBAR Format for Communicating with Client's Physician

S Situation "Dr. Preston, this is Wendy Obi, evening nurse on 4G at St. Simeon Hospital, calling about Mr. Lakewood, who's having trouble breathing."

  B Background "Kyle Lakewood, DOB 7/1/60, a 53-year-old man with chronic lung disease, admitted 12/25, who has been sliding downhill × 2 hours. Now he's acutely worse: his vital signs are heart rate 92 bpm, respiratory rate 40 breaths/min with gasping, blood pressure 138/94 mm Hg, oxygenation down to 72%."

  A Assessment "I don't hear any breath sounds in his right chest. I think he has a pneumothorax."

  R Recommendation "I need you to see him right now. I think he needs a chest tube."

Adapted from Leonard M, Graham S, Bonacum D: The human factor: the critical importance of effective teamwork and communication in providing safe care, *Qual Saf Health Care* 13(Suppl 1):i85-i90, 2004.

EXERCISE 4-1	**Using Standardized Communication Formats**

Purpose: To practice the situation, background, assessment, recommendation (SBAR) technique.

Case Study

Mrs. Robin, date of birth January 5, 1950, is a preoperative client of Dr. Hu's. She is scheduled for an abdominal hysterectomy at 9 a.m. She has been NPO (fasting) since last midnight. She is allergic to penicillin. The night nurse reported she got little sleep and expressed a great deal of anxiety about this surgery immediately after her surgeon and anesthesiologist examined her at the time of admission. Preoperative medication consisting of atropine was administered at 8:40 instead of 8:30 as per order. Abdominal skin was scrubbed with Betadine per order, and an intravenous (IV) drip of 1 L 0.45 saline was started at 7 a.m. in her left forearm. She has a history of chronic obstructive pulmonary disease, controlled with an albuterol inhaler, but has not used this since admission yesterday.

Directions

In triads, organize this information into the SBAR format. Student no. 1 is giving report. Student no. 2 role-plays the nurse receiving report. Student no. 3 acts as observer and evaluates the accuracy of the report.

EXERCISE 4-2	**Telephone Simulation: Conversation between Nurse and Physician about a Critically Ill Client**

Purpose: To increase your telephone communication technique using structured formats.

Procedure

Read case and then simulate making a phone call to the physician on call. It is midnight.

Case

Ms. Babs Pointer, date of birth January 14, 1942, is 6 hours post-op for knee reconstruction, complaining of pain and thirst. Her leg swelling has increased 4 cm in circumference, lower leg has notable ecchymosis spreading rapidly. Temperature 99° F; respiratory rate 20 breaths/min; pedal pulse absent.

Discussion/Written Paper

Record your conversation for later analysis. In your analysis, write up an evaluation of this communication for accurate use of situation, background, assessment, recommendation (SBAR) format, effectiveness, and clarity.

EXERCISE 4-3	**SBAR for Change of Shift Simulation**

Purpose: To practice use of situation, background, assessment, recommendation (SBAR).

Procedure

In post conference have Student A be the day-shift nurse reporting to Student B, who is acting as the evening nurse. Practice reporting on their assigned clients' conditions or simulate four or five postoperative clients' status. Use the SBAR format.

Discussion

Have the entire post conference group of students critique the advantages and disadvantages of using this type of communication.

physicians about emergent changes in client condition (Krautscheid, 2008). And its use has been shown to help develop a mental schema that facilitates rapid decision-making by nurses (Vardaman et al., 2012). This format sets expectation about what will be communicated to other members of the health care team (see Figure 4-1).

TJC, the Institute for Health Care Improvement, and AACN all support the use of SBAR as a desirable structured communication format. (TJC requires hospitals develop a standardized handoff format.) Thus, we consider the SBAR tool as a best practice protocol. In addition to using SBAR when there is a change in a client's health status, this communication format is used between shifts between nurse colleagues, between nurses and physicians during rounds, transfers, and handoffs from one care setting or unit to another. Some suggest that agencies conduct annual SBAR competency validations.

A distinct advantage of using SBAR or other standardized communication tools between physicians and nurses is that it decreases professional differences in communication styles. In a study by Compton and colleagues (2012), 78% of physicians surveyed stated they receive enough information to make clinical decisions.

In addition to communication with professional colleagues at regular intervals or when a client's condition changes, nurses are accountable for orally informing ancillary clinical staff about the meaning of changes in the client's condition. They are responsible for appropriately supervising their care of the client and for questioning unclear or controversial orders made by a physician.

Several authors speculate that use of SBAR leads to creation of cognitive schemata in staff. Use of this structured format enable less-experienced nurses to give as complete reports as experienced nurses.

Use of electronic SBAR format when transferring clients to another unit or during change of shift report has been shown to enhance the amount, consistency, and comprehensiveness of information conveyed, yet to not take any longer than traditional shift report (Cornell and Gervis, 2013; Wentworth et al., 2012).

CREW RESOURCE MANAGEMENT-BASED TOOLS

Crew resource management (CRM) is another communication tool similar to SBAR, which was adapted from aviation. It provides rules of conduct for communication, especially during handoff care transitions. Just prior to an event such as surgery, all members of the team stop and summarize what is happening. Each team member has an obligation to voice safety concerns.

Briefing. In team situations, such as in the operating room, the team may use another sort of standardized format: a briefing. The leader (the surgeon, in this case) presents to the team a brief overview of what procedure is about to happen, identifies roles and responsibilities, plans for the unexpected, and increases each member's awareness of the situation. The leader asks anyone who sees a potential problem to speak up. In this manner, the leader "gives permission" for every team member to speak up. This can include the client also, as many clients will not speak unless specifically invited to do so. A debriefing is usually led by someone other than the leader. It occurs toward the end of a procedure and is a "recap" or summary as to what went well or what might be changed (Bonacum, 2009). This is similar to the feedback nurses ask clients to do after they have presented some educational health teaching, which verifies that the client understood the material.

Debriefing. Debriefing occurs after a surgery or critical incident. It is a callback or review during which each team member has an opportunity to voice problems that arose, identify what went well, and suggest changes that can be made.

Client Safety Outcomes

Mortality rates have decreased using this tool in the surgical area. Staff identify adverse events that were avoided due to the information communicated during the briefing (Bagian, 2010). Use of structured handoff tools increases perceptions of adequate communication (Jukkala et al., 2012).

TEAM TRAINING MODELS

Teamwork is described in Chapter 24 on continuity of the physician-nurse communication.

The majority of reported errors have been found to stem from poor teamwork and poor communication (McCaffery et al., 2012). An effective team has clear, accurate communication understood by all. All team members work together to promote a climate of client safety. To improve interdisciplinary health team collaboration and communication, it is recommended that physicians and nurses jointly share communication training and team building sessions to develop an "us" rather than "them" work philosophy. When clashes occur, differences need to be settled. Specific conflict resolution techniques are discussed in Chapter 23.

Ideally, the health care team would provide the client with more resources, allow for greater flexibility, promote a "learning from each other" climate, and promote collective creativity to problem solving. Use of standardized communication tools fosters collaborative practice by creating shared communication expectations. Obstacles to effective teamwork include lack of time, culture of autonomy, heavy workloads, and different terminologies and communication styles held by each discipline. Building in redundancy cuts errors but takes extra time, which can be irritating.

TEAMSTEPPS MODEL

One prominent model is Team Strategies and Tools to Enhance Performance and Patient Safety (TeamSTEPPS). This program emphasizes improving client outcomes by improving communication using evidence-based techniques. Communication skills include briefing and debriefing, conveying respect, clarifying team leadership, cross-monitoring, situational monitoring feedback, assertion in a climate valuing everyone's input, and use of standard communication formats such as SBAR and Comprehensive Unit-based Safety Program (CUSP) (AHRQ, CUSP, 2008). Creating a team culture means each member is committed to

- Open communication with frequent timely feedback
- Protecting others from work overload
- Asking for and offering assistance

AHRQ's CUSP was designed to implement teamwork and communication. It is a multifaceted strategy to help create a culture of safety, urging health care workers to use communication tools. CUSP incorporates team training with strategies to translate research into staff's evidence-based practice (Weaver et al., 2013).

TeamSTEPPS with "I PASS the BATON." Regarding handoffs, AHRQ's TeamSTEPPS program (2008b) recommends that all team members use the "I PASS the BATON" mnemonic during any transition by staff in client care. Table 4-3 explains this communication strategy.

Veterans Administration Clinical Team Training Program. The Department of Veterans Affairs has

TABLE 4-3		I PASS the BATON
I	Introduction	Introduce yourself and your role
P	Patient	State patient's name, identifiers, age, sex, location
A	Assessment	Present chief complaint, vital signs, symptoms, diagnosis
S	Situation	Current status, level of certainty, recent changes, response to treatment
S	Safety concerns	Critical laboratory reports, allergies, alerts (e.g., falls)
the		
B	Background	Comorbidities, previous episodes, current medications, family history
A	Actions	State what actions were taken and why
T	Timing	Level of urgency, explicit timing and priorities
O	Ownership	State who is responsible
N	Next	State the plan: what will happen next, any anticipated changes

Developed by the U.S. Department of Defense: Department of Defense patient safety program: healthcare communications toolkit to improve transitions in care. Falls Church, VA: TRICARE Management Activity, 2005.

developed a multidisciplinary program for building teams. Based on principles from aviation's CRM, it is an entire program infused with techniques and standardized care strategies to improve open communication. One example is the concept of "assertive inquiry," modeled on aviation CRM, under which any member of the crew is empowered to speak up if they have a safety concern.

CLIENT SAFETY OUTCOMES OF TEAM TRAINING PROGRAMS

Multiple studies tend to demonstrate increased satisfaction, primarily from nurses, when team communication strategies are implemented. In a review of findings from multiple studies, Weaver found moderate support that improvements in client safety are associated with CUSP.

NURSING TEAMWORK

The traditional client report from one nurse handing over care to another nurse needs to be accurate, specific, and clear, and allow time for questions to foster a culture of client safety. Team training is a tool to increase collaboration between physicians and nurses. Use of teams is a concept that has been around for years within medical and nursing professions. For example, medicine has used medical rounds to share information among physicians. Nursing has end-of-shift reports, when responsibility is handed over to the next group of nurses. Using SBAR or any other standardized communication format for reports, especially if these reports are at the bedside, results in a safer environment for your clients, includes clients as active team members, and has been shown not to increase report duration (Woods et al., 2008).

INTERDISCIPLINARY ROUNDS AND TEAM MEETINGS

Contemporary health care teams use "interdisciplinary **rounds**" to increase communication among the whole team—physicians, pharmacists, therapists, nurses, and dieticians. This strategy may increase communication and positively affect client outcome. For example, daily discharge multidisciplinary rounds have been correlated with decreased length of hospital stay.

Interdisciplinary "team" meetings can be used daily or weekly to explore common goals, concerns, and options; smooth problems before they escalate into conflicts; or provide support. Lower on the scale are *clinical teaching rounds,* where a physician once weekly teaches nurses, which has the goal of encouraging physician communication with the nursing staff.

A **huddle** is a brief, informal gathering of the team to decide on a course of action. Huddles reinforce the existing plan of care or inform team members of changes to the plan. A team huddle can be called by any team member.

Callouts and **time-outs** allow staff to stop and review. As mentioned earlier, TJC mandates that staff working in surgery have a time-out in which all team members review the details of the surgery about to take place to prevent wrong client, wrong site surgeries.

STANDARDIZED HANDOFF TOOLS

Many formats are available to foster complete, organized transfer of information, including electronic handoff checklists. In addition to the checklists already described, TJC released SHARE, a targeted solutions tool.

S = Standardize crucial content: give client's history, key current data

H = Hardwire your system: develop or use standardized tools, checklists

A = Allow opportunities for questions: use critical thinking, share data with entire team

R = Reinforce: common goal, member accountability

E = Educate: team training on use of standardized handoffs with real-time feedback

Client Safety Outcomes

All these strategies to improve interdisciplinary communication break down barriers, increase staff satisfaction (Rosenthal, 2013), decrease night pager calls to residents, and hopefully help improve the quality of care.

TECHNOLOGY-ORIENTED SOLUTIONS CREATE A CLIMATE OF CLIENT SAFETY

Health information technologies (HITs) are a key tool for increasing safety, as well as a means to decrease health care costs and increase quality of care (Parsons, 2013). HITs, text messaging, and dedicated smart phones are some of the technological innovations discussed in Chapters 25 and 26, as are clinical decision support systems, electronic clinical pathways and care plans, and computerized registries or national databanks that monitor treatment.

Electronic transmission of prescriptions involves sending medication orders directly to the client's pharmacy in the community. This can help decrease errors caused by misinterpretation of handwritten scripts.

Radiofrequency identification (RFID), which puts a computer chip in identity cards or even into some people, is an emerging technology allowing you to locate a certain nurse, identify a patient, or even locate an individual medication. RFID may be able to be incorporated into the nurse's handheld computer.

Prevention of misidentification of the client is an obvious error prevention strategy. Before administering medication, the nurse needs to verify client allergies, use another nurse to verify accuracy for certain stock medications, and re-verify the client's identity. TJC's best practice recommendation is to check the client's name band and then ask the client to verbally confirm his or her name and give a second identifier such as date of birth.

Use of technology such as *bar-coded name bands* offers protection against misidentification (AHRQ, n.d.[c]). Some bar-coded name bands include the client's picture, as well as name, date of birth, and bar code for verification of client identity.

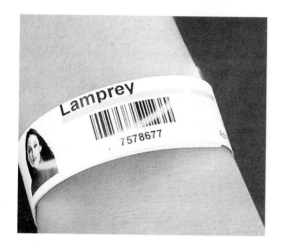

Whiteboards have long been used at the central nursing station to list the census, the staff assigned to care, in delivery suites to list labor status, in surgical suites to track procedures and staff. Now we have electronic whiteboards, and clients are invited to add to information displayed on them.

Client Safety Outcomes

Many agencies, including the Veterans Administration (VA) hospital system, have used bar codes for years. When a new medication is ordered by a physician, it is transmitted to the pharmacy, where it is labeled with the same bar code as is on the client's name band. The nurse administering that medication must first verify both codes by scanning with the battery-operated bar-code reader, just as a grocery store employee scans merchandise. In the VA, this resulted in a 24% decrease in medication administration errors (Wright and Katz, 2005). In a similar fashion, bar-coded labels on laboratory specimens prevent mix-ups.

OTHER SPECIFIC NURSING EFFORTS

FOLLOWING SAFETY POLICIES

Implementing unit-based safety programs, such as CUSP and following policy helps decease errors and improve efficiency of care. Measures to improve efficiency may also increase the time you have for communication with clients. Examples of safety redundant process are the two identifiers required before administering a procedure or medicine, or use of the two challenge rule.

Work-arounds are shortcuts. Nurses under pressure of time constraints have sometimes developed shortcuts commonly known as "work-arounds." These are nonapproved methods to expedite one's work. An example is printing an extra set of bar codes for all your clients who are scheduled to receive medication at 10 a.m., and scanning them all at once rather than scanning each client's bar-code name band in his room.

Client Safety Outcomes

Deviating from safety protocols inherently introduces risks. While in the short term, some time may be saved, in the long run, mistakes cost millions of dollars each year, harm clients, and put you at risk for liability or malpractice suits.

TRANSFORMING CARE AT THE BEDSIDE

Begun in 2003, Transforming Care At the Bedside (**TCAB;** pronounced *tee-cab*) is an Institute for Healthcare Improvement initiative funded by the Robert Wood Johnson Foundation to improve client safety and the quality of hospital bedside care by empowering nurses at the bedside to make system changes (Robert Wood Johnson Foundation, 2008; Stefancyk, 2009).

This program has four core concepts to improve care:

1. Create a climate of safe, reliable patient care. Uses practices, such as brainstorming and retreats for staff nurses, to develop better practice and better communication ideas. One example is nurses initiate presentation of the client's status to physicians at morning rounds, using a standard format. Another strategy is to empower staff nurses to make decisions.

2. Establish unit-based vital teams. Interdisciplinary, supportive care teams foster a sense of increased professionalism for bedside nurses. This together with better nurse-physician communication should positively affect client outcomes.

3. Develop client-centered care. This ensures continuity of care and respects family and client choices.

4. Provide value-added care. This eliminates inefficiencies, for example, by placing high-use supplies in drawers in each client's room.

Client Safety Outcomes

Evaluation in more than 60 project hospitals showed that units using this method cut their mortality rate by 25% and reduced nosocomial infections significantly. Nurse-physician collaboration and communication was improved, with both physicians and nurses voicing increased satisfaction. Nurses said that overall they felt empowered (Stefancyk, 2008a; 2008b).

CLIENT-PROVIDER COLLABORATIONS

Communicating with clients about the need for them to participate in their care planning. This is a goal set in 2009 by TJC. Goal 13 states, "Encourage patients' active involvement in their own care as a patient safety strategy," which includes having clients and families report their safety concerns. Clients and their families should be specifically invited to be an integral part of the care process. Another strategy is to provide more opportunities for communication.

EMPHASIZE TO CLIENTS THAT THEY ARE VALUED MEMBERS OF THE HEALTH TEAM

Let your client know he or she is expected to actively participate in his or her care. Safe care is a top goal shared by client and care provider. Empowering your client to be a collaborator in his or her own care enhances error prevention. Emphasize this provider-client partnership and increase open communication through bedside rounds, bedside change of shift handoffs, and client access to their own records. This is the second step in a communication model described by Fleischman and Rabatin (2008). In building the relationship, to establish rapport, participants follow the mnemonic PEARLS (*p*artnership; *e*mpathy; *a*pology, such as "sorry you had to wait"; *r*espect; *l*egitimize or validate your client's feelings and concerns with comments such as "many people have similar concerns"; *s*upport).

CONDUCT DAILY CLIENT BRIEFINGS

Physicians have long used hospital rounds to briefly speak with each of their patients. Some supervising nurses have begun this practice, especially at change of shift report. This allows the client to be included in the information exchange. With rapid development technology as described in Chapter 26, bedside rounds

should become even more efficient. Use of computer tablets may obviate the need to push the heavy cart around with the unit computer attached. New electronic trends, such as electronic clinical pathways, are becoming used as client care plans, allowing each client to know today's goals.

USE WRITTEN MATERIALS

In one hospital system, written pamphlets are given to clients on admission, instructing them to become partners in their care. A nurse comes into the client's room at a certain time each day, sits, and makes eye contact. Together, nurse and client make a list of today's goals, which are written on a whiteboard in the client's room (Runy, 2008). As part of safety and communication, awareness of language barriers can be signaled to everyone entering the room by posting a logo on the chart, and room or bed. Use of interpreters and information materials written in the client's primary language may also reduce risk.

ASSESS CLIENT'S LEVEL OF HEALTH LITERACY

As mentioned, it is important to make verbal and written information as simple as possible. As a nurse, you need to assess the health literacy level of each client. Provide privacy to avoid embarrassment. Obtain feedback or teach-backs to determine the client's understanding of teaching: Simplify, clarify, verify!

Client Safety Outcomes

We need more data about client involvement effects on safety. Evidence does show increases in client satisfaction after changing to a model of bedside report (Radtke, 2013). AHRQ advises clients to speak up if they have a question or concern, to ask about test results rather than to assume that "no news is good news." Placing information such as fall prevention posters in the room of an at-risk client have been reported by agencies to reduce the number of falls.

SUMMARY

Major efforts to transform the health care system are ongoing. We maximize client safety by minimizing errors made by all health care workers. Because miscommunication has been documented to be a most significant factor in occurrence of errors, this chapter focused on communication solutions. It described some individual and system solutions.

ETHICAL DILEMMA | What Would You Do?

You are a new nurse working for hospice, providing in-home care for Ms. Wendy, a 34-year-old with recurrent spinal cancer. At a multidisciplinary care planning conference 2 months ago, Dr. Chi, oncologist, and Dr. Spenski, family physician, hospice staff, and Ms. Wendy agreed to admit her when her condition deteriorated to the point that she would require ventilator assistance. Today, however, when you arrive at her home, she states a desire to forego further hospitalization. Her family physician is a personal friend and agrees to increase her morphine to handle her increased pain, even though you feel that such a large dose will further compromise her respiratory status.

1. What are the possibilities for miscommunication?
2. What steps would you take to get the health care team "on the same page"?

DISCUSSION QUESTIONS

1. Examine Table 4-1 and give one example you have seen for each of the "best practice" communication solutions provided.
2. Use the SBAR exercises given. What was the easiest part? Or the hardest? Many schools actually have students telephone physicians and role-play a scenario. Have you?

REFERENCES

Abrahamson KA, Fox RL, Doebbeling BN: Facilitators and barriers to clinical practice guidelines use among nurses, *Am J Nurs* 112(7): 26–35, 2012.

Agency for Healthcare Research and Quality (AHRQ):
- AHRQ [a]. National healthcare quality report.2005. www.ahrq.gov/qual/nhqr05/nhrq05.htm Author. Accessed 7/1/14.
- AHRQ [b]. Medical errors: the scope of the problem: an epidemic of errors. Author. www.ahrq.gov/research/findings/factsheets/errors-safety/improving-quality/index.html. Accessed 7/1/14.
- AHRQ. 2009. Patient safety initiative: building foundations, reducing risk. Patient Safety Goals Available online: www.ahrq.gov/qual/pscongrpt/psinisum.htm. Accessed February 28, 2009.
- AHRQ [c]. Mistaken identity www.ahrq.gov/ [search 'mistaken identity']Author.
- AHRQ. Comprehensive unit-based safety program (CUSP). 2008. Using a comprehensive unit-based safety program to prevent healthcare-associated infections tool.
- http://www.ahrq.gov/professionals/quality-patient-safety/cusp/index.htm. Accessed 1/7/14.
- AHRQ. 2008. Patient safety and quality: an evidence-based handbook for nurses. Hughes, RG [ed]. Agency for Healthcare Research and Quality: Rockville, MD [AHRQ pub no. 08-0043]

- AHRQ. 2008. Publication No. 06-0020-3. TeamSTEPPS [trademark], pocket guide Author: Rockville, MD. http://teamstepps.ahrq.gov/: Agency for Healthcare Research and Quality's Patient Safety Network : PSNet (http://PSNet.ahrq.gov/collection.aspx) [search by name]
- PSNet:Checklists. http://psnet.ahrq.gov/primer.aspx?primerID=14. Accessed 7/1/14. PSNet: Error Disclosure. http://psnet.ahrq.gov/Primer.aspx?primerID=2. Accessed 7/1/14.
- PSNet: Handoffs and Signouts. http://psnet.ahrq.gov/primer.aspx?primerID=9. Accessed 7/1/14.
- PSNet: Medication Errors. http://psnet.ahrq.gov/primer.aspx?primerID=23. Accessed 7/1/14.
- PSNet: Nursing and Patient Safety. http://psnet.ahrq.gov/primer.aspx?primerID=22. Accessed 7/1/14.
- PSNet: Physician Work Hours and Patient Safety. http://psnet.ahrq.gov/primer.aspx?primerID=19. Accessed 7/1/14.
- PSNet: Root Cause Analysis. http://psnet.ahrq.gov/primer.aspx?primerID=10. Accessed 7/1/14.
- PSNet: Safety Culture. http://psnet.ahrq.gov/primer.aspx?primerID=5. Accessed 7/1/14.
- PSNet: Systems Approach. http://psnet.ahrq.gov/primer.aspx?primerID=21. Accessed 7/1/14.

Amer KS: *Quality and Safety for Transformational Nursing: Care Competencies*, Boston, 2013, Pearson Publishing.

American Association of Colleges of Nursing (AACN):
- AACN. 2006a. Hallmarks of quality and patient safety: recommended baccalaureate competencies and curricular guidelines to ensure high-quality and safe patient care. *J Prof Nurs* 22 (6), 329–330.Available online: www.aacn.org or http://qsen.org/competencydomains/safety Accessed.
- AACN. 2006b. Safety. http://www.aacn.nche.edu/publications/white-papers/hallmarks-quality-safety Accessed 7/1/14.Bagian JP. 2010. Medical team communication training before, during and after surgery improves patient outcomes, *JAMA* 304(5), 1693-1700.

Barnsteiner J, Disch J: A just culture for nurses and nursing students, p. 407–416. In Disch J, Barnsteiner J, editors: *Second Generation QSEN: An Issue of Nursing Clinics*, Philadelphia, 2012, Saunders/Elsevier.

Bonacum D: CSP, CPHQ, CPHRM, Vice President, Safety Management, *Kaiser Foundation Health Plan, Inc*, 2009 [Kaiser Permanente]: Personal interview February 25.

Brickell TA, McLean C: Emerging issues & challenges for improving patient safety in mental health: A qualitative analysis of expert peer perspective, *Patient Saf* 7(1):39–44, 2011.

Compton J, Copeland K, Flanders S, Cassity C, et al.: Implementing SBAR across a large multihospital health system, *Jt Comm J Qual Patient Saf* 38(6):261–268, 2012.

Cornell P, Gervis MT: Improving shift report focus and consistency with the Situation, Background, Assessment, Recommendation protocol, *J Nurs Admin* 43(7/8):422–428, 2012.

Cronenwett L, G. Sherwood J, Barnsteiner, et al.: Quality and safety education for nurses, *Nurs Outlook* 55(3):122–131, 2007.

De Meester K, Verspuy M, Monsieurs KG, Van Bogaert P: SBAR improves nurse-physician communication and reduces unexpected death: A pre and post intervention study, *Resuscitation 2013 Sep* 84(9):1192–1196, 2013. Epub 2013 Mar 26 http://dx.doi.org/10.1016/j.resuscitation.2013.03.016.

Denham CR: SSBAR for patients, *J Patient Saf* 4(1):38–48, 2008.

Denholm B: Time-out checklist, *AORN* 98(1):87–90, 2013.

Elder NC, Brungs SM, Nagy M, et al.: Nurses' perceptions of error communication and reporting in the intensive care unit, *J Patient Saf* 4:162–168, 2008.

Fleischman A, Rabatin J. 2008. Provider-Patient Communication. Conference materials supplied by Mayo Health Care System Medical Continuing Education Department MN: Rochester, obtained May 27

Fleischmann JA: *Medical Vice President of Franciscan Skemp, Mayo HealthCare System*, LaCrosse, WS, 2008, Personal interview May 29.

Hartnell N, MacKinnon N, Sketris I, Fleming M: Identifying, understanding and overcoming barriers to medication error reporting in hospitals: A focus group study, *BMJ Qual Saf* 21(5):361–368, 2012.

Haw C, Cahill C: A computerized system for reporting medication events in psychiatry: The first two years of operation, *J Psychiatr Mental Health Nurs* 18:308–315, 2011.

Henkind JR, Sinnett JC: Patient care, square-rigger sailing, and safety, *JAMA* 300(14):1691–1693, 2008.

Hospital Safety Score: *Latest Hospital Safety Scores Show Incremental Progress in Patient Safety* U.S. State Rankings, 2013, New Letter Grades Shift. Accessed 7/17/13 www.hospitalsafetyscore.org/latest-hospital-safety-scores-show-incremental-progress.

Hughes RG, 2008. Editor. Patient safety and quality: an evidence-based handbook for nurses vols. 1–3 2008 Agency for Healthcare Research and Quality: Rockville, MD April [AHRQ Publication No. 08–0043]

The Joint Commission (TJC)
- TJC. 2008. Behaviors that undermine culture of safety. Sentinel Event Alert Issue 40. Available online: http://www.jointcommission.org/sentinelevent_alert_issue_40_behaviors_that_undermine_a_culture_of_safety/. Accessed 7/1/14
- TJC. 2007. Preventing medication errors. In RA Porche' [ed]. Front Line of Defense: The Role of Nurses in Preventing Sentinel Events. [2nd ed]. Oakbrook Terrace, Il.
- TJC Safety Goals. www.jcipatientsafety.org/
- TJC. 2006. Root causes of sentinel events Author: www.jointcommission.org/SentinelEvants/Statistics/
- TJC. Sentinel event statistics. www.jointcommission.org/sentinel_event_statistics_quarterly/

The Joint Commission International with Robert Wood Johnson Foundation. 2010. The Future of Nursing. Author. www.nap.edu/catalog.php?record_id=12956/ 7/1/14.The Joint Commission International, WHO Solutions. ww.jointcommissioninternational.org/24839/ Accessed Sept. 1, 2013.

Jukkala AM, James D, Autrey P, Azuero A, et al.: Developing a standardized tool to improve nurse communication during shift report, *J Nurs Care Qual* 27(3):240–246, 2012.

Kaboli PJ: Medication reconciliation, *Arch Intern Med* 172(19): 1069–1070, 2012.

Institute of Medicine (IOM): *To Err Is Human: Building a Safer Health System*, Washington, DC, 2000, The National Academies Press.

Krautscheid LC: Improving communication among healthcare providers: preparing student nurses for practice, *Int J Nurs Educ Sch* 5(1), 2008 article 40.

Leonard M, Bonacum D: *SBAR application and critical success factors of implementation. Kaiser Permanente Health Care System presentation.* Rochester, MN, 2008, Pulmonary and Critical Care Medicine, Mayo Healthcare System May 2008, by Dr. Rabatin Jeff, Consultant.

McCaffery R, Hayes RM, Cassell A, Miller-Reyes S, et al.: The effect of an educational program on attitudes of nurses and medical residents towards the benefits of positive communication and collaboration, *J Adv Nurs* 68(2):293–301, 2012.

National Patient Safety Foundation (NPSF, nd). www.npsf.org/category/updates-news-press/research-news/for-patients-consumers/patients-andconsumers-key-facts-about-patient-safety

Parsons A. 2013. Webinar on translating electronic data. AHRQ webinar event #998 908 862. Accessed August, 29.

Quality and Safety Education for Nurses (QSEN, 2013): www.qsen.org/

Radtke K: Improving patient satisfaction with nursing communication using bedside shift report, *Clin Nurse Spec* 27(1):19–25, 2013.

Rideout D: "Just Culture" encourages error reporting, improves patient safety, *OR Manger* 29(7):1, 2013.

Ring L, Fairchild RM: Leadership and patient safety: A review of the literature, *J Nurs Reg* 4(1):52–56, 2013.

Rosenthal L: Enhancing communication between nightshift RNs and hospitalists, *J Nurs Admin* 43(2):59–61, 2013.

Runy LA: The nurse and patient safety, *Hosp Health Netw.* 2008 Nov 82(11):5, 2008 . p following 42, 1. Accessed January 6, 2009.

Saintsing D, Gibson LM, Pennington AW: The novice nurse and clinical decision-making: How to avoid errors, *J Nurs Manag* 19:354–359, 2011.

Schroeder MJ: Looking to improve your bedside report? Try SBAR, *Nursing Made Incredibly Easy* 9(5):53–54, 2011.

Singh H, Thomas E, Peterson L, et al.: Medical errors involving trainees, *Arch Intern Med* 167(19):2030–2036, 2007.

Semel ME, Resch S, Haynes AB, Funk LM, et al.: Adopting a surgical safety checklist could save money and improve the quality of care in U.S. hospitals, *Health Aff (Millwood)* 29:1593–1599, 2010.

Stefancyk AL: Transforming care at the bedside: transforming care at Mass General, *Am J Nurs* 108(9):71–72, 2008a.

Stefancyk AL: Transforming care at the bedside: nurses participate in presenting patients in morning rounds, *Am J Nurs* 108(11):70–72, 2008b.

Stefancyk AL: Transforming care at the bedside: high-use supplies at the bedside, *Am J Nurs* 109(2):33–35, 2009.

Robert Wood Johnson Foundation. 2008. The Transforming Care At the Bedside (TCAB) Toolkit. http://www.rwjf.org/en/research-publications/find-rwjf-research/2008/06/the-transforming-care-at-the-bedside-tcab-toolkit.html.

World Health Organization (WHO): WHO Collaborating Centre on Patient Safety Solutions. http://www.who.int/patientsafety/solutions/patientsafety/collaborating_centre/en/.

Vardaman JM, Cornell P, Gondo MB, Amis JM, et al.: Beyond communication: The role of standardized protocols in a changing health care environment, *Health Care Manage Rev* 37(1):88–97, 2012.

Weaver SJ, Lubomksi LH, Wilson RF, Pfoh ER, et al.: Promoting a Culture of Safety as a patient safety strategy: A systematic review, *Ann Intern Med* 158(5 Part 2):369–374, 2013.

Wentworth L, Diggins J, Bartel D, Johnson, et al.: SBAR: Electronic hand-off tool for noncomplicated procedural patients, *J Nurs Care Qual* 27(2):125–131, 2012.

Woods DM, Holl JL, Angst D, et al.: Improving clinical communication and patient safety: clinician-recommended solutions, *J Healthcare Qual* 30(5):4354, 2008.

Wright AA, Katz IT: Bar coding and patient safety, *N Eng J Med* 353(4):329–331, 2005.

Yee KC, Wong MC, Turner P: Understanding how clinical judgement and communicative practices interact with the use of an electronic clinical handover system, *Stud Health Technol Inform* 188:168–173, 2013.

Zbar RI, Taylor LD, Canady JW, et al.: The disruptive physician: righteous Maverick or dangerous Pariah? *Plast Reconstr Surg* 123(1):409–415, 2009.

CHAPTER 5

Developing Therapeutic Communication Skills

Elizabeth C. Arnold

OBJECTIVES

At the end of the chapter, the reader will be able to:

1. Describe the concept of therapeutic communication.
2. Describe theoretical frameworks used in therapeutic communication.
3. Differentiate characteristics of social versus therapeutic communication.
4. Apply concepts of client-centered communication.
5. Discuss active listening responses used in therapeutic communication.
6. Describe the use of verbal responses as a communication strategy.
7. Describe other forms of communication formats used in health alliances.

C hapter 5 focuses on the communication principles, skills, and strategies that nurses need to support, educate, and empower clients to effectively cope with personal health-related issues. The chapter reviews the components and purposes of effective communication, using a client-centered focus. Applications describe empathetic active listening responses and common communication strategies used in nurse-client relationships.

Therapeutic communication is the primary means through which the health care team, clients, and families collaboratively consider care options, plan treatment approaches, reach consensus about treatment decisions, conduct treatment activities, and evaluate clinical outcomes. Therapeutic communication takes place in the present moment in health care encounters, but discussions can have a profound impact on achieving clinical outcomes and a client's future health status. Effective communication is essential to achieving Quality and Safety Education for Nurses (QSEN) nursing competencies fundamental to client-centered care and team collaboration in clinical practice (Cronenwett et al., 2007). The significance of effective communication skills in quality health practice is reflected in The Joint Commission Standards (2010) and Institute of Medicine (IOM) reports. Health care is largely communication dependent and is closely linked to client safety. Using planned communication strategies therapeutically is a *learned* skill, which requires study and practice for proficiency and professional self-confidence.

BASIC CONCEPTS

CONCEPTS OF THERAPEUTIC COMMUNICATION

DEFINITION

Therapeutic communication is defined as a dynamic interactive process consisting of words and actions, and entered into by a clinician and client for the purpose of achieving identified health-related goals. Originally conceptualized by Jurgen Ruesch (1961), communication skills are essential drivers for developing therapeutic relationships and facilitating interdisciplinary collaborative communication with clients and families. Fundamental forms of health communication include verbal and written words and nonverbal communicative behaviors.

Contemporary thinking holds that verbal and non-verbal communication should be treated as an integrated communication construct (Stewart, 2011; Knapp and Colleagues, 2014). In face-to-face interactions, nurses have a rich range of visual and vocal behavioral information from which to consider client-centered responses. Embracing *both* verbal and nonverbal expressions of a message provides more complete understanding. Verbal and nonverbal can also communicate more than one message at a time (Knapp and Colleagues, 2014).

VERBAL COMMUNICATION

Verbal communication refers to language communication; Words are the most consciously used form of communication. Wachtel (2011) states "words are the medium of relationships" (p. 3). Words are comprised of language symbols, which allow people to create, reflect on, and interpret reality. Each word symbolically represents an idea, a concrete phenomenon, or thing (West and Turner, 2009). Words are the primary means through which the health care team and client organize data about human clinical problems, explain diagnosis, explore different options, make meaning of experiences, and dialogue with each other.

How words are put together and delivered in conversation matters. The meaning of words resides in the person who uses them, not in the words themselves. When language or word connotations differ between clinicians and clients, meanings change. Words cannot be erased, although they can be explained, or modified. Verbal expressions should be clear, complete, concrete, and easily understandable. Choice of words is important. Words should neither overstate nor understate the meaning of a situation. Straightforward easily understood messages are trustworthy. Vague messages are not. As you pay close attention to your client's verbal expression, and forms of language, noting and mirroring them increases recognition of content.

Words are not the sole source of meaning. Nadzam (2009) notes, "Communication is not just about what a person says, but how he or she says it" (p. 184). Nurses should be sensitive to what is left out of the message, as well as to what is included. The client's personal voice tonal quality (whiny, angry, surprised), hesitations, rapidity or slowness of speech, and forcefulness of verbal expression are dimensions of communication, which can be so strong, so weak, or so distracting, that its delivery overshadows the meaning of the message.

NONVERBAL (BEHAVIORAL) COMMUNICATION

Schmid (2001) notes, "language always has a non-verbal dimension expressed by the body" (p. 226). *Nonverbal communication* refers to physical expressions, and behaviors not expressed in words. It involves four categories: *kinesics* (movements, body position and tension), *proxemics* (space between clinician and client), *paralanguage* (vocal tones, rate, rhythm, volume), and *autonomic physical responses* (blushing, sweating). Over 50% of interpersonal communication is nonverbal (Burgoon et al., 2009).

Nonverbal behaviors help clinicians grasp the emotional meanings of messages. Nurses use body language, for example, with leaning forward, frequent eye contact, and attentive facial expressions to signal full attention on the client. People use nonverbal communication simultaneously with words in everyday conversations; neither dimension is discrete or independent of the other (Stewart, 2011). Nonverbal physical communication behaviors can have different cultural meanings for the person demonstrating them, or observing them in interactions. Examples are presented in the application section.

Metacommunication (see Chapter 6) refers to how nonverbal cues are used to enhance or negate the meaning of words. In addition to observable nonverbal behavior, client choices about clothing, personal and religious items, hairstyle and hygiene, and voluntary use of gestures inform, add to, and complete verbal messages. Behavioral communication is influenced by life circumstances, culture, and immediate context, so it is susceptible to misinterpretation, and requires validation.

PURPOSE OF CLIENT-CENTERED COMMUNICATION

The complexity of care and current emphasis on team collaboration create new communication opportunities and challenges. The overarching purpose of client-centered communication is to promote individualized quality of health outcomes within a shortened time frame, at less cost. To accomplish this goal, you need to know about the health disruption from the client's perspective. A simple statement—"I wonder if you could tell me what this illness (injury) has been like for you"—can provide clients with the opening they need to tell their story of it.

Clinicians depend on communication to support clients in learning new self-management skills, lessen client anxiety, and provide comfort to clients and families (Street et al., 2009). Communication influences the completeness of diagnostic information and compliance with treatment. The dialogue between clinicians and clients is a major factor in client satisfaction with care. "Good" clinical experiences from a client perspective involve meaningful human communication encounters in which the client's human needs and values are respected and the humanity of the clinician is transparent (Snellman et al., 2012). In "negative" clinical encounters, a client experiences a communication disconnect, which interferes with trust and shared decision making. Poor communication is implicated as a primary contributing factor in clinical safety errors (Woods, 2006).

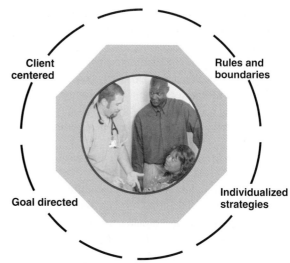

Figure 5-1   Characteristics of therapeutic communication.

THEORETICAL PERSPECTIVES

The word "communication" derives from the Latin word, meaning *to share*; Hargie (2011) defines *interpersonal communication* "as a process that is transactional, purposeful, multidimensional, irreversible and (possibly) inevitable" (p. 42). Basic theoretical communication components, involving sender, receiver, message, and channels (see Chapter 1) apply to therapeutic communication.

A transactional model of communication with its circular social system communication structure fits well with the more egalitarian emphasis in client-centered communication. A transactional model posits that communication is context bound. The communicators mutually, and continuously influence each other throughout a conversation. In a transactional encounter, two or more individuals build a shared meaning through concurrent sending and receiving of messages, and negotiating their meaning. Both sender and receiver are responsible for the effectiveness of their communication (West and Turner, 2011) The transactional model offers a standardized framework for considering the current emphasis on joint care planning and shared decision making in health care. It allows for the weaving of a shared reality developed and evolved through multiple communications. Figure 5-1 displays a transactional communication skill model that nurses can use as a theoretical foundation for client-centered communication.

CLIENT-CENTERED COMMUNICATION

Client or patient-centered care, and associated teamwork and collaboration are identified as QSEN nursing competencies (Cronenwett et al., 2007). These competencies require a broader span of communication proficiency. Client-centered communication goes beyond finding out about a client's health problems and developing a problem-focused solution. Its purpose is to understand and incorporate a client's worldview, values, and preferences, as part of client assessment and as the foundation for mutually determined tailored health interventions. Personal ways of relating to others, physical and emotional conditions, concurrent life events, culture, and place in the life cycle are unique factors to consider in communication approaches. Appendix E in The Joint Commission's *The Road Map for Hospitals* (2010) provides a compilation of resources geared to support the communication needs of special populations.

Integration of client- and family-centered care principles in client-centered communication and collaborative interdisciplinary team partnering with clients represents a major change in health care deliverables. Clients are assuming new roles as stakeholders, critical informants, and active collaborators in contemporary health care. They expect to be listened to, involved in their own care, and able to choose between treatment options as a final decision maker. Transparent teamwork, incorporating client values and preferences into treatment, and actively involving them in care decisions empowers clients who must assume an active role in self-management of their health and well-being.

The centrality of client-centered two-way communication has become a key factor in client satisfaction with specific ratings for nurse-client communication—and medicare reimbursement based on results. Survey questions directly related to nurse-client communication include the following:

- "How often did nurses treat you with courtesy and respect?
- How often did nurses listen carefully to you?
- How often did nurses explain things in a way that you could understand?" (Lang, 2012, p. 114).

Illness, or injury is a major event in a client and family's life. Client-centered care stresses listening to understand the meaning a client gives to his or her health problems. Accepting a client's personalized interpretation of why a health problem has occurred, the values and behaviors it challenges, and its impact on self and others is critical input. A respectful dialogue between nurse and client is essential to learning about each client as a "person" as the basis for care. Client-centered communication requires an ongoing exchange of ideas focused on understanding what it is like to be *this* person in *this* situation with *this* illness (McGilton et al., 2012). Each client and family has its unique set of values, patterns of behavior, and preferences that must be taken into account. Exercise 5-1 introduces a role play as a format for exploring the nature of client-centered communication processes.

Epstein and Street (2007) identify six core, overlapping functions of client (patient)-centered communication needed to achieve beneficial health outcomes.

- Fostering healing relationships
- Exchanging information
- Responding to emotions
- Managing uncertainty
- Making decisions
- Enabling patient self-management (p. 17)

Talking about complex health problems with a trained health professional *and* being a core member of a collaborative care team allows clients and families to hear themselves, as they share information. Clients and families are expected to take an active role in sorting through options and making reasoned decisions guided by professional input. Professional feedback helps clients realistically sort out priorities and determine the actions they want to take to achieve health goals.

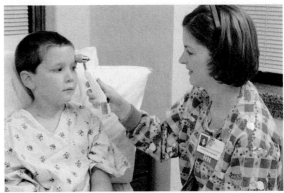

Whether you are sitting or standing, your posture should be relaxed, with the upper part of your body inclined slightly toward the client.

FACTORS AFFECTING CLIENT-CENTERED COMMUNICATION

Contextual Factors

Communication occurs within a personal, social, and environmental context. Personal and environmental contextual factors, referred to as "noise" influence the flow of therapeutic communication. *Noise* factors refer to *any* distraction that interferes with being able to pay full attention to the discussion (Weiten et al., 2009). Distractions can originate in the environment or internally in the nurse, the client, or both. Impediments to communication occur in *clients* when they are:

- Preoccupied with pain, physical discomfort, worry, or contradictory personal beliefs
- Unable to understand the nurse's use of language or terminology
- Struggling with an emotionally laden topic
- Feeling defensive, insecure, or judged
- Confused by the complexity of the message—too many issues, tangential comments
- Deprived of privacy, especially if the topic is a sensitive one
- Have sensory or cognitive deficits that compromise receiving accurate messages

Semantic noise occurs when the words and phrases used by either the client or the clinician are familiar to the sender but not to the receiver. Lack of understanding is a key contributor to noncompliance. Examples include medical terminology, street language used to

---

EXERCISE 5-1   Initial Client-Centered Communication Interview

Purpose: To help students use client-centered interview strategies.

Procedure

1. Develop a one-paragraph case scenario of a client situation that you are familiar with, before class.
2. Break into dyads, with one student taking the role of client, the other the nurse.
3. Conduct an initial client-centered 5-minute assessment interview using one of the group's scenarios, with the author of the paragraph taking the role of the nurse and the other student taking the client role. Be sure to include questions about values, beliefs, preferences.
4. Reverse roles, and repeat the interview process with the second student's scenario.

Discussion

1. In what ways were client-centered communication strategies used in this role-play?
2. How awkward was it for you in the nursing role to incorporate queries about the client's preferences, values, and so on?
3. What parts of the interview experience were of greatest value to you when you assumed the client role?
4. If you were conducting an assessment interview with a client in the future, what modifications might you make?
5. How could you use what you learned from doing this exercise in future nurse-client interviews?

---

describe drug abuse, and abstract words with several meanings.

Noise interference within the *nurse* can relate to:

- Preoccupation with personal agendas
- Being in a hurry to complete physical care
- Making assumptions about client motivations
- Cultural stereotypes and biases
- Defensiveness or personal insecurity about being able to help the client
- Thinking ahead to the next question
- Emotional overreaction to certain client behaviors or personal characteristics

Environmental noise can involve anything in the external environment, for example: competing sound from TV audio, cell phones, other conversations, coughing or hiccupping of other clients, noises in the hall, poor lighting, intravenous (IV) alarms, interruptions, and irritating smells such as cigarette smoke or heavy perfume. Each can compromise a nurse or client's full attention on a clinical interaction.

Interpersonal Space and Timing Issues

Privacy, space, and timing are other aspects to consider. Clients need privacy, free from interruption, and with adequate space requirements to fully engage in meaningful conversations. Hall (1959) in his seminal work refers to time, and interpersonal space as "the silent language." Therapeutic conversations typically take place within a social distance (3 to 4 feet is optimal). Culture, personal preference, and the topic influence client personal space needs. Highly anxious clients may need more physical space, whereas clients experiencing a sudden physical injury or undergoing a painful procedure may appreciate having the nurse in closer proximity. Sitting at eye level with bedridden clients enhances connectivity.

Timing affects communication effectiveness. Planning communication for periods when the client is able to participate physically and emotionally is time-efficient, plus respectful of client needs. Some people function better in the morning, others later in the day. The client's condition, medication, metabolic fluctuations, and variations in energy levels, influence a client's ability to participate in dialogue. Nonverbal behavior can sometimes cue the nurse about emotional readiness, and available energy.

Professional Self-Reflection

Self-reflection is a prerequisite for effective communication. Mindfulness of personal behaviors and values allows nurses to recognize the sometimes unintentional effects their words or behaviors have on the communication process. Biases concerning cultural differences, sexual preferences, alcoholism, teenage pregnancy, or any other value-laden behavior affects communication. Nurses may feel intimidated by clients who have higher social status, education, or influence, and respond in subtle ways to these differences. Caring for clients who refuse to comply with treatment or who have given up can be a communication challenge. Self-awareness allows nurses to value the person despite personal feelings about a client's behavior or problem, and to maintain the patience, neutrality, and understanding needed for therapeutic communication.

Nurses have an ethical and professional responsibility to resolve personal issues that could potentially affect client-centered communication.

Active Listening

Active listening is a communication concept, which embodies an intentional empathetic form of listening for understanding collaboratively constructed meanings. There is a commitment to full attention on the client, as well as on the topic. This means temporarily suspending your own reactions as you *listen for understanding*. Active listening contributes to fewer incidents of misunderstanding, more accurate information, and stronger health related relationships. Rather than listening to a one-sided narrative as a basis for problem exploration, the process of interactive dialogue represents a joint opportunity to consider new facts—leading to different possibilities, choices, and options. Active listening allows both communicators to offer presence and bear witness to one another in the telling of the client's story (Kagan, 2008). Genuine positive regard and clear, concise listening responses are fundamental basics for empathetic nursing conversations. Language that appreciates a person's culture, spiritual beliefs, and educational level capture the client's attention. Communication that disregards or diminishes client or family input as being less important than that of the health care provider's opinions demonstrates lack of understanding.

SOCIAL VERSUS CLIENT-CENTERED THERAPEUTIC COMMUNICATION

At first glance, it may appear that effective therapeutic client-centered communication does not require specialized study—that it is simply a health-related application of social dialogue. This is not true. Significant communication differences exist between social and therapeutic communicative exchange of ideas and feelings, starting with the purpose, focus, and scope of communication activities. Client-centered communication has a therapeutic intent and differs from "social chitchat" because its purpose is always to promote the client's personal development and improve health outcomes (Peplau, 1960, p. 964).

Unlike social conversations, therapeutic discussions have defined interpersonal boundaries related to time, topics, and clinician self-disclosure. In social conversations it is customary to respond to someone's story with a personal experience. Clinicians need to

limit self-disclosure, use it sparingly, and only if it furthers the goals of a clinical encounter. Whereas spontaneous recommendations and global reassurance are freely given in social conversations, clinicians avoid giving advice in clinical conversations. Instead, they provide as much detailed coaching information as each client needs, keeping in mind that clients are ultimately responsible for self-management of their health issues.

Whereas social communication carries ethical responsibilities for privacy, there are no legal constraints. By contrast, federal privacy regulations, and professional standards govern sharing of therapeutic conversations; and Health Insurance Portability and Accountability Act (HIPAA) regulations *ensure* privacy of client information. They control who has jurisdiction and access to private information and limit information to only those within designated informational boundaries (Bylund et al., 2012).

Clients vary in their ability to effectively communicate their feelings, preferences, and concerns (Epstein and Street, 2007). Effective communicators recognize differences in client communication patterns and that similar ideas can be expressed in a variety of ways. They modify communicative behaviors and message delivery accordingly, taking into account client conversational needs, preferences, and values, and differences in power role relationships.

Developing an Evidence-Based Practice

Svavarsdottir E, Sigurdardottir A. Benefits of a brief therapeutic conversation intervention for families of children and adolescents in active cancer treatment, *Oncol Nurs Forum* 40(5):E346-E357, 2013.

Purpose: This research was designed to test the effectiveness of a two- to three-session brief therapeutic conversation intervention related to perceived family support and expressive family functioning.

Study Design and Methods: The study design was quasi-experimental, with a group pre- and posttest. The sample consisted of 19 parent caregivers of children in active cancer treatment. After completing baseline data questionnaires, participants attended two family therapeutic conversation intervention sessions, spaced 4 and 8 weeks apart. A third session was offered to those who needed it 1 week later.

Results: Family caregivers perceived significantly higher family support, significantly higher expressive family functioning, and significantly higher emotional communication after the intervention.

Application to your clinical practice: This research supports the benefit of using brief therapeutic conversation interventions with family caregivers of children and adolescents with cancer using simple communication strategies.

APPLICATIONS

APPLYING CONCEPTS OF CLIENT-CENTERED COMMUNICATION

Health care, viewed as a shared partnership where the client is an equal stakeholder, and valued partner in ensuring quality health care is relatively new. *Client-centered communication* is a critical component in creating and sustaining a shared partnership through words and actions. Nurses play a key role in providing a safe accepting environment for clients and in collaborating with their health team.

A prepared organized communicator is more effective. Effective communicators draw from a large range of skills, based on knowledge and experience (Adler et al., 2010). Flexibility in your approach depends on mindful forethought about the clinical situation your client presents. Before meeting with your client, review chart information and your knowledge of standard clinical data. Consult if needed with health team members. This preparation allows you to pick up on subtle data that clients may not recognize as being germane to their clinical situation. Responses to client questions are more likely based on solid evidence-based clinical findings, taking into account personalized client data. A knowledgeable clinician inspires confidence and invites collaboration with clients and health team members.

BUILDING RAPPORT

Building rapport through communication is an art, which begins with a genuine desire to know the client as a person, as well as a client. This approach encourages you and the client to conjointly construct the meaning of a health experience as a basis for intervention. Exercise 5-2, Establishing Rapport: "What Makes Me Comfortable," allows you to reflect on communication features relevant to facilitating rapport.

No single communication strategy serves the needs of all clients equally well. Even the most effective communicators perform more skillfully in some situations and less so in others. Some clients work better with providers who are warmly expressive; others need a more reserved objective approach (Egan, 2013). Not all clients can put their concerns easily into words; some clients lack awareness. Some client issues elicit powerful personal emotions in either the client or the nurse, which make talking about them more difficult. Respecting different ways of communicating and relating to clients *as they are*, not as you think they should be, advances rapport. When clients feel valued and accepted, they are better able to organize their thoughts and are more likely to reveal things that otherwise might not come to mind.

EXERCISE 5-2	Establishing Rapport: "What Makes Me Comfortable"

Purpose: To help students identify personal communication features, which make it easier for people to establish rapport in new situations.

Procedure

In groups of three to five students, each student should individually describe a firsthand interpersonal situation in which you felt comfortable with people you were meeting for the first time.
1. Individually, write down the factors that you feel accounted for your comfort in communicating with people in this situation. What made the situation different from other first encounters?
2. Share your findings with the other members in your student group.

Discussion
1. What words, actions, attitudes contributed to your feelings of comfort? Which of the three was most important to your comfort?
2. Were there any common communication features that facilitated initial rapport?
3. How could you use findings from this exercise to facilitate connection with new clients?

A client-centered communication process starts with the first encounter. Entering the client's space with an open, welcoming facial expression, respectful tone, and direct eye contact demonstrates your interest and intent to know the person behind the symptoms. Your posture should be open and attentive. An unhurried, welcoming, and respectful approach eases client anxiety. Greet the client by name, "Good morning, Mr. Jacks, how are you today?" Next, introduce yourself, "I'm Marilyn Hawkins, a registered nurse, and I will be taking care of you today. I'd like to ask you some questions so we can better help you. Is that OK with you?"

Initial assessments (history taking) require immediate intimate sharing of client information that normally would not be shared in initial interactions. Communication to obtain a health history is more structured than everyday health dialogues. O'Gara and Fairhurst (2004) identify a five-stage strategy to maximize history taking. Strategies involve:

1. Asking open-ended questions
2. Listening, and noticing nonverbal behaviors
3. Communicating empathy
4. Establishing and addressing concerns
5. Agreeing with plans

ASKING QUESTIONS

A client-centered interview begins with encouraging clients to tell the story of their illness (Platt and Gaspar, 2001). This format helps nurses integrate personal with medical perspectives. Using short unambiguous listening responses focused on current health issues, and client concerns offer the best means of helping clients tell their story. You will get a better idea of how clients communicate and what clients consider most important about their clinical situation with relevant queries. In addition to using a "here and now" approach, avoid asking more than one question at a time and allow enough time for the client to fully answer. Related follow-up questions to clarify or help clients expand on what has been introduced can be helpful. A simple way to do this is to ask for an example. Questions fall into different categories: open ended, focused, and closed ended.

OPEN-ENDED QUESTIONS

Open-ended questions permit clients to express health problems and needs in their own words. They are especially helpful at the start of a relationship when the nurse's objective is to gather information, and to get to know the client as a person. You are more likely to elicit a client's values, preferences, and ways of thinking about their illness if you allow them latitude in telling their story through open-ended questions. Sharing the personal meanings of an illness rather than identifying a diagnosis or listing discrete symptoms helps the client and nurse link the context of a health disruption with symptoms and provides more complete information.

An open-ended question is similar to an essay question on a test. It is open to interpretation and cannot be answered by "yes," "no," or a one-word response. Open-ended questions ask the client to think and reflect on their situation. They help connect relevant elements of the client's experience without influencing the direction of the response (e.g., relationships, impact of the illness on self or others, environmental barriers, potential resources). Open-ended questions are used to elicit the client's thoughts and perspectives without influencing the direction of an acceptable response. Open-ended questions focus on "what" or "how." Here are some examples:

"Can you tell me what brought you to the clinic (hospital) today?"

" I wonder if you could tell me a little about yourself?"

"What has it been like for you since the accident?"

"Where would you like to begin today?"

"What can I do to help you?"

Start with simple general questions, and move to inquiries about more complex information once initial rapport is established. Open-ended questions can be answered with a variety of responses; they are used to identify and expand on client strengths and preferences, as well as concerns. Ask about the client's spiritual or philosophical beliefs and values. Incorporate questions about the client's support systems including level of support and availability. Environmental, economic, and legal factors are a consideration, when related to the client's health and well-being. At the end of an interaction, you can provide a short summary, followed by asking, "Is there anything else you would like to add?" This final query can provide relevant information that might otherwise be overlooked. Exercise 5-3 provides practice with the use of open-ended questions.

EXERCISE 5-3	Asking Open-Ended Questions

Purpose: To develop skill in the use of open-ended questions to facilitate information sharing.

Procedure

1. Break up into pairs. Role-play a situation in which one student takes the role of the facilitator and the other the sharer. (If you are in the clinical area, you may want to choose a clinical situation.)
2. As a pair, select a topic. The facilitator begins asking open-ended questions.
3. Dialogue for 5 minutes on the topic.
4. In pairs, discuss perceptions of the dialogue and determine which questions were comfortable and open ended. The facilitating student should reflect

on the comfort level experienced with asking each question. The sharing student should reflect on the efficacy of the listening responses in helping to move the conversation toward his or her perspective.

Discussion

As a class, each pair should contribute examples of open-ended questions that facilitated the sharing of information. Compile these examples on the board. Formulate a collaborative summation of what an open-ended question is and how it is used. Discuss how open-ended questions can be used sensitively with uncomfortable topics.

FOCUSED QUESTIONS

Focused questions require a specific short response rather than a yes or no answer. More specific than open-ended questions, focused questions help clients describe specific details about an illness such as when the symptoms began, what other symptoms are present, pain level, or what the client has done to date to resolve the health problem. They are used when more detail is needed to have a complete picture.

Focused questions can help clients prioritize immediate concerns, for example, "Of all the concerns we have talked about today, which do you see as being the most difficult for you?" They assist overtalkative clients bent on providing excessive details to focus on immediate health issue priorities. For example, "I'm impressed with your careful notes. I was wondering if you could also tell me a little more about..." Circular questions are a form of focused questions, which give attention to the interpersonal context in which an illness occurs. These are used to explore the impact of a health disruption on family functioning and relationships with significant others. Clients with limited verbal skills sometimes respond better to focused questions because they require less interpretation. Examples of focused questions include:

"Could you tell me more about the pain in your arm?"

"Can you give me a specific example of what you mean by... ?"

CLOSED-ENDED QUESTIONS

Closed-ended questions require a yes or no or single phrase response. They are used in emergency situations, when the goal is to obtain information quickly, and the context, or client's emotional reactions are of secondary importance in the immediate situation. Examples of closed-ended questions include:

"Does the pain radiate down your left shoulder and arm?"

"When was your last meal?"

EMPATHETIC LISTENING FOR UNDERSTANDING

Therapeutic communication requires a special kind of listening, referred to as active or empathetic listening, the goal of which is shared understanding and a positive health care experience. Active listening involves both intrapersonal and interpersonal processes. Myers (2000) suggests, "Any actual dialogue has an inner, subjectively experienced component" (p. 151). As a person listens, talks, or responds, an intrapersonal process related to personalized reactions to the message, and level of understanding occurs. Box 5-1 identifies what the nurse listens for in client-centered conversations.

THEMES

Listening for themes requires observing and understanding what the client is not saying, as well as what the person actually reveals. Emotional objectivity in making sense of client themes is essential. "Objectivity here refers to seeing what an experience is for another person, not how it fits or relates to other experiences, not what causes it, why it exists, or what purposes it serves. It is an attempt to see attitudes and concepts, beliefs and values of an individual as they are to him at the moment he expresses them—not what they were or will become" (Moustakas, 1974, p. 78).

Identifying the underlying themes presented in a therapeutic conversation can relieve client anxiety and provides direction for individualized nursing interventions. For example, the client may say to the nurse, "I'm worried about my surgery tomorrow."

This is one way of framing the problem. If the same client presents his concern as "I'm not sure I will make it through the surgery tomorrow," the underlying theme of the communication changes from a generalized worry to a more personal theme of survival. Alternatively, a client might say, "I don't know whether my husband should stay tomorrow when I have my surgery. It is going to be a long procedure, and he gets so worried." The theme (focus) expresses her concern about her relationship with her husband. In each communication, the client expresses a distinct theme of concern related to a statement, but the emphasis in each requires a different response. Exercise 5-4 provides practice in intensifying themes.

INFERENCES AND DATA CUES

Inferences and data cues are a different source of information about a client's message. An *inference* is an educated guess about the meaning of an observed behavior or statement. To ensure that the inference represents a correct interpretation of an observation or statement, you need to validate it with the client. For example, if a client is withdrawn and distractible, the nurse might "conclude" that the client is struggling with an internal emotional issue. To validate this inference, you could comment, "You seem withdrawn, as though something is troubling you. Is that true for you right now?" Exercise 5-5 offers an opportunity to develop skills in interpreting nonverbal cues.

| **BOX 5-1** | **What the Nurse Listens For** |

- Content themes
- Communication patterns
- Discrepancies in content, body language, and vocalization
- Feelings, revealed in a person's voice, body movements, and facial expressions
- What is not being said, as well as what is being said
- The client's preferred representational system (auditory, visual, tactile)
- The nurse's own inner responses
- The effect communication produces in others involved with the client

---

| **EXERCISE 5-4** | **Listening for Themes** |

Purpose: To help students identify underlying themes in messages.

Procedure
1. Divide into groups of three to five students.
2. Take turns telling a short story about yourself—about growing up, important people or events in your life, or significant accomplishments (e.g., getting your first job).
3. As each student presents a story, take mental notes of the important themes. Write them down so you will not be tempted to change them as you hear the other students. Notice nonverbal behaviors accompanying the verbal message. Are they consistent with the verbal message?
4. When the story is completed, each of the other people in the group shares his or her observations with the sharer.

5. After all students have shared their observations, validate their accuracy with the sharer.

Discussion
1. Were the underlying themes recorded by the group consistent with the sharer's understanding of his or her communication?
2. As others related their interpretations of significant words or phrases, did you change your mind about the nature of the underlying theme?
3. Were the interpretations of pertinent information relatively similar or significantly different?
4. If they were different, what implications do you think such differences have for nurse-client relationships in nursing practice?
5. What did you learn from doing this exercise?

Data cues are defined as small pieces of data that would not reveal much when taken by themselves. When considered within a total assessment picture, they are important information about the client's frame of mind. For example, hesitancy, anger, or nervousness about a certain topic or switching topics are data cues, needing fuller exploration. The client who declares that he is ready for surgery and seems calm at first glance may be sending a very different message through the tense muscles the nurse accidentally touches. Environmental cues such as a half-eaten lunch or noncompliance with treatment also provide data cues about distress. Verbalizing an incongruent data cue helps clients recognize unexpressed feelings. When considering data cues, consider the context factors that contribute to them.

OBSERVING NONVERBAL BEHAVIORS

Nonverbal cues can act as conversation regulators, for example by increasing or decreasing eye contact (Knapp and Hall, 2014). Active listening includes thoughtful observation of different forms of nonverbal communications, which are presented in Box 5-2.

Behavioral reactions that the nurse feels are out of proportion to the situation provide nonverbal data bits that need further exploration. Examples include
- Complete calm before major surgery
- Excessive anger or little emotionality where some would be expected
- Noncompliance with treatment
- Verbal agreement with no follow through; guarded or defensive verbalizations

EXERCISE 5-5	Observing for Nonverbal Cues

Purpose: To develop skill in interpreting nonverbal cues.

Procedure
1. Watch a dramatic movie (that you haven't seen before) with the sound off for 10 minutes.
2. As you watch the movie, write down the emotions you see expressed, the associated nonverbal behavior, and your interpretations of the meaning and the other person's response.

Discussion
In a large group, share your observations and interpretations of the movie scene. Discussion should focus on the variations in the interpretations of the nonverbal language. Discuss ways in which the nurse can use inferences and data cues to gain a better understanding of the client. Time permitting, the movie segment could be shown again, this time with the sound. Discuss any variations in the interpretations without sound versus with verbal dialogue. Discuss the importance of validation of nonverbal cues.

BOX 5-2	Functional Nonverbal Cues

Emblems: Gestures or body motions having a generalized verbal interpretation (e.g., handshaking, baby waving bye-bye, sign language, nodding your head).

Illustrators: Actions that accompany and exemplify the meaning of the verbal message. Illustrators are used to emphasize certain parts of the communication (e.g., smiling, a stern facial expression, pounding the fist on a table). Illustrators usually are not premeditated.

Affect displays: Facial presentation of emotional affect. Similar to the illustrators, the sender has more control over their display (e.g., a reproving look, an alert expression, a smile or a grin, a sneer). Affect displays have a larger range of meaning and act to support or contradict the meaning of the verbal message. Sometimes the generalized affect is not related to a specific message (e.g., a depressed client may have a retarded emotional affect throughout the relationship that has little to do with the communicated message).

Regulators: Nonverbal activities that adjust the course of the communication as the receiver gives important information to the sender about the impact of the message on the sender. Regulators include nodding, facial expressions, some hand movements, and looking at a watch.

Adaptors: Characteristic, repetitive, nonverbal actions that are client specific and of long duration. They give the nurse information about the client's usual response to difficult emotional issues. Sample behaviors include a psychogenic tic, nervous foot tapping, blushing, and twirling the hair.

Physical characteristics: Nonverbal information about the client that can be gleaned from the outward appearance of the person (e.g., skin tone, descriptions of height and weight and relation to body shape, body odor, physical appearance [dirty hair, unshaven, teeth missing or decayed]).

Adapted from Blondis M, Jackson B: (1982) Nonverbal communication with patients: back to the human touch (pp. 9–5), ed 2, New York, Wiley.

Conversely, if *you* begin to experience strong positive, or negative feelings about a client stimulated by, but unrelated to the reality of a client's situation, this may be an intrapersonal response requiring self-awareness to regain empathetic objectivity.

OBSERVING COMMUNICATION PATTERNS

Observing the client's communication pattern provides a different type of information. Some clients exaggerate information; others characteristically leave out highly relevant details. Some talk a lot, using dramatic language and multiple examples; others say very little and have to be encouraged to provide details. Evaluation of the client's present overall pattern of interaction with others includes strengths and limitations, family communication dynamics, and developmental and educational levels. Culture and customary ways of dealing with emotions influence communication patterns in ways you may not fully understand. Being respectful of the client's communication pattern builds trust and demonstrates positive regard.

Case Example

AJ is a client with chronic mental illness. She frequently interrupts and presents with a loud, ebullient opinion on most things. This is AJ's communication pattern. To engage successfully with her, you would need to accept her way of communicating as a part of who she is, and gently guide her without getting lost in opinion detail.

USING ACTIVE LISTENING RESPONSES

A key component of client-centered care is the clinician's capacity to communicate in ways that convey and support understanding of client needs (McGilton et al., 2012). Empathetic active listening responses are designed to mutually explore, and expand the meaning of a client's message. Full attention is on each client and what matters to them. Listening responses ask about *different aspects* of client health concerns, and take into account the client's values, preferences, and expectations related to treatment goals, priorities, and attitudes about treatment suggestions. Queries should include open-ended questions such as "What is important to you now?" or "What are you hoping will happen with this treatment?"

Empathetic listening responses demonstrate the nurse's commitment to help clients carry health care discussions to a deeper level. Minimal verbal cues, clarification, restatement, paraphrasing, reflection, summarization, silence, and touch are examples of skilled listening responses nurses can use to guide therapeutic interventions Examples are presented in Table 5-1.

MINIMAL CUES

Minimal cues are defined as brief, encouraging phrases and nonverbal prompts, which communicate interest. By not detracting from the client's

TABLE 5-1	Listening Responses
Listening Response	**Example**
Minimal cues and leads	Body actions: smiling, nodding, leaning forward
	Words: "mm," "uh-huh," "oh really," "go on"
Clarification	"Could you describe what happened in sequence?" "I'm not sure I understand what you mean." Can you give me an example?"
Restatement	"Are you saying that… (repeat client's words)?" "You mean… (repeat client's words)?"
Paraphrasing	Client: "I can't take this anymore. The chemo is worse than the cancer. I just want to die."
	Nurse: "It sounds as though you are saying you have had enough."
Reflection	"It sounds as though you feel guilty because you weren't home at the time of the accident." "You sound really frustrated because the treatment is taking longer than you thought it would."
Summarization	"Before moving on, I would like to go over with you what we've accomplished thus far."
Silence	Briefly pausing, but continuing to use attending behaviors after an important idea, thought, or feeling
Touch	Gently rubbing a person's arm during a painful procedure

message and giving permission to tell the story as the client sees it, minimal cues promote client comfort in sharing intimate information. Short phrases such as "Go on" or "And then?" or "Can you say more about… ?" are useful prompts. Minimal physical cues, for example, leaning toward the client, nodding, smiling, are used to accentuate words and to connect with people nonverbally, as well as verbally. Exercise 5-6 involves making inferences about nonverbal behavioral cues.

CLARIFICATION

Clarification is a listening response, used to ask clients for more information or for elaboration on a point. The strategy is useful when parts of a client's communication are ambiguous or not easily understood. Failure to ask for clarification when part of the communication is poorly understood means that the nurse will act on incomplete or inaccurate information. For example, you could say, "May I tell you what I have

understood so far, and see if you think I understand your situation?

Clarification listening responses are expressed as a question or statement followed by restatement or paraphrasing part of the communicated message; for example, "You stated earlier that you were concerned about your blood pressure. Can you tell me more about what concerns you." The tone of voice with a clarification response should be neutral, not accusatory or demanding. Practice this response in Exercise 5-7.

RESTATEMENT

Restatement is an active listening strategy used to broaden a client's perspective, or when the nurse needs to provide a sharper focus on a specific part of the communication. Restating a self-critical or irrational part of the message in a questioning manner focuses the client's attention on the possibility of an inaccurate or global assertion. Restatement is

---

EXERCISE 5-6	Minimal Cues and Leads

Purpose: To practice and evaluate the efficacy of minimal cues and leads.

Procedure
1. Initiate a conversation with someone outside of class and attempt to tell the person about something with which you are familiar for 10 minutes.
2. Make note of all the cues that the person puts forth that either promote, or inhibit conversation.
3. Now try this with another person and write down the different cues and leads you observe as you are speaking and your emotional response to them (e.g., what most encouraged you to continue speaking).

Discussion
As a class, share your experience and observations. Different cues and responses will be compiled on the board. Discuss the impact of different cues and leads on your comfort and willingness to share about yourself. What cues and leads promoted communication? What cues and leads inhibited sharing?

Variation
This exercise can be practiced with a clinical problem simulation in which one student takes the role of the professional helper and the other takes the role of client. Perform the same scenario with and without the use of minimum encouragers. What were the differences when encouragers were not used? Was the communication as lively? How did it feel to you when telling your story when this strategy was used by the helping person?

EXERCISE 5-7	Using Clarification

Purpose: To develop skill in the use of clarification.

Procedure
1. Write a paragraph related to an experience you have had.
2. Place all the student paragraphs together and then pick one (not your own).
3. Develop clarification questions you might ask about the selected paragraph.

Discussion
Share with the class your chosen paragraph and the clarification questions you developed. Discuss how effective the questions are in clarifying information. Other students can suggest additional clarification questions.

particularly effective when the client overgeneralizes or seems stuck in a repetitive line of thinking. To challenge the validity of the client's statement directly could be counterproductive, whereas repeating parts of the message in the form of a query serves a similar purpose without raising defenses; for example, "Let me see if I have this right…" (Coulehan et al., 2001).

PARAPHRASING

Paraphrasing is a listening response, which focuses on the *cognitive* component of a message. It is used to check whether the nurse's translation of the client's words represents an accurate interpretation of the message. The strategy takes the essential information expressed in the client's original message and presents it in a shorter, more specific form, without losing its meaning. The focus is on the core elements of the original statement: "In other words, what I think I hear you saying is," or "let me understand, are you saying that….?" Exercise 5-8 provides an opportunity to see the influence of paraphrasing and reflection on communication.

Case Example

Client: "I don't know about taking this medicine the doctor is putting me on. I've never had to take medication before, and now I have to take it twice a day.
Nurse: It sounds like you don't know what to expect from taking the medication.

REFLECTION

Reflection is a listening response, focused on the *emotional* implications of a message. This listening response helps the client clarify important feelings and experience them with their appropriate intensity in relation to a particular situation or event. There are several ways to use reflection, for example:

- Reflection on vocal tone: "I can sense anger and frustration in your voice as you describe your accident."
- Linking feelings with content: "It sounds like you feel _____ because _____."
- Linking feelings with previous experiences, "It seems as if this experience reminds you of feelings you had with other health care providers where you didn't feel understood."
- Reflection on possible outcomes: "Can you tell me a little about what you were hoping for?"

Reflective responses give clients permission to have feelings and help them identify underlying feelings that may be getting in the way of productive solutions. Sometimes students feel they are putting words into the client's mouth when they "choose" an emotion from their perception of the client's message. This would be true if you were choosing an emotion out of thin air, but not when you empathetically relate it to the client's situation. Suggesting an underlying feeling from the client's narrative, without interpreting its meaning broadens perspective. Exercise 5-9 provides practice in using summarization as listening response.

EXERCISE 5-8	Role Play Practice with Paraphrasing and Reflection

Purpose: To practice use of paraphrasing and reflection as listening responses.

Procedure
1. The class forms into groups of three students each. One student takes the role of client, one the role of nurse, and one the role of observer.
2. The client shares with the nurse a recent health problem he or she encountered, and describes the details of the situation and the emotions experienced. The nurse responds, using paraphrasing and reflection in a dialogue that lasts at least 5 minutes. The observer records the statements made by the helper. At the end of the dialogue, the client writes his or her perception of how the helper's statements affected the conversation, including what comments were most helpful. The helper writes a

short summary of the listening responses he or she used, with comments on how successful they were.

Discussion
1. Share your summary and discuss the differences in using the techniques from the helper, client, and observer perspectives.
2. Discuss how these differences related to influencing the flow of dialogue, helping the client feel heard, and the impact on the helper's understanding of the client from both the client and the helper positions.
3. Identify places in the dialogue where one form of questioning might be preferable to another.
4. How could you use this exercise to understand your client's concerns?
5. Were you surprised by any of the summaries?

EXERCISE 5-9	Practicing Summarization

Purpose: To provide practice in summarizing interactions.

Procedure
1. Choose a partner for a pair's discussion.
2. For 5 minutes, discuss a medical ethics topic such as euthanasia, heroic life support for the terminally ill, or "Baby Doe" decisions to allow malformed babies to die if the parents desire.
3. After 5 minutes, both partners must stop talking until Participant A has summarized what Participant B has just said to Participant B's satisfaction, and vice versa.

Discussion
After both partners have completed their summarizations, discuss the process of summarization, answering the following questions:
1. Did knowing you had to summarize the other person's point of view encourage you to listen more closely?
2. Did the act of summarizing help clarify any discussion points? Were any points of agreement found? What points of disagreement were found?
3. Did the exercise help you to understand the other person's point of view?
4. How did you determine which points to focus on in your summarization?

EXERCISE 5-10	Active Listening

Purpose: To develop skill in active listening and an awareness of the elements involved.

Procedure
1. Class divides into pairs. Each pair will take a turn reflecting on and describing an important experience they have had in their lives. The person who shares should describe the details, emotions, and outcomes of his or her experience. During the interaction, the listening partner should use listening responses such as clarification, paraphrasing, reflection, and focusing, as well as attending cues, eye contact, and alert body posture to carry the conversation forward.

2. After the sharing partner finishes his or her story, the listening partner indicates understanding by (a) stating in his or her own words what the sharing partner said and (b) summarizing perceptions of the sharing partner's feelings associated with the story and asking for validation. If the sharing partner agrees, then the listening partner can be sure he or she correctly utilized active listening skills.

Discussion
In the large group, have pairs of students share their discoveries about active listening. As a class, discuss aspects of nursing behavior that will foster active listening in client interactions.

SUMMARIZATION

Summarization is an active listening skill used to pull several ideas and feelings together, either from one interaction, or a series of interactions, into a few succinct sentences. It provides focus in a conversation and can serve as a bridge to a different topic or idea for further reflection. Summarization statements can be followed by a comment seeking validation, such as "Tell me if my understanding of this agrees with yours." Exercise 5-10 can provide insight into the use of summarization as a listening response.

SILENCE

Silence, when used purposefully, is a powerful listening response. Intentional pauses allow clients to think.

When a client falls silent, it can mean many things: Something has touched the client, the client is angry or does not know how to respond, or the client is thinking. By pausing briefly after presenting a key idea and before proceeding to the next topic, you can encourage a client to notice its vital elements. A verbal comment to validate meaning is helpful. A short pause also lets the nurse step back momentarily and process what he or she has heard before responding. Silence can be used to emphasize important points that you want the client to reflect on.

Not all listening responses are helpful. Nurses need to recognize when their responses are interfering with objectivity or inviting premature closure. Table 5-2 provides definitions of negative listening responses that block communication.

TABLE 5-2	Negative Listening Responses	
Category of Response	**Explanation of Category**	**Examples**
False reassurance	Using pseudocomforting phrases in an attempt to offer reassurance	"It will be okay." "Everything will work out."
Giving advice	Making a decision for a client; offering personal opinions; telling a client what to do (using phrases such as "ought to," "should")	"If I were you, I would…" "I feel you should…"
False inferences	Making an unsubstantiated assumption about what a client means; interpreting the client's behavior without asking for validation; jumping to conclusions	"What I think you really mean is …." "Subconsciously, you may be blaming your husband for the accident."
Over generalizing	Using absolute terms, which eliminate other possibilities, such as "all, no one, every one, always, never"	Virtually every stereotype is an example of an overgeneralization
Moralizing	Expressing your own values about what is right and wrong, especially on a topic that concerns the client	"Abortion is wrong." "It is wrong to refuse to have the operation even at your age."
Value judgments	Conveying your approval or disapproval about the client's behavior or about what the client has said using words such as "good," "bad," or "nice." Using high arousal words. Disapproving or irritated tone of voice.	"I'm glad you decided to…" "That really wasn't a nice way to behave." "She's a good patient."
Social responses	Polite, superficial comments that do not focus on what the client is feeling or trying to say; use of clichés	"Hospital rules, you know?" "Just do what the doctor says." "It's a beautiful day."

VERBAL RESPONSES

Active listening and verbal responses are inseparable from each other. Each strategy informs and reinforces the other. With shorter time frames for client contact, verbal responses are critical components of therapeutic dialogue. Most clients are not looking for brilliant answers from the nurse. Rather they desire and need relevant feedback and support that suggests a compassionate understanding of their particular dilemma. No matter what level of communication exists in the relationship, the same needs—"hear me," "touch me," "respond to me," "feel my pain and experience my joys with me"—are fundamental themes. When clients seem out of sorts or angry, they usually are expressing something about themselves and their own pain. This knowledge can help you look for clues to the underlying dynamic, including giving the client more space and understanding. (Rosenberg and Gallo-Silver. 2011). Nurses are significant connection points for each client. For clients, knowing they are not alone

and that a knowledgeable clinician wants to take time to understand and assist them in a meaningful way, lightens the burden of illness or injury.

Verbal responses are used to teach, encourage, support, and provide and gather information related to goal achievement. Professional verbal communication leads to better quality health care decisions (Bylund et al., 2012). Each client's needs are different but regardless of the details, being authentically present is a critical dimension of creating rapport and understanding. Tailored information and support combined with empathetic listening makes a significant difference in client engagement and satisfaction. Appropriate instructive communication is critical for effective decisions and informed consent. Exercise 5-2 is designed to increase the student's understanding of communication strategies using a client-centered focus.

Gaining specific knowledge about their medical and psychological conditions *empowers* clients to better self-manage chronic disorders and build healthy lifestyles. Nurses use observation, validation, and patterns of knowing to gauge the effectiveness of their verbal interventions. On the basis of a client's reaction, the nurse may decide to use simpler language or to try a different strategy in collaborative discussion.

When providing information, avoid overloading the client with too many ideas or details at the same time. This strategy allows clients time to better process and respond to different ideas. People can absorb only so much information at one time, particularly if they are tired, fearful, or discouraged. Repeating key ideas and reinforcing information with concrete examples facilitates understanding and provides an additional opportunity for the client to ask questions. Pay attention to response cues from the client, which support understanding, or reflect a need for further attention in the form of additional explanation or change in direction. If you find you are doing most of the talking, you need to back up and use listening responses to elicit the client's perspective.

Verbal response strategies used in client-centered communication include matching responses (mirroring), focusing, presenting reality, metaphors, humor, reframing, feedback, and validation. These strategies are designed to strengthen the coping abilities of the client, alone or in relationship with others.

MATCHING RESPONSES

Lang (2012) proposes "matching the patient's initial demeanor, disposition, and rhythm is the fastest, simplest, and most powerful way to establish rapport" (p. 117). Regardless of content, the nurse's verbal responses should match the client's message related to level of depth, meaning, and language. Verbal responses should neither expand nor diminish the meaning of the client's remarks. If the client makes a serious statement, the nurse should not respond with a flip remark; a superficial statement does not warrant an intense response. Irate, demanding clients need a firm, assertively calm tone to help them deescalate. Responses that encourage a client to explore feelings about limitations or strengths, at a slightly deeper but related level of conversation, tend to meet with more success. Children, and adults need different levels of listening response language (Weldon et al. 2014). Remember that the child is observing and listening carefully even if it doesn't appear that way. Always provide interpersonal space for further discussion and confirm what the client understands. Note the differences in the nature of the following responses to a client in the following case example.

Case Example

> Client: I feel so discouraged. No matter how hard I try, I still can't walk without pain on those parallel bars.
>
> Nurse: You want to give up because you don't think you will be able to walk again?
>
> At this point, it is unclear that the client wants to give up, so the nurse's comment expands on the client's meaning without having sufficient data to support it. It is possible that this is what the client means; it is not the only possibility. The next response focuses only on the negative aspects of the client's communication and ignores the client's comment about his or her efforts.
>
> Nurse: So you think you won't be able to walk independently again?
>
> Finally, the nurse addresses both parts of the client's message and makes the appropriate connection, and invites the client to validate the nurse's perception.
>
> Nurse: It sounds to me as if you don't feel your efforts are helping you regain control over your walking.

USING SIMPLE CONCRETE LANGUAGE

Before framing any message, observe the client to determine receptivity, and the ability to accurately interpret the meaning of your message. Notice the client's level of anxiety and potential culture or language issues. Use simple, clear-cut concrete words, keeping the client's culture as well as developmental and educational level in mind. Because we are so familiar with our native language, most of us tend to talk faster than someone with English as a second language can respond to with ease. Clients with low literacy also respond better to short uncomplicated explanations. Speaking with a general spirit of inquiry and concern for the client is more likely to get the client's attention. Address core issues in a concise manner, taking into account the guidelines for effective verbal message delivery, listed in Box 5-3.

Avoid using medical jargon, and complex abstract terms that clients may have trouble understanding. Unless clients can associate new ideas with familiar words and ideas having personalized meaning, the nurse might as well be talking in a different language. Clients may not tell their nurse that they do not understand for fear of offending the nurse or revealing personal deficits. Giving information that fails to

BOX 5-3	Guidelines to Effective Verbal Communication

- Define unfamiliar terms and concepts.
- Match content and delivery with each client's developmental and educational level, experiential frame of reference, and learning readiness.
- Keep messages clear, concrete, honest, and simple to understand.
- Put ideas in a logical sequence of related material.
- Relate new ideas to familiar ones when presenting new information.
- Repeat main ideas.
- Reinforce key points with vocal emphasis and pauses.
- Keep language as simple as possible; use vocabulary familiar to the client.
- Focus only on essential elements; present one idea at a time.
- Use as many sensory communication channels as possible for key ideas.
- Make sure that nonverbal behaviors support verbal messages.
- Seek feedback to validate accurate reception of information.

take into account a client's previous experiences, or assumes that clients have knowledge they do not possess, tends to fall on deaf ears. Frequent validation with the client related to content helps reduce this problem.

ESTABLISHING FOCUS

In the past, nurses had more time with clients. Today nurses must make every second count. Nurses and clients need to select the most pressing health care needs for attention. Focus on what is essential to know, rather than what might be nice to know. This requires planning and sensitivity to client need and preferences. Klagsbrun (2001) describes focusing as a useful strategy to help clients identify their most important concern, and connect emotional feelings with factual concerns.

Case Example

"Mr. Solan, you have given me a lot to think about here, but I would like to hear more about how you are handling the surgery tomorrow. You mentioned that you were feeling afraid. Most people are concerned. I wonder if it would be helpful to talk more about this."

PRESENTING REALITY

Presenting reality to a client who is misinterpreting it can be helpful. To ensure that the client does not perceive that the nurse is criticizing the client's perception of reality you can use a simple statement such as the following. "I know that you feel very strongly about _____, but I don't see it that way." This is an effective way for the nurse to express a different interpretation of the situation. Another strategy is to put into words the underlying feeling implied but not directly stated. For example, you might say, "I can see that you are really upset. It must feel as if no one is paying attention to your situation and that must be frustrating for you"

GIVING FEEDBACK

Feedback is a response message related to specific client behaviors and words. Nurses give, and ask, for client feedback to ensure mutual understanding. Feedback can focus on the content, the relationship between people and events, the feelings generated by the message, or parts of the communication that are not clear. Feedback should be specific and focused on observed behavior. Analyzing a client's motivations make clients defensive.

Feedback should be a two-way interactive process. Feedback responses reassure the client that the nurse is fully attentive to what the client is communicating. When it offers a neutral mirror, clients are able to view a problem or behavior from a different perspective. Feedback is most relevant when it only addresses the topics under discussion and does not go beyond the data presented by the client. Feedback provided to nurses about their health teaching, helps them to individualize teaching content and methodology to better facilitate the learning process.

Effective feedback is specific rather than general. Telling a client he or she is shy or easily intimidated is less helpful than saying, "I noticed when the anesthesiologist was in here that you didn't ask her any of the questions you had about your anesthesia tomorrow. Would it be okay with you to look at what you would like to know, and how you can get the information you need?" With this response, the nurse provides precise information about an observed behavior and offers a solution. The client is more likely to respond with validation or correction, and the nurse can provide specific guidance.

Feedback should be to the point, consistent with the situation, and delivered with empathy. It takes different forms, for example, as observations of nonverbal behaviors: "You seem (angry, upset, confused, pleased, sad, etc.)." It can be a direct question: "How do you feel about what I just said?" or "I'm curious what your thoughts are about what I just told you." If the client does not have any response, you can suggest that the client can respond later, "Many people do find they have reactions or questions about [the issue] after they have had a chance to think about it. I would be glad to discuss this further if this occurs with you."

Not all feedback is equally relevant, nor is it uniformly accepted. Benchmarks for deciding whether feedback is appropriate relates to: "Does the feedback advance the goals of the relationship?" and "Does the feedback consider the individualized needs of the client?" If the answer to either question is "no," then the feedback may be accurate, but inappropriate.

Timing of feedback is important. Feedback given as soon as possible after observing a behavior is more effective then when presented after a time lapse. Other factors (e.g., a client's readiness to hear feedback, privacy, and the availability of support from others) contribute to effectiveness. Providing feedback about behaviors over which the client has little control increases the client's feelings of low self-esteem and leads to frustration. Instead, seek the reasons behind the behavior and build your response in positive ways that acknowledge feelings and perceptions as well as "facts."

Case Example

Client: I can't talk to anyone around here. All you people seem to care about is the money, not the patient.

Nurse: It sounds like you are feeling frustrated and all alone right now.

Effective feedback is clear, honest, and reflective. Feedback supported with realistic examples is believable, whereas feedback without documentation to support it can lack credibility. Nonverbal feedback registers the other's reaction to the sender's message through facial expressions such as surprise, boredom, or hostility. When you receive nonverbal messages suggesting uncertainty, concern, or inattention, use a listening response to fully inquire about what the client is having trouble understanding. Feedback can have a surprise twist leading to an unexpected conclusion, as shown in the following case example.

Case Example

An obese mother in the hospital was feeding her newborn infant 4 ounces of formula every 4 hours. She was concerned that her child vomited a considerable amount of the undigested formula after each feeding. Initially, the nursing student gave the mother instructions about feeding the infant no more than 2 ounces at each feeding in the first few days of life, but the mother's behavior persisted, and so did that of her infant. During a client-centered discussion with the client, the student discovered that her client's mother had fed her 4 ounces right from birth with no problem, so she considered this the norm. The nurse did not challenge the mother's perception, but gave her support and information in seeing the uniqueness of her child and understanding what the infant was telling her through his behavior. The client began to feel comfortable and confident in feeding her infant a smaller amount of formula consistent with his needs.

Validation

Validation is a special form of feedback, used to ensure that both participants have the same basic understanding of messages. Simply asking clients whether they understand what was said is not an adequate method of validating message content. Validation can provide new information that helps the nurse frame comments that match the client's need.

Case Example

It was Jovan's third birthday. There was a party of adults (his mother and father; his grandparents; his great-uncle and great-aunt; and me, his aunt) because Jovan was the only child in the family. While we were sitting and chatting, Jovan was running around and playing. At a moment of complete silence, Jovan's great-uncle asked him solemnly: "Jovan, who do you love the best?" Jovan replied, "Nobody!" Then Jovan ran to me and whispered in my ear: "You are Nobody!" (Majanovic-Shane, 1996, p. 18-19).

OTHER FORMS OF COMMUNICATION

TOUCH

Touch, the first of our senses to develop, and the last to leave, provides a nurturing form of communication and validation. How you touch a client in providing everyday nursing care communicates caring. The positive effects of touch are well documented.

Touch stimulates comfort, security, and decreases pain (Sundin and Jansson, 2003; Herrington and Chiodo, 2014). For example, gentle massage of a painful area helps clients relax. Holding the hand of a client with dementia can reduce agitation. Gently rubbing a client's forehead or stroking the head is comforting to most very ill clients. Touch comforts and stimulates newborns. Intentional comforting touch benefits the nurse, as well as the client (Connor and Howett, 2009).

Touch is a powerful listening response as a way of expressing empathy to clients in vulnerable health situations (Rasmark et al, 2014). A hand placed on a frightened mother's shoulder or a reassuring squeeze of the hand can speak far more eloquently than words in times of deep emotion. Clients in pain, those who feel unacceptable to others because of altered appearance, lonely and dying clients, and those experiencing sensory deprivation or feeling confused respond positively to the nurse who is unafraid to enter their world and touch them. Children and the elderly are especially comforted by touch (Bush, 2001).

Touch has multiple cultural meanings and people vary in their interpretation of it as a form of communication. It is a valued form of communication in some cultures. In others, touch is reserved for religious purposes, or is seldom used as a form of communication, for example in Asian cultures (Samovar, Porter, & McDaniel, 2013). If the client is paranoid, out of touch with reality, verbally inappropriate, or mistrustful, touch is contraindicated as a listening response because the client may misinterpret it as an invasion of personal space.

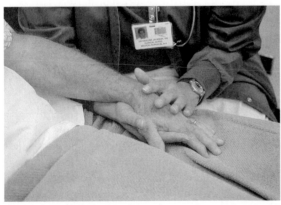

Touch can be an important form of communication.

Case Example

Mr. Brown (to nurse taking his blood pressure): I can't stand that medicine. It doesn't sit well. (He grimaces and holds his stomach.)

Nurse: Are you saying that your medication for lowering your blood pressure upsets your stomach?

Mr. Brown: No, I just don't like the taste of it.

Validation can be observational rather than expressed through words. For example, when the client independently exercises, or takes medication as directed.

Case Example

"I found out that if I held Sam's hand he would lie perfectly still and even drift off to sleep. When I sat with him, holding his hand, his blood pressure and heart rate would go down to normal and his intracranial pressure would stay below 5. When I tried to calm him with words, there was no response—he [had] a blood pressure of 160/90!" (Chesla, 1996, p. 202).

METAPHORS AND ANALOGIES

A key goal of communication is to promote client understanding and decision making. Complex medical conditions or relationships between health disruptions and treatment, can compromise comprehension. Metaphors and analogies use figurative language to help clients and families process difficult new information by connecting abstract concepts with familiar images from ordinary life experience. For example, Arroliga and colleagues (2002) describe chronic lung disease as "emphysema is like having lungs similar to 'swiss cheese,'" and the airways in asthma are like "different sized drainpipes that can get clogged up and need to be unclogged" (p. 377). In several research studies, clinician use of analogies resulted in higher client ratings of communication and better understanding (Casarett et al., 2010).

In health care situations, metaphors need to be used carefully. Periyakoil (2008) suggests that using war or sports metaphors with clients experiencing advanced metastatic cancer sometimes has an unintended impact when the client can no longer "fight the valiant battle" or "win" the game by playing according to prescribed moves.

HUMOR

Humor is a powerful therapeutic communication technique when used for a specific therapeutic purpose. Appropriate humor grabs the attention of the client, and humanizes the nurse-client relationship. Clients appreciate humor; they wish nurses would use it, and respond to humor more often in health care settings (McCreaddie and Payne, 2014). Humor allows taboo topics to be raised without creating hostility or discomfort.

Humor and laughter have healing purposes. Laughter generates energy and activates β-endorphins, a neurotransmitter that creates natural highs and reduces stress hormones. The surprise element in humor can cut through an overly intense situation and put it into perspective. Humorous remarks are best delivered as simple statements that contain positive kernels of truth and are conveyed with calmness. Humor recognizes the incongruities in a situation, or an absurdity present in human nature or conduct as illustrated below (McCreaddie and Wiggins, 2008.

Case Example

Karen, the mother of 4-year-old Megan, had just returned from a long shopping trip in which she had purchased several packages of paper towels. While she was in another room, Megan took everything out of four kitchen drawers, put them on the floor, and put the paper towels in the drawers. Her mother expressed her anger to Megan in no uncertain terms. As she was leaving the kitchen, she heard Megan say to herself, "Well, I guess she didn't like that idea." Karen's anger was effectively interrupted by her daughter's innocent humorous remark.

Humor is most effective when rapport is well established and a level of trust exists between the nurse and client. Not all clients will respond to the same types of humor. When using humor as a strategy, you need to take into consideration the capacity of each client's age, culture, gender and worldview to appreciate its use.

When humor is used, it should focus on the idea, event, or situation, or something other than the client's personal characteristics. Humor that ridicules is not funny. Some clients respond well to humor; others are insulted or perplexed by it. Humor is less effective when the client is tired or emotionally vulnerable. Instead, that client may need structure and calming support.

Humor should fit the situation, not dominate it. The following factors contribute to its successful use:

- Knowledge of the client's response pattern
- An overly intense situation

- Timing
- Situation that requires an imaginative or paradoxical solution
- Gearing the humor to the client's developmental level
- Focus on incongruities in a situation or circumstance, rather than client characteristics

REFRAMING

Bandler and Grindler (1997) define **reframing** as "changing the frame in which a person perceives events in order to change the meaning" (p. 1). Reframing offers a different positive interpretation designed to broaden the client's perspective; they should accentuate client strengths. The new frame must fit the current situation *and* be understandable to the client; otherwise, it will not work. Reframing a situation is helpful when blame is a component of a family's response to the client's illness, for example, with alcoholism. Helping a family view the alcoholism as a disease rather than as a reaction to family members permits necessary detachment.

USING TECHNOLOGY IN COMMUNICATION

Uses of technology in health care communication are the focus in Chapters 25 and 26. For this chapter, a reminder suffices that electronic communication begins when the nurse comes online or begins speaking to the client on the phone (Sharpe, 2001). From that point forward, the nurse needs to follow defined standards of nursing care, using communication principles identified in this chapter. At the end of each telehealth encounter, nurses need to provide their clients with clear directions and contact information should additional assistance be required. Confidentiality, and protection of identifiable client information are as essential in telehealth communications as they are in face-to-face communications.

Telemonitoring is emerging as a viable means to support the home care management of chronic diseases. It works best when clients are able to develop an ongoing relationship with their professional caregivers (Fairbrother and Colleagues, 2013). Although technology can never replace face-to-face time with clients, the emergence of voice mail, e-mail, and telehealth virtual home visits help connect clients with care providers and provide critical information. For example, routine laboratory results, appointment scheduling, and links to information on the Web can be transmitted through technology.

Technology allows clients to use the Internet as a communication means to share common experiences with others who have a similar disease condition, to consult with experts about symptoms and treatment, to learn up-to-date information about their condition, and accessible health care services. Nurses can be helpful to their clients in making productive use of the web, and helping them assess the relevance of web site health information.

SUMMARY

This chapter discusses client-centered communication strategies nurses can use with clients across clinical settings. Communication is identified as a primary means of helping clients achieve mutually negotiated health goals. Empathetic active listening response is an intentional response evidenced as paraphrasing, reflection, clarification, silence, summarization, and touch. These strategies provide a communication bridge to understanding and negotiating meaning between clinicians and clients. Nonverbal behaviors and paralanguage are sources of information about the meaning of communication; validation is required to ensure accuracy. Open-ended questions allow clients to express ideas and feelings as they are experiencing them. Focused, and closed-ended questions are appropriate in emergency clinical situations, when precise information is needed quickly. Nurses ideally use verbal communication strategies consistent with a client's communication patterns in terms of level, meaning, and language. Other strategies include use of metaphors, reframing, humor, confirming responses, feedback, and validation. Feedback provides a client with needed information.

ETHICAL DILEMMA | What Would You Do?

You have been working with a young client on a mental health unit. Over the course of the rotation, you have established a trusting relationship, and she has made a lot of progress. She tells you in confidence that she has a small kitchen knife hidden in her room. She shows it to you, and tells you how special it is because her mother gave it to her. She begs you to keep her confidence, and assures you that she would never use it. Her symptoms would not suggest a suicide risk. You want to maintain her trust and she is due to be discharged. What should you do?

REFLECTIVE DISCUSSION QUESTIONS

- In what ways do individual client-centered encounters and effective team collaboration intersect to meet client needs?
- What are some ways you can demonstrate that you value a client's individual experience in the health care setting?

REFERENCES

Adler R, Rosenfeld L, Proctor R: *Interplay: The Process of Interpersonal Communication*, New York, 2010, Oxford University Press.

Arroliga A, Newman S, Longworth DL, et al.: Metaphorical medicine: using metaphors to enhance communication with patients who have pulmonary disease, *Ann Intern Med* 137(5 Part 1):376–379, 2002.

Bandler R, Cahill J, Grindler J, 1997 *Reframing.* Science and Behavior Books: Palo Alto, CA

Burgoon JK, Guerrero LK, Floyd K: *Nonverbal Communication*, Boston, MA, 2009, Allyn and Bacon.

Bush E: The use of human touch to improve the well-being of older adults: a holistic nursing intervention, *J Holist Nurs* 19(3):256–270, 2001.

Bylund CL, Peterson EB, Cameron KA: A practitioner's guide to interpersonal communication theory: An overview and exploration of selected theories, *Patient Educ Couns* 87(3):261–267, 2012.

Casarett D, Pickard A, Fishman J, et al.: Can metaphors and analogies improve communication with seriously ill patients? *J Palliat Med* 13(3):255–260, 2010.

Chesla C: Reconciling technologic and family care in critical-care nursing, *Image J Nurs Sch* 28(3):199–203, 1996.

Connor A, Howett M: A conceptual model of intentional comfort touch, *J Holist Nurs* 27(2):127–135, 2009.

Coulehan J, Platt FW, Egener B, et al.: Let me see if I have this right…: words that help build empathy, *Ann Intern Med* 135:221–227, 2001.

Cronenwett L, Sherwood G, Barnsteiner J, Disch J, Johnson J, Mitchell P, Sullivan D, Warren J: Quality and safety education for nurses, *Nurs Outlook* 55(3):122–131, 2007.

Egan G: *The Skilled Helper: A Problem Management and Opportunity Development Approach to Helping*, 10th ed. Belmont CA, 2013, Brooks Cole, Cenage Learning.

Epstein R, StreetJr RL, (2007) *Patient-centered communication in cancer care: promoting healing and reducing suffering* National Cancer Institute: Bethesda, MD (NIH Publication No. 07–6225)

Fairbrother P, Ure J, Hanley J, Clughan L, Denvir M, McKinstry: Telemonitoring for chronic heart failure: the views of patients and health care professionals—a qualitative study, *J Clin Nurs* 23:132–144, 2013.

Hall E: *The silent language*, New York, 1959, Doubleday.

Hargie O: *Skilled Interpersonal Communication: Research, Theory and Practice*, London and New York, 2011, Routledge.

Herrington C, Chiodo L: Human touch effectively and safely reduces pain in the newborn intensive care unit, *Pain Manag Nurs* 15(1):107–115, 2014.

Kagan P: Feeling listened to: a lived experience of human becoming, *Nurs Sci Q* 21(1):59–67, 2008.

Klagsbrun J: Listening and focusing: holistic health care tools for nurses, *Nurs Clin North Am* 36(1):115–130, 2001.

Knapp M, Hall J, Horgan T: *Nonverbal Communication in Human Inter-action*, Boston MA, 2014, Wadsworth Cengage Learning.

Lang E: A better patient experience through better communication, *J Radiol Nurs.* 31:114–119, 2012.

Majanovic-Shane A., (1996) *Metaphor: a propositional comment and an invitation to intimacy* Paper presented at the Second Conference for Sociocultural Research, Geneva, Switzerland September 1996 Paper Available online: www.mendeley.com/profiles/ana-marjanovic-Shane/

McCreaddie M, Payne S: Humor in health-care interactions: a risk worth taking, *Health Expect* 17(3):332–344, 2014.

McCreaddie M, Wiggins S: The purpose and function of humour in health, health care and nursing: A narrative review, *J Adv Nurs* 61(6):584–595, 2008.

McGilton K, Sorin-Peters R, Sidani S, et al.: Patient-centered com-munication intervention study to evaluate nurse-patient interactions in complex continuing care, *BMC Geriatr* 12:61, 2012.

Moustakas C, (1974) *Finding yourself: finding others* Prentice Hall: Englewood Cliffs, NJ

Myers S: Empathetic listening: reports on the experience of being heard, *J Humanist Psychol* 40(2):148–174, 2000.

Nadzam D: Nurses' role in communication and patient safety, *J Nurs Care Qual* 24(3):184–188, 2009.

O'Gara P, Fairhurst W: Therapeutic communication part 2: strategies that can enhance the quality of the emergency care consultation, *Accid Emerg Nurs* 12(3):201–207, 2004.

Peplau H: Talking with patients, *Am J Nurs* 60(7):964–966, 1960.

Periyakoil V: Using metaphors in medicine, *J Palliat Med* 11(6): 842–844, 2008.

Platt FW, Gaspar DL: Tell me about yourself"; the patient-centered interview, *Ann Intern Med* 134(11):579–585, 2001.

Rasmark G, Richt B, Rudebeck C: Touch and relate: body experience among staff in habilitation services, *Int J Qual Stud Health Well-Being* 9:21901, 2014.

Rosenberg S, Gallo-Silver L: Therapeutic communication skills and student nurses in the clinical setting, *Teach Learn Nurs* (6):2–8, 2011.

Ruesch J, (1961) *Therapeutic communication* Norton: New York.

Samovar L, Porter R, McDaniel E, Roy C: *Communication between Cultures, 8th* ed., Boston MA, 2013, Wadsworth Cengage Learning.

Schmid PF: Authenticity: the person as his or her own author. Dialogi-cal and ethical perspectives on therapy as an encounter relationship. And beyond. In *Rogers' therapeutic conditions: Evolution, theory and practice*, 1. Ross-on-Wye, UK, 2001, PCCS Books, pp 213–228.

Sharpe C, (2001) *Telenursing: nursing practice in cyberspace* Auburn House: Westport, CT

Snellman I, Gustafsson C, Gustafsson LK: Patients' and caregivers' attributes in a meaningful care encounter: Similarities and notable differences, *ISRN Nurs. Article ID* 320145:1–9, 2012.

Street R, Makoul G, Arora N, Epstein R: How does communication heal? Pathways linking clinician-patient communication to health outcomes, *Patient Educ Couns* 74(3):295–301, 2009.

Stewart J: *Bridges not walls: A Book about Interpersonal Communication*, 11th ed., Boston MA, 2011, McGraw Hill.

Sundin K, Jansson L: "Understanding and being understood" as a creative caring phenomenon: in care of patients with stroke and aphasia, *J Clin Nurs* 12:57–116, 2003.

The Joint Commission: *Advancing Effective Communication, Cultural Competence, and Patient-and Family-Centered Care: A Roadmap for Hospitals*, Oakbrook Terrace, IL, 2010, The Joint Commission.

Wachtel P: *Therapeutic Communication*, New York, NY, 2011, The Guilford Press.

Weldon J, Langan K, Miedema A, Myers J, Oakie A: Overcoming language barriers for pediatric surgical patients and their family members, *AORN Journal* 99(5):616–629, 2014.

Weiten W, Lloyd M, S.Dun S, et al.: *Psychology applied to modern life: adjustment in the 21st century*, Belmont CA, 2009, Wadsworth Cengage Learning.

West R, Turner L: *Understanding Interpersonal Communication: Making Choices in Changing Times*, Enhanced second edition, Boston MA, 2011, Wadsworth.

West R, Turner L: *Introducing Communication Theory: Analysis and Application*, 4th ed., , New York, 2009, McGraw Hill.

Woods M: "How Communication complicates the patient safety move-ment," *Patient Safety & Quality Healthcare*, May/June. http://www.psqh.com/mayjusn06/dun.html, 2006.

CHAPTER 6

Variation in Communication Styles

Kathleen Underman Boggs

OBJECTIVES

At the end of the chapter, the reader will be able to:

1. Describe the component systems of communication, describing congruence between verbal and nonverbal messages.
2. Discuss influence of gender and culture on professional communication.
3. Identify five communication style factors that influence the nurse-client relationship.
4. Discuss how metacommunication messages may affect client responses.
5. Cite examples of body cues that convey nonverbal messages.
6. Discuss application of research studies for evidence-based clinical practice.

This chapter explores styles of communication that serve as a basis for building a relationship to provide patient-centered care. Communication is an underlying component of all six of the prelicensure competencies identified in the Quality and Safety Education for Nurses project, as introduced in Chapter 2 (www.QSEN.com). Effective communication has been shown to produce better health outcomes, greater client satisfaction, and increased client understanding. Style is defined as the manner in which one communicates. It is important to learn as much as possible about your own communication style (Rogers, 2012). Some of us tend to be more assertive, more forceful, and even dominant in our relationships, imposing our desires on others, while others seek more of an equal partnership, bargaining or negotiating in a give and take fashion. At the other end of the personal style spectrum, some individuals tend to withdraw or even put all of the other person's desires ahead of their own needs. In developing a style suitable to professional nurse-client or nurse-team-client relationships, we modify our personal style to fit our professional role. As learners, students are monitored in the clinical setting as we demonstrate expected communication styles which convey warmth, trustworthiness, and respectful assertiveness as we use our newly acquired therapeutic communication skills (Rosenberg and Gallo-Silver, 2011).

Verbal style includes pitch, tone, and frequency. Nonverbal style includes facial expression, gestures, body posture and movement, eye contact, distance from the other person, and so on. These nonverbal behaviors are clues clients provide to us to help us understand their words. Sharpening our observational skills helps us gather data needed for nursing assessments and interventions. Both of us, client and nurse, enter this new relationship with our own specific style of communication.

Some individuals depend on a mostly verbal style to convey their meaning, whereas others rely on nonverbal strategies to send the message. Some communicators emphasize giving information; others have as a priority the conveying of interpersonal sensitivity. Longer nurse-client relationships allow each person to better understand the other person's communication style.

BASIC CONCEPTS

METACOMMUNICATION

Communication is a combination of verbal and non-verbal behaviors integrated for the purpose of sharing information. Within the nurse-client relationship, any exchange of information between two individuals also carries messages about how to interpret the communication.

Metacommunication is a broad term used to describe all of the factors that influence how the message is perceived (Figure 6-1). It is a message about how to interpret what is going on. Metacommunicated messages may be hidden within verbalizations or be conveyed as **nonverbal** gestures and expressions. The following case example should clarify this concept.

Case Example: Student Nurse Sydney

Some studies find greater compliance to requests when they are accompanied by a metacommunication message that demanded a response about the appropriateness of this request:

Student (smiling): Hi, I am Sydney. We nursing students are trying to encourage community awareness in promoting environmental health and are looking for people to hand out fliers. Would you be willing?

(Metacommunication): I realize that this is a strange request, seeing that you do not know who I am, but I would really appreciate your help. I am a nice person.

In this metacommunicated message about how to interpret meaning, the student nurse used both verbal and nonverbal cues. She conveyed a verbal message of caring to her white, middle-class client by making appropriate, encouraging responses, and a nonverbal message by maintaining direct eye contact, presenting a smooth face without frowning, and using a relaxed, fluid body posture without fidgeting.

In a professional relationship, verbal and nonverbal components of communication are intimately related. A student studying American Sign Language for the deaf was surprised that it was not sufficient merely to make the sign for "smile," but rather she had to actually show a smile at the same time. This congruence helped convey her message. You can nonverbally communicate your acceptance, interest, and respect for your client.

VERBAL COMMUNICATION

Words are symbols used by people to think about ideas and communicate with others. Choice of words is influenced by many factors (e.g., your age, race, socioeconomic group, educational background, and sex) and by the situation in which the communication is taking place.

The interpretation of the meaning of words may vary according to the individual's background and experiences. It is dangerous to assume that words have the same meaning for all persons who hear them. Language is useful only to the extent that it accurately reflects the experience it is designed to portray. Consider, for example, the difficulty an American has communicating with a person who speaks only Vietnamese, or the dilemma of the young child with a limited vocabulary who is trying to tell you where it hurts. Our voice can be a therapeutic part of treatment.

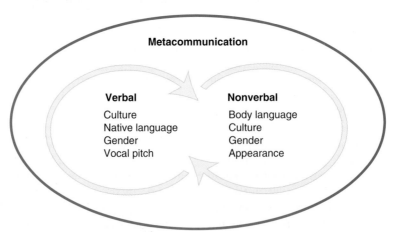

Figure 6-1   Factors in communication styles.

Case Example: Mrs. Garcia

For weeks while giving care to Mrs. Garcia, a 42-year-old unconscious woman, her nurse used soothing touch and conversation. She also encouraged the client's husband to do the same. When the woman later regained consciousness, she told the nurse that she recognized her voice.

MEANING

There are two levels of meaning in language: denotation and connotation. Both are affected by one's culture. **Denotation** refers to the generalized meaning assigned to a word; **connotation** points to a more personalized meaning of the word or phrase. For example, most people would agree that a dog is a four-legged creature, domesticated, with a characteristic vocalization referred to as a bark. This would be the denotative, or explicit, meaning of the word. When the word is used in a more personalized way, it reveals the connotative level of meaning. "What a dog" and "His bark is worse than his bite" are phrases some people use to describe personal characteristics of human beings, rather than a four-legged creature. We need to be aware that many communications convey only a part of the intended meaning. Do not assume that the meaning of a message is the same for the sender and the receiver until mutual understanding is verified. To be sure you are getting your message across, ask for feedback.

VERBAL STYLE FACTORS THAT INFLUENCE NURSE-TO-CLIENT PROFESSIONAL COMMUNICATION

The following six **verbal** styles of communication are summarized in Table 6-1:

1. *Moderate pitch and tone in vocalization.* The oral delivery of a verbal message, expressed through tone of voice, inflection, sighing, and so on, is referred to as **paralanguage.** It is important to understand this component of communication because it affects how the verbal message is likely to be interpreted. For example, you might say, "I would like to hear more about what you are feeling" in a voice that sounds rushed, high-pitched, or harsh. Or you might make this same statement in a soft, unhurried voice that expresses genuine interest. In the first instance, the message is likely to be misinterpreted by the client, despite your good intentions. Your caring intent is more apparent to the client in the second instance. Voice inflection (pitch and tone), loudness, and fast rate either supports or contradicts the content of the verbal message. Ideas may be conveyed merely by emphasizing different portions of your statement. When the tone of voice does not fit the words, the message is less easily understood and is less likely to be believed. Some, especially when upset, communicate in an emotional rather than intellectual manner. A message conveyed in a firm, steady tone is more reassuring than one conveyed in a loud, emotional, abrasive, or uncertain manner. In contrast, if you speak in a flat, monotone voice when you are upset, as though the matter is of no consequence, you confuse the client, making it difficult for him to respond appropriately.

2. *Vary vocalizations.* In some cultures, sounds are punctuated, whereas in other cultures, sounds have a lyrical or singsong quality. We need to orient ourselves to the characteristic voice tones associated with other cultures.

3. *Encourage client involvement.* Professional styles of communication have changed over time. We now partner with our clients in promoting their optimal health. We expect and encourage our clients to assume responsibility for their own health. Consequently, provider-client communication

TABLE 6-1	Styles That Influence Professional Communications in Nurse-Client Relationships	
Verbal	**Nonverbal**
Moderates pitch and tone	Allows therapeutic silences; listens
Varies vocalizations	Uses congruent nonverbal behaviors
Encourages client involvement	Uses facilitative body language
Validates client's worth	Uses touch appropriately
Advocate for client as necessary	Proxemics—respects client's space
Appropriately provides needed information: briefly and clearly, avoiding slang	Attends to client's nonverbal cues

has changed. Paternalistic, "I'll tell you what to do" styles are no longer acceptable.

4. *Validate client's worth.* Styles that convey "caring" send a message of individual worth that sustains the relationship with the client. For example, clients prefer providers who use a "warm" communication style to show caring, give information, and to allow them time to talk about their own feelings. Confirming responses validate the intrinsic worth of the person. These are responses that affirm the right of the individual to be treated with respect. They also affirm the client's autonomy (i.e., his or her right, ultimately, to make his or her own decisions). Disconfirming responses, in contrast, disregard the validity of feelings by either ignoring them or by imposing a value judgment. Such responses take the form of changing the topic, offering reassurance without supporting evidence, or presuming to know what a client means without verifying the message with the client. More-experienced nurses use more confirming communication. These communication skills are learned.

5. *Advocate for client when necessary.* Our personalities affect our style of social communication; some of us are naturally shy. But in our professional relationships, it often becomes necessary that we take on an assertive style of communicating with other health providers or agencies to obtain the best care or services for our client.

6. *Provide needed information appropriately.* Providing accurate information to our client in a timely manner in understandable amounts is discussed throughout this book. In our social conversations there often is a rhythm: "you talk—I listen," then "I get to talk, you listen." However, in professional communications, the content is more goal focused. Self-disclosure from the nurse needs to be limited. Telling a client your problems is not appropriate.

NONVERBAL COMMUNICATION

The majority of person-to-person communication of the meaning of our message is **nonverbal**. All our words are accompanied by nonverbal cues that offer meaning about how to interpret the message (Cruz et al., 2011). Think of the most interesting lecturer you ever had. Did this person lecture by making eye contact? Using hand gestures? Moving among the

students? Learners generally are most interested in lecturers whose nonverbal actions convey enthusiasm.

The function of nonverbal communication is to give us cues about what is being communicated. We nonverbally give meaning about the purpose or context of our message, as well as increasing the accuracy and efficiency of its impact on the listener. Some of these nonverbal cues we send are conveyed by our tone of voice, our facial expression, and body gestures or movement. Skilled use of nonverbal communication through therapeutic silences, use of congruent nonverbal behaviors, body language, touch, proxemics, and attention to client nonverbal cues such as facial expression can improve your relationship and build rapport with a client.

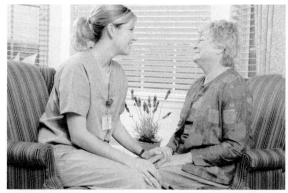

Emotional meanings are communicated through body language, particularly facial expression.

NONVERBAL STYLE FACTORS THAT INFLUENCE NURSE-TO-CLIENT PROFESSIONAL COMMUNICATION

We need to be aware of the position of our nonverbal messages as we talk to our client. Awareness of the position of our hands, the look on our face, and our body movements gives cues to our client (Levy-Storms, 2008). It is important to use attending behaviors such as leaning forward slightly, to convey to the client that his or her conversation is worth listening to. Think of the last time an interviewer kept fidgeting in his seat, glanced frequently at his wall clock or shuffled his papers. How did this make you feel? What nonverbal message was being conveyed? Table 6-1 summarizes the following six nonverbal behaviors of a competent nurse:

1. *Allow silences.* In our social communications, we often become uncomfortable if conversation lags. There is a tendency to rush in to fill the void. But in our professional nurse-client communication, we

use silence therapeutically, giving our clients needed time to think about things.

2. *Use congruent nonverbal behaviors.* Nonverbal behavior should be congruent with the message and reinforce it. If you knock on your instructor's office door to seek help, do you believe her when she says she would love to talk if you see her grimace and roll her eyes at her secretary? In another example, if you smile while telling your nurse-manager that your assignment is too much to handle, the seriousness of the message is negated. Try to give nonverbal cues that are congruent with the message you are verbally communicating. When nonverbal cues are incongruent with the verbal information, messages are likely to be misinterpreted. When your verbal message is inconsistent with the nonverbal expression of the message, the nonverbal expressions assume prominence and are generally perceived as more trustworthy than the verbal content. You need to comment on any incongruences to help your client. For example, when you enter a room to ask Mr. Sala if he is having any postoperative pain, he may say "No," but he grimaces and clutches his incision. After you comment on the incongruent message, he may admit he is having some discomfort. Can you think of a clinical situation in which you changed the meaning of a verbal message by giving nonverbal "don't believe what I say" cues?

3. *Use facilitative body language. Kinesics* is an important component of nonverbal communication. Commonly referred to as **body language**, it is defined as involving the conscious or unconscious body positioning or actions of the communicator. Words direct the content of a message, whereas emotions accentuate and clarify the meaning of the words. Some nonverbal behaviors such as tilting your head or facing your client at an angle promote communication.

   - **Posture.** Leaning forward slightly communicates interest and encourages your client to keep the conversation going. Keep your arms relaxed with palms open, knees unlocked and body loose, not tight and tense. Turning away indicates lack of interest, while directly and closely facing, crossing your arms and staring unblinkingly, or jabbing your finger in the air suggests aggression.
   - **Facial expression.** Six common facial expressions (surprise, sadness, anger, happiness/joy, disgust/contempt, and fear) represent global, generalized interpretations of emotions common to all cultures. Facial expression either reinforces or modifies the message the listener hears. The power of the facial expression far outweighs the power of the actual words. So try to maintain an open, friendly expression without being boisterously cheerful. Avoid furrowed forehead or a distracted or bored expression.
   - **Eye contact.** Making direct eye contact with your client generally conveys a positive message. Most clients interpret direct eye contact as an indication of your interest in what they have to say, although there are cultural differences.
   - **Gestures.** Some gestures such as affirmative head nodding help facilitate conversation by showing interest and attention. Use of open-handed gestures can also facilitate your nurse-client communication. Avoid folding arms across chest or fidgeting.

4. *Touch.* Touching a client is one of the most powerful ways you have to communicate nonverbally. Within a professional relationship, affective touch can convey caring, empathy, comfort and reassurance. When a nurse touches clients, this contact can be perceived by the client as either an expression of caring or negatively as a threat. Care must be taken to abide by the client's cultural proscriptions about the use of touch. This varies across cultures. An example would be the proscription some Muslim men and Orthodox Jewish men follow against touching women outside of family members. They might be uncomfortable shaking the hand of a female health care provider. In another example, some Native Americans use touch in healing, so that casual touching may be taboo.

The vast majority of clients report feeling comforted when a professional health provider touches them (Atenstaedt, 2012). The "best" type of touch cited by clients is holding their hand (Kozlowska and Doboszynska, 2012). All nurses caring directly for clients use touch to assess and to assist. We touch to help our client walk, roll over in bed, and so on. However, just as you are careful about invading the client's personal space, you are careful about when and where on the body you touch your clients. Your use of touch can elicit misunderstanding if your client perceives it as invasive or inappropriate. Gender of the nurse nuances the client's perception of the meaning of being touched. The findings of Harding and colleagues (2008) suggest that in our culture, whereas a woman's touch is seen as a normal expression of caring, we have sexualized male touching. This is a potential problem for male nurses. Therapeutic touch is discussed in Chapter 5.

5. *Proxemics.* We can use physical space to improve our interactions with clients. **Proxemics** refers to a client's perception of what is a proper distance to be maintained between the client and others. Use of space communicates messages. You've heard the phrase "Get out of my face" used when someone stands too close, often interpreted as an attempt to intimidate.

- Each culture proscribes expectations for appropriate distance depending on the context of the communication. For example, the Nonverbal Expectancy Violations Model defines "proper" social distance for an interpersonal relationship as 1.5 to 4 feet in Western cultures. Americans tend to become uncomfortable if someone stands closer than 3 feet. The interaction's purpose determines appropriate space, so that appropriate distance in space for intimate interaction would be zero distance, with increased space needed for personal distance, social distance, and public distance. In almost all cultures, zero distance is shunned except for loving or caring interaction. In giving physical care, nurses enter this "intimate" space. Care needs to be taken when you are at this closer distance, lest the client misinterpret your actions. Violating the client's sense of space can be interpreted as threatening.

6. *Attend to Client's Nonverbal Body Cues.*
- *Posture.* Often, the emotional component of a message can be indirectly interpreted by observing the client's body language. Rhythm of movement and body stance may convey a message about the speaker. For example, when a client speaks while directly facing you, this conveys more confidence than if the client turns his or her body away from you at an angle. A slumped, head-down posture and slow movements might give you an impression of lassitude or low self-esteem, whereas the client's erect posture and decisive movements suggest confidence and self-control. Rapid, diffuse, agitated body movements may indicate anxiety. Forceful body movements may symbolize anger. When clients bow their heads or slump their bodies after receiving bad news, it conveys sadness. Can you think of other cues your client's body posture might give you?

- *Facial expression.* Facial characteristics such as frowning or smiling add to the verbal message conveyed. Almost instinctively, we use facial expression as a barometer of another person's feelings, motivations, approachability, and mood. From infancy, we respond to the expressive qualities of another's face, often without even being aware of it. Therefore, assessing clients' facial expression together with their other nonverbal cues may reveal vital information that will affect the nurse-client relationship. Observing your client's facial expressions can signal his or her feelings. For example, a worried facial expression and lip biting may suggest an anxious client. Absence of a smile in greeting or grimacing may convey a message about how ill the client feels.

- *Eye contact.* Research suggests that individuals who make direct eye contact while talking or listening create a sense of confidence and credibility, whereas downward glances or averted eyes signal submission, weakness, or shame. In addition to conveying confidence, maintaining direct eye contact communicates honesty. Failure to maintain eye contact, known as *gaze aversion,* is perceived by adults and children as a nonverbal cue meaning that the person is lying to you. If your client's eyes wander around during a conversation, you may wonder if he is being honest. Even young children are more likely to attribute lying to those who avert their gaze.

- *Gestures.* Movements of his extremities may give cues about your client. Making a fist could convey how angry he is, just as use of stabbing, abrupt hand gestures may suggest distress, while hugging arms (self-embracing gestures) might suggest fear.

Assessing the extent to which the client uses these nonverbal cues to communicate emotions helps you communicate better. Studies repeatedly show us that failure to acknowledge nonverbal cues is often associated with inefficient communication by the health provider.

It is best if we verify our assessment of the meaning of our client's nonverbal behaviors. Body cues, although suggestive, are imprecise. When communication is limited by the client's health state, pay even closer attention to nonverbal cues. Pain, for example, can be assessed through facial expression even when the client is only partially conscious.

Case Example: Mr. Geeze

Mr. Geeze smiles but narrows his eyes and glares at the nurse. An appropriate comment for the nurse to make might be, "I notice you are smiling when you say you would like to kill me for mentioning your fever to the doctor. It seems that you might be angry with me."

COMMUNICATION ACCOMMODATION THEORY

Howard Giles theorized that people adapt or adjust their speech, vocal patterns (diction, tone, rate of speaking), dialect, word choice, and gestures to accommodate others. This theory suggests it is desirable to adjust one's speech to our conversational partners to help facilitate our interaction, to increase our acceptance, and to increase trust and rapport. This is known as *convergence.* Convergence is thought to increase the effectiveness of your communication.

Accommodation can occur unconsciously or can be a conscious choice. For example, when speaking to a child you might deliberately assume a more assertive, commanding style to get the child to obey. Choice of a distinctly different style is known as *divergence*. Conversely, you might choose convergence when you want to teach a client something about his or her disease condition. You might attempt to match the client's speed and speech cadence. You definitely adapt or accommodate by choosing to match your vocabulary to his or hers in an effort to be better understood. In general, if the person choosing to use convergence has more power in the relationship, he or she may be perceived as being patronizing. This needs to be guarded against as it determines subsequent behavior (Giles, n.d.). This theory assumes people are communicating in a rational manner. During a conflict, people can become unreasonable or even irrational—not a time to choose use of an accommodation style.

EFFECTS OF SOCIOCULTURAL FACTORS ON COMMUNICATION

Communication is also affected by such style factors as age cohort, gender, cultural background, ethnicity, social class, and location. Of course, not every

nurse cohort-member communicates in the manner described. These are broad generalizations as described in the literature.

AGE COHORT AND GENERATIONAL DIVERSITY

According to the Department of Health and Human Services, today's nursing workforce members now span four generations. As might be expected, members of different generations hold differing work motivation, personal values and attitudes, and have differing communication styles and preferences. Differences exist in communication styles and preferences, especially the style of interacting with authority figures, as well as differences in learning styles and commitment to the organization (Keepnews et al., 2010; QSEN, n.d.). If ignored, generational differences can become a source of conflict in the workplace.

Each age cohort, born approximately every 20 years, has some communication style characteristics in common, which differentiate their group from prior generations. Communication Accommodation Theory, as described earlier, has been used to explore intergenerational communication problems. In considering the generation gap, beliefs about communication and goals for interactions differ between cohorts. For example, Accommodation theory has been used to explore ageism, the negative evaluation of elderly by those who are younger. In society, youth may deliberately choose divergence, purposely amplifying differences, such as talking more rapidly, using slang, or emphasizing difference in values. In health care settings, studies of the generation gap and ageism stereotypes has found miscommunication outcomes in intergenerational interactions between physicians and clients. Individuals have been seen as more likely to use a patronizing style, while clients are less likely to respond assertively to ageist language if in a hospital setting.

Wieck and colleagues (2010) and other nursing authors stress the importance of this issue to job satisfaction and for the retention of new graduates. Brunetto and colleagues (2012) advocate for recognition of intergenerational differences and suggest integrating these into supervisor-subordinate communications on nursing units. Although some hospitals still forbid use of smart phones, Larson (2011) suggests younger nurses might prefer digital communication (via secure texting), while nurses from an older generation might prefer face-to-face communication. A study by Robinson and colleagues (2012) found younger nurses more likely to be abstract learners, using inductive reasoning, while older nurses are more concrete and rely more on intuitive, experienced-based strategies.

The newest nursing graduates may have been born since the mid-1990s and are said to belong to "the millennium generation" known as Generation Z. Prior generations are commonly labeled Y and X. A trend toward decreased commitment to the employing organization has been noted with each generation. Younger nurses and physicians were raised in the digital age and rely on the Internet and social medial for information, social interaction, and communication. It is said they have broader knowledge, tend to multitask, like instant gratification, use of communication devices such as "smart phones," and desire to work, learn, and study whenever they want. The nursing literature suggests that agencies and supervisors need to determine a person's preferred method of communication. People learn and communicate best if they are engaged in their preferred style.

While there clearly is a need for more research to substantiate the just-mentioned assertions, suggestions for adapting intergenerational communication from the authors cited in this chapter have been compiled in Box 6-1.

| BOX 6-1 | Adapting Communication to Differing Intergenerational Styles |

- Develop awareness of differences in intergenerational communication styles.
- Assess preferred interpersonal and communication style of every staff member (affective in-person vs. electronic; introverted vs. extroverted; people oriented vs. task oriented).
- Understand each member's expectations and learn how each defines "good communication."
- Build on strengths, adapting communication to preferred style (perhaps extra orientation on use of electronics for older generations, with increased opportunities for digital communication for younger nurses).
- Support manager-to-staff effective communication to ensure receipt of the message that management wants to develop the individual's full potential, while clarifying expectations for performance.
- Identify personal motivators such as sincere and regular praise, social recognition, increased responsibilities, and so forth.
- Emphasize that we all are committed to the same goal to deliver high-quality care.

GENDER

Communication patterns are integrated into gender roles defined by an individual's culture. Gender differences in communication studies have been shown to be greatest in terms of use and interpretation of nonverbal cues. This may reflect gender differences in intellectual style, as well as culturally reinforced standards of acceptable role-related behaviors. Of course, there are wide variations within the same gender.

We are now questioning whether traditional ideas about male and female differences in communication are as prevalent as previously thought. Is there really a major difference in communication according to gender? According to many reports, there is no major difference.

What is factual and what is a stereotype? More health care communication studies need to be done before we will really know. Because traditional thinking about gender-related differences in communication content and process in both nonverbal and verbal communication are being revised, consider critically what you read.

Traditionally, female individuals in most cultures were said to tend to avoid conflict and to want to smooth over differences. They were said to demonstrate more effective use of nonverbal communication and to be better decoders of nonverbal meaning. Feminine communication was thought to be more person centered, warmer, and more sincere. Studies show that women tend to use more facial expressiveness, smile more often, maintain eye contact, touch more often, and nod more often. Women have a greater range of vocal pitch and also tend to use different informal patterns of vocalization than men. They use more tones signifying surprise, cheerfulness, and unexpectedness. Women tend to view conversation as a connection to others.

Traditionally, male individuals in Western cultures were thought to communicate in a more task-oriented, direct fashion, demonstrate greater aggressiveness, and boast about accomplishments. They also have been viewed as more likely to express disagreement. Studies show that men prefer a greater interpersonal distance between themselves and others, and that they use gestures more often. Men are more likely to maintain eye contact in a negative encounter, although overall they maintain less direct eye contact; they use less verbal communication than women in interpersonal relationships. Men are more likely to initiate an interaction, talk more, interrupt more freely, talk louder, disagree more, use hostile verbs, and talk more about issues.

Gender Differences in Communication in Health Care Settings

It has been suggested that more effective communication occurs when the provider of the care and the client are of the same gender, although this was not found to be true in some studies. In professional health care settings, women have been noted to use more active listening, using encouraging responses such as "Uh-huh," "Yeah," and "I see," and to use more supportive words.

CULTURE

Although there is clear evidence that effective communication is related to better client health outcomes, greater client satisfaction, and better compliance, there is less evidence showing how cultural competency directly affects health outcomes. Yet authors such as Engelbretson (2011) stress the need for us to become culturally competent. To communicate as a culturally competent professional, you need to develop an awareness of the values of a specific client's culture and adapt your style and skills to be compatible with that culture's norms. Chapter 7 deals in depth with intercultural communication concepts.

LOCATION

Clients in urban areas have reported poorer communication by their health care providers. One factor that might affect these results is that rural clients tend to be cared for by the same "usual" providers. In a clinic or other busy location, lack of privacy certainly affects the style, as well as the content of your communication.

Developing an Evidence-Based Practice

Fisher MJ, Broome ME. Parent-Provider communication during hospitalization, *J Pediatr Nurs* 26(1):1-12, 2011.

This small study of hospitalized children used a case study methodology to examine communications across the parent-nurse-physician triads of three children in order to compare the perceptions of each. Semistructured interview questions were used.

Results: Findings focused on three themes: the importance of providing simple, clear, reciprocal communication in a caring manner; the benefits of sustaining a nurturing interpersonal relationship with parents; and identified behaviors, which sustain a positive communication experience. Specific behaviors that promoted positive communication included expressions of warmth, listening to and taking the parents' experiences seriously; promptness; and consistent assignment of heath care providers.

Application to your clinical practice: Because of the small size and the methodology of this study, it is difficult to make generalizations. Interestingly, the authors discuss the effectiveness of triad participation in medical rounds, which include the physician, the nurse, and the parents, as well as the ill child. The triad approach is unique and may provide a model for your future clinical practice, in which you provide client-centered communication as part of your client-centered care. According to prior studies, parents expect honest, factual frequent communications without an overwhelming amount of conflicts in information or incongruence between verbal and nonverbal behavior. Findings are consistent with multiple other studies and with the principles described in this book.

APPLICATIONS
KNOWING YOUR OWN COMMUNICATION STYLE

The style of communication you use can influence your clients' behavior and their compliance with treatment. Evidence suggests clients are dissatisfied with poor communication more than other aspects of their care. Exercises in prior chapters should give you basic skills used in the nurse-client relationship, but you bring your own communication style with you, as does your client. Because we differ widely in our personal communication styles, it is important for you to identify your style and to understand how to modify it for certain clients. How does your affective style come across? Do your clients view you as empathetic, caring and reassuring? Experienced nurses adapt their innate social style so their professional communication fits the client and the situation. Personality characteristics influence your style. For example, would you be described as more shy or assertive? One nurse might be characterized as "bubbly," whereas another is thought of as having a "quiet" manner. Similarly, clients have various styles. You need to make modifications so your style is compatible with client needs. Think about the potential for incompatibility in the following case.

Case Example: Mr. Michaels

Nurse (in a firm tone): Mr. Michaels, it is time to take your medicine.

Mr. Michaels (complaining tone): You are so bossy.

Empathetic communication is crucial to your nursing care and may improve your client's outcome (McMillian and Shannon, 2011). Recognize how others perceive you. Consider all the nonverbal factors that affect a client's perception of you. Your gender, manner of dress, appearance, skin tone, hairstyle, age, role as a student, gestures, or confident mannerisms may make a difference. Exercise 6-1 may increase your awareness of gender bias.

The initial step in identifying your own style may be to compare your style with that of others. Ask yourself, "What makes a client perceive a nurse either as authoritarian or as accepting and caring?" The Exercise 6-2 video may help you to compare your style with that of others.

Adapt your communication style as necessary.

Develop an awareness of alternative styles that you can comfortably assume if the occasion warrants. Next, it is important to figure out whether some other factors influence whether your style is appropriate for a particular client. How might the other person's age, race, socioeconomic status, or gender affect their response to you? We need to continually work to update our communication competencies. Internal organizational communication is rapidly becoming electronic. For example, Baird and colleagues (2012) describes how a particular hospital system found it more effective to communicate changes via e-mails that were electronically tracked. Digital communication eliminates pretty much all the nuances communicated nonverbally.

INTERPERSONAL COMPETENCE

Nurse-client communication processes are based on the nurse's interpersonal competence. **Interpersonal competence** develops as the nurse comes to understand the complex cognitive, behavioral, and cultural factors that influence communication. This understanding, together with the use of a broad range of communication skills, helps you interact with your client as he or she attempts to cope with the many demands placed on him or her by the environment. Good communication skills are associated with competency. Competent communication skills are identified as one of the attributes of expert nurses who were perceived as having clinical credibility. In dealing with the client in the sociocultural context of the health care system, two kinds of abilities are

---

EXERCISE 6-1	Gender Bias

Purpose: To create discussion about gender bias.

Procedure
In small groups, read and discuss the following comments that are made about care delivery on a geriatric psychiatric unit by staff and students: "Male staff tend to be slightly more confident and to make quicker decisions. Women staff are better at the feeling things, like conveying warmth."

Discussion
1. Were these comments made by male or female staff?
2. How accurate are they?
3. Can you truly generalize any attribute to all male and female individuals?

EXERCISE 6-2	Self-Analysis of Video Recording

Purpose: To increase awareness of students' own style.

Procedure
With a partner, role-play an interaction between nurse and client. Video record or use the video capacity of your cell phone to record a 1- to 2-minute interview with the camera focused on you. The topic of the interview could be "identifying health promotion behaviors" or something similar.

Discussion
What posture did you use? What nonverbal messages did you communicate? How did you communicate them? Were your verbal and nonverbal messages congruent?

required: social cognitive competency and message competency.

Social cognitive competency is the ability to interpret message content within interactions from the point of view of each of the participants. By embracing the client's perspective, you begin to understand how the client organizes information and formulates goals. This is especially important when your client's ability to communicate is impaired by mechanical barriers such as a ventilator. Clients who recovered from critical illnesses requiring ventilator support reported fear and distress during this experience.

Message competency refers to the ability to use language and nonverbal behaviors strategically in the intervention phase of the nursing process to achieve the goals of the interaction. Communication skills are used as a tool to influence the client to maximize his or her adaptation. Think how it feels when your client sees you smile and hears you say, "That's impressive; you have successfully self-injected your insulin!"

STYLE FACTORS THAT INFLUENCE RELATIONSHIPS

The establishment of trust and respect in an interpersonal relationship with client and family is dependent on open, ongoing communication style. Having knowledge of communication styles is not sufficient to guarantee successful application. You need to understand how the materials discussed in this chapter interrelate. For example, providers who sit at client's eye level, at optimal distance **(proxemics)**, without furniture between them (special configuration) will likely have more eye contact and use more therapeutic touching. Box 6-2 contains suggestions to improve your own professional style of communicating.

SLANG AND JARGON

Different age groups even in the same culture may attribute different meanings to the same word. For example, an adult who says, "That's cool," might be referring to the temperature, whereas a teenager might convey his satisfaction by using the same phrase. In health care, the "food pyramid" is understood by nurses to represent the basic nutritional food groups needed for health; however, the term may have limited meaning for individuals not in the health professions.

MEDICAL JARGON

Beginning nursing students often report confusion while learning all the medical terminology required for their new role. Remembering our own experiences, we can empathize with clients who are attempting to understand the **medical jargon** involved in health care. Careful explanations help clients overcome this communication barrier. For successful communication, words used should have a similar meaning to both individuals in the interaction. An important part of the communication process is the search for a common vocabulary so that the message sent is the same as the one received. Consider the oncology nurse who develops a computer databank of cancer treatment terms. When admitting Mr. Michaels as a new client, the nurse uses an existing template model on her computer to create an individualized terminology sheet with just the words that would be encountered by him during his course of chemotherapy treatment.

BOX 6-2	Suggestions to Improve Your Communication Style

- Adapt yourself to your client's cultural values.
- Use nonverbal communication strategies, such as:
  - Maintain eye contact.
  - Display pleasant, animated facial expressions.
  - Smile often.
  - Nod your head to encourage the client to continue talking.
  - Maintain attentive, upright posture and sit at his or her level, leaning forward toward the client slightly.
  - Attend to proper proximity and increase space if client shows signs of discomfort, such as gaze aversion, leg swinging, or rocking.
- Use touch with client if appropriate to the situation.
- Use active listening and respond to client's cues.
- Use verbal strategies to engage your client.
  - Use humor, but avoid gender jokes.
  - Attend to proper tone and pitch, avoiding being overly loud.
  - Avoid using jargon.
  - Use nonjudgmental language and open-ended questions.
  - Listen and avoid jumping in too soon with problem solving.
  - Verbalize respect for client.
  - Ask permission before addressing client by his first name.
  - Convey caring comments.
  - Use confirming, positive comments.

RESPONSIVENESS OF PARTICIPANTS

How responsive the participants are affects the depth and breadth of communication. Reciprocity affects not only the relationship process, but also client outcomes. Some clients are naturally more verbal than others. It is easier to have a therapeutic conversation with extroverted clients who want to communicate. You will want to increase the responsiveness of less verbal clients and enhance their communication responsiveness. Verbal and nonverbal approval encourages clients to express themselves. Elsewhere, we discuss skills that promote responsiveness such as active listening, demonstration of empathy, and acknowledgment of the content and feelings of messages. Sometimes acknowledging the difficulty your client is having expressing certain feelings, praising efforts, and encouraging use of more than one route of communication helps. Such strategies demonstrate interpersonal sensitivity. Listening to the care experience of a client, responding to verbal or nonverbal cues, and avoiding "talking down" encourages communication and may improve compliance with the treatment regimen. Exercise 6-3 will help you practice using confirming responses.

ROLES OF PARTICIPANTS

Paying attention to the **role relationship** of the communicators may be just as important as deciphering the content and meaning of the message. The relationships between the roles of the sender and of the receiver influence how the communication is likely to be received and interpreted. The same constructive criticism made by a good friend and by one's immediate supervisor is likely to be interpreted differently, even though the content and style are quite similar. Communication between subordinates and supervisors is far more likely to be influenced by power and style than by gender. When roles are unequal in terms of power, the more powerful individual tends to speak in a more dominant style. This is discussed in Chapter 23.

CONTEXT OF THE MESSAGE

Communication is always influenced by the environment in which it takes place. It does not occur in a vacuum but is shaped by the situation in which the interaction occurs. Taking time to evaluate the physical setting and the time and space in which the contact takes place, as well as the psychological, social, and cultural characteristics of each individual involved, gives you flexibility in choosing the most appropriate context.

INVOLVEMENT IN THE RELATIONSHIP

Relationships generally need to develop over time because communication changes with different phases of the relationship. Uitterhoeve and colleagues (2008) validated prior research showing that nurses respond to less than half of client concerns, and tend to focus on physical care whereas ignoring client's social emotional care. In these days of managed care, nurses working with hospitalized clients have less time to develop a relationship, whereas community-based nurses may have greater opportunities. To begin to explore ethical problems in your nursing relationships, consider the ethical dilemma provided.

ADVOCATE FOR CONTINUITY OF CARE

We have learned that a client's perception of positive health care communication is higher when they consistently relate to the same individuals who provide their care. These providers were more likely to listen to them, to explain things clearly, to spend enough time with them, and to show them respect. Because physicians and nurses communicate differently with clients, it is crucial that these professionals pool their information.

EXERCISE 6-3	Confirming Responses

Purpose: To increase students' skills in using confirming communication.

Procedure
Change these disconfirming, negative messages into positive, confirming, caring comments.
1. "Three of your 14 blood sugars this week were too high. What did you do wrong?"
2. "Your blood pressure is dangerously high. Are you eating salty foods again?"
3. "You gained five pounds this week. Can't you stick to a simple diet?"

Discussion
Suggest better rephrasing to communicate the same message. Was it relatively easy to send a positive, confirming message?

SUMMARY

Communication between nurse and client or nurse and another professional involves more than an exchange of verbal and nonverbal information. As our population becomes more diverse, we are challenged to provide patient-centered care that is sensitive to our client's culture, race, ethnicity, gender, and sexual orientation. Suggestions for improving your communication style are provided. Professional communication, like personal communication, is subtly altered by changes in pitch of voice and use of accompanying facial expressions or gestures. This chapter explores factors related to effective styles of verbal and nonverbal communication. Cultural and gender differences associated with each of these three areas of communication are discussed. For professionals, maintaining congruence is important. Style factors that affect the communication process include the responsiveness and role relationships of the participants, the types of responses and context of the relationships, and the level of involvement in the relationship. Confirming responses acknowledge the value of a person's communication, whereas disconfirming responses discount the validity of a person's feelings. More nonverbal strategies to facilitate nurse-client communication are discussed in later chapters.

ETHICAL DILEMMA   What Would You Do?

Katy Collins, RN, is a new grad who learns that a serious error has occurred on her unit that harmed a client. She realizes that if staff continue to follow the existing protocol, there is a risk this error will occur again. In a team meeting led by an administrator, Katy raises this issue in a tentative manner. The leader speaks in a loud, decisive voice and states he wants input from the staff nurses. However, he glances at the clock, gazes over her head, and maintains a bored expression. Katy gets the message that the administration wants to smooth over the error, bury it, and go on as usual, rather than using resources and time to correct the underlying problem.

1. What ethical principle is being violated in this situation?
2. What message does the administrator's behavior convey?
3. Is his verbal and nonverbal message congruent?
4. What would you do if you were in Katy's place?

DISCUSSION QUESTIONS

1. Discuss the Ethical Dilemma provided. Is the verbal congruent with the nonverbal message? How would you change the nonverbal to make it more congruent with the verbal message?
2. Use Exercise 6-1 to discuss the influence of gender on communication.
3. In a loud, commanding voice, a nurse tells an immediate postoperative client to take deep breaths every 20 minutes despite the pain it causes. Describe three possible reactions that might occur. What would you do to make this intervention more effective?

REFERENCES

Atenstaedt R: Touch in the consultation, *Br J Gen Pract* 62(596):147–148, 2012.

Baird BK, Funderburk A, Whitt M, Wilbanks P: Structure strengthens nursing communication, *Nurse Leader* 10(2):1–3, 2012. www.nursingconsult.com/nursing/journals/1541-4612/.

Brunetto Y, Farr-Wharton R, Shacklock K: Communication, training, well-being, and commitment across nurse generations, *Nurs Outlook* 60:7–15, 2012.

Giles, H. (n.d.) Communication Accommodation Theory. www.public.iastate.edu/~mredmond/SpAccT.htm. Accessed 8/2/13.

Cruz M, Roter D, Cruz RF, Wieland M, Cooper LA, Larson S, Pincus HA: Psychiatrist-patient verbal and nonverbal communications during split-treatment appointments, *Psychiatr Serv* 62(11):1361–1368, 2011.

Engelbretson J: Clinically applied medical ethnography: Relevance to cultural competence in patient care, *Nurs Clin North Am* 46:145–154, 2011.

Harding T, North N, Perkins R: Sexualizing men's touch: male nurses and the use of intimate touch in clinical practice, *Res Theory Nurs Pract* 22(2):88–102, 2008.

Keepnews DM, Brewer CS, Kovner CT, Shin JH: Generational differences among newly licensed registered nurses, *Nurs Outlook* 58:155–163, 2010.

Kozlowska L, Doboszynska A: Nurses' nonverbal methods of communicating with patients in the terminal phase, *Int J Palliat Nurs* 18(1):40–46, 2012.

Larson J. Communication skills: Moving beyond basics. NurseZone.com. http://www.nursezone.com/nursing-news-events/more-features/Communication-Skills-Moving-Beyond-the-Basics_37646.aspx. 2011.

Levy-Storms L: Therapeutic communication training in long-term institutions: recommendations for future research, *Patient Educ Couns* 73:8–21, 2008.

McMillian LR, Shannon D: Program evaluation of nursing school instruction in measuring students' perceived competence to empathically communicate with patients, *Nurs Educ Perspect* 32(3):150–154, 2011.

Quality and Safety Education for Nurses (QSEN). (n.d.) Teamwork & Collaboration (QSEN competencies: online teaching modules). www.QSEN.org/. Accessed 6/1/13.

Robinson J, Scollan-Koliopoulos M, Kamienski M: Generational differences and learning style preferences in nurses from a large metropolitan medical center, *J Nurs Staff Dev* 28(4):166–172, 2012.

Rogers R: Leadership communication styles: A descriptive analysis of health care professionals, *J Healthc Leader* 2012(4):47–57, 2012.

Rosenberg S, Gallo-Silver L: Therapeutic communication skills and student nurses in the clinical setting, *Teach Learn Nurs* 6(2):1–8, 2011. www.jtln.org/.

Uitterhoeve R, deLeeuw J, Bensing J, et al.: Cue-responding behaviors of oncology nurses in video-simulated interviews, *J Adv Nurs* 61(1):71–80, 2008.

Wieck KL, Dols J, Landrum P: Retention priorities for the intergenerational nurse workforce, *Nurs Forum* 45(1):7–17, 2010.

Intercultural Communication

Elizabeth C. Arnold

OBJECTIVES

At the end of the chapter, the reader will be able to:
1. Define culture and related terms.
2. Discuss the concept of intercultural communication.
3. Describe the concept of cultural competence.
4. Apply the nursing process to the care of culturally diverse clients.
5. Discuss characteristics of selected cultures as they relate to the nurse-client relationship.

Chapter 7 describes intercultural communication principles and strategies nurses can use to provide culturally sensitive client and family-centered care. Included are social and cultural factors associated with the nation's four major cultural groups.

BASIC CONCEPTS

DEFINITIONS

Culture is a complex social concept, which encompasses socially transmitted communication styles, family customs, political systems, and ethnic identity held by a particular group of people. Alexander (2008) suggests "Each individual, family, and community represents a unique blend of overlapping and intersecting cultural elements in which the whole is greater than the sum of the parts" (p. 416). In health care, culture provides a relevant context for therapeutic communication, shared decision making, and client-centered care. Embedded cultural considerations in health care delivery enhance client-centered compliance with treatment. Most people belong to more than one culture, so the concept of culture can extend beyond a specific ethnic background or country of origin (Betancourt, 2004). "Culture" is a term also applied to professional and organizational systems, subgroups within a dominant culture, including religious denominations and lifestyle orientations.

CULTURAL PATTERNS

Culture is a crucial filter through which people "learn how to be in the world, how to behave, what to value, and what gives meaning to existence" (Schim and Doorenbos, 2010, p. 256). Cultural patterns are socially transmitted through family, and other social institutions. They are an essential part of personal identity. People pass down social customs ("the way we do things"), cultural beliefs, values, and language, from one generation to the next (Giger et al, 2007). Cultures evolve, but vestiges from the past can still influence behavior and communication in the present.

Cultural patterns influence health-related beliefs, attitudes, values, and behaviors (Kleinman and Benson, 2006). Traditions affect client preferences and how people process and interpret the information they receive. Social factors such as class and literacy further distinguish individual response patterns within a culture (Wiener, McConnell and Colleagues, 2013). Decisions to seek professional health care services are strongly influenced by socio-cultural and family contexts, especially for minority populations (Scheppers et al., 2006). Exercise 7-1, Cultural Authenticity, offers you an opportunity to reflect on your own cultural heritage.

| EXERCISE 7-1 | Cultural Authenticity |

Purpose: To help students appreciate the importance of understanding your own culture as a basis for understanding culture relationships in health care.

Procedure
1. Write a one-page story about your own culture and/or ethnic background as you understand it.
2. Describe in what ways family and social customs or culture-bound traditions have influenced your sense of personal development, career and leisure choices, opportunities, values, and so forth.
3. Discuss how personal understanding of your cultural background has changed over time.

4. Identify how knowing about one's own culture informs cultural sensitivity to others in health care situations.
5. Briefly answer the question, "Does my story represent my cultural authenticity?"

Discussion
1. Share your culture story in small groups of three to four students.
2. As a class, discuss how personal culture can influence health behaviors.
3. Identify common themes.
3. Discuss how culturally authentic knowledge prevents unconscious projection of a personal cultural context on a client from a different culture.

CULTURAL DIVERSITY

Cultural diversity refers to variations between cultural groups. People tend to notice differences related to language, mannerisms, and behaviors in people of different cultures, in ways that do not happen with people from their own culture (Spence, 2001). Lack of exposure to and understanding of people from other cultures reinforces stereotypes and creates prejudice.

Diversity also exists *within* a culture. In fact, more differences can exist among individuals within a culture than between cultural groups related to educational and socioeconomic background, age, gender, and life experiences (Drench et al., 2009). Consider your nursing class. Which would be more appropriate—to consider your class as having a homogenous or a heterogeneous culture?

Within the same culture, individuals with radically different philosophies, social patterns, and sanctioned behaviors coexist, sometimes peacefully and other times in conflict with each other. Consider, for example, the wide political divergence between extreme liberals and conservatives, differences between faith beliefs, the very poor and the very rich. Other influences from the sociocultural environment include differences in response patterns to illness, health promotion behaviors, and societal supports (IOM, 2002a). Negative stereotypes about minorities as consumers and comments from minority populations about health care options available to them and provider discrimination persist. Despite historic legislation designed to make quality health care

| BOX 7-1 | Points of Cultural Diversity in Health Care |

- People's feelings, attitudes, and behavioral standards
- Ways of living, language, and habits
- How people relate to others, including attitudes about health professionals
- Nutrition and diet
- Personal views of what is right and wrong
- Perspectives on health, illness, and death, including appropriate rituals
- Hearing about and discussing negative health information
- Decisional authority, role relationships, and truth-telling practices
- Child-rearing practices
- Use of advance directives, informed consent, and client autonomy (Calloway, 2009; Carrese and Rhodes, 2000; Karim, 2003; Searight and Gafford, 2005)

opportunities available to everyone, progress is slow and attitudes play a role in ending unequal treatment for minority populations. Box 7-1 identifies points of cultural diversity.

Culture diversity is an issue within the nursing profession. Minority nurses account for only 16.8% of the professional nursing workforce (Isaacson, 2014). Having a common understanding of health care influences the quality of care across health disciplines too. Currently minorities comprise only about 3% of medical school faculty and about 17% of public health officers (Betancourt et al, 2003). Exercise 7-2 provides

EXERCISE 7-2	Diversity in the Nursing Profession

Purpose: To help students learn about the experience of nurses from a different ethnic group.

Procedure

1. Each student will interview a registered nurse from an ethnic minority group different from their own ethnic origin.
2. The following questions serve as an interview guide:
   a. In what ways was your educational experience more difficult or easier as a minority student?
   b. What do you see as the barriers for minority nurses in our profession?
   c. What do you see as the opportunities for minority nurses in our profession?
   d. What do you view as the value of increasing diversity in the nursing profession for health care?
   e. What do you think we can do as a profession and personally to increase diversity in nursing?
3. Write a one- to two-page narrative report about your findings to be presented in a follow-up class.

Discussion

1. What were the common themes that seemed to be present across narratives?
2. In what ways, if any, did doing this exercise influence your thinking about diversity?
3. Did you find any of the answers to the interview questions disturbing, or surprising?
4. How could you use this exercise in becoming culturally competent?

an opportunity to study components of cultural diversity within the profession.

WORLDVIEW

Concepts such as cultural and spiritual beliefs are closely linked to the concept of worldview. Although related, they are not the same. **Worldview** is defined as, "the way people tend to look out upon their world or their universe to form a picture or value stance about life or the world around them" (Leininger and McFarland, 2006, p. 15). Whereas culture identifies the social characteristics of a society, a person's worldview describes an individual's perceptions of his or her reality within a society. A teenager and an older adult can have similar beliefs about their culture, but their worldviews would be dissimilar because of their experiential age difference. Clients with different worldviews can have different goals and health concerns. The worldview of a significant number of immigrants to this country would likely differ because their unique complex social and health needs would mirror their country of origin, rather than the United States.

How Culture Is Learned

We are born *into* a culture, however culture is not an inborn characteristic. Initially culture is primarily learned through family, and then through other social institutions such as school, church affiliations, and community contacts (Giger, 2013). As children learn language from their primary care givers, and later refine language skills in school, they integrate the cultural attitudes, meanings, values, and thought patterns that inform their words.

Immigrants acquire a cultural identity through a two-step interpersonal process in which a person transitions from his or her traditional cultural beliefs and values, toward full adoption of the values and beliefs of the dominant culture. **Acculturation** describes how immigrants from a different culture initially learn the behavior norms and values of another dominant culture, and begin to adopt its behaviors and language patterns. The acculturation process can be stressful because of competing pressures to reconcile aspects of a familiar cultural identity with a need to adopt new customs essential to functioning effectively in the adopted culture (Marsiglia, et al, 2013). Client centered assessment should include level of acculturation related to explanatory models of illness, level of health literacy, traditional health behaviors and their potential impact on health care matters (Hardin, 2014). Trust is an important factor. **Assimilation** takes place as the individual from a different culture fully accepts and adopts the behaviors, customs, and values of the mainstream culture as part of his or her social identity. In order to become fully assimilated, immigrants must conform and adapt to the norms of the adopted cultures. By the third generation, many immigrants may have little knowledge of their traditional culture and language or allegiance to their original heritage (Bacallao and Smokowski, 2005; Schwartz et al., 2006). Efforts to understand and influence health behaviors of culturally diverse clients is best achieved at the community level (Huff and Kline, 2008).

Table 7-1 summarizes selected descriptors of concepts related to culture.

LINKED CONCEPTS

Ethnicity describes a person's awareness of a shared cultural heritage with others based on common racial, geographic, ancestral, religious or historical bonds. People develop a sense of identity associated with that heritage and the cultural legacy passes from generation to generation. Ethnicity creates a sense of belonging and inspires strong commitment to associated values and practices. Research indicates that ethnicity is an important aspect of a person's social identity (Malhi et al., 2009).

Ethnicity represents a sociopolitical construct, different from race and physical characteristics (Ford and Kelly, 2005). People with similar skin color and features can have a vastly different ethnic heritage, for example, Jamaican versus African American descent. Ethnicity can reflect spiritually-based values and membership, for example, the Amish (Donnermeyer and Friedrich, 2006). A relevant question to ask yourself and to reflect on with your client is what does it mean for you to be a member of a particular culture (for example, a Latino American, or an Asian American)?

Ethnocentrism

Neuliep (2005) proposes that "ethnocentrism is essentially descriptive, not necessarily pejorative" (p. 206). In some instances milder form of ethnocentrism can be an advantage in encouraging patriotism. Taking pride in one's culture is appropriate, but when a person fails to respect the value of other cultures, it is easy to develop stereotypes and prejudice. Ethnocentrism can foster the belief that one culture has the right to impose its standards of "correct" behavior and values on another. Prejudice can be directed to an ethnic group as a whole or toward an individual associated with the group. The deadly consequences of prejudice were evidenced in the persecution of innocent people during Hitler's regime. Strong prejudice continues today with terrorist attacks and targeted violence embedded in ethnocentric views and extreme sectarian differences.

A variation of ethnocentrism labels people who differ from the mainstream in personal ways as being inferior (Canales and Howers, 2001). The Institute of Medicine (IOM, 2003) identifies economic status and social class as components of diversity related to health risk and treatment outcomes. Other examples include physical or mental disability, sexual orientation, ageism, morbid obesity, and unusual physical or personal characteristics.

TABLE 7-1	Definitions Associated with Culture
Concept	**Definition**
Subculture	A smaller group of people living within the dominant culture with a distinct lifestyle, shared beliefs, and expectations that set them apart from the mainstream (Drench et. al., 2009). Example: Amish, Mormons
Ethnicity	Group of people who share a common social identity based on ancestral, national, or cultural experiences (Day-Vines et al., 2007).
Ethnocentrism	Belief that one's own culture is superior to all others, and should be the norm (Lewis, 2000).
Cultural relativism	Concept that each culture is unique and should be judged only on the basis of its own values and standards (Aroian and Faville, 2005).

Adapted from: Aroian K, Faville K: Reconciling cultural relativism for a clinical paradigm: what's a nurse to do? *J Prof Nurs* 21(6):330, 2005; Day-Vines N, Wood S, Grothaus T, et al: Broaching the subjects of race, ethnicity and culture during the counseling process, *J Couns Dev* 85:401-409, 2007; Drench M, Noonan A, Sharby N, et al: *Psychosocial aspects of health care*, ed 2, Upper Saddle River, NJ, 2009, Pearson Prentice Hall.

Case Example

"I knew a man who had lost the use of both eyes. He was called a blind man. He could also be called an expert typist, a conscientious worker, a good student, a careful listener, and a man who wanted a job. But he couldn't get a job in the department store order room where employees sat and typed orders, which came over the phone. The personnel man was impatient to get the interview over. "But you are a blind man," he kept saying, and one could almost feel his silent assumption that somehow the incapability in one aspect made the man incapable in every other. So blinded by the label was the interviewer that he could not be persuaded to look beyond it" (Allport, 1979, p. 178).

Cultural Relativism

Cultural relativism holds that each culture is unique and its merits should be judged only on the basis of its own values and standards. Behaviors viewed as unusual from outside a culture can make perfect sense when they are evaluated within a cultural context (Aroian and Faville, 2005).

Case Example

Benjamin Franklin's Comments on Native Americans

"Savages we call them, because their Manners differ from ours, which we think the Perfection of Civility; they think the same of theirs. Perhaps if we could examine the Manners of Different Nations with Impartiality, we should find no people so rude, as to be without any Rules of Politeness; nor any so polite, as not to have some Remains of Rudeness" (Benjamin Franklin, quoted in Jandt, 2003, p. 76).

Exercise 7-3 looks at how culture shapes our values and perceptions.

INTERCULTURAL COMMUNICATION

Intercultural communication refers to conversations taking place between people from different cultures. The concept embraces differences in perceptions, language, and nonverbal behaviors, and recognition of different interpretive contexts (Samovar et al., 2008). It is a primary means of sharing meaning and developing relationships between people of different cultures. Effective intercultural interactions take place within "transcultural caring relationships" (Pergert et al., 2007, p. 18). This means that the client's *perception* of his or her relationship with the nurse can be just as important as the words used in the communication.

Case Example

A Chinese first-time mother, tense and afraid as she entered the transition phase of labor, spoke no English. Her husband spoke very little, and saw birthing as women's work. Callister (2001) relates, "The nurse could feel palpable tension that filled the room. The nurse could not speak Chinese either, but she tried to convey a sense of caring, touching the woman, speaking softly, modeling supportive behavior for her husband and helping her to relax as much as possible. The atmosphere in the room changed considerably with the calm competence and quiet demeanor of the nurse. Following the birth …, the father conveyed to her how grateful he was that she spoke Chinese. She tactfully said, 'Thank you, but I don't speak Chinese.' He looked at her in amazement and said with conviction, 'You spoke Chinese.' The language of the heart transcends verbal communication" (p. 212).

Language

Successful outcomes depend on developing a common understanding and inclusion of issues and values that facilitate treatment (Purnell et al., 2008). Linguistic rules, language structures, and meanings vary among cultures. Different languages create, and express different personal realities. Understanding vocabulary and grammar is not enough. Language cultural competence requires "knowing what to say, and how, when, where, and why to say it" (Hofstede et al., 2002, p. 18).

Within the same language, words can have more than one meaning. For example, the words *hot, warm,* and *cold* can refer to temperature, or to impressions of strong personal characteristics, or responses to new ideas (Sokol and Strout, 2006). Idioms are particularly problematic because they represent a nonliteral expression of an idea. For example, Neulip (2015) describes a common use of the word "bomb" to indicate a strong

EXERCISE 7-3	Values and Perceptions Associated with Different Cultures

Purpose: To help students appreciate values and generalized perceptions associated with different cultures.

Procedure
1. Select a specific ethnic culture.
2. Interview someone from that culture and ask them to tell you about their culture related to family values, religion, what is important in social interaction, health care beliefs, and end-of-life rituals.
3. Write a short report on your findings.
4. Share your written report with your classmates.

Discussion
1. What important values did you uncover?
2. In what ways did the person's answers agree or disagree with the generalized cultural characteristics of the culture?
3. What did you learn from doing this exercise that you could use in your clinical practice with culturally diverse clients?

performance on an exam. In the US, the word bomb is used to express doing poorly on an examination. Nonverbal behaviors, particularly gestures and eye contact, can have very different meanings in various cultures. What is appropriate in one culture can be thought of as discourteous or insulting in another culture (Anderson and Wang, 2008).

Even when a client speaks good English, it is best to use clear simple language rather than complex words and to speak more slowly. Despite having relatively strong verbal skills in an adopted language, many clients with English as a second language lack the complex vocabulary in English needed to quickly grasp what is being said. Think about your own experiences learning a foreign language in school. You probably were more comfortable expressing yourself in simple terms basically because you didn't have the more complex vocabulary needed to understand language nuances and multiple meanings. You could attend to the conversation better when the words were spoken slowly with spacing between words. Frequent checks for understanding facilitate communication with culturally diverse clients.

High Context versus Low Context Communication Style

Understanding the implications of differences between high and low context culturally based communication styles is an important dimension of intercultural communication. Drawn from Hall's original work (1976), high context cultures prefer an indirect communication style in which much of the shared information is *implicit*. High context communication styles are associated with collectivistic cultures; they are characterized by a "we" consciousness and a strong stress on group loyalty and harmony. Relationship is more important than task in communication (Hofstede, 2011). Trust is a critical dimension in communication, and the words are not as important as the tone of voice and perception of interpersonal relations. Asia, Africa, and South America and parts of the Middle East are considered high context collective cultures. In low context individualistic cultures, Hofstede suggests, the "task prevails over relationship" (p. 11). Information is reality based and *explicitly* conveyed. Precise words are taken literally and lead to mutually determined actions. North American and Western European cultures are considered low context cultures.

Developing an Evidence-Based Practice

Underwood S, Buseh A, Kelber S, Stevens P, Townsend L. Enhancing the participation of African Americans in health-related genetic research: findings of a collaborative academic and community based research study, *Nurs Res Pract* 2013:749563, 2013. http://dx.doi.org/10.1155/2013/749563. Epub December 4, 2013.

Purpose: This exploratory study sought to identify factors associated with the participation of African Americans in health-related research. The study was guided by a framework related to the influence of knowledge, beliefs, and perceptions about genetics on enhancing African American participation in health related genetic research.

Results: Findings indicated that knowledge, beliefs, and perceptions about genetics, and provider involvement were associated with willingness to participate in health-related genetic research ($P < 0.05$). The study also showed that 88.7% of the 212 African American participants who had not previously been involved in a health-related research study reported they had never been asked.

Application to your clinical practice: As professionals working in an increasingly multicultural society, nurses need to develop clinical strategies and innovative research to further examine factors that could be used to enhance minority participation in health related research.

APPLICATIONS

IMPORTANCE OF CULTURE IN HEALTH CARE COMMUNICATION

Samovar and colleagues (2014) note, "The forces of globalization have created an environment where cross-cultural awareness and intercultural communication competence are daily necessities" (p. 3). Knowledge of cultural differences, and specialized development of multicultural interpersonal communication skills should be part of every nurse's essential tool box. We currently live in a global society, created by changes in immigration patterns and instant technological connectivity. Most industrialized nations are becoming multiethnic with majority population percentages becoming significantly smaller. Minority populations represent a critical and expanding component of health care consumers in our nation.

The Institute of Medicine (2002b, 2003) identifies ineffective communication as a significant source of unequal care and health outcomes among minority populations in the United States. Your ability to communicate and function effectively with culturally diverse clients has a lot to do with personal values and beliefs from your personal cultural background. Self-awareness and careful reflection can help you appreciate how these factors influence communication with clients from different cultures. Another component of effective intercultural communication relates to developing knowledge of common cultural patterns associated with different cultures, and worldviews.

HEALTH DISPARITIES

An overarching goal in *Healthy People 2020* is "to achieve health equity, eliminate disparities, and improve the health of all groups." This document defines a **health disparity** as "a particular type of health difference that is closely linked with social, economic, and/or environmental disadvantage."

Health disparities, coupled with lack of easy access to health care are a major health issue globally, and nationally. In 2002 the Institute of Medicine reported that people of color and ethnic minorities received a lower quality of care even when insurance and income were considered. This phenomena has been shown in a number of research studies (Giger, 2013). The *National Healthcare Disparities Report* (U.S. Department of Health and Human Services [DHHS], 2007) confirms that minority status accounts for major differences and inequality in the quality of health care related to access, screenings, and level of care. The National Center for Health Statistics (2007) indicates that ethnic and racial minorities, which make up 30% of the adult population and almost 40% of the U.S. population younger than 18, have greater mortality and morbidity rates (Edwards, 2009; National Center for Health Statistics, 2007). Increasing the number of culturally diverse nurses within the profession has been identified as key to increasing cultural responsiveness in health care (Lowe and Archibald, 2009). By 2050 ethnic minorities are expected to become a numerical majority (Sue and Sue, 2003; Geiger, 2013).

CULTURAL COMPETENCE

Cultural competence is defined as "a set of cultural behaviors and attitudes integrated into the practice methods of a system, agency, or its professionals that enables them to work effectively in cross cultural situations" (Sutton, 2000, p. 58). The concept represents a process, not an event. The Institute of Medicine (IOM, 2003) and the American Association of Colleges of Nursing (AACN, 2008) identify cultural competence as an essential skill set required for professional nurses and other health care providers.

Developing competence begins with self-awareness of your own cultural values, attitudes, and perspectives, followed by developing knowledge and acceptance of cultural differences in others (Gravely, 2001; Leonard and Plotnikoff, 2000). Value judgments are hard to eliminate, particularly those outside of awareness. Self-awareness allows you to own your own biases and not project them onto clients.

Cultural sensitivity is an integral part of competence. The Office of Minority Health (DHHS, 2001) defines *cultural sensitivity* as "the ability to be appropriately responsive to the attitudes, feelings, or circumstances of groups of people that share a common and distinctive racial, national, religious, linguistic, or cultural heritage" (p. 131). Cultural sensitivity emphasizes an openness to different cultural beliefs and values, with a corresponding willingness to incorporate the client's cultural values in care whenever possible. Cultural sensitivity facilitates care and self-management of health conditions. It is hard for clients to overlook a significant tradition. When health recommendations conflict with their worldview, clients are less likely to follow them. Cultural sensitivity is key to safe care (Knoerl, 2011).

Nurses demonstrate cultural sensitivity by using neutral words, categorizations, and behaviors, which are respectful of the client's culture, and avoiding those which could be interpreted as offensive (AACN, 2008). A valuable way to learn about another person's culture is to spend time with them and to ask questions about what is important to them about their culture (Jandt, 2003).

Minority populations, especially new immigrants, have special problems with access and continuity. They often are marginalized economically, occupationally, and socially in ways that adversely affect their access to mainstream health care. Accessing health care can be so frustrating that they give up when they meet even small obstacles. A secondary issue is a lack of knowledge and experience with how to obtain services. Undocumented immigrants have an added burden of fearing deportation if their legal status is revealed (Chung et al., 2008). Nurses can help clients successfully navigate the health care system. Clients also appreciate providers who orient them to the clinical setting and set the stage for a comfortable encounter.

CARE OF THE CULTURALLY DIVERSE CLIENT

By 2050, minority groups are projected to make up 54% of the population in the United States (Florczak, 2013). This section describes the integration of cultural sensitivity into the assessment, diagnosis and treatment planning, implementation, and evaluation of client-centered professional nursing care. Having knowledge and an accepting attitude about the health traditions associated with different cultures increases client comfort and engagement with caregivers. Hulme (2010) distinguishes between the folk domain and alternative health care remedies. She emphasizes the need to understand the client's health care traditions which are "specific to—and fundamentally a part of—an individual's culture" (p. 276).

BUILDING RAPPORT

When meeting a client for the first time, you should introduce yourself, and identify your role.

- Pronounce the client's name correctly. Always ask if you are not sure. Calling the client by title and last name shows respect.
- Speak clearly and spend time with the client before asking assessment questions to make the client or family comfortable.
- Avoid assumptions or interpretations about what you are hearing without validating the information.
- Allot more time to conduct a health assessment, to accommodate language needs and cultural interpretations.
- Take the position of interested co-learner when inquiring about cultural values and standards of behavior.
- Inquire about individual perceptions, as well as cultural explanatory models associated with the illness and preferences for treatment.
- Explain treatment procedures at every opportunity and alert clients ahead of time of potential discomfort.
- Ask permission for and explain the necessity for any physical examination or use of assessment tools.

THEORETICAL FRAMEWORKS

Madeleine Leininger's Theory of Culture Care (Leininger and McFarland, 2006) is recognized as the first major theory-based approach to describe the nature of culture in health care. Leininger believes that nurses must have knowledge about diverse cultures to provide care that fits the client; today this would be viewed as an essential component of client-centered care. Her sunrise model is composed of "enablers," which help explain each person's cultural environmental context, language, and ethnohistory. Enabling factors reflect the person's worldview and a person's social and culture structures. Each influences verbal and nonverbal expressions, patterns, and understandings of health and health practices.

PURNELL'S MODEL

Larry Purnell (2008) considers cultural competence from a macro level (global society, community, family, and the person). Micro levels, consisting of 12 interconnected domains at the individual level, are identified in Table 7-2.

Using Purnell's domains as a framework for understanding individual differences allows for a comprehensive cultural assessment leading to a culturally congruent, individualized, patient-centered approach to client care. Understanding the client's cultural explanation for the health problem is essential, as different cultures frame illness and its cause in various ways. For example, in Asian cultures, depression is characterized as "sadness," rather than a mental disorder. It is not uncommon for Asian and Arab Israeli women to believe that breast cancer is God's will or fate (Baron-Epel et al., 2009; Kim and Flaskerud, 2008). Table 7-3 provides sample questions to assess client preferences when the client is from a different culture.

CULTURAL IMPLICATIONS IN CLIENT-CENTERED DECISION MAKING

National health reform expectations for client-centered care call for a shared client-centered understanding of illness, diagnosis, and prognosis. This expectation may require adaptation with some clients. For example, certain cultures have strong beliefs about providing direct disclosure of diagnosis and prognosis to clients.

TABLE 7-2	Purnell's Domains of Cultural Assessment
Domains of Cultural Assessment	**Sample Areas for Inquiry**
Personal heritage	Country of origin, reasons for migration, politics, class distinctions, education, social and economic status
Communication	Dominant language and dialects, personal space, body language and touch, time relationships, greetings, eye contact
Family roles and organization	Gender roles; roles of extended family, elders, head of household; family goals, priorities, and expectations; lifestyle differences
Workforce issues	Acculturation and assimilation, gender roles, temporality, current and previous jobs, variance in salary and status associated with job changes
Bioecology	Genetics, hereditary factors, ethnic physical characteristics, drug metabolism
High-risk health behaviors	Drugs, nicotine and alcohol use, sexual behaviors
Nutrition	Meaning of food, availability and food preferences, taboos associated with food, use of food in illness
Pregnancy and childbearing	Rituals and constraints during pregnancy, labor and delivery practices, newborn and postpartum care
Death rituals	How death is viewed, death rituals, preparation of the body, care after death, use of advance directives, bereavement practices
Spirituality	Religious practices, spiritual meanings, use of prayer
Health care practices	Traditional practices, religious health care beliefs, individual versus collective responsibility for health, how pain is expressed, transplantation, mental health barriers
Health care practitioners	Use of traditional and/or folk practitioners, gender role preferences in health care

Adapted from Purnell JD, Paulanka BJ: *Transcultural health care: a culturally competent approach*, ed 3, Philadelphia, 2008, F.A. Davis; Purnell, J.D. (2009). *Guide to culturally competent health care*, ed 2, Philadelphia, 2009, F.A. Davis.

TABLE 7-3	Assessing Client Preferences When the Client Is from a Different Culture
Areas to Assess	**Sample Assessment Questions**
Explanatory models of illness	"What do you think caused your health problem? Can you tell me a little about how your illness developed?"
Traditional healing processes	"Can you tell me something about how this problem is handled in your country? Are there any special cultural beliefs about your illness that might help me give you better care? Are you currently using any medications or herbs to treat your illness?"
Lifestyle	"What are some of the foods you like? How are they prepared? What do people do in your culture to stay healthy?"
Type of family support	"Can you tell me who in your family should be involved with your care? Who is the decision maker for health care decisions?"
Spiritual healing practices and rituals	"I am not really familiar with your spiritual practices, but I wonder if you could tell me what would be important to you so we can try to incorporate it into your care plan."
Cultural norms about personal care	"A number of our patients have special needs around personal care, of which we are not always aware. I am wondering if this is true for you and if you could help me understand what you need to be comfortable."
Truth-telling and level of disclosure	Ask the family about cultural ways of talking about serious illness. In some cultures, the family knows the diagnosis/prognosis, which is not told to the ill person (e.g., Hispanic, Asian).
Ritual and religious ceremonies at time of death	Ask the family about special rituals and religious ceremonies at time of death.

Cultural norms may dictate that the family be notified first. Asian and Hispanic cultures traditionally prefer family-centered decision making about care for a family member with a terminal diagnosis (Kwak and Haley, 2005). The family then decides when and if the disclosure should be made to the client. This contingency comes up often enough to warrant your full attention to its implications for care.

Before discussing important health matters, ask the client who should be involved. Careful, unhurried discussion and inclusion of family members in decision-making processes can be helpful. Although informed consent forms require full disclosure, the cultural acceptability of autonomous informed consent can be an ethical issue when interacting with clients who hold different cultural values (Calloway, 2009). When the family is authorized by the client to discuss diagnosis and make treatment decisions, the client's preference should be honored. Exploration of each client's preferences about disclosure should take place early in the clinical relationship.

WORKING WITH LANGUAGE BARRIERS

Clients from different cultures often identify language barriers as the most frustrating aspect of communicating in health care situations. Limited language proficiency is a fundamental barrier to client safety and a client's full participation in learning self-management strategies. For example, in addition to obtaining knowledge about cultural differences, health providers must learn from their clients how these differences influence treatment decisions (Vaughn et al., 2009).

Even if the client speaks relatively good English, always allow additional time for processing. People with English as a second language tend to think and process information in their native language, translating back and forth from English. Language also involves subtleties of meaning (IOM, 2002a, p. 232). Internal interpretation of a message is often accompanied by visual imagery reflecting the person's cultural beliefs and experiences. (This can change the meaning of the original message, with neither party having awareness of the differences in interpretation.) Sometimes the nurse is aware only that the client seems to be taking more time than usual, or seems more anxious. It is important to speak slowly and clearly; use simple words; and avoid slang, technical jargon, and complex sentences.

VALIDATION

Validation is an important communication strategy with culturally diverse clients, as word meanings are not the same even within a culture (Giger, 2012). In many cultures, there is a tendency to view health professionals as authority figures, treating them with deference and respect. This value can be so strong that a client will not question the nurse or in any way indicate mistrust of professional recommendations. They just do not follow the professional advice. Using teach-back and having clients repeat process instructions improves comprehension.

USE OF INTERPRETERS

Federal law (Title VI of the Civil Rights Act) mandates the use of a *trained* interpreter for any client experiencing communication difficulties in health care settings because of language. Interpreters should have a thorough knowledge of the culture, as well as the language. Interpreters should be carefully chosen, keeping in mind variations in dialects, as well as differences in the sex and social status of the interpreter and the client if these factors are likely to be an issue. There are quality assurance and ethical issues associated with the use of untrained interpreters such as family, friends, or ancillary staff. They may not be familiar with medical terminology or may unintentionally misrepresent the meaning of a message. The client may or may not want a relative, friend, or nonprofessional staff to "know their business" or have access to subjective information (Messias et al., 2009). Box 7-2 provides guidelines for the use of interpreters in health care interviews.

TIME ORIENTATION

Culturally, clock time versus activity time can reflect cultural standards (Galanti, 2008). This can be a

BOX 7-2	Guidelines for Using Interpreters in Health Care

- Whenever possible, the translator should not be a family member.
- Orient the translator to the goals of the clinical interview and expected confidentiality.
- Look directly at the client when either you or the client is speaking.
- Ask the translator to clarify anything that is not understood by either the nurse or the client.
- After each completed statement, pause for translation.

major issue when appointments, or medications are involved. Precise time frames are important in low context cultures (North America and Western Europe). People are accustomed to setting, and meeting exact time commitments for appointments and taking medications. In high context cultures, individuals do not consider commitment to a future appointment as important as attending to what is happening in the moment. Contrast the difference in time orientation of a clock-conscious German person with that of his Italian counterpart in the following case example.

Case Example

Germans and Swiss love clock-regulated time, for it appears to them as a remarkably efficient, impartial, and very precise way of organizing life—especially in business. For Italians, on the other hand, time considerations will usually be subjected to human feelings. "Why are you so angry because I came at 9:30?" an Italian asks his German colleague. "Because it says 9 a.m. in my diary," says the German. "Then why don't you write 9:30 and then we'll both be happy?" is a logical Italian response. The business we have to do and our close relations are so important that it is irrelevant at what time we meet. The meeting is what counts (Lewis, 2000, p. 55).

COMMUNICATION PRINCIPLES

Culturally diverse clients respond better to health care providers who ask about and incorporate knowledge of client social circumstances and cultural values into care Knoerl, (2011). Framing interventions that the client recognizes as familiar and valid, and openly discussing differences in backgrounds, norms, and health practices builds trust. Exercise 7-4 provides experience with culture assessment interviews.

The LEARN model is also used to frame clinical teaching and coaching encounters with culturally diverse clients.

- *Listen carefully* to client perceptions and the words the client uses. Ask the client to describe the illness or injury, how it occurred, and what the client believes caused it.
- *Explain what the client needs to understand* about his or her condition or treatment, incorporating client's words and explanatory models. Remember the client is a person first, and a member of a different culture second.
- *Acknowledge cultural differences between nurse and client viewpoints, without devaluing the client's viewpoint.* Respect cultural sources of health care, and incorporate culturally acceptable treatments and interventions when possible. Ask

| EXERCISE 7-4 | Key Informant Cultural Assessment Exercise |

Purpose: To provide practice with assessment related to cultural information.

Procedure
Each person is a key informant about your own culture. Pair off with another student. Interview your student partner about his or her cultural background related to the questions below. Guide the interview process, so that you address all questions.
1. Where did your family originate?
2. What are the cultural values held in your family?
3. What do you believe about the gender roles of men and women? Are your beliefs different or consistent with those of your parents?
4. How much physical distance do you need for comfort in social interactions?
5. Who are the decision makers in your family, and to whom do you look to for guidance in important matters?
6. What are your definitions of health and well-being?

7. If you needed health care, how would you respond to this need, and what would be your expectations?
8. In a health care situation, what would be the role of your family?
9. In a health care situation, how important would religion be, and what would you need for spiritual comfort?
10. What do you like, and dislike about your cultural background?

Discussion
1. What was it like to be the interviewer? The interviewee?
2. How difficult was it for you to really identify some of the behaviors and expectations that are part of your cultural self?
3. Were you surprised with any of your answers? If so, in what ways?
4. How can you use this exercise in communicating with clients from culturally diverse backgrounds?

about cultural and family treatment considerations. Use frequent validation to ensure cultural
appropriateness of provider assumptions.

- *Recommend what the client should do.* Frame
treatment suggestions using a culturally acceptable care process. Invite client participation in
developing a plan that is culturally authentic as
well as therapeutic.
- *Negotiate with the client to culturally adapt constructive self-management strategies, based on client input.* Negotiation of cultural acceptability
is fundamental to client compliance. Familiarity
with formal and informal sources of health care
such as churches, shamans, medicine men and
women, curanderos, and other faith healers provides additional client support.

INFORMED CONSENT AND CLIENT AUTONOMY

Issues of informed consent need to be reframed within
a cultural context (Calloway, 2009). Without full disclosure, consent forms are not valid.

Philosophical differences about end-of-life care
exist between Western values and those of the four
major minority groups. Many minority clients believe
in prolonging life and are reluctant to use advance
directives (Thomas, 2001). Exercise 7-5 provides an
opportunity to explore the role of cultural sensitivity
in care planning.

KEY CULTURAL GROUPS

Wilson (2011) notes, "domains such as family roles,
health care practices, religion, and communication

are essential attributes that define an individual's culture" (p. 222). These attributes provide a framework
for identifying common cultural features of the four
major minority cultures in the United States as discussed in the following sections. There is not a single
"national" culture. Culture plays a significant role in
shaping people's health related beliefs, values, and
behaviors (Betancourt, 2004). As you review each
culture overview, keep in mind that cultural descriptors should be treated as generalized impressions.
Galanti (2008) distinguishes between generalizations, which can be helpful, and stereotypes, which
overlook individual variants in culture values leading
to an inaccurate descriptor.

Case Example

"An example is the assumption that Mexicans have large
families. If I meet Rosa, a Mexican woman, and I say to
myself, "Rosa is Mexican; she must have a large family," I
am stereotyping her. But if I think Mexicans often have
large families and wonder whether Rosa does, I am making a generalization" (Galanti, 2008, p. 7).

HISPANIC/LATINO CULTURE

Hispanic Americans account for 16.7% of the population (Office of Minority Health and Health and
Health Equity [OMHHE], n.d.), making them the
largest minority group in the United States. This figure
is projected to increase to 29% by 2050. Identifying
themselves as Hispanics, or Latinos, this population
is more racially diverse and represents a wider range
of cultures than other minority groups. Within the

EXERCISE 7-5	Applying Cultural Sensitivity to Care Planning

Purpose: To practice cultural sensitivity in care planning.

Procedure
This can be done in small, even-numbered groups
rather than as an individual exercise.
1. Out of class, create a written clinical scenario
based on a culturally diverse client you have
cared for recently. Identify ethnic or cultural factors present in the client's nursing needs.
2. Trade scenarios with another student.
3. Write what should be included in a culturally
sensitive care plan.
4. Discuss each of the care plans and make any
revisions.

Discussion
1. What were the areas of agreement and disagreement about the care plan?
2. What questions would you need to ask to clarify
needs?
3. In developing the plan, did you find any additional
needs?
4. How could you use this exercise to improve your
clinical practice?

Hispanic/Latino populations are Mexican Americans (Chicanos), Puerto Ricans, Cubans, individuals from the Dominican Republic, and South or Central America (Hardin, 2014).

Current growth of the Hispanic population in the United States consists mainly of first-generation and younger immigrants with lower socioeconomic status (SES) and undocumented legal status. Many do not speak English or do not speak it well enough to negotiate the U.S. health care system. Implementation of bilingual and ESOL education programs in schools acknowledges the significance of the growth in the Hispanic population and social repositioning of diversity as a fact of life in the United States.

Family and Gender Roles

Familismo is a strong value in the Hispanic/Latino community. Ayon and colleagues (2010) describe *familismo* as having a strong family loyalty with corresponding responsibilities for ensuring its stability. The "family" includes immediate and extended family members; it is considered a protective factor in promoting the mental health and individual well being of family members. Familismo can extend to helping immigrant family members adjust and navigate the new health care system if resident family members are included in health care visits. The family is the center of Hispanic life and serves as a primary source of emotional support. Hispanic clients are "family members first, and individuals second" (Pagani-Tousignant, 1992, p. 10). Family units tend to live in close proximity with each other and close friends are considered a part of the family unit. Asking about "who" the "family" is for the client, especially in clinical situations involving life transitions, and who needs to be present is important assessment information. Family opinions are sought in decision-making processes. Families show their love and concern in health care situations by pampering the client.

Gender roles are rigid, with the father viewed as head of the household and primary decision maker. Latino women are socialized to serve their husbands and children without question (*la sufrida*, or the long-suffering woman; Pagani-Tousignant, 1992). The nurse needs to be sensitive to gender-specific cultural values in treatment situations.

Religion

Hispanic clients are predominantly Roman Catholic. Latino families have strong cultural values and beliefs about the sanctity of life. Receiving the sacraments is important, and calls for family celebration. The final sacrament in the Roman Catholic Church, anointing of the sick, offers comfort for clients and families. Faith in God is closely linked with the Hispanic population's understanding of health care problems (Zapata and Shippee-Rice, 1999). Their relationship with God is an intimate one, which may include personal visions of God or saints. This should not be interpreted as a hallucination. Hispanic clients view health as a gift from God, related to physical, emotional, and social balance (Kemp, 2004). Many believe that illness is the result of a great fright (*susto*), or falling out of favor with God. "Santeros" are folk healers whose healing powers derive from the power of the saints. Santeros may prescribe lighting of candles or incense, as well as herbs and ointments, which are purchased from a spiritual pharmacy.

Health Beliefs and Practices

Latinos have a lower prevalence for chronic disorders in general than the nation's overall population, with the exception of diabetes (Livingston et al., 2008). They are less likely to have a regular health provider and use the formal health care system episodically, as a short-term problem-solving strategy for health problems. Many are illegal immigrants, making them ineligible for health insurance. A source of health care outside the family is the use of *curanderos* (local folk healers and herb doctors) for initial care. The *curandera* uses a combination of prayers, healing practices, medicines, and herbs to cure illness (Amerson, 2008).

Latino clients may identify a "hot-cold balance," referring to a cultural classification of illness resulting from an imbalance of body humors, as essential for health. When a person loses balance, illness follows (Juckett, 2005). "Cold" health conditions are treated with hot remedies, and vice versa. Mental illness is not addressed as such. Instead, a Hispanic client will talk of being sad *(triste)*. Modesty is important to Hispanic women. Women may be reluctant to express their private concerns in front of their children, even adult children.

It is not uncommon for clients to share medications with other family members. Aponte (2009) suggests that nurses should ask Hispanic clients about the use of folk medicine and explain, if needed, the reason and importance of sharing this information with the nurse. A proactive prevention approach tailored to the health care needs of this minority population is essential.

Communication and Social Interaction Patterns

Spanish is the primary language spoken in all Latin American countries except Brazil (Portuguese) and Haiti (French). Hispanics are an extroverted people who value interpersonal relationships. Hispanic clients trust feelings more than facts. Strict rules govern social relationships (*respecto*), with higher status being given to older individuals, and to male over female individuals. Nurses are viewed as authority figures, to be treated with respect. Clients hesitate to ask questions, so it is important to ask enough questions to ensure that your clients understand their diagnosis and treatment plan (Aponte, 2009).

Hispanic clients look for warmth, respect, and friendliness (*personalismo*) from their health care providers. It is important to ask about their well-being and to take extra time with finding out what they need. They value smooth social relations, and avoid confrontation and criticism (*simpatia*). Hispanic people are sensitive and easily hurt.

The Latino culture is a high context culture from a communication perspective. Hispanic clients need to develop trust (*confianza*) in the health care provider. They do this by making small talk before getting down to the business of discussing their health problems. Knowing the importance of *confianza* to the Hispanic client allows nurses to spend initial time engaging in general topics before moving into assessment or care (Knoerl, 2007).

AFRICAN AMERICAN CULTURE

African Americans account for approximately 14.2% of the U.S. population (OMHHE, n.d.), making them the second largest minority group in the nation. Purnell and colleagues (2008) note, "Black or African American refers to people having origins in any of the black racial groups of Africa, and includes Nigerians and Haitians or any person who self-designates this category regardless of origin" (p. 2). Although African Americans are represented in every socioeconomic group, approximately one-third of them live in poverty (Spector, 2004).

For too many, their cultural heritage traces back to cultural oppression. This unfortunate legacy colors the expectations of African Americans with health care issues, and explains the mistrust many African Americans have about the American health care system (Eiser and Ellis, 2007; Wilson, 2011). African Americans need to experience feeling respected by their caregivers to counteract the sense of powerlessness and lack of confidence they sometimes feel in health care settings.

The African American worldview consists of four fundamental characteristics:

- *Interdependence:* feeling interconnected and as concerned about the welfare of others as of themselves
- *Emotional vitality:* expressed with intensity and animation in lifestyle, dance, language, and music
- *Harmonious blending:* "going with the flow" or natural rhythm of life
- *Collective survival:* sharing and cooperation is essential to everyone surviving and succeeding (Parham et al., 2000)

Family and Gender Roles

The family is considered the "primary and most important tradition in the African American community" (Hecht et al., 2003, p. 2). Women are often considered the head of the family, consistent with vestiges of a matriarchal tradition in many African villages. Many low-income African American children grow up in extended families.

African American older women are referred to as "the backbone" of the African American family and community (Carthron et al., 2014). They assume multiple roles in church and community, and often assume caregiving responsibilities for working parents. Including grandparents, particularly grandmothers, is useful when caring for African American clients in the community (Purnell et al., 2008).

African Americans depend on kinship networks for support. Loyalty to the extended family is a dominant value, and family members rely on each other for emotional and financial support (Sterritt and Pokorny, 1998). The combination of strong kinship bonds and the value of "caring for one's own" are important aspects of the African American culture. Caring for less fortunate family members is viewed as a resource strength of African American families (Littlejohn-Blake and Darling, 1993). Family members want to be involved when one of their members is ill: It is not unusual to have five or six people descend on a client's hospital room. When planning interventions, taking advantage of kinship bonds and incorporating family as supportive networks can greatly enhance the quality of care.

Religion and Spiritual Practices

Spirituality is a very important deep dimension of all aspects of life. Faith represents a *personal connected* relationship with God, or a higher being, experienced as an essential life support. Honoring God, self, and others is important for personal health (Lewis et al., 2007). The church serves the dual purpose of providing a structure for meeting spiritual needs and functioning as a primary social, economic, and community life center. Chambers (1997) explains, "Since its inception, the black church has been more than a place of worship for African-Americans. It is where the community has gathered to lobby for freedom and equal rights" (p. 42). African American political leaders (e.g., Jesse Jackson and Dr. Martin Luther King, Jr.) are revered as influential church leaders. Major religions include Christianity (predominantly Protestant), Islam, and Pentecostal.

Christianity is often associated with evangelical expression. Prayer and the "laying on of hands" are important to many African American clients (Purnell et al., 2008). Because of the central meaning of the church in African American life, incorporating appropriate clergy as a resource in treatment is a useful strategy. Readings from the Bible and gospel hymns are sources of support during hospitalization. Barton-Burke and colleagues (2010) suggest that care interventions should address the client's spiritual needs.

Islam in America is considered a religious tradition rather than a political movement. African Americans account for approximately 30% of the U.S. Muslim population. Islam influences all aspects of life. Muslim clients are expected to follow the Halal (lawful) diet, which calls for dietary restrictions on eating pork or pork products and drinking alcohol (Rashidi and Rajaram, 2001).

Health Beliefs and Practices

African Americans suffer more health disparities than any other minority population (Hopp and Herring, 2014). African Americans have higher rates of hypertension, adolescent pregnancy, diabetes, heart disease, and stroke, and male African Americans have a significantly greater chance of developing cancer and of dying of it (Spector, 2004). Lower income African American clients statistically are less likely to use regular preventive health services. Because of cost, many African Americans use emergency departments as a major health care resource (Lynch and Hanson, 2004).

African Americans tend to rely on informal helping networks in the community, particularly those associated with their churches, until a health problem becomes a crisis. Purnell and colleagues (2008) advise engagement of the extended family system, particularly grandmothers, in providing support and health teaching when working with African American clients in the community.

Communication and Social Interaction

Establishing trust is essential for successful communication with African American clients. They are more willing to participate in treatment when they feel respected and are treated as treatment partners in their health care. Allowing clients to have as much control over their health care as possible reinforces self-efficacy and promotes self-esteem. Recognizing and respecting African American values of interdependence, emotional vitality, and collective survival helps facilitate confidence in health care. Awareness of community resources in the African American community and incorporation of informal care networks such as the church, neighbors, and extended family can help provide culturally congruent continuity of care.

ASIAN AMERICAN

As of 2010, Asian Americans were estimated to make up 4.8% of the U.S. population and represented the fastest growing minority group (Hoeffel et al, 2012; OMHEE, n.d.) of all major ethnic groups. Asians and Pacific Islanders comprise more than 32 ethnic groups, among them people from China, the Philippines, Japan, Vietnam, Laos, Cambodia, and India (Hardin, 2014). Even within the same geographic grouping, significant cultural differences exist. For example, in India, there are more than 350 "major languages," with 18 being acknowledged as "official languages," and a complex caste system defines distinctive behavioral expectations for gender roles within the broader culture (Chaudhary, 2004).

Asian cultures value hard work, education, and going with the flow of events. There is an emphasis on politeness and correct behavior. The appropriate cultural behavior is to put others first, and to not create problems. This standard can lead to vagueness in communication that is not always understandable to cultures using a direct communication style. Traditionally, Asian clients exercise emotional restraint in communication, stoicism with pain, and controlled facial expressions. Interpersonal conflicts are not directly addressed, and challenging an expert is not allowed (Chen, 2001). Jokes and humor are usually not appreciated because "the Confucian and Buddhist preoccupation with truth, sincerity, kindliness and politeness automatically eliminates humour techniques such as sarcasm, satire, exaggeration and parody" (Lewis, 2000, pp. 20-21).

Family and Gender Roles

Asian families traditionally live in multigenerational households, with extended family providing important social support. Individual privacy is uncommon. The Asian culture places family before individual welfare. Family members will sacrifice their individuality if needed for the good of the family. The need to avoid "loss of face" by acting in a manner that brings shame to the individual is paramount, because loss of face brings shame to the whole family, including ancestors.

The "family" may consist of the nuclear family, grandparents, and other relatives living together; or a broken family in which some family members are in the United States and other nuclear family members still live in their country of origin (Gelles, 1995). There is family pressure on younger members to do well academically, and the behavior of individual members is considered within the context of its impact on the family as a whole. Family members are obligated to assume a great deal of responsibility for each other, including ongoing financial assistance. Older children are responsible for the well-being of younger children.

Family communication takes place through prescribed roles and obligations, taking into account family roles, age, and position in the family. The husband (father) is the primary authority and decision maker. He acts as the family spokesperson in crisis situations. Elders in the Asian community are highly respected and well taken care of by younger members of the family (Pagani-Tousignant, 1992). The wisdom of the elders helps guide younger family members on many life issues, including major health decisions (Davis, 2000).

The family is a powerful force in maintaining the religious and social values in Asian cultures. "Good health" is described as having harmonious family relationships and a balanced life (Harrison et al., 2005). Tradition strongly regulates individual behavior. Traditional Chinese culture does not allow clients to discuss the full severity of an illness; this creates challenges for mutual decision making based on full disclosure that is characteristic of Western health care. Family members take an active role in deciding whether a diagnosis should be disclosed to a client. They frequently are the recipients of this information before the client is told of the diagnosis, prognosis, and treatment options.

Religion and Spiritual Practices

Religion plays an important role in Asian society, with religious beliefs tightly interwoven into virtually every aspect of daily life. Referred to as "Eastern religions," major groups include Hindus, Buddhists, and Muslims.

Hinduism is not a homogeneous religion, but rather a living faith and philosophical way of life with diverse doctrines, religious symbols, and moral and social norms (Michaels, 2003). Being a Hindu provides membership in a communal society. Hinduism represents a pragmatic philosophy of life that articulates harmony with the natural rhythms of life, and "right" or "correct" principles of social interaction and behavior. The *veda* refers to knowledge passed through many generations from ancient sages, which combined with Sanskrit literature provides the "codes of ritual, social and ethical behavior, called dharma, which that literature reveals" (Flood, 1996, p. 11). Hindus are vegetarians: It is against their religion to kill living creatures. Sikhism is a reformed variation of Hinduism in which women have more rights in domestic and community life.

Buddhism represents a philosophical approach to life that identifies fate, referred to as the four noble truths. Buddhists believe:

1. All life is suffering.
2. Suffering is caused by desire or attachment to the world.
3. Suffering can be extinguished by eliminating desire
4. The way to eliminate desire is to live a virtuous life (Lynch and Hanson, 2004).

Buddhists follow the path to enlightenment by leading a moral life, being mindful of personal thoughts and actions, and by developing wisdom and understanding. Buddhists pray and meditate frequently. They eat a vegetarian diet, and alcohol, cigarettes, and drugs are not permitted.

The Muslim religion (Islam) is a way of life. Muslims adhere to the Quran/Koran, the holy teaching of Muhammad. Faith, prayer, giving alms, and making a yearly pilgrimage to Mecca are requirements of the religion. Identified as an Eastern monotheistic religion, Islam is practiced throughout the world. Followers are called Muslims. Allah is identified as a higher power or God. Muhammad is his prophet. Muslims submit to Allah and follow Allah's basic rules about everything from personal relationships to business matters, including personal matters such as dress and hygiene. Islam has strong tenets that affect health care, an important one being that God is the ultimate healer.

Dietary restrictions center on consuming Halal (lawful) food. Excluded from the diet are pork and pork products, and alcohol. In the hospital, Muslims can order Kosher food because it meets the requirements for Halal (Davidson et al., 2008). The Muslim client values physical modesty, and the family may request that only female staff care for female family members. Physical contact, eye contact, touch, and hugs between members of the opposite sex who are not family are avoided (McKennis, 1999).

Muslims believe death is a part of Allah's plan, so to fight the dying process with treatment is wrong. They believe that the dying person should not die alone. A close relative should be present, praying for God's blessing or reading the Quran/Koran. Once the person actually dies, it is important to perform the following: turn the body toward Mecca; close the person's mouth and eyes, and cover the face; straighten the legs and arms; announce the death to relatives and friends; bathe the body (with men bathing men and women bathing women); and cover the body with white cotton (Servodido and Morse, 2001).

Health Care Beliefs and Practices

Health is based on the ayurvedic principle, which requires harmony and balance between yin and yang, as the two energy forces required for health (Louie, 2001). A blockage of qi, defined as the energy circulating in a person's body, creates an imbalance between yin (negative energy force) and yang (positive energy force), resulting in illness (Chen, 2001). Yin represents the female force, containing all the elements that represent darkness, cold, and weakness. Yang symbolizes the male elements of strength, brightness, and warmth. Ayurveda emphasizes health promotion and disease prevention.

The influence of Eastern health practices and alternative medicine is increasingly incorporated into the health care of all Americans. Many complementary and alternative medical practices in the United States (acupuncture, botanicals, and massage and therapeutic touch) trace their roots to Eastern holistic health practices. Acupressure and herbal medicines are among the traditional medical practices used by Asian clients to reestablish the balance between yin and yang. In some Asian countries, healers use a process of "coining," in which a coin is heated and vigorously rubbed on the body to draw illness out of the body. The resulting welts can mistakenly be attributed to child abuse if this practice is not understood. Traditional healers, such as Buddhist monks, acupuncturists, and herbalists, also may be consulted when someone is ill.

Asian clients typically respond better to a formal relationship and an indirect communication style characterized by polite phrases and marked deference. They work better with well-defined boundaries and clear expectations (Galanti, 2008). The client waits for the information to be offered by the nurse as the authority figure. Sometimes this gets interpreted as timidity. A better interpretation is that the client is deferring to the health professional's expertise.

Sometimes it is difficult to tell what Asian clients are experiencing. Facial expressions are not as flexible, and words are not as revealing as those of people in other cultures. Asian clients may not request pain medication until their pain is quite severe (Im, 2008). Asking the client about pain and offering medication as normal clinical management usually is needed.

Health care concerns specifically relevant to this population include a higher-than-usual incidence of tuberculosis, hepatitis B, and liver cancer (OMHHE, n.d.). People with mental health issues do not seek early treatment because of shame and the lack of culturally appropriate mental health services (Louie, 2001).

Asian men may have a difficult time disclosing personal information to a female nurse unless the nurse explains why the data are necessary for care, because in serious matters, women are not considered as knowledgeable as men. Asian clients may be reluctant to be examined by a person of the opposite sex, particularly if the examination or treatment involves intimate areas.

Social Interaction Patterns

Communication behaviors in the Asian culture are characterized by mutuality, respect, and honesty (Chen, 2007). Health care providers are considered health experts, so they are expected to provide specific advice and recommendations (Lynch and Hanson, 2004). Asian clients prefer a polite, friendly, but formal approach in communication. They appreciate clinicians willing to provide advice in a matter-of-fact, concise manner. Always ask what a behavior means to a client, as misinterpretations can easily occur

Asian clients favor harmonious relationships. Confrontation is avoided; clients will nod and smile in agreement, even when they strongly disagree (Cross and Bloomer, 2010; Xu et al., 2004). Nurses need to ask open-ended questions and clarify issues throughout an interaction. If you use questions that require a yes or no answer, the answer may reflect the client's polite deference rather than an honest response. Explain treatment as problem solving, ask the client how things are done in his or her culture, and work with your Asian client to develop culturally congruent solutions (McLaughlin and Braun, 1998).

NATIVE AMERICAN CLIENTS

Native Americans account for 1.7% of the U.S. population (OMHHE, n.d.). American Indians and Alaska natives trace their origins to the original populations of North, Central, and South America. There are more than 500 federally recognized tribes, and another 100 tribes or bands that are state-recognized but are not recognized by the federal government. Native Americans include First or Original Americans, American Indians, Alaskan Natives, Aleuts, Eskimos, Metis (mixed blood), or Amerindians. Most will identify themselves as members of a specific tribe (Garrett and Herring, 2001). Tribal identity is maintained through regular powwows and other ceremonial events. Like other minority groups with an oppressed heritage, the majority of Native Americans are poor and undereducated, with associated higher rates of social and health problems (Hodge et al, 2014).

Family and Gender Roles

The family is highly valued by Native Americans. Multigenerational families live together in close proximity. When two individuals marry, the marriage contract implicitly includes attachment and obligation to a larger kinship system (Red Horse, 1997). Both men and women feel a responsibility to promote tribal values and traditions through their crafts and traditional ceremonies. However, women are identified as their culture's standard bearers. A Cheyenne proverb graphically states, "A nation is not conquered until

the hearts of its women are on the ground. Then it is done, no matter how brave its warriors nor how strong their weapons" (Crow Dog and Erdoes, 1990, p. 3), and Cheshire (2001) notes, "It is the women—the mothers, grandmothers and aunties—that keep Indian nations alive" (p. 1534).

Gender roles are egalitarian, and women are valued. Being a mother and auntie gives a social standing as a life giver related to the survival of the tribe (Barrios and Egan, 2002). Because the family matriarch is a primary decision maker, her approval and support may be required for compliance with a treatment plan (Cesario, 2001).

Native American culture is high context. Identifying and including from the outset all those who will be taking an active part in the care of the client recognizes the communal nature of family involvement in health care. For the Native American client, this may include members of an immediate tribe or its spokesperson.

Spiritual and Religious Practices

The religious beliefs of Native Americans are strongly linked with nature and the earth. There is a sense of sacredness in everyday living between "grandmother earth" and "grandfather sky" that tends to render the outside world extraneous (Kavanagh et al., 1999, p. 25).

Health Beliefs and Practices

Native Americans suffer from greater rates of mortality from chronic diseases such as tuberculosis, alcoholism, diabetes, and pneumonia. Domestic violence, often associated with alcoholism, is a significant health concern. Pain assessment is important, because the Native American client tends to display a stoic response to pain (Cesario, 2001). Health concerns of particular relevance to the Native American population are unintentional injuries (of which 75% are alcohol related), cirrhosis, alcoholism, and obesity. Homicide and suicide rates are significantly greater for Native Americans (Meisenhelder et al., 2000).

Illness is viewed as a punishment from God for some real or imagined imbalance with nature. Native Americans believe illness to be divine intervention to help the individual correct evil ways, and spiritual beliefs play a significant role in the maintenance and restoration of health (Cesario, 2001; Meisenhelder et al., 2000). Spiritual ceremonies and prayers form an important part of traditional healing activities, and healing practices are strongly embedded in religious beliefs. Recovery occurs after the person is cleansed of "evil spirits."

Medical help is sought from tribal elders and shamans (highly respected spiritual medicine men and women) who use spiritual healing practices and herbs to cure the ill member of the tribe (Pagani-Tousignant, 1992). For example, spiritual and herbal tokens or medicine bags placed at the bedside or in an infant's crib are essential to the healing process and should not be disturbed (Cesario, 2001). Native Americans view death as a natural process, but they fear the power of dead spirits and use numerous tribal rituals to ward them off.

Social Interaction Patterns

Respect is a core value in American Indian and Alaska Native cultures (Hodges et al, 2014). Building a trusting relationship with the health care provider is important to the Native American client. They respond best to health professionals who stick to the point and do not engage in small talk. Conversely, they love story telling and appreciate humor.

Nurses need to understand the value of nonverbal communication and taking time in conversations with Native American clients. Direct eye contact is considered disrespectful. Listening is considered a sign of respect and essential to learning about the other (Kalbfleisch, 2009). The client is likely to speak in a low tone. Native Americans are private people who respect the privacy of others and prefer to talk about the facts rather than emotions about them.

Native Americans live in "present" time. They have little appreciation of scheduled time commitments, which in their mind do not necessarily relate to what needs to be achieved. For Native Americans, being on time or taking medication with meals (when three meals are taken on one day and two meals are eaten on another day) has little relevance (Kavanagh et al., 1999). Understanding time from a Native American perspective decreases frustration. Calling the client before making a home visit or to remind the client of an appointment is a useful strategy.

Verbal instructions delivered in a story-telling format is more familiar to Native Americans (Hodge et al., 2002). Preferred learning style is observational and oral; charts, written instructions, and pamphlets are not well received. Native Americans are experiential learners, but their cultural posture may not show the same type of engagement commonly seen in client education.

Case Example

When the nurse is performing a newborn bath demonstration, the Native American mother is likely to watch from a distance, avoid eye contact with the demonstrator, ask few or no questions, and decline a return demonstration. This learning style should not be seen as indifference or lack of understanding. Being an experiential learner, the Native American woman is likely to assimilate the information provided and simply give the newborn a bath when it is needed (Cesario, 2001, p. 17).

POVERTY

Poverty is a difficult, but important sociocultural concept, particularly in today's uncertain economy. Commitment to the health of vulnerable populations, and the elimination of health disparities is identified as one of the five competencies required to provide culturally competent care; it is an overarching goal for *Healthy People 2020*.

Recent research suggests that socioeconomic status SES "drives health disparities more than minority status" (Barton-Burke, et al. 2010, p. 158). The plight of those who fall below the poverty line is significant enough to warrant special consideration of their needs in health care settings. Raphael (2009) notes, "Poverty is not only the primary determinant of children's intellectual, emotional, and social development but also an excellent predictor of virtually every adult disease known to medicine" (p. 10).

People living in poverty have to think carefully about seeking medical attention for anything other than an emergency situation. The emergency department becomes a primary health care resource, and health-seeking behaviors tend to be crisis oriented. Things that most of us take for granted, such as food, housing, clothing, the chance for a decent job, and the opportunity for education, are not available, or are insufficient to realistically meet needs. People at the poverty level have to worry on a daily basis about how to provide for basic human needs. Usually they are less educated and have more limited knowledge of healthy lifestyle-promoting activities.

Lack of essential resources is associated with political and personal powerlessness (Reutter et al., 2009). The idea that the poor can exercise choice, or make a difference in their lives, is not necessarily part of their worldview. People living in poverty overlook opportunities simply because life experience tells them that they cannot trust their own efforts to produce change. They want, but do not really expect their health providers to help. This mindset prompts people living in poverty to avoid and distrust the health care system for anything other than emergencies. If they are treated less favorably than people with money or good insurance, this further exacerbates their sense of helplessness in the health care system. Care strategies require a proactive, persistent, client-oriented approach to helping clients and families self-manage health problems.

Respect for the human dignity of the poor client is a major component of proactive care. This means that the nurse pays strict attention to personal biases and stereotypes so as not to distort assessment data or impede caring implementation of nursing interventions. It means treating each client as "culturally unique" with a set of assumptions and values regarding the disease process and its treatment, and acting in a nonjudgmental manner that respects the client's cultural integrity (Haddad, 2001). Ethics become particularly important in client situations requiring informed consent, health care decision making, involvement of family and significant others, treatment access and care choices, and decisions about end-of-life care.

SUMMARY

This chapter explores the intercultural communication that takes place when the nurse and client are from different cultures. Culture is defined as a common collectivity of beliefs, values, shared understandings, and patterns of behavior of a designated group of people. Culture needs to be viewed as a human structure with many variations in meaning.

Related terms include cultural diversity, cultural relativism, subculture, ethnicity, ethnocentrism, and ethnography. Each of these concepts broadens the definition of culture. Intercultural communication is defined as a communication in which the sender of a message is a member of one culture and the receiver of the message is from a different culture. Different languages create and express different personal realities.

A cultural assessment is defined as a systematic appraisal of beliefs, values, and practices conducted to determine the context of client needs and to tailor nursing interventions. It is composed of three progressive, interconnecting elements: a general assessment, a problem-specific assessment, and the cultural details needed for successful implementation.

Knowledge and acceptance of the client's right to seek and support alternative health care practices dictated by culture can make a major difference in compliance and successful outcome. Health care professionals sometimes mistakenly assume that illness is a single concept, but illness is a personal experience, strongly colored by cultural norms, values, social roles, and religious beliefs. Interventions that take into consideration the specialized needs of the client from a culturally diverse background follow the mnemonic LEARN: Listen, Explain, Acknowledge, Recommend, and Negotiate.

Some basic thoughts about the traditional characteristics of the largest minority groups (African American, Hispanic, Asian, Native American) living in the United States relating to communication preferences, perceptions about illness, family, health, and religious values are included in the chapter. The culture of poverty is discussed.

ETHICAL DILEMMA   What Would You Do?

Antonia Martinez is admitted to the hospital and needs immediate surgery. She speaks limited English, and her family is not with her. She is frightened by the prospect of surgery and wants to wait until her family can be with her to help her make the decision about surgery. As a nurse, you feel there is no decision to be made: She must have the surgery, and you need to get her consent form signed now. What would you do?

DISCUSSION QUESTIONS

1. In what ways does your own culture influence the way you think and feel and act toward someone of another culture?
2. Think of a person or a client from another culture, and describe how you think that this person perceives or responds to you as someone from a different culture.

REFERENCES

Alexander G: Cultural competence models in nursing, *Crit Care Nurs Clin North Am* 20:415–421, 2008.
Allport G: *The nature of prejudice*, Reading, MA, 1979, Addison-Wesley.

American Association of Colleges of Nursing: *The essentials of baccalaureate education for professional nursing practice.* Retrieved from http://www.aacn.nche.edu/educationresources/BaccEssentials08.pdf, 2008.

American Association of Colleges of Nursing: *The essentials of master's education on nursing.* Retrieved from http://www.aacn.nche.edu/education resources/Masters Essentials11.pdf, 2011.

Amerson R: Reflections on a conversation with a curandera, *J Transcult Nurs* 19(4):384–387, 2008.

Anderson P, Wang H: Beyond language: nonverbal communication across cultures. In Samovar L, Porter R, McDaniel E. (editors) Intercultural Communication: A Reader. ed. 12, Belmont CA, Wadsworth, 2008.

Aponte J: Addressing cultural heterogeneity among Hispanic subgroups by using Campinha-Bacote's model of cultural competency, *Holist Nurs Pract* 23(1):3–12, 2009. quiz 13–14.

Aroian K, Faville K: Reconciling cultural relativism for a clinical paradigm: what's a nurse to do? *J Prof Nurs* 21(6):330, 2005.

Ayon C, Marsiglia F, Bermudez-Parsai M: Latino family mental health: exploring the role of discrimination and familismo, *J Community Psychol* 38(6):742–756, 2010.

Bacallao M, Smokowski P: "Entre dos mundos" (between two worlds): bicultural skills with Latino immigrant families, *J Prim Prev* 26(6):485–509, 2005.

Baron-Epel O, Friedman N, Lernau O O, et al.: Fatalism and mammography in a multicultural population, *Oncol Nurs Forum* 36(3):353–361, 2009.

Barrios PG, Egan M: Living in a bicultural world and finding the way home: native women's stories, *Affilia* 17:206–228, 2002.

Barton-Burke M, Smith E, Frain J, Loggins C: Advanced cancer in underserved populations, *Semin Oncol Nurs* 26(3):157–167, 2010.

Betancourt J: Cultural competence—marginal or mainstream movement, *N Engl J Med* 35(10):953–955, 2004.

Betancourt J, Green A, Carrillo J: Defining cultural competence: A practical framework for addressing racial/ethnic disparities in health and health care, *Public Health Reports* 118:293–302, 2003.

Black P: A guide to providing culturally appropriate care, *Gastrointest Nurs* 6(6):10–17, 2008.

Callister L: Culturally competent care of women and newborns: knowledge, attitude, and skills, *J Obstet Gynecol Neonatal Nurs* 30(2):209–215, 2001.

Calloway S: The effect of culture on beliefs related to autonomy and informed consent, *J Cult Divers* 16(2):68–70, 2009.

Canales M, Howers H: Expanding conceptualizations of culturally competent care, *J Adv Nurs* 36(1):102–111, 2001.

Carrese JA, Rhodes LA: Bridging cultural differences in medical practice, *J Gen Intern Med* 15:92–96, 2000.

Carthron D, Bailey D, Anderson R: The "invisible caregiver": multi-caregiving among diabetic African American grandmothers, *Geriatr Nurs* 35:S32–S36, 2014.

Cesario S: Care of the Native American woman: strategies for practice, education and research, *J Obstet Gynecol Neonatal Nurs* 30(1):13–19, 2001.

Chambers V, Higgins C: Say amen, indeed, *American Way* 30(4):38–43, 102–105. 1997.

Chaudhary N: *Listening to culture: constructing reality from every day talk,* Thousand Oaks CA, 2004, Sage Publications, Inc.

Chen GM, editor: Communication and culture in global context [Special issue], *Intercult Comm Stud* 16(1):1–262, 2007.

Chen YC Chinese values, health and nursing. *J Adv Nurs* 36(2): 270–273, 2001.

Cheshire T: Cultural transmission in urban American Indian families, *Am Behav Sci* 44(9):1528–1535, 2001.

Chung R, Bernak F F, Otiz C D, et al.: Promoting the mental health of immigrants: a multicultural/social justice perspective, *J Couns Dev* 86:310–317, 2008.

Cross W, Bloomer M: Extending boundaries: clinical communication with culturally and linguistically diverse mental health clients and carers, *Int J Ment Health Nurs* 19:268–277, 2010.

Crow Dog M, Erdoes R R: *Lakota woman,* New York, 1990, Grove Weidenfeld.

Davidson J, Boyer M, Casey D, et al.: Gap analysis of cultural and religious needs of hospitalized patients, *Crit Care Nurs Q* 31(2):119–126, 2008.

Davis R: The convergence of health and family in the Vietnamese culture, *J Fam Nurs* 6(2):136–156, 2000.

Day-Vines N, Wood S, Grothaus T, et al.: Broaching the subjects of race, ethnicity and culture during the counseling process, *J Couns Dev* 85:401–409, 2007.

U.S. Department of Health and Human Services (DHHS): Healthy People 2020: Disparities. Available at http://healthypeople.gov/2020/about/Disparities About.aspx, 2010.

Donnermeyer J, Friedrich L: Amish society: an overview reconsidered, *J Multicult Nurs* 12(3):36–43, 2006.

Drench M, Noonan A, Sharby N, et al.: *Psychosocial aspects of health care,* ed 2, Upper Saddle River, NJ, 2009, Pearson Prentice Hall.

Edwards K: Disease prevention strategies to decrease health disparities, *J Cult Divers* 16(1):3–4, 2009.

Eiser A, Ellis G: Cultural competence and the African American experience with health care: the case for specific content in cross-cultural education, *Acad Med* 82:176–183, 2007.

Flood G: *An introduction to Hinduism,* Cambridge, 1996, Cambridge University Press.

Florczak K: Culture: fluid and complex, *Nursing Science Quarterly* 26(1):12–13, 2013.

Ford M, Kelly P: Conceptualizing and categorizing race and ethnicity in health services research, *Health Serv Res* 40 (5 pt 2):1658–1675, 2005.

Galanti G: *Caring for patients from different cultures,* ed 4, Philadelphia, 2008, University of Pennsylvania Press.

Garrett M, Herring R: Honoring the power of relations: counseling Native adults, *J Humanist Couns Educ Dev* 40(20):139–140, 2001.

Gelles R: *Contemporary families,* Thousand Oaks, CA, 1995, Sage.

Giger, J. N (2013). Transcultural nursing: Assessment and intervention. 6th ed. Mosby.

Giger J, Davidhizar R, Purnell L, et al.: American Academy of Nursing Expert panel Report: developing competence to eliminate health disparities in ethnic minorities and other vulnerable populations, *J Transcult Nurs* 18(2):95–102, 2007.

Gravely S: When your patient speaks Spanish—and you don't, *RN* 64(5):64–67, 2001.

Haddad A: Ethics in action, *RN* 64(3):21–22, 2001. 24.

Hall E: *Beyond Culture,* Garden City NY, 1976, Doubleday.

Hardin S: Ethnogeriatrics in critical care, *Crit Care Nurs N Am* 26:21–30, 2014.

Hoeffel E, Rastogi S, Kim M, Shahid H: The Asian population: 2010 census briefs. www.census.gov/rpod/cen2010/briefs/c2010br-11pdf, 2012 (Issued, March 2012)>.

Harrison G, Kagawa-Singer M, Foerster S, et al.: Seizing the moment, *Cancer* 15(104–112 Suppl):2962–2968, 2005.

CDC (Page last updated March 14, 2014) *Healthy People 2020 Social Determinants of Health* http://www.cdc.gov/socialdeterminants/Definitions.html.

Hecht G, Ronald L, L Jackson L, et al.: *African American communication: identity and cultural interpretation,* Mahwah, NJ, 2003, Erlbaum.

Hodge F, Rodriguez'g Hodge C: Health and disease of American Indian and Alaska Native Populations: An overview. In Huff R, Kline M, editors: *Promoting health in multicultural populations, 2nd ed*, Thousand Oaks, CA, 2014, Sage Publications, pp 270–291.

Hodge FS A, Pasqua A, Marquez C, et al.: Utilizing traditional storytelling to promote wellness in American Indian communities, *J Transcult Nurs* 13(1):6–11, 2002.

Hofstede G, Pedersen P, Hofsted GH, et al.: *Exploring culture: exercises, stories, and synthetic cultures*, Yarmouth, ME, 2002, Intercultural Press, Inc.

Hofstede G: Dimensionalizing cultures: The Hofstede Model in context, *Online Readings in Psychology and Culture* 2(1), 2011. http://dx.doi.org/10.9707/2307-0919.1014.

Hopp J, Herring RP: Promoting health among Black Americans: An overview. In Huff R, Kline M, editors: *Promoting health in multicultural populations, 2nd ed*, Thousand Oaks, C, 2014, Sage Publications, pp 238–269.

Hulme P: *Cultural considerations in evidence-based practice* 21(3):271–280, 2010.

Im E: The situation specific theory of pain experience for Asian American cancer patients, *Adv Nurs Sci* 31(4O):319–331, 2008.

Institute of Medicine: *The future of nursing: Leading change, advancing health*, Washington, DC, 2011, National Academy Press.

Institute of Medicine (IOM): *Unequal treatment: confronting racial and ethnic disparities in health care*, Washington, DC, 2003, National Academy Press.

Institute of Medicine (IOM): *Speaking of health: assessing health communication strategies for diverse populations*, Washington DC, 2002a, National Academy Press.

Institute of Medicine (IOM): *Unequal Treatment. What healthcare providers need to know about racial and ethnic disparities in healthcare*, Washington, D.C, 2002b, National Academy Press. Author.

Isaacson M: Clarifying concepts: cultural humility or competence, *J Prof Nurs* 30:251–258, 2014.

Jandt F: *An introduction to intercultural communication: identities in a global community*, Thousand Oaks, CA, 2003, Sage Publications.

Juckett G: Cross cultural medicine, *Am Fam Physician* 1(72):2189–2190, 2005.

Kalbfleisch P: Effective health communication in native populations in North America, *J Lang Soc Psychol* 28(2):158–173, 2009.

Karim K: Informing cancer patients: truth telling and culture, *Cancer Nurs Pract* 2:23–31, 2003.

Kavanagh K, Absalom K, Beil W, et al.: Connecting and becoming culturally competent: a Lakota example, *Adv Nurs Sci* 21(3):9–31, 1999.

Kemp C: *Mexican & Mexican-Americans: health beliefs & practices*, Cambridge, 2004, Cambridge University Press.

Kim S, Flaskerud J: Does culture frame adjustment to the sick role? *Issues Ment Health Nurs* 29:315–318, 2008.

Kleinman A, Benson P: Anthropology in the clinic: the problem of cultural competency and how to fix it, *PLoS Med* 3:1672–1675, 2006.

Kline and Huff: *Health promotion in multicultural populations*. In Kline M, Huff R, editors: ed 2, Thousand Oaks, CA, 2008, Sage Publications.

Knoerl (AM): Cultural considerations and the Hispanic cardiac client, *Home Health Care Nurse* 25(2):82–86, 2007.

Knoerl AM, Esper K, Hasenau S: Cultural sensitivity in patient health education, *Nurs Clin North Am* 46(3):335–340, 2011.

Kwak J, Haley W: Current research findings on end-of-life decision making among racially or ethnically diverse groups, *Gerontologist* 45(5):634–641, 2005.

Leininger M, McFarland R, editors: *Culture care diversity and universality: a worldwide nursing theory*, Sudbury, MA, 2006, Jones and Bartlett.

Leonard B, Plotnikoff G: Awareness: the heart of cultural competence, *AACN Clin Issues* 11(1):51–59, 2000.

Lewis R: *When cultures collide: managing successfully across cultures*, London, 2000, Nicholas Brealey Publishing.

Lewis L, Hankin S, Reynolds D, Ogedegbe G: African American spirituality: a process of honoring God, others and self, *J Holist Nurs* 25(1):16–23, 2007.

Livingston G, Minushkin S, Cohn D: Hispanics and Health Care in the United States: Access, Information and knowledge, *Pew Hispanic Center and Robert Wood Johnson Foundation*, 2008. www.pewhispanic.org/files/reports/91.pdf.

Littlejohn-Blake S, Darling CA: Understanding the strengths of African American families, *J Black Stud* 23(4):460–471, 1993.

Louie K: White paper on the health status of Asian-Americans and Pacific Islanders and recommendations for research, *Nurs Outlook* 49:173–178, 2001.

Lowe J, Archibald C: Cultural diversity: The intention of nursing, *Nursing Forum* 44(1):11–18, 2009.

Lynch E, Hanson M: *Developing cross-cultural competence: a guide for working with children and families*, ed 3, Baltimore, MD, 2004, Paul H. Brookes Publishing Co.

Malhi R, Boon S, Rogers T, et al.: "Being Canadian" and "being Indian": subject positions and discourses used in South Asian-Canadian women's talk about ethnic identity, *Culture Psychol* 15(2):255–283, 2009.

Marsiglia F, Booth J: Cultural Adaptation of Interventions in Real Practice Settings. Draft submitted for: *Bridging the Research & Practice Gap Symposium*, Houston, 2013.

McKennis A: Caring for the Islamic patient, *AORN J* 69(6):1185–1206, 1999.

McLaughlin L, K: Asian and Pacific Islander cultural values: considerations for health care decision-making, *Health Soc Work* 23(2):116–126, 1998.

Meisenhelder M, Bell J, Chandler E, et al.: Faith, prayer, and health outcomes in elderly Native Americans, *Clin Nurs Res* 9(2):191–204, 2000.

Messias D, McDowell L, Estrada R: Language interpreting as social justice work: Perspectives of formal and informal healthcare interpreters, *Adv Nurs Sci* 32(2):128–143, 2009.

Michaels A: *Hinduism: past and present*, Princeton, NJ, 2003, Princeton University Press.

Neuliep J: *Intercultural Communication: A Contextual Approach*, Thousand Oaks, CA, 2015, Sage Publications.

U.S. Department of Health and Human Services (DHHS): *National standards for culturally and linguistically appropriate services in health care*, Washington, DC, 2001, Author. Available online www.omhrc.gov/assets/pdf/checked/finalreport.pdf. Accessed, July 3, 2014.

Office of Minority Health and Health Equity (OMHHE). (n.d.) Available at http://www.cdc.gov/minorityhealth. Accessed July 3, 2014

Pagani-Tousignant C: *Breaking the rules: counseling ethnic minorities*, Minneapolis, MN, 1992, The Johnson Institute.

Parham TA, White JL, Ajamu A, et al.: *The psychology of Blacks: an African centered perspective*, Upper Saddle River, NJ, 2000, Prentice Hall.

Pergert P, Ekblad S, Enskar K, et al.: Obstacles to transcultural caring relationships: experiences of health care staff in pediatric oncology, *J Pediatr Oncol Nurs* 24(6):314–328, 2007.

Purnell L, Purnell JD, Paulanka BJ, et al.: *Transcultural health care: A culturally competent approach*, ed 3, Philadelphia, PA, 2008, F.A. Davis.

Purnell JD: *Guide to culturally competent health care*, ed 2, Philadelphia PA, 2009, F.A. Davis.

Raphael D: Poverty, human development, and health in Canada: research, practice, and advocacy dilemmas, *Can J Nurs Res* 41(2):7–18, 2009.

Rashidi A, Rajaram S: Culture care conflicts among Asian-Islamic immigrant women in US hospitals, *Holist Nurs Pract* 16(1):55–64, 2001.

Red Horse J: Traditional American Indian family systems, *Fam Syst Health* 15(3):243–250, 1997.

Reutter L, Stewart M, Veenstra G, et al.: Who do they think we are anyway? Perceptions and responses to poverty stigma, *Qual Health Res* 19(3):297–311, 2009.

Samovar L L, Porter R R, McDaniel E E, et al.: *Intercultural communication: a reader*, ed 12, Belmont, CA, 2008, Wadsworth.

Samovar L, Porter R, McDaniel E, Roy C: *Intercultural Communication. A Reader*, 14th ed, Boston, MA, 2014, Cenage Learning.

Scheppers E, Dongen E, Dekker J, Geertzen J, Dekker J: Potential barriers to the use of health services among ethnic minorities: a review, *Fam Pract* 23(3):325–348, 2006.

Schim S, Doorenbos A: A three-dimensional model of cultural congruence: Framework for intervention, *J Soc Work End Life Palliat Care* 6(3-4):256–270, 2010.

Schwartz S, Montgomery M, Briones E: The role if identity in acculturation among immigrant people: theoretical propositions, empirical questions, and applied recommendations, *Hum Dev* 49:1–30, 2006.

Searight H, Gafford J: Cultural diversity at the end of life: issues and guidelines for family physicians, *Am Fam Physician* 71:3, 2005.

Servodido C, Morse E: End of life issues, *Nurs Spectr* 11(8DC):20–23, 2001.

Sokol R, Strout S: A complete theory of human emotion: the synthesis of language, body, culture and evolution in human feeling, *Cult Psychol* 12(10):115–123, 2006.

Spector R: *Cultural diversity in health and illness*, ed 8, Upper Saddle River, NJ, 2012, Pearson Prentice Hall.

Spence D: Prejudice, paradox, and possibility: nursing people from cultures other than one's own, *J Transcult Nurs* 12(2):100–106, 2001.

Sterritt P, Pokorny M: African American caregiving for a relative with Alzheimer's disease, *Geriatr Nurs* 19(3):127–128, 133–134. 1998.

Sue DW, Sue S: *Counseling the culturally diverse: theory and practice*, ed 4, New York, 2003, Wiley.

Sutton M: Cultural competence, *Fam Pract Manag* 7(9):58–62, 2000.

Thomas N: The importance of culture throughout all of life and beyond, *Holist Nurs Pract* 15(2):40–46, 2001.

Underwood S, Buseh A, Kelber S, et al.: Enhancing the participation of African Americans in health-related genetic research: Finding of a collaborative academic and community based research study, *Nurs Res Pract. 2013* 2013:749563, 2013, . http://dx.doi.org/10.1155/2013/749563. Epub 2013 Dec 4.

U.S. Department of Health and Human Services (DHHS): *National standards for cultural and linguistically appropriate services in health care*, Washington, DC, 2001, final report Author.

U.S. Department of Health and Human Services (DHHS): *2006 National Healthcare Disparities Report*, Rockville, MD, 2007, Author.

Vaughn L, Jacquez F, Baker R: Cultural health attributions, beliefs, and practices: Effects on health care and medical education, *Open Med Educ J* 2:64–74, 2009.

Weiner L, McConnell D, Latella L, Ludi E: Cultural and religious considerations in pediatric palliative care. *Palliat Support Care* 11(1):47–67, 2013.

Wilson L: Holistic care to African Americans, *Nurs Clin North Am* 46:219–232, 2011.

Xu Y, Davidhizar R, J, Giger J, et al.: What if your nursing student is from an Asian culture, *J Cult Divers* 12(1):5–12, 2004.

Zapata J, Shippee-Rice R: The use of folk healing and healers by six Latinos living in New England, *J Transcult Nurs* 10(2):136–142, 1999.

WEB RESOURCES

http://www.diversityrx.org.
http://www.minorityhealth.hhs.gov.
http://www.ceh.org.au.
http://www.hispanichealth.org.

Therapeutic Communication in Groups

Elizabeth C. Arnold

OBJECTIVES

At the end of the chapter, the reader will be able to:

1. Define group.
2. Identify the characteristics of small group communication.
3. Describe the stages of small group development.
4. Discuss theory-based concepts of group dynamics.
5. Apply group concepts in therapeutic groups.
6. Compare and contrast different types of therapeutic groups.
7. Apply concepts of group dynamics to work groups.
8. Discuss differences in small group communication versus team communication.

Chapter 8 focuses on small group communication in contemporary health care. The chapter identifies theory-based concepts related to small group dynamics and process and describes group role functions as a foundation for interactive applications in clinical and work groups. The chapter concludes with a discussion of applications to team communication.

BASIC CONCEPTS

DEFINITIONS OF GROUP

Rothwell (2013) defines a *group* as "a human communication system composed of three or more individuals, interacting for the achievement of some common goal(s) who influence and are influenced by each other" (p. 36). Unlike communication in dyad relationships, there are multiple inputs and responses to each conversational segment. Group relationships are interdependent. In this way, group communication shares a key characteristic with system concepts (see Chapter 1). It is impossible to take into account the behavior of one group member without considering its influence on the behavior and responses of other group members. Group "cultures" develop

through shared images, values, and meanings. Over time, a group culture emerges, supported by stories, myths, and metaphors about the group, and how it functions.

PRIMARY AND SECONDARY GROUPS

"Membership in groups is inevitable and universal" states Johnson and Johnson (2012, p. 2). A group is a social unit, which can satisfy a person's need for belongingness. Groups are categorized as primary or secondary. Primary groups are formed early in life, characterized by an informal structure and close personal relationships. Primary groups have a lifelong influence on self-identity and social behaviors. Group membership is automatic (e.g., in a family) voluntarily chosen because of a common interest (e.g., long-term friendship), and open ended.

Secondary groups represent less personalized, time-limited relationships with an established beginning and end. They differ from primary groups in purpose and function as they have a prescribed structure, a designated leader, and specific goals (Forsyth, 2010). When the group completes its task or achieves its goals, the group disbands. People join secondary groups to meet personally established goals, to develop knowledge and

EXERCISE 8-1	Groups in Everyday Life

Purpose: To help students gain an appreciation of the role group communication plays in their lives.

Procedure
1. Write down all the groups in which you have been a participant (e.g., family; scouts; sports teams; community, religious, work, and social groups).
2. Describe the influence membership in each of these groups had on the person you are today.
3. Identify the ways in which membership in different groups was of value in your life.

Discussion
1. How similar or dissimilar were your answers from those of your classmates?
2. What factors account for differences in the quantity and quality of your group memberships?
3. How similar were the ways in which membership enhanced your self-esteem?
4. If your answers were dissimilar, what makes membership in groups such a complex experience?
5. Could different people get different things out of very similar group experiences?
6. What implications does this exercise have for your nursing practice?

skills, or because it is required by the larger community system to which the individual belongs. Work groups, social action, and health-related therapeutic or support groups are good examples. Exercise 8-1 presents the role that group communication plays in a person's life.

GROUP COMMUNICATION IN HEALTH CARE

Group counseling, psychoeducation, work groups, and interdisciplinary teams functioning within a larger health care system setting rely on group communication as an essential component of contemporary health care delivery. In your nursing program, group communication provides an important foundation for working together in clinical groups, completing group projects, and for reflective experiential learning.

Joseph Pratt, a physician, first introduced the value of group communication as a therapeutic tool for clients in medical settings. He found that his tuberculosis (TB) patients improved dramatically when exposed to regular group-based classes. Group therapy for psychological issues developed during World War II when it was used as a primary treatment modality to treat soldiers for war-related stress. Outcomes were so successful that mental health professionals continued to use group therapy to treat people with psychological problems. Jacob Moreno later developed psychodrama as an experiential form of group therapy and introduced sociometry as a way to diagram group participation. Samuel Slavson introduced the idea of using therapeutic activity groups for disturbed children (Rutan et al., 2007), and many others contributed to the development of group communication as a treatment modality for psychological problems and general medical issues.

The changing landscape in health care delivery places a renewed emphasis on developing proficiency in small group communication skills. Nurses are expected to interact with professionals from different professional backgrounds and to function as part of a well-coordinated team unit to provide quality health care delivery. Interprofessional education and practice collaboration, now a global initiative in health care, uses small group communication as a primary form of interaction.

In 2011 the Institute of Medicine (IOM) made specific recommendations for nursing and other health programs to include collaborative interprofessional training opportunities. Interprofessional group learning formats use group communication concepts and simulated group experiences to help students to develop critical thinking about difficult clinical problems. Clinical simulations prepare students experientially to work together in prototype situations similar to those they will encounter in actual practice. As students share information, question and negotiate with each other in simulated clinical scenarios, they develop team-building skills. Reflective group discussions are a critical component of the team learning processes (Michaelsen and Sweet, 2008).

CHARACTERISTICS OF SMALL GROUP COMMUNICATION

GROUP PURPOSE

Group purpose provides the rationale for a group's existence (Powles, 2007). Purpose provides direction for group decisions, and influences the type of communication and activities required to meet group goals.

TABLE 8-1	Therapeutic Group Type and Purpose
Group	**Purpose**
Therapy	Reality testing, encouraging personal growth, inspiring hope, strengthening personal resources, developing interpersonal skills
Support	Giving and receiving practical information and advice, supporting coping skills, promoting self-esteem, enhancing problem-solving skills, encouraging client autonomy, strengthening hope and resiliency
Activity	Getting people in touch with their bodies, releasing energy, enhancing self-esteem, encouraging cooperation, stimulating spontaneous interaction, supporting creativity
Health education	Learning new knowledge, promoting skill development, providing support and feedback, supporting development of competency, promoting discussion of important health-related issues

For example, the purpose of group therapy would be to improve interpersonal functioning, and behavior, whereas in a work group, the purpose would relate to support a specific work-related issue. The purpose of a health team would be to deliver quality care. Purposes of different group types are presented in Table 8-1.

GROUP GOALS

Group goals define expected therapeutic outcomes in a client group, or a defined work result indicating goal achievement. Goals serve as benchmarks for successful achievement. Matching group goals with client needs and characteristics is essential in counseling and therapeutic groups. In work groups, the match is between group expertise and goal requirements. Specific goals need to be clearly understood by all group members; goals need to be achievable, measurable, and within the capabilities of group membership. A good match energizes a group; members develop commitment and perceive the group as having value.

GROUP SIZE

Group purpose dictates group size. Client-centered therapeutic groups consist of six to eight members. With fewer than five members, deep sharing tends to

be limited. If one or more members are absent, group interaction can become intense and uncomfortable for remaining members. Powles (2007) argues "the threesome rarely leads to solid group formation or a productive group work" (p. 107). Education-focused groups, such as medication, psychoeducation, diagnosis, skill training, and treatment groups can have 10 or more members. Membership on interdisciplinary teams should reflect the essential number of health care professionals needed to coordinate and share care responsibility for a common client population.

GROUP MEMBER COMPOSITION

Careful selection of group members should be based on a person's capacity to derive benefit from the group and to contribute to group goals (Yalom and Leszcz, 2005). *Functional similarity* is defined as choosing group members similar enough—intellectually, emotionally, and experientially to interact with each other in a meaningful way. An older highly educated adult placed in a therapy group of young adults having limited verbal and educational skills, or a single adolescent girl placed in a group of boys can be a group casualty or scapegoat, simply because of personal characteristics beyond their control. In a different group, with clients of similar intellectual, emotional, and life experiences, treatment outcomes might be different. Group therapy is contraindicated for acutely psychotic, suicidal, paranoid, excessively hostile or impulsive clients. Functional similarity is not the same as interpersonal attraction or having similar interpersonal characteristics. Differences in interpersonal style are advantageous as they help clients learn a broader range of behavioral responses.

In work groups, functional similarity is thought of as choosing members with comparable interests, complementary knowledge, and essential skills to achieve group goals (Hinds et al., 2000). A functional match produces a higher level of group performance and member satisfaction. A certain interpersonal compatibility is desirable, as this can enhance task interdependence and the desire to work together as a group. Exercise 8-2 provides an opportunity to explore the concept of functional similarity.

GROUP NORMS

Group norms refer to the unwritten behavioral rules of conduct expected of group members. Norms provide needed predictability for effective group functioning

EXERCISE 8-2	Exploring Functional Similarity

Purpose: To provide an experiential understanding of functional similarity.

Procedure
1. Break class into groups of four to six people.
2. One person should act as a scribe.
3. Identify two characteristics or experiences that all members of your group have in common other than that you are in the same class.
4. Identify two things that are unique to each person in your group (e.g., only child, never moved from the area, born in another country, unique skill or life experience).

5. Each person should elaborate on both the common and different experiences.

Discussion
1. What was the effect of finding common ground with other group members?
2. In what ways did finding out about the uniqueness of each person's experience add to the discussion?
3. Did anything in either the discussion of commonalities or differences in experience stimulate further group discussion?
4. How could you use what you have learned in this exercise in your clinical practice?

EXERCISE 8-3	Identifying Norms

Purpose: To help identify norms operating in groups.

Procedure
1. Divide a piece of paper into three columns.
2. In the first column, write the norms you think exist in your class or work group. In the second column, write the norms you think exist in your family. Examples of norms might be as follows: no one gets angry, decisions are made by consensus, assertive behaviors are valued, missed sessions and lateness are not tolerated.

3. Share your norms with the group, first related to the school or work group and then to the family. Place this information in the third column.

Discussion
1. What were some of the differences in existing norms for school and work and family?
2. Were there any "universal" norms on either of your lists?
3. Was there more or less consistency in overall student responses about class and work group norms and family norms? If so, what would account for it?

and make the group safe for its members. There are two types of norms: universal and group specific.

Universal norms are explicit behavioral standards, which must be present in all groups for effective outcomes. Examples include confidentiality, regular attendance, and not socializing with members outside of the group (Burlingame et al., 2006). Unless group members believe that personal information will not be shared outside the group setting (confidentiality), trust will not develop. Regular attendance at group meetings is critical to group stability and goal achievement. Even if the member is a perfect fit with group goals, he or she must fully commit to regular attendance. Personal relationships between group members outside of the group also threaten the integrity of the group.

Group-specific norms are constructed by group members. They represent the shared beliefs, values and unspoken operational rules governing group functions (Rothwell, 2013). Norms help define member interactions. Often they are implicit. Examples include the group's tolerance for lateness, use of humor, or confrontation, and talking directly to other group members rather than about them. Exercise 8-3 can help you develop a deeper understanding of group norms.

GROUP ROLE POSITIONS

A person's role position in the group corresponds with the status, power, and internal image that other members in the group have of the member. Group members assume, and/or are ascribed roles that influence their communication and the responses of others. They usually have trouble breaking away from roles they have been cast in despite their best efforts. For example, people will look to the "helper" group member for advice, even when that person lacks expertise or personally needs the group's help. The identified "helper" member may suffer because they do not always receive the help they need. Other times, group members "project" a role position onto a particular group member that represents a hidden agenda or an unresolved

EXERCISE 8-4	Headbands: Group Role Expectations

Purpose: To experience the pressures of role expectations on group performance.

Procedure

1. Break the group up into a smaller unit of six to eight members. In a large group, a small group performs while the remaining members observe.
2. Make up mailing labels or headbands that can be attached to or tied around the heads of the participants. Each headband is lettered with directions on how the other members should respond to the role. Examples:
   - Comedian: laugh at me
   - Expert: ask my advice
   - Important person: defer to me
   - Stupid: sneer at me
   - Insignificant: ignore me
   - Loser: pity me
   - Boss: obey me
   - Helpless: support me
3. Place a headband on each member in such a way that the member cannot read his or her own label, but the other members can see it easily.
4. Provide a topic for discussion (e.g., why the members chose nursing, the women's movement) and instruct each member to interact with the others in a way that is natural for him or her. Do not role-play, but be yourself. React to each member who speaks by following the instructions on the speaker's headband. You are not to tell each other what the headbands say, but simply to react to them.
5. After about 20 minutes, the facilitator halts the activity and directs each member to guess what his or her headband says, and then to take it off and read it.

Discussion

Initiate a discussion, including any members who observed the activity. Possible questions include the following:

1. What were some of the problems of trying to "be yourself" under conditions of group role pressure?
2. How did it feel to be consistently misinterpreted by the group—to have them laugh when you were trying to be serious or ignore you when you were trying to make a point?
3. Did you find yourself changing your behavior in reaction to the group treatment of you—withdrawing when they ignored you, acting confident when they treated you with respect, giving orders when they deferred to you?

Modified from Pfeiffer J, Jones J: *A handbook of structured experiences for human relations training*, vol VI, La Jolla, CA, 1977, University Associate Publishers.

issue for the group as a whole (Gans and Alonso, 1998). Projection is largely unconscious, but it can be destructive to group functioning (Moreno, 2007). For example, if the group as a whole seems to scapegoat, ignore, defer to, or consistently idealize one of its members, this group projection can compromise the group's effectiveness because of the unrealistic focus on one group member. Exercise 8-4 considers group role position expectations.

GROUP DYNAMICS

Group dynamics is a term originally used by Kurt Lewin (Forsyth, 2010) to describe the communication processes and behaviors occurring during the life of the group. They represent a complex blend of individual and group characteristics that interact with each other to achieve a group purpose. Bernard et al (2008) categorized the primary forces operating in groups as individual dynamics (member variables), interpersonal dynamics (group communication variables) and group as a whole dynamics related to purpose, norms, etc.

These are displayed in Figure 8-1. The group leader is charged with integrating these multiple variables into a workable group process.

GROUP PROCESS

Group process refers to the structural development of small group relationships. Bruce Tuckman's (1965; Tuckman and Jensen, 1977) five-stage model of small group development (forming, storming, norming, performing, and adjourning) provides the most commonly used framework describing the structural development and relationship process of small groups. Stages of group development are applicable to work groups as well as therapeutic groups. Each sequential phase of group development has its own set of tasks, which build and expand on the work of previous phases.

Forming

The forming phase begins when members first come together as a group. Members enter group relationships as strangers to each other. The leader orients the group

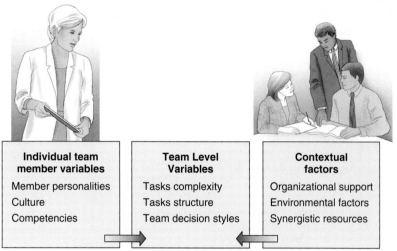

Figure 8-1   Factors affecting group dynamics.

to the group's purpose and asks members to introduce themselves. The information each person shares about themselves should be brief and relate to personal data relevant to achieving the group's purpose.

During the forming phase, universal norms (group ground rules) for attendance, participation, and confidentiality are defined. Getting to know each other, finding common threads in personal or professional experience, and acceptance of group goals and tasks are initial group goals. Members have a basic need for acceptance, so communication is more tentative than it will be later when members know and trust each other.

Storming

The storming phase focuses on power and control issues. Members use testing behaviors around boundaries, communication styles, and personal reactions with other members and the leader. Characteristic behaviors include disagreement with the group format, topics for discussion, the best ways to achieve group goals, and comparisons of member contributions. Although the storming phase is uncomfortable, successful resolution leads to the development of group-specific norms.

Norming

In the norming phase, individual goals become aligned with group goals. Group-specific norms help create a supportive group climate characterized by dependable fellowship and purpose. These norms make the group "safe," and members begin to experience the cohesiveness of the group as "their group." The group holds its

members accountable and challenges individual members who fail to adhere to expected norms.

Cohesiveness is recognized as the foundation for group identity. It develops as group-specific behavioral standards established by members are accepted as operational norms. Sources of cohesiveness include shared goals, working through and solving problems, and the nature of group interaction.

Performing

Most of a group's "work" gets accomplished in the performing phase. This phase of group development is characterized by interdependence, full acceptance of each member as a person of value, and cohesion. Members feel loyal to the group and engaged in its work. They are comfortable taking risks and are invested enough in each other and the group process to offer constructive comments.

Adjourning Phase

Tuckman introduced the adjourning phase as a final phase of group development at a later date (Tuckman and Jensen, 1977). This phase is characterized by reviewing what has been accomplished, reflecting on the meaning of the group's work together, and making plans to move on in different directions.

GROUP ROLE FUNCTIONS

Functional roles differ from positional roles group members assume in that they relate to the type of member contributions needed to achieve group goals.

BOX 8-1	Task and Maintenance Functions in Group Dynamics

Task Functions: Behaviors Relevant to the Attainment of Group Goals

- **Initiating:** Identifies tasks or goals; defines group problem; suggests relevant strategies for solving problem
- **Seeking information or opinion:** Requests facts from other members; asks other members for opinions; seeks suggestions or ideas for task accomplishment
- **Giving information or opinion:** Offers facts to other members; provides useful information about group concerns
- **Clarifying, elaborating:** Interprets ideas or suggestions placed before group; paraphrases key ideas; defines terms; adds information
- **Summarizing:** Pulls related ideas together; restates key ideas; offers a group solution or suggestion for other members to accept or reject
- **Consensus taking:** Checks to see whether group has reached a conclusion; asks group to test a possible decision.

Maintenance Functions: Behaviors That Help the Group Maintain Harmonious Working Relationships

- **Harmonizing:** Attempts to reconcile disagreements; helps members reduce conflict and explore differences in a constructive manner
- **Gatekeeping:** Helps keep communication channels open; points out commonalties in remarks; suggests approaches that permit greater sharing
- **Encouraging:** Indicates by words and body language unconditional acceptance of others; agrees with contributions of other group members; is warm, friendly, and responsive to other group members
- **Compromising:** Admits mistakes; offers a concession when appropriate; modifies position in the interest of group cohesion
- **Setting standards:** Calls for the group to reassess or confirm implicit and explicit group norms when appropriate
  Note: Every group needs both types of functions and needs to work out a satisfactory balance of task and maintenance activity.

Modified from Rogers C: The process of the basic encounter group. In Diedrich R, Dye, HA, editors: *Group procedures: purposes, processes and outcomes,* Boston, 1972, Houghton Mifflin.

Benne and Sheats (1948) described constructive role functions as the behaviors members use to move toward goal achievement (task functions) and behaviors designed to ensure personal satisfaction (maintenance functions).

TABLE 8-2	Nonfunctional Self-Roles	
Role	**Characteristics**	
Aggressor	Criticizes or blames others, personally attacks other members, uses sarcasm and hostility in interactions	
Blocker	Instantly rejects ideas or argues an idea to death, cites tangential ideas and opinions, obstructs decision making	
Joker	Disrupts work of the group by constantly joking and refusing to take group task seriously	
Avoider	Whispers to others, daydreams, doodles, acts indifferent and passive	
Self-confessor	Uses the group to express personal views and feelings unrelated to group task	
Recognition seeker	Seeks attention by excessive talking, trying to gain leader's favor, expressing extreme ideas, or demonstrating peculiar behavior	

Modified from Benne KD, Sheats P: Functional roles of group members, *J Soc Issues* 4(2):41-49, 1948.

Balance between task and maintenance functions increases group productivity. When task functions predominate, member satisfaction decreases, and a collaborative atmosphere is diminished. When maintenance functions override task functions, members have trouble reaching goals. Members do not confront controversial issues, so the creative tension needed for successful group accomplishment is compromised. Task and maintenance role functions found in successful small groups are listed in Box 8-1.

Benne and Sheats also identified nonfunctional role functions. *Self-roles* are roles a person unconsciously uses to meet self-needs at the expense of other members' needs, group values, and goal achievement. Self-roles, identified in Table 8-2, detract from the group's work and compromise goal achievement by taking time away from group issues and creating discomfort among group members.

APPLICATIONS TO HEALTH-RELATED GROUPS

In clinical settings the health-related group purpose and goals dictate group structure, membership, and format. For example, a medication group would have an educational purpose. A group for parents with critically ill children would have a supportive design, while a therapy group would have restorative healing functions. Activity groups are used therapeutically with children and with chronically mentally ill clients who may have difficulty fully expressing themselves verbally. Exploration of personal feelings would be limited and related to the topic under discussion in an education group. In a therapy group, such probing would be encouraged.

GROUP MEMBERSHIP

Therapeutic and support groups are categorized as closed or open groups, and as having homogeneous or heterogeneous membership (Corey, 2013). *Closed therapeutic* groups have a selected membership with an expectation of regular attendance for an extended time period. Group members may be added, but their inclusion depends on a match with group-defined criteria. Most psychotherapy groups fall into this category. *Open* groups do not have a defined membership. Most community support groups are open groups. Individuals come and go depending on their needs. One week the group might consist of 2 or 3 members and the next week 15 members. Some groups, such as Alcoholics Anonymous, have "open" meetings that anyone can attend and "closed" meetings, which only alcoholic members can attend.

Having a homogeneous or heterogeneous membership identifies member characteristics. *Homogeneous* groups share common characteristics, for example, diagnosis (e.g., breast cancer support group) or a personal attribute (e.g., gender, or age). Twelve-step programs for alcohol or drug addiction, eating disorders, and gender-specific consciousness-raising groups are familiar examples of homogeneous groups. Psychoeducation (e.g., medication groups) groups often have a homogeneous membership related to particular medications or diagnosis.

Heterogeneous groups represent a wider diversity of member characteristics and personal issues. Members vary in age, gender, and psychodynamics. Most psychotherapy and insight-oriented personal growth groups have a heterogeneous membership.

CREATING A SAFE ENVIRONMENT

Privacy and freedom from interruptions are key considerations in selecting an appropriate location. A sign on the door indicating the group is in session is essential for privacy. Seating should be comfortable and arranged in a circle so that each member has face-to-face contact with other members. Being able to see facial expressions and to respond to several individuals at one time is essential to effective group communication. Often group members choose the same seats in therapy groups. When a member is absent, that seat is left vacant.

Therapy groups usually meet weekly. Support groups meet at regular intervals, often monthly. Educational groups meet for a predetermined number of sessions, and then disband. Unlike individual sessions, which can be convened spontaneously in emergency situations, therapeutic groups meet only at designated times. Most therapeutic and support groups meet for 60 to 90 minutes on a regular basis with established, agreed-on meeting times. Groups that begin and end on time foster trust and predictability.

GROUP LEADERSHIP

Two assumptions support the function of group leadership: (1) group leaders have a significant influence on group process; and (2) most problems in groups can be avoided or reworked productively if the leader is aware of and responsive to the needs of individual group members, including the needs of the leader (Corey and Corey, 2008).

Effective leadership behaviors require adequate preparation, professional attitudes and behavior, responsible selection of members, and an evidence-based approach. Personal characteristics demonstrated by effective group leaders include commitment to the group purpose; self-awareness of personal biases and interpersonal limitations, careful preparation for the group, and with the group, and an open attitude toward group members. Knowledge of group dynamics, training, and supervision are additional requirements for leaders of psychotherapy groups. Health education group leaders need to have expertise on the topic for discussion.

Throughout the group's life, the group leader models an attitude of caring, objectivity, and integrity. Effective leaders are good listeners; they can adapt their leadership style to fit the changing needs of the group. They respectfully support the integrity of group members as equal partners in meeting group goals. Successful leaders trust the group process enough to know that group members can work through conflict and difficult situations. They know that even mistakes can be used for discussion to promote group member growth (Rubel and Kline, 2008).

Informal power is given to members who best clarify the needs of the other group members, or who move the group toward goal achievement. They are not always the group members making the most statements. Some individuals, because of the force of their personalities, knowledge, or experience, will emerge as informal leaders within the group.

Case Example

Al is a powerful informal leader in a job search support group. Although he makes few comments, he has an excellent understanding of, and sensitivity to the needs of individual members. When these are violated, Al speaks up and the group listens.

Other group members recognize emergent informal leaders as being powerful and their comments are equated with those of the designated leader. Ideally, group leadership is a shared function of all group members, with many opportunities for different informal leaders to divide up responsibility for achieving group goals.

CO-LEADERSHIP

Co-leadership represents a form of shared leadership found primarily in therapy groups. It is desirable for several reasons. The co-leader adds another perspective related to processing group dynamics. Co-leaders provide a wider variety of responses and viewpoints that can be helpful to group members. When one leader is under fire, it can increase the other's confidence, knowing that in-group support and an opportunity to process the session afterward is available.

Respecting and valuing each other, with sensitivity to a co-leader's style of communicating is characteristic of effective co-leadership (Corey and Corey, 2008). Problems can arise when co-leaders have different theoretical orientations or are competitive with each other. Needing to pursue solo interpretations rather than explore or support the meaning of a co-leader's interventions is distracting to the group. Yalom and Leszcz (2005) stated: "You are far better off leading a solo group with good supervision than being locked into an incompatible co-therapy relationship" (p. 447).

Co-leaders should spend sufficient prep time together prior to meeting with a therapy group to ensure personal compatibility, and having the same understanding of the group purpose. Co-leaders need to process group dynamics together, preferably after each meeting. Processing group dynamics allows leaders to consider different meanings, to evaluate what happened in the group session and what might need to be addressed in order to productively move the group ahead.

Developing an Evidence-Based Practice

Mitchell R, Parker V, Giles M, Boyle B: The ABC of health care team dynamics: understanding complex affective, behavioral, and cognitive dynamics in interprofessional teams, *Health Care Manage Rev* 39(1):1-9, 2014.

Purpose: The purpose of this study was to explore the impact of interprofessional team composition on team dynamics, related to conflict and open-mindedness. Using a cross-sectional correlational design, survey data from 218 team members of 47 interprofessional teams in an acute care setting were analyzed to investigate two moderated mediation pathways.

Results: Study results demonstrated a significant relationship between interprofessional composition and affective conflict for teams rated highly for individualized professional identification.

Practice Implications: Study results indicate the need for developing a shared group identity with reinforcement of shared values related to client care as a means of improving interprofessional team communication dynamics.

APPLICATIONS

THERAPEUTIC GROUPS

Counselman (2008) refers to the power of a group being able to resonate with a member's experience, change behaviors, and strengthen emotions as being unparalleled. "Group demonstrates that there truly are multiple realities" (p. 270). Group communication is more complex than individual communication because each member brings to the group a different set of perspectives, perception of reality, communication style, and personal agenda. Instead of immediately responding to individual members, group leaders can broaden potential for different options by engaging group responses. The leader relates to the group as a whole,

TABLE 8-3	Therapeutic Factors in Groups
Installation of hope	Occurs when members see others who have overcome problems and are successfully managing their lives
Universality	Sharing common situations validates member experience; decreases sense of isolation: "Maybe I am not the only one with this issue."
Imparting information	New shared information is a resource for individual members, and stimulates further discussion and learning of new skills.
Imitative behavior	Members learn new behaviors through observation, and modeling of desired actions, and gain confidence in trying them, e.g., managing conflict, receiving constructive criticism.
Socialization	Group provides a safe learning environment in which to take interpersonal risks and try new behaviors.
Interpersonal learning	Group acts as a social microcosm; focus is on members learning about how they interact, and getting constructive feedback and support from others.
Cohesiveness	Sense of we-ness. Emphasizes personal bonds and commitment to the group. Members feel acceptance and trust from others. Cohesiveness serves as the foundation for all curative factors.
Catharsis	Expression of emotion that leads to receiving support and acceptance from other group members.
Corrective recapitulation of primary family	Allows for recognition and handling of transference issues in therapy groups. This helps group members to avoid repeating destructive interaction patterns in the "here and now."
Altruism	Providing help and support to other group members enhances personal self-esteem.
Existential factors	Highlights primary responsibility for taking charge of one's life, and the consequences of their actions; creating a meaningful existence.

Adapted from Yalom I, Leszcz M: *The theory and practice of group psychotherapy*, ed 5, New York, 2005, Basic Books.

instead of with only one person, and ties member comments or themes together. Making connections among multiple realities offers different possibilities to individual clients to learn about, and test out new interpersonal communication skills. Yalom and Leszcz's therapeutic factors (2005) presented in Table 8-3 offer the most influential construct of evidence-based features associated with effective group therapy.

APPLICATIONS IN THERAPEUTIC GROUPS

PRE-GROUP INTERVIEW

Adequate preparation of group members in pre-group interviews enhances the effectiveness of therapeutic groups (Corey, 2007; Yalom and Leszcz, 2005). A pre-group interview makes the transition into the group easier as group members have an initial connection with the leader and an opportunity to ask questions before committing to the group. Reservations held by either the leader or potential group member are handled beforehand. The description of the group and its members should be short and

simple, as this information will be repeated in initial meetings.

FORMING PHASE

How well leaders initially prepare themselves and group members has a direct impact on building the trust needed within the group (Corey and Corey, 2008). The forming phase in therapeutic groups focuses on helping clients establish trust in the group and with each other. Communication is tentative. Members are asked to introduce themselves and share a little of their background or their reason for coming to the group. An introductory prompt such as, "What would you most like to get out of this group?" helps the clients link personal goals to group goals.

In the first session, the leader introduces group goals. Clear group goals may need to be restated as the group progresses, but they are particularly important to frame the group in its initial session. The leader clarifies how the group will be conducted and what the group can expect from the leader and each other in achieving group goals. It is helpful to ask clients in round robin fashion about their personal expectations and to allow time for questions. Orienting statements may need to be restated in subsequent early sessions, especially if there is a lot of anxiety in the group.

The leader introduces universal behavioral norms such as confidentiality, regular attendance, and mutual respect (Corey and Corey, 2008). Confidentiality is harder to implement with group formats because members are not held to the same professional ethical standards as the group leader. However, for the integrity of the group, all members need to commit to confidentiality as a universal group norm (Lasky and Riva, 2006).

STORMING PHASE

The leader plays an important facilitative role in the storming phase by accepting differences in member perceptions as being normal and growth producing. By affirming genuine strengths in individual members, leaders model handling conflict with productive outcomes. Linking constructive themes while identifying the nature of the disagreement is an effective modeling strategy. Members who test boundaries through sexually provocative, flattery, or insulting remarks should have limits set promptly. Refer to the work of the group as being of the highest priority, and tactfully ask the person to align remarks with the group purpose. Working through conflicts allows members to take stands on their personal preferences without being defensive, and to compromise when needed. Conflict issues in groups are informants of what is important to group members and how individual members handle difficult emotions. Resolution leads to development of cohesion.

NORMING PHASE

Once initial conflict is resolved in the storming phase, the group moves into the norming phase. Group-specific norms develop spontaneously through group member interactions and represent the group's shared expectations of its members. The group leader encourages member contributions and emphasizes cooperation in recognizing each person's talents related to group goals. Successful short-term groups focus on "here and now" interactions, giving practical feedback, sharing personal thoughts and feelings, and listening to each other (Corey and Corey, 2008).

Cohesion begins to develop as sharing of feelings deepens the trust in the group as a safe place.

Cohesion describes the emotional bonds members have for each other and underscores the level of member commitment to the group (Yalom and Leszcz, 2005). Research suggests that cohesive groups experience more personal satisfaction with goal achievement and that members of such groups are more likely to join other group relationships. In a cohesive group, members demonstrate a sense of common purpose, caring commitment to each other, collaboration in problem solving, a sense of feeling personally valued, and a team spirit (Powles, 2007). See Box 8-2 for communication principles that facilitate cohesiveness.

PERFORMING PHASE

The performing phase is similar to the working phase in individual relationships; members focus on problem solving and developing new behaviors. The leader is responsible for keeping the group on task to accomplish group goals and maintaining a supportive group environment. If group members seem to be moving off track, asking open-ended questions or verbally observing group processes can restore forward movement. Modeling respect, empathy, appropriate self-disclosure, and ethical standards helps ensure a supportive group climate. Working together and participating in another person's personal growth allows members to experience one another's personal strengths and the collective caring of the group. Of all the possibilities that can happen in a group, feeling affirmed and respected by other group members is most highly valued by individual members.

Because members function interdependently, they are able to work through disagreements and difficult issues in ways that are acceptable to the

| BOX 8-2 | Communication Principles to Facilitate Cohesiveness |

- Group tasks should be within the membership's range of ability and expertise.
- Comments and responses should be nonevaluative, focused on behaviors rather than on personal characteristics.
- The leader should point out group accomplishments and acknowledge member contributions.
- The leader should be empathetic and teach members how to give effective feedback.
- The leader should help group members view and work through creative tension as being a valuable part of goal achievement.

individual and the group. Effective group leaders trust group members to develop their own solutions, but call attention to important group dynamics when needed. This can be introduced with a simple statement such as, "I wonder what is going on here right now" (Rubel and Kline, 2008). Feedback should be descriptive and specific to the immediate discussion. As with other types of constructive feedback, it should focus only on modifiable behaviors. Think about how you can word your message so that it helps a member better understand the impact of a behavior, make sense of an experience, and grow from the experience.

Monopolizing

Monopolizing is a negative form of power communication used to advance a personal agenda without considering the needs of others. When one member monopolizes the conversation, there are several ways the leader can respond. Remember it may not be intentional, but rather a member's way of handling anxiety. Acknowledging a monopolizer's contribution and broadening the input with a short question, such as, "Has anyone else had a similar experience?" can redirect attention to the larger group. Looking in the direction of other group members as the statements are made encourages alternative member responses. If a member continues to monopolize, the leader can respectfully acknowledge the person's comment and refocus the issue within the group directly, "I appreciate your thoughts, but I think it would be important to hear from other people as well. What do you think about this, Jane?" or "We don't have much time left,

I wonder if anyone else has something they need to talk about."

ADJOURNING PHASE

The final phase of group development, termination or adjournment, ideally occurs when the group members have achieved desired outcomes. The termination phase is about task completion and disengagement. The leader encourages the group members to express their feelings about one another with the stipulation that any concerns the group may have about an individual member or suggestions for future growth be stated in a constructive way. The leader should present his or her comments last and then close the group with a summary of goal achievement. By waiting until the group ends to share closing comments, the leader has an opportunity to soften or clarify previous comments, to connect cognitive and feeling elements that need to be addressed. The leader needs to remind members that the norm of confidentiality continues after the group ends (Mangione et al., 2007). Referrals are handled on an individual as needed basis. Exercise 8-5 considers group closure issues.

TYPES OF THERAPEUTIC GROUPS

Individuals tend to act in groups as they do in real life. The group provides a microcosm of social dynamics. Through group participation, clients can learn how others respond to them in a safe learning environment. The group provides an opportunity for individual members to practice new and different interpersonal skills (interpersonal learning).

EXERCISE 8-5	Group Closure Activities

Purpose: To develop closure skills in small group communication.

Procedure
1. Focus your attention on the group member next to you and think about what you like about the person, how you see him or her in the group, and what you might wish for that person as a member of the group.
2. After five minutes, your instructor will ask you to tell the person next to you to use the three themes in making a statement about the person. For example, "The thing I most like about you in the

group is . . ."; "To me you represent the _____ in the group"; and so on.
3. When all of the group members have had a turn, discussion may start.

Discussion
1. How did you experience telling someone about your response to him or her in the group?
2. How did you feel being the group member receiving the message?
3. What did you learn about yourself from doing this exercise?
4. What implications does this exercise have for future interactions in group relationships?

The term *therapeutic*, as it applies to group relationships, refers to more than treatment of emotional and behavioral disorders. In today's health care arena, short-term groups are designed for a wide range of different client populations as a first-line therapeutic intervention to either remediate problems or prevent them (Corey and Corey, 2013). Therapeutic groups offer a structured format that encourages a person to experience his or her natural healing potential (instillation of hope) and achieve higher levels of functioning. Other group members provide ideas and reinforce individual group members' resolve.

Therapeutic groups provide reality testing. People under stress lose perspective. Other group members can gently challenge cognitive distortions, carried over from previous damaging relationships (corrective recapitulation of primary family relationships). Because of the nature of a therapy group, group members can say things to the client that friends and relatives are afraid to say—and they are able to do so in a compassionate, constructive way. It becomes difficult for a troubled member to deny or turn aside the constructive observations and suggestions of five to six caring people who know and care about the member.

INPATIENT THERAPY GROUPS

Therapy groups in inpatient settings are designed to stabilize the client's behavior enough for them to functionally transition back into the community. Groups focus on "here and now group interaction" as the primary vehicle of treatment (Beiling et al., 2009). Because hospitalizations are brief, clients attend focused therapy groups on a daily basis. When situations cannot be changed, psychotherapy groups help clients accept that reality and move on with their lives by empowering and supporting their efforts to make constructive behavioral changes. The value of a short-term process group is the immediate interaction. Deering (2014) suggests allowing a theme to emerge and then using it to stimulate interaction about possible ways to handle difficult issues. A hidden benefit of group therapy is the opportunity to experience giving as well as receiving help from others. Helping others is important, especially for people with low self-esteem, who feel they have little to offer others.

Leading Groups for Psychotic Clients

Staff nurses are sometimes called upon to lead or co-lead unit-based group psychotherapy on inpatient units (Clarke et al., 1998). Other times, staff nurses participate in community group meetings comprised mostly of psychotic clients.

Because the demands of leadership are so intense with psychotic clients, co-leadership is recommended. Co-therapists can share the group process interventions, model healthy behaviors, offset negative transference from group members, and provide useful feedback to each other. Every group session should be processed immediately after its completion.

A directive, but flexible leadership approach works best with psychotic clients. Active encouragement of group comments related to relevant concrete topics of potential interest facilitates communication. This strategy is more effective than asking clients to share their feelings. For example, the leader could ask the group to discuss how to handle a simple behavior in a more productive way. This type of discussion allows clients to feel more successful with contributions. Full attention on the speaker, and offering commendations for member effort as well as contributions is useful. Other members can be encouraged to provide feedback, and the group can choose the best solution.

Before the group begins, the leader should remind individual members that the group is about to take place. Some clients may want to leave the group before it ends. Viewed as anxiety, the leader can gently encourage the client to remain for the duration of the group. A primary goal in working with psychotic clients is to respect each person as a unique human being, with a potentially valuable contribution. Although their needs are disguised as symptoms, you can help clients "decode" a psychotic message by uncovering the underlying theme, and translating it into understandable language. Or, the leader might ask, "I wonder if anyone in the group can help us understand better what John is trying to say." Keep in mind how difficult it is for the psychotic client to tolerate close interaction, and how necessary it is to interact with others if the client is to succeed in the outside environment.

Therapeutic Groups in Long-Term Settings

Therapeutic groups in long-term settings offer opportunities for socially isolated individuals to engage with others. Common types of groups include reminiscence, reality orientation, resocialization, remotivation groups, and activity groups.

Reminiscence Groups

Reminiscence groups focus on life review, and/or pleasurable memories (Stinson, 2009). They are not designed as insight groups, but rather to provide a supportive, ego-enhancing experience. Each group member is expected to share a few memories about a specific weekly group focus (holidays, first day of school, family photos, songs, favorite foods, pets, etc.). The leader encourages discussion. Depending on the cognitive abilities of members, the leader will need to be more or less directive. Sessions are held on a weekly basis and meet for an hour.

Reality Orientation Groups

Used with confused clients, reality orientation groups help clients maintain contact with the environment and reduce confusion about time, place, and person. Reality orientation groups are usually held each day for 30 minutes. Nurses can use everyday props such as a calendar, a clock, and pictures of the seasons to stimulate interest. The group should not be seen as an isolated activity; what occurs in the group should be reinforced throughout the 24-hour period. For example, on one unit, nurses placed pictures of the residents in earlier times on the doors to their bedrooms.

Resocialization Groups

Resocialization groups are used with confused elderly clients who are too limited to benefit from a remotivation group, but still need companionship and involvement with others. Resocialization groups focus on providing a simple social setting for clients to experience basic social skills again, for example, eating a small meal together. Although the senses and cognitive abilities may diminish in the elderly, basic needs for companionship, interpersonal relationships, and a place where one is accepted and understood remain the same throughout the life span. Improvement of social skills contributes to an improved sense of self-esteem.

Remotivation Groups

Remotivation groups are designed to stimulate thinking about activities required for everyday life. Originally developed by Dorothy Hoskins Smith for use with chronic mental patients, remotivation groups represent an effort to reach the unwounded areas of the patient's personality (i.e., those areas and interests that have remained healthy). Remotivation groups focus on tapping into strengths through discussions of realistic scenarios that stimulate and build confidence. They are successfully used in long-term settings, substance use prevention, with the chronically mentally ill and in combination with recreational therapy (Dyer and Stotts, 2005). Group members focus on a defined everyday topic, such as the way plants or trees grow, or they might consist of poetry reading or art appreciation. Visual props engage the participant and stimulate more responses.

THERAPEUTIC ACTIVITY GROUPS

Activity groups offer clients a variety of self-expressive opportunities through creative activity rather than through words. They are particularly useful with children and early adolescents (Aronson, 2004). The nurse functions as group leader, or as a support to other disciplines in encouraging client participation. Activity groups include the following:

- *Occupational therapy* groups allow clients to work on individual projects or to participate with others in learning life skills. Examples are cooking, making ceramics, or activities of daily living groups. Tasks are selected for their therapeutic value as well as for client interest. Life skills groups use a problem-solving approach to interpersonal situations.
- *Recreational therapy groups* offer opportunities to engage in leisure activities that release energy and provide a social format for learning interpersonal skills. Some people never learned how to build needed leisure activities into their lives.
- *Exercise or movement therapy groups* allow clients to engage in structured exercise. The nurse models the exercise behaviors, either with or without accompanying music and encourages clients to participate. This type of group works well with chronically mentally ill clients.
- *Art therapy groups* encourage clients to reveal feelings through drawing or painting. It is used in different ways. The art can be the focus of discussion. Children and adolescents may engage in a combined group effort to make a mural. Clients are able to reveal feelings through expression of color and abstract forms that they have trouble putting into words.
- *Poetry and bibliotherapy groups* select readings of interest and invite clients to respond to literary

works. Sluder (1990) describes an expressive therapy group for the elderly in which the nurse leader first read free verse poems and then invited the clients to compose group poems around feelings such as love or hate. Clients then wrote free verse poems and read them in the group. In the process of developing their poetry, clients got in touch with their personal creativity.

SELF-HELP AND SUPPORT GROUPS

Self-help and support groups provide emotional and practical support to clients and/or families experiencing chronic illness, crises, or the ill health of a family member. Held mostly in the community, peer support groups are led informally by group members rather than professionals, although often a health professional acts as an adviser. Criteria for membership is having a particular medical condition (e.g., cancer, multiple sclerosis) or being a support person (family of an Alzheimer victim). Self-help groups are voluntary groups, led by consumers and designed to provide peer support for individuals and their families struggling with mental health issues. Support groups have an informational function in addition to social support (Percy et al., 2009). Nurses are encouraged to learn about support group networks in their community. Exercise 8-6 offers an opportunity to learn about them.

Self-help groups are often associated with hospitals, clinics, and national health organizations. They provide a place for people with serious health care problems to interact with others experiencing similar physical or emotional problems.

EDUCATIONAL GROUPS

Community health agencies provide education groups to impart important knowledge about lifestyle changes needed to promote health and well-being and to prevent illness. Family education groups provide families of clients with the knowledge and skills they need to care for their loved ones.

Educational groups are time-limited group applications (e.g., the group might be held as four 1-hour sessions over a 2-week period or as an 8-week, 2-hour seminar). Examples of primary prevention groups are childbirth education, parenting, and stress reduction.

Medication groups offer clients and families effective ways to carry out a therapeutic medication regimen, while learning about a particular disorder. A typical sequence would be to provide clients with information about:

- Their disorder and how the medication works to reduce symptoms
- Medications including purpose, dosage, timing, side effects, what to do when the client does not take the medication as prescribed
- What to avoid while on the medication (e.g., some medications cause sun sensitivity)
- Tests needed to monitor the medication

Giving homework, written instructions, and materials to be read between sessions helps if the medication group is to last more than one session. Allowing sufficient time for questions and encouraging an open informal discussion of the topic, mobilizes client energy to share concerns and fears that might not otherwise come to light.

EXERCISE 8-6	**Learning about Support Groups**

Purpose: To provide direct information about support groups in the community.

Procedure
1. Directly contact a support group in your community. (Ideally, students will choose different support groups so that a variety of groups are shared.)
2. Identify yourself as a nursing student and indicate that you are looking at community support groups. Ask for information about the group (e.g., the time and frequency of meetings, purpose and focus of the group, how a client joins the group, who sponsors the group, issues the group might discuss, and fee, if any).
3. Write a two-paragraph report including the information you have gathered and describe your experience in asking for the support group information.

Discussion
1. How easy was it for you to obtain information?
2. Were you surprised by any of the informants' answers?
3. If you were a client, would this information inform your decision to join the support group? If not, what else would be important to you?
4. What did you learn from doing this exercise that might be useful in your nursing practice?

DISCUSSION GROUPS

Functional elements appropriate to discussion groups are found in Table 8-4.

Careful preparation, formulation of relevant questions, and use of feedback ensure that personal learning needs are met in discussion groups. Discussion group topics often include prepared data and group-generated material, which then is discussed in the group. Before the end of each meeting, the leader or a group member should summarize the major themes developed from the content material.

Group participation on an equal basis should be a group expectation. Although the level of participation is never quite equal, discussion groups in which only a few members actively participate are disheartening to group members and limited in learning potential. Referred to as "social loafing," when individual group members fail to do their part of the work, and skip or come late to group project meetings, it can be frustrating for other group members (Aggarwal, and O'Brien,

2008). Because the primary purpose of a discussion group is to promote the learning of all group members, other members are charged with the responsibility of encouraging the participation of more silent members. Cooperation, not competition, needs to be developed as a conscious group norm for all discussion groups. Strategies can include allowing more room for more reticent members by asking for their thoughts or opinions. Sometimes, when verbal participants keep quiet, the more reticent group member begins to speak. Exercise 8-7 provides an opportunity to explore potential group participation issues.

GROUP PRINCIPLES APPLIED TO PROFESSIONAL WORK GROUPS

Unlike therapeutic groups, task and work groups do not emphasize personal behavior change as a primary focus (Gladding, 2011). Health care organizations use work groups to identify problems, plan and implement changes to improve client work care, and engage in strategies to more effectively with each other. Work groups (e.g., standing committees, ad hoc task forces, and quality circles) accomplish a wide range of tasks related to organizational goals. They allow health professionals, staff, and involved stakeholders to more quickly develop and implement new evidence-based initiatives. Involvement of stakeholders helps ensure the needed buy-in for recommendation acceptance.

Work groups are part of a larger organizational system, with a work-related political culture. The small group operates as an adaptive open system (Beebe and Masterson, 2014, Tubbs, 2011). All aspects of group work should incorporate the values, norms, general mission, and philosophy of the larger work system. Task group activities must be congruent with the goals of the larger system (Mathieu et al., 2008). Group strategies, group activities, and methods of evaluation should be consistent with the organizational ethos and the goals of the larger organizational system to achieve maximum success.

Work groups are concerned with content and process. The content (task) is predetermined by organizational parameters or the charge given to the group. Effective group leaders need to have a strong working knowledge of task expectations and their relationship to existing content. Having sufficient available resources in terms of time, money, information, and member expertise is essential to achieving successful outcomes.

TABLE 8-4	Elements of Successful Discussion Groups
Element	**Rationale**
Careful preparation	Thoughtful agenda and assignments establish a direction for the discussion and the expected contribution of each member.
Informed participants	Each member should come prepared so that all members are communicating with relatively the same level of information and each is able to contribute equally.
Shared leadership	Each member is responsible for contributing to the discussion; evidence of social loafing is effectively addressed.
Good listening skills	Concentrates on the material, listens to content. Challenges, anticipates, and weighs the evidence; listens between the lines to emotions about the topic.
Relevant questions	Focused questions keep the discussion moving toward the meeting objectives.
Useful feedback	Thoughtful feedback maintains the momentum of the discussion by reflecting different perspectives of topics raised and confirming or questioning others' views.

| EXERCISE 8-7 | Addressing Participation Issues in Professional Discussion Groups |

Purpose: To provide an opportunity to develop response strategies in difficult group participation issues.

Procedure

A class has been assigned a group project for which all participants will receive a common group grade. Develop a group understanding of the feelings experienced in each of the following situations, as well as a way to respond to each. Consider the possible consequences of your intervention in each case.

1. Don tells the group that he is working full time and will be unable to make many group meetings. There are so many class requirements that he is not sure he can put much effort into the project, although he would like to help and the project interests him.
2. Martha is very outspoken in the group. She expresses her opinion about the choice of the group project and is willing to make the necessary contacts. No one challenges her or suggests another project. At the next meeting, she informs the group that the project is all set up and she had made all the arrangements.
3. Joan promises she will have her part of the project completed by a certain date. The date comes, and Joan does not have her part completed.

Discussion

1. What are some actions the participants can take to initiate a win-win solution, and move the group forward?
2. How can you use this exercise as a way of understanding and responding effectively in group projects?

| TABLE 8-5 | Characteristics of Effective and Ineffective Work Groups |

Effective Groups	Ineffective Groups
Goals are clearly identified and collaboratively developed.	Goals are vague or imposed on the group without discussion.
Open, goal-directed communication of feelings and ideas is encouraged.	Communication is guarded; feelings are not always given attention.
Power is equally shared and rotates among members, depending on ability and group needs.	Power resides in the leader or is delegated with little regard to member needs. It is not shared.
Decision making is flexible and adapted to group needs.	Decision making occurs with little or no consultation. Consensus is expected rather than negotiated based on data.
Controversy is viewed as healthy because it builds member involvement and creates stronger solutions.	Controversy and open conflict are not tolerated.
There is a healthy balance between task and maintenance role functioning.	There is a one-sided focus on task or maintenance role functions to the exclusion of the complementary function.
Individual contributions are acknowledged and respected. Diversity is encouraged.	Individual resources are not used. Conformity and being a "company person," is rewarded. Diversity is not respected.
Interpersonal effectiveness, innovation, and problem-solving adequacy are evident.	Problem-solving abilities, morale, and interpersonal effectiveness are low and undervalued.

Group membership should reflect stakeholders and key informants with the different skill sets needed to accomplish group goals. Essential member matching with task requirements includes matching with:

- Group goals
- Identified expectations for group achievement
- Availability and meeting schedule
- Capacity for ensuring deliverables

Task groups usually take place within specified time frames and need consistent administrative support to flourish. Table 8-5 lists characteristics of effective versus ineffective work groups.

LEADERSHIP STYLES

A flexible leadership style seems to work best for most groups. Effective leadership develops from leader characteristics, situational features, and member inputs working in tandem with each other. Different groups require different leadership behaviors. Leadership is contingent on a proper match between a group situation and the leadership style. Three types of leadership styles found in groups are authoritarian, democratic, and laissez-faire. Leaders demonstrating an **authoritarian leadership** style take full responsibility for group direction and control group interaction. Authoritarian leadership styles work best when the group needs a strong structure to function and there is limited time to reach a decision. **Democratic leadership** is a form of participative leadership, which involves members in active discussion and shared decision making (Rothwell, 2013). Democratic leaders are goal-directed but flexible. They offer members a functional structure while preserving individual member autonomy. Group members feel ownership of group solutions. **Laissez-faire leadership** is a disengaged form of leadership. The leader avoids making decisions, and is minimally present emotionally or otherwise in the group even in crisis situations. Groups with laissez-faire leadership are likely to be less productive and satisfying to group members.

Another way to look at leadership styles in professional group life is by using a situational framework (Blanchard et al 2013). This format requires group leaders to match their leadership style to the situation, and the maturity of the group members. A situational leadership style can be particularly adaptive in organizational group life when a new project is the object of group focus. The situational leader varies the amount of direction and support a group needs based on the complexity of the task and the follower's experience and confidence with achieving task or group goals.

Group maturity involves two forms of maturity: job maturity and psychological maturity related to the work. Job maturity refers to the level of group member work abilities, skills, and knowledge. Psychological job maturity refers to the group member feelings of confidence, willingness, and motivation. The capacity and readiness of situational maturity plays a role in type of preferred leadership style to accomplish goals. A basic assumption is that leadership should be flexible and adapted to group needs. Hershey and Blanchard describe four leadership styles, matched to employee's maturity level in a particular work situation and dependent on their need for structure and direction.

- Telling: high structure, low consideration
- Selling: high structure, high consideration
- Participating: high consideration, low structure
- Delegating: low consideration, low structure

Effective leaders adapt to the amount of structure required by changes in the group's maturity in working together. As the group matures, leaders turn more of the responsibility for the group to its members. Decision making is collaborative. The leader seeks member input, acts as discussion facilitator, and seeks consensus.

Leader and Member Responsibilities

Leadership tasks in work groups include:

- Forming the group structure and establishing the agenda for each meeting
- Clarifying the group's tasks and goals (providing background data and material if needed)
- Notifying each member of meeting dates, times, and place
- Keeping group members focused on tasks
- Adhering to time limits
- Concluding each meeting with a summarization of progress

Each member has accountability for the overall functioning of the group and the achievement of group goals. Group members should take responsibility for coming prepared to meetings, demonstrating respect for other members' ideas, and taking an active participatory role in the development of viable solutions. Affirming the contributions of team members helps build cohesion and investment in ensuring productive outcomes.

WORK GROUP DYNAMICS
Pre-Group Tasks

Successful work groups do not just happen. Before the group starts, participants should have a clear idea of what the group task commitment will entail in terms of time, effort, and knowledge—and be willing to commit to the task. Group members should have enough in common to engage in meaningful communication, relevant knowledge of the issues, and/or expertise needed for resolution, a willingness to make a contribution to the group solution, and the ability to complete the task. The group leader should come to each meeting prepared with a clear agenda, an overview of key issues, and member concerns. You can invite members to submit agenda items and involve others in developing an agenda.

Forming

Even if members are known to each other, it is useful to have each person give a brief introduction that includes his or her reason for being part of the work group. The leader should explain the group's purpose and structural components (e.g., time, place, and commitment) and ask for buy-in. Member responsibilities should be outlined clearly with time for questions. A task group with vague or poorly understood goals or structure breeds boredom or frustration, leading to power struggles and inadequate task resolution.

Norming

To be successful, group norms should support accomplishment of stated goals. In general, all data developed within the group context should be kept confidential until officially ready for publication. Otherwise the "grapevine" can distort information and sabotage group efforts. Members should be accountable for regular attendance. If administrative staff is part of the group membership, they should attend all, or designated meetings. Few circumstances are more threatening to a work-related group than having a supervisor enter and exit the task group at will.

Performing

Most of the group's work gets accomplished in the performing phase, including development of recommendations and preparation of final reports. Leader interventions should be consistent, well defined, and supportive as the group works to fulfill its charge.

Brainstorming

Brainstorming is a commonly employed strategy used to generate solutions during the performing phase. Guidelines for brainstorming include:

- Entertaining all ideas without censure
- Testing the more promising ideas for relevance
- Exploring consequences of each potential solution
- Identifying human and instrumental resources, including availability
- Achieving agreement about best possible solutions Exercise 8-8 provides an opportunity to experience brainstorming.

Group Think

Extreme cohesiveness can result in a negative group phenomena, referred to as group think. Originally defined by Janis (1971, 1982), **group think** occurs when the approval of other group members becomes so important that group members support a decision they fundamentally do not agree with, just for the

---

| EXERCISE 8-8 | **Brainstorming: Selecting Alternative Strategies** |

Purpose: To help students use a brainstorming process for considering and prioritizing alternative options.

Procedure

You have two exams within the next 2 weeks. Your car needs servicing badly. Because of all the work you have been doing, you have not had time to call your mother, and she is not happy. Your laundry is overflowing the hamper. Several of your friends are going to the beach for the weekend and have invited you to go along. How can you handle it all?

1. Give yourself 5 minutes to write down all the ideas that come to mind for handling these multiple responsibilities. Use single words or phrases to express your ideas. Do not eliminate any possibilities, even if they seem farfetched.
2. In groups of three or four students, choose a scribe and share the ideas you have written down. Discuss relevant pros and cons of each idea.
3. Select the three most promising ideas.
4. Develop several small, concrete, achievable actions to implement these ideas.
5. Share the small group findings with the class group.

Discussion

1. In what ways were the solutions you chose similar or dissimilar to those of your peers?
2. Were any of your ideas or ways of achieving alternative solutions surprising to you or to others in your group?
3. What did you learn from doing this exercise that could help you and a client generate possible solutions to seemingly impossible situations?

sake of harmony. Individual members are afraid to express conflicting ideas and opinions for fear of being excluded from the group. The group exerts pressure on members to act as one voice in decision making. Realistic evaluation of issues does not occur because group members minimize conflict in an effort to reach consensus. Warning signs of group think are listed in Box 8-3. Group think can create irrational decisions and dissatisfaction with goal achievement. Figure 8-2 displays the characteristics.

Norms that allow members to:
- Hold different opinions from other group members

BOX 8-3   Warning Signs of Group Think

1. Illusion of invulnerability
2. Collective rationalization that disregards warnings
3. Belief in inherent morality of the decision
4. Stereotyped or negative views of people outside of group
5. Direct pressure on dissenters to not express their concerns
6. Self-censorship—individual members with doubts do not express them
7. Illusion of unanimity in which majority view is held to be unanimous
8. Self-appointed "mindguards" within the group who withhold data that would be problematic or contradictory

Adapted from Janis I: *Groupthink: psychological studies of policy decisions and fiascoes*, ed 2, New York, 1982, Houghton Mifflin.

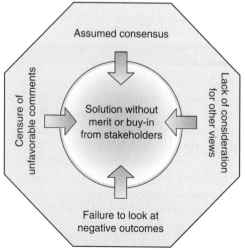

Figure 8-2   Characteristics of group think.

- Seek fresh information and outside opinions
- Act as "devil's advocate" about important issues

Adjourning Phase

Termination in work groups takes place when the group task is accomplished. The leader should summarize the work of the group, allow time for processing level of goal achievement, and identify any follow-up. Work groups need to disband once the initial charge is satisfied. They should not simply move on into a never-ending commitment without negotiation and the agreement of participants to continue with another assignment.

GROUPS VERSUS TEAMS

In 2003 the IOM report, *Health Professions Education: A Bridge to Quality*, identified the development and implementation of collaborative, multiskilled interdisciplinary teams as a key priority in contemporary health care delivery. Tubbs (2011) distinguishes between a group and a team by suggesting that a group connotes a more general term and that a team represents stronger cohesiveness and closeness than a group. Whereas Forsyth maintains that teams are fundamentally groups having similar characteristics of interdependence, structure, and ways of interacting, there are notable differences. The level of team interaction cannot be fully explained through group dynamics because team communication occurs within a continuous action-oriented relationship, using multiple formal and informal formats.

Team diversity increases team performance (Lundsmen et al, 2010).

A health care team can be defined as a coordinated group of professionals with complementary skills, who are mutually committed to specific performance goals, with shared accountability for goal achievement (Beebe and Masterson, 2014; Forsyth, 2010; Katzenbach and Smith, 1993). Communication and information sharing on interdisciplinary teams is a complex and multifaceted process.

There are many types of teams in health care organizations:
- *work teams* (e.g., surgical, primary care emergency),
- *parallel teams* (e.g., designated team to respond to cardiac arrest or to complete transitional transfers)

- *project teams* that work together on a single deliverable project.
- *management teams* that oversee the work of others (Taplin et al, 2013).

A health care team is an **embedded team**, meaning that it is "nested in and embedded with organizations in multiple ways and at multiple levels" (Seibold et al., 2014, p. 328). On an embedded team, members are expected to develop shared meanings related to established health goals, achieve consensus and constructively manage conflict, coordinate their actions, and offer interpersonal support to each other. Implementation takes place through actions related to specified health goals. Communication takes place through electronic channels, as well as in face-to-face contacts during meetings.

Each health care team is unique with its own set of purpose, member composition, and methods of communication (Mitchell et al., 2012). Team members, trained in different aspects of health care "seek to deliver coordinated care through a complex maze of roles, structures, regulations, and contexts with the goal of achieving optimal health outcomes for patients" (Villagran and Baldwin, 2014, p. 362). The team provides a professional interpersonal context for delivering synergistic quality client- and family-centered health care. Interdependence is evidenced in working together and collaborating to actively coordinate activities related to providing excellent clinical care. Team roles, functions, and contributions are interconnected and reinforce each other in completing the work of the team. The action component of team functions requires ongoing member interaction and coordinated actions to achieve desired clinical outcomes. Discussion in team meetings focuses on collaborative problem solving and decision making, with the goal of achieving effective coordination and implementation of quality client-centered care. The client and family are considered part of the health team.

All teams go through the stages of development described earlier for groups. Initially, team members have to build trust in each other and in the team process by getting to know each other and agreeing on common team-based goals and objectives. On interprofessional teams, this requires a broader knowledge than discipline-specific expectations. Team members are tasked with becoming knowledgeable about expected roles and expectations required to achieve client-centered clinical outcomes. Trust begins to develop as group members address personal concerns that could impede team effectiveness, and then develop norms to facilitate working together as a team. This stimulates an increase in team cohesion and leads to the trust needed for shared decision-making and the open communication required for productive team functioning.

Group member composition is different for interprofessional health care teams than for task or other types of work groups. The team brings together people with individual skills and abilities to complete coordinated and collaborative specialized tasks related to common client-centered health goals; the number of members varies and team composition needs to reflect specific health-related goals. Each team requires a stronger interdependent and adaptive commitment to the team's common purpose (Gladding, 2011).

Successful outcomes depend on team members combining and adapting their individual inputs to meet team goals as a unit. To accomplish the team's mission, it is critical that each member understands the various professional philosophies, training requirements, and role responsibilities of every other health team member, and that they trust each other's capabilities to achieve identified client-centered health goals. Differences are just as important as similarities in working together as a team. Professional roles and skills differ for each health profession, as does the professional socialization process for each clinical discipline. Just as with a sports team, different player roles complement each other and strengthen the team's ability to function as a single unit. Leadership is shared and can shift depending on the situation. Differences between groups and teams are outlined in Table 8-6.

SUMMARY

Chapter 8 looks at the ways in which a group experience enhances clients' abilities to meet therapeutic self-care demands, provides meaning, and is personally affirming. The rationale for providing a group experience for clients is described. Group dynamics include individual member commitment, functional similarity, and leadership style. Group concepts related to group dynamics consist of purpose, norms, cohesiveness, roles, and role functions. Tuckman's phases of group development—forming, storming, performing, and adjourning—provide guidelines for group leaders.

TABLE 8-6	Differences between Groups and Teams	
Working Group	**Team**
Strong, clearly focused leader	Shared leadership role
Individual accountability	Individual and mutual accountability
The group's purpose is the same as the broader organizational mission	Specific team purpose that the team itself delivers
Individual work products	Collective work products
Runs efficient meetings	Encourages open-ended discussion and active problem-solving meetings
Measures its effectiveness indirectly by its influence on others (e.g. financial performance of the business)	Measures performance directly by assessing collective work products
Discusses, decides, and delegates	Discusses, decides, and does real work together

Reprinted with permission from Katzenbach J, Smith D: The discipline of teams, *Harv Bus Rev*, 113, March/April 1993. Reprint number 93201.

In the forming phase of group relationships, the basic need is for acceptance. The storming phase focuses on issues of power and control in groups. Behavioral standards are formed in the norming phase that will guide the group toward goal accomplishment, and the group becomes a safe environment in which to work and express feelings. Most of the group's work is accomplished during the performing phase. Feelings of warmth, caring, and intimacy follow; members feel affirmed and valued. Finally when the group task is completed to the satisfaction of the individual members, or of the group as a whole, the group enters an adjourning (termination) phase. Different types of groups found in health care include therapeutic, support, educational, and discussion focus groups.

ETHICAL DILEMMA   What Would You Do?

Mrs. Murphy is 39 years old and has had multiple admissions to the psychiatric unit for bipolar disorder. She wants to participate in group therapy but is disruptive when she is in the group. The group gets angry with her monopolization of their time, but she says she has just as much right as a group member to talk if she chooses. Mrs. Murphy's symptoms could be controlled with medication, but she refuses to take it when she is "high" because it makes her feel less energized. How do you balance Mrs. Murphy's rights with those of the group? Should she be required to take her medication? How would you handle this situation from an ethical perspective?

DISCUSSION QUESTIONS

1. How would you describe the differences between a work task group and a collaborative health care team?
2. How do "active listening" strategies differ in group communication versus individual communication?
3. What do you see as potential ethical issues in group communication formats?

REFERENCES

Aronson S: Where the wild things are: the power and challenge of adolescent group work, *Mt Sinai J Med* 71(3):174–180, 2004.

Aggarwal P, O'Brien CL: Social loafing on group projects: Structural antecedents and effects on student satisfaction, *J Market Educ* 30(3):255–264, 2008.

Beebe SA, Masterson JT: *Communicating in Small Groups: Principles and Practices*, 10th ed, Boston, 2012, Pearson.

Beebe S, Masterson J: *Communicating in small groups: principles and practices*, ed 11, Pearson, 2014.

Benne KD, Sheats P: Functional roles of group members, *J Soc Issues* 4(2):41–49, 1948.

Beiling P, McCabe R, Antony M: *Cognitive-Behavioral Therapy in Groups*, New York, 2009, Guilford Press.

Bernard H, Birlingame G, Flores P, Greene L, Joyce A, et al.: Clinical practice guidelines for group psychotherapy, *Int J Group Psychother* 58(4):455–542, 2008.

Blanchard K, Zigarmi P, Zigarmi D: *Leadership and the one minute manager Updated*, New York, NY, 2013, Harper Collins.

Burlingame G, Strauss B, Joyce A, MacNair-Semands R, Mackenzie K, Ogrodniczuk J, et al.: *Core Battery—Revised*, New York, 2006, American Group Psychotherapy Association.

Clarke D, Adamoski E, Joyce B: In-patient group psychotherapy: the role of the staff nurse, *J Psychosoc Nurs Ment Health Serv* 36(5):22–26, 1998.

Corey M, Corey B: *Groups: process and practice*. 9th ed., Pacific Grove CA, 2013, Brooks/Cole.

Counselman E: Reader's forum: Why study group therapy? *International Journal of Group Psychotherapy* 58(2):265–272, 2008.

Deering CG: Process oriented groups: alive and well? *Int J Group Psychother* 64(2):164–179, 2014.

Dyer J, Stotts M: *Handbook of Remotivation Therapy*, Binghampton, NY: The Haworth clinical Practice Press, 2005.

Forsyth D: *Group Dynamics*, 5th ed, Belmont, CA, 2010, Wadsworth Cengage Learning.

Gans J, Alonso A: Difficult patients: their construction in group therapy, *Int J Group Psychother* 48(3):311–326, 1998.

Gladding S: *Groups: A Counseling Specialty*, 6th ed, Merrill, 2011.

Hinds P, Carley K, Krackharat D, Wholey D: Choosing work group members: Balancing similarity, competence, and familiarity, *Organ Behav Hum Decis Process* 81(2):226–251, 2000.

Institute of Medicine (IOM): *Report on Health Professions Education: A Bridge to Quality*, Washington DC, 2003, National Academies Press.

Institute of Medicine (IOM): *The Future of Nursing: Leading Change, Advancing Health*, Washington, DC, 2011, National Academies Press.

Janis I: Groupthink, 1971, *Psychol Today* 5:43–46, 1971, 74–76.

Janis Irving: *Groupthink: Psychological Studies of Policy Decisions and Fiascoes*, 2nd ed, New York, 1982, Houghton Mifflin.

Johnson D, Johnson F: *Joining Together: Group Theory and Group Skills*, 11th ed., Edinburgh Gate, 2012, England: Pearson Education Limited.

Katzenbach J, Smith J: The discipline of teams, *Harv Bus Rev*, 1993.

Lasky G, Riva M: Confidentiality and privileged communication in group psychotherapy, *Int J Group Psychother* 56(4):455–476, 2006. 2006.

Lumsden G, Lumsden D, Wiethoff C: *Communicating in Groups and Teams*, 5th ed, Boston, MA, 2010, Cengage Learning, Inc.

Mangione L, Forti R, Iacuzzi C: Ethics and endings in group psychotherapy: Saying good-bye and saying it well, *International J Group Psychother* 57(1):25–40, 2007.

Mathieu J, Maynard T, Rapp T, Gilson L: Team effectiveness A review of recent advancements and a glimpse into the future, *J Manage* 34:410–476, 2008.

Michaelsen LK, Sweet M: Team-Based Learning: Small Group Learning's Next Big Step. (eds). *New Directions in Teaching and Learning*, 2008.

Mitchell P, Wynia M, Golden R, et al: Core Principles and Values of Effective Team-Based Health Care: A Discussion Paper. Institute of Medicine, Washington, DC.

Moreno KJ: Scapegoating in Group Psychotherapy, *Int J Group Psychother* 57(1):93–104, 2007.

Percy C, Gibbs T, Potter L, Boardman S: Nurse-led peer support group: experiences of women with polycystic ovary syndrome, *J Adv Nurs* 65(10):2046–2055, 2009.

Powles W: Reader's forum: Reflections on "what is a group?", *Int J Group Psychother* 57(1):105–113, 2007.

Seibold D, Hollingshead A, Yoon K: Chapter 13: Embedded teams and embedding organizations. (2014). In Putnam L, Mumby D, editors: *The Sage Handbook of Organizational Communication*, 3rd ed, Thousand Oaks, CA, 2014, Sage Publications.

Rogers C: The process of the basic encounter group. In Diedrich R, Dye HA, editors: *Group procedures: purposes, processes and outcomes*, Boston, 1972, Houghton Mifflin.

Rothwell D: *In Mixed Company*, Boston MA, 2013, Wadsworth Cengage Learning.

Rubel D, Kline W: An exploratory study of expert group leadership, *J Special Group Work* 3(2):138–160, 2008.

Rutan JS, Stone W, Shay J: *Psychodynamic Group Psychotherapy*, New York, 2007, The Guilford Press.

Sluder H: The write way: using poetry for self-disclosure, *J Psychosoc Nurs Ment Health Serv* 28(7):26–28, 1990.

Stinson C: Structured group reminiscence: an intervention for older adults, *J Contin Educ Nurs* 40(11):521–528, 2009.

Taplin S, Foster M, Shortell S: Organizational leadership for building effective health care teams, *Ann Fam Med* 11(3):279–281, 2013.

Tubbs S: *A Systems Approach to Small Group Interaction*, 11th ed, Boston, 2011, McGraw Hill.

Tuckman B: Developmental sequence in small groups, *Psychological Bulletin* 63(6):384–399, 1965.

Tuckman B, Jensen M: Stages of small-group development revisited, *Group Organ Manag* 2(4):419–427, 1977.

Villagran M, Baldwin P: Chapter 22: Health care team communication. In *The Routledge Handbook of Language and Health Communication*, New York, 2014, Routledge.

Yalom I, Leszcz M: *The theory and practice of group psychotherapy*, 2005, ed 5, New York, 2005, Basic Books.

WEB RESOURCES

American Group Psychotherapy Association: www.groupsinc.org

American Society of Group Psychotherapy and Psychodrama (ASGPP): www.asgpp.org

Association for Specialists in Group Work
- Professional Training Standards: www.asgw.org/PDF/training_standards.pdf
- Best Practices Guidelines: www.asgw.org/PDF/best_Practices.pdf
- Principles for Diversity Competent Group Workers: www.asgw.org/PDF/Principles_for_Diversity.pdf

Self Concept in Professional Interpersonal Relationships

Elizabeth C. Arnold

OBJECTIVES

At the end of the chapter, the reader will be able to:
1. Define self-concept.
2. Describe the features of and functions of self-concept.
3. Identify theoretical frameworks associated with self-concept.
4. Identify functional health patterns and nursing diagnoses related to self-concept pattern disturbances.
5. Apply the nursing process in caring for clients with self-concept pattern disturbances related to body image, personal identity, and role performance.
6. Use therapeutic interventions related to self-esteem issues.
7. Recognize and apply therapeutic responses to meet client spiritual needs in health care.

Chapter 9 focuses on self-concept as a key dynamic in health communication and therapeutic relationships. The chapter identifies theoretical frameworks related to self-concept, and its development. The "Application" section discusses communication strategies nurses can use with clients to enhance positive self-concept and increase self-esteem in health care.

BASIC CONCEPTS

DEFINITION

Self concept represents peoples' complex reflection of their cultural heritage, their environment, their upbringing and education, their basic personality traits, and cumulative life experiences. Hypothesized as a multidimensional systems construct, it consists of personal beliefs, values, and attitudes (schemas and possible selves), which a person holds about who he or she is in relation to self-perceptions and others. The self-concept has personal physical, emotional, social, and spiritual dimensions, linked to functional well-being and quality of life.

Self-concept mirrors personal life experiences and incorporates the reflected appraisals of important people in a person's life. Self-identity usually incorporates a person's ethnic identity (Bailey, 2003). A healthy self-concept reflects attitudes, emotions, and values, which are realistic, congruent with each other, and consistent with a meaningful purpose in life. Figure 9-1 identifies characteristics of a healthy self-concept.

SIGNIFICANCE OF SELF-CONCEPT IN HEALTH CARE

A strong sense of self has been described as noteworthy protective factor in coping with chronic illness (Mussato et al., 2014). When people experience a major health disruption, it stimulates a significant alteration in the way they think, feel, and value their sense of self and the way they communicate with others in their immediate environment.

Case Example

I once interviewed a patient with advanced cancer. Tears came to his eyes as he told me about how he had to leave his job, couldn't run around with his grandchildren, couldn't do the things he loved, not like he used to, nope, not anymore. A single diagnosis had inflicted such profound devastation (Yurkiewicz, 2011).

Self-concept creates and reflects a person's personal reality in many aspects of life, but particularly in personal and work relationships, careers, life choices, and as a determinant of what is important to each person. Choices, congruent with self-concept, feel true; those that are not consistent with personally determined self-concepts create doubt and uncertainty. McCormick and Hardy (2008) observe, "Identity, the definition of one's self, is the heart of one's life" (p. 405). Some life choices are voluntary; others are not.

FEATURES AND FUNCTIONS OF SELF-CONCEPT

Cunha and Goncalves (2009) refer to the self as an open *system*, one that is fluid and dynamic. A person's self-concept consists of multiple self-images, which coexist in a person's consciousness. Different aspects of the self-concept become visible, depending on the situation in which people find themselves (Prescott, 2006). For example, a star athlete might be a marginal student. Which is the true self-image or

are both valid? Self-concepts help people make sense of their past, experience who they are in the present, and imagine what they are capable of becoming physically, emotionally, intellectually, socially, and spiritually in relationship with others in the future (Lee and Oyserman, 2009).

Over the course of a lifetime, the self-concept changes and develops in complexity. Hunter (2008) noted, "As one ages, the 'self' develops and becomes a more and more unique entity formed by personal experiences and personally developed values and beliefs" (p. 318). Exercise 9-1 provides an opportunity for you to practice self-awareness by examining your self-concept.

Self-Fulfilling Prophecies

Self-concepts help individuals make personal sense of their past, as it relates to the present and as it might be in the future (Lee and Oyserman, 2009). **Possible selves** is a term used to explain the future-oriented component of self-concept. Expectations and personal hope are part of the possible self. They are a valuable influence in goal setting and motivation, especially if they lead to realistic actions. For example, a nursing student might think, "I can see myself becoming a nurse practitioner." Such thoughts help the novice nurse work harder to achieve professional goals.

Concepts of negative possible selves can become a self-fulfilling prophecy (Markus and Nurius, 1986). For example, Martha receives a performance evaluation indicating a need for improved self-confidence. Viewing the criticism as a negative commentary on her "self," she performs awkwardly and freezes when asked questions in the clinical area.

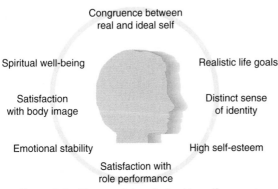

Congruence between real and ideal self

Spiritual well-being

Realistic life goals

Satisfaction with body image

Distinct sense of identity

Emotional stability

High self-esteem

Satisfaction with role performance

Figure 9-1   Characteristics of a healthy self-concept.

EXERCISE 9-1   Who Am I?

Purpose: To help students understand some of the self-concepts they hold about themselves.

Procedure
1. Spend 10 to 15 minutes reflecting about how you would define yourself if you had to do so, using only **three one-word** descriptors. There are no right or wrong answers.
2. Pick the one descriptor that you believe defines yourself best.
3. In small groups of four to six students, share your results.

Discussion
1. Were you surprised with any of your choices?
2. How hard was it to pick the one best descriptor out of the five?
3. How did you describe yourself? Could your self-descriptors be categorized or prioritized in describing your overall self-concept?
4. What did you learn about the process of examining your self-concept from doing this exercise?
5. How could you use this information in professional interpersonal relationships with clients?

DEVELOPMENT OF SELF-CONCEPT

At birth, people do not possess a self-concept. The external social context into which the child is born and personal caretaking relationships contribute greatly to self-understandings that shape a person's self-concept. Self-concept represents a blending of perceptions related to what life has presented to each person and how each person responds to it. Consider differences in the life experience and socialization of Prince George in London versus a child born into poverty with both parents working to make ends meet. What implications do you see for the development of each child's self-concept? Life experiences, significant relationships, opportunities, and setbacks influence how people define themselves throughout life.

Jackson (2014) notes, "Our sense of self is socially constructed" (p. 130). Social environment plays an important role in shaping and supporting personal self-concepts. A stable home environment, sports participation, academic success, religious institutions, professional opportunities, praise for successful accomplishments, supportive parents and mentors, tend to encourage the development of a positive self-concept. Factors such as poverty, chaotic upbringing, early loss of a parent, lack of educational opportunities, and adverse life events contribute to development of negative self-concepts. Some people with unfortunate social circumstances develop a dynamic self-concept as a reaction to their circumstances. They are interested in making their environment better and serve as role models to others about what is possible against all odds. Others with more fortunate life circumstances develop negative self-concepts or overinflated positive self- concepts with little grounding in reality.

When life "throws a health-related curve ball," nurses play a critical role in helping clients reframe a potentially incapacitating sense of self into one with more hope and broader options. They can help clients revisit personal strengths, consider new possibilities, incorporate new information, and seek out appropriate resources as a basis for making good clinical decisions and taking constructive actions. Even a nurse's "supportive presence" can give a client a reason to hope. Adler and colleagues (2012) note that a physician's belief as to whether a client will recover or not, can influence a client's true health state.

SELF-CONCEPT IN INTERPERSONAL RELATIONSHIPS

Self-concept is formed in relationship with others (Guerrero et al., 2014). When two people communicate, each person's perceptions are influenced by his or her own self-concepts and level of self-esteem. Sometimes referred to as an "affective margin of distortion," the factors presented in Figure 9-2 can implicitly influence interpersonal interactions.

A clear cultural identity is positively related to self-concept clarity and self-esteem (Usborne and Taylor, 2010). Understanding fundamental differences in cultural worldview orientation helps nurses frame supportive self-concept interventions in ways that support ethnocultural variations (see Chapter 7). In general, Western cultures tend to be individualistic, whereas Asian cultures see the individual as part of a collective group.

Case Example

From a North American perspective, a collective answer to the "who am I" question is that "I am a bounded, autonomous whole." The solution to this question from a Japanese perspective is "I am a member or a participant of a group" (Oyserman and Markus, 1998, p. 110).

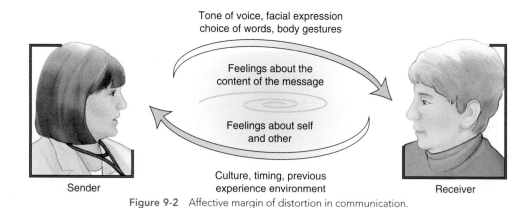

Figure 9-2 Affective margin of distortion in communication.

GENDER

Gender refers to "socially constructed and enacted roles and behaviors that occur in a historical and cultural context, and that vary across societies and over time" (Leerdam et al., 2014, p. 53). Gender self-perceptions evolve from socially learned behaviors and are supported with distinctions in dress and role expectations. Even children in kindergarten distinguish between girls wearing dresses and liking dolls, and boys liking rough play and playing active games (Martin and Ruble, 2010). Despite progressive sociological changes, subtle gender differences are still evidenced in social expectations, career options, pay differentials, and so forth. They exist in how people are treated, what is important to them, and in how men and women are socialized to respond to verbal and nonverbal cues in communication.

SELF-CONCEPT CLARITY

Self-concept clarity is defined as "the extent to which the contents of one's self-beliefs are clearly and confidently defined, internally consistent, and temporally stable" (Blazek and Besta, 2012, p. 1). During midlife, women in particular can experience greater self-clarity and identity integration (Arnold, 2005; Stewart et al., 2001). In later life, social role changes related to retirement, loss of a spouse, and limiting medical or economic circumstances influence self-concept clarity (Lodi-Smith and Roberts, 2010).

Although cognitive awareness of the self-concept is never fully complete, the Johari Window provides a disclosure/feedback model to help people learn more about their self-concept (Luft and Ingham, 1955). The model consists of four areas:

1. Open self (arena): what is known to self and others
2. Blind self: what is known by others but not by self
3. Hidden self (façade): what is known by self but not by others
4. Unknown self: what is unknown to self and also unknown to others

The larger the open self-box is, the more one knows about oneself and the more flexibility a person has to realistically interpret and constructively cope with challenging health situations. Increasing the open area through asking for and receiving feedback (decreasing blind self) and using self-disclosure (decreasing the hidden self) contribute to self-awareness. Decreasing the unknown area through self-discovery, new observations by others, and mutual illumination of experiences increases the open area. The larger the open self-box is, the more one knows about oneself and the more flexibility a person has to realistically interpret and constructively cope with challenging health situations.

Developing self-awareness is critical for nurses. A nurse's unfavorable self-impressions of a client can unintentionally limit a client's sense of self-esteem. Communicating requires a well-defined, straightforward unbiased self-concept, which allows nurses to more authentically connect with clients.

THEORETICAL FRAMEWORKS

SELF-CONCEPT FRAMEWORKS

William James (1890) was the first major theorist to describe self-concept as an important idea in psychology. He makes a distinction between "the I and the me: the I is equated with the self-as-knower and the me is equated with the self-as-known" (Konig, 2009, p. 102). The "I" refers to what we cognitively and emotionally think about ourselves, and the "me" refers to the content of those observations for example perception of personal characteristics, activity preferences, capabilities, and values.

The self is a central construct in humanistic and psychodynamic theories of personality. Both approaches argue that our self-concept develops out of, and is influenced by, social interactions with others. Carl Rogers (1951) defined the *self* as "an organized, fluid, but consistent conceptual pattern of perceptions of characteristics and relationships or the 'I' and the 'me' together with values attached to these concepts" (p. 498). When the "actual self" and the "ideal self" (how a person would ideally like to be) are similar, the person is likely to have a positive self-concept and self-esteem. Rogers believed that all individuals want to achieve their human potential. He equated having a coherent well-integrated self-concept with being mentally healthy and well adjusted (Diehl and Hay, 2007). Harry Stack Sullivan (1953) referred to self-concept as a self-system that people develop to (1) develop a consistent image of self, (2) protect themselves against feeling anxiety, and (3) maintain their interpersonal security. During early childhood, people develop self-concepts of a good me (resulting from reward and approval experiences), a bad me (resulting from punishment and disapproval experiences), and a not me (resulting from anxiety-producing experiences that are dissociated by the person as not being a part of his or her self-concept). Having a therapeutic relationship can help clients develop a different more positive sense of self.

George Mead applies a sociological approach to the study of self-concept. The self-concept affects and is influenced by how people experience themselves in relation to others (Elliott, 2008). Mead's model emphasizes the influence of culture, moral norms, and language in framing self-concepts through interpersonal interactions (symbolic interactionism).

ERIKSON'S THEORY OF PSYCHOSOCIAL DEVELOPMENT

Erik Erikson's (1968, 1982) theory of psychosocial self-development is a well-known model. Central to his framework is the concept of personal identity. He believed that "identity formation neither begins nor ends with adolescence: it is lifelong development" (Erikson, 1959, p. 122). Personality develops in complexity as a person recognizes and responds to evolving developmental challenges (psychosocial crises) during the life cycle. As people pass through ascending stages of ego development, with mastery of each developmental task, a personalized sense of identity evolves. Many of the conflicted behaviors seen in adolescence reflect a teen's testing of different roles as they seek to establish a strong comfortable personal identity Although individuals mature physically and psychosocially sequentially in the same order, they do so at different speeds, in line with their environment, culture, and genetic makeup, (Myers, 2012).

The first four stages of Erikson's model serve as building blocks for his central developmental task of establishing a healthy ego identity (identity vs. identity diffusion). Diehl and Hay (2007) note, "Successful resolution of this particular developmental task is believed to be an important cornerstone for successful social and emotional development in middle age and later adulthood" (p. 1258). Developmental tasks in adulthood include finding a meaningful occupation, establishing committed relationships, contributing to the welfare of family and others, and sharing one's wisdom with the larger community. In later adulthood, a well-lived life results in a sense of integrity about oneself and satisfaction with that life. Life review reveals few regrets, even when confronting death. Failure to successfully complete tasks associated with a developmental stage results

in a reduced capacity to effectively negotiate later stages and a weakened self-concept. Erikson stages of ego stage development are outlined in Table 9-1.

Erikson believes that stage development is never final. Individuals have the potential to successfully rework developmental stages at a later time. Nurses use Erikson's model to analyze age appropriateness of behavior from an ego development perspective. For example, a teenager giving birth is still coping with issues of self-identity, rather than generativity. Exercise 9-2 focuses on applying Erikson's concepts to client situations.

Developing an Evidence-Based Practice

Ponsford J, Kelly A, Couchman G: Self-concept and self-esteem after acquired brain injury: a control group comparison, *Brain Inj* 28(2):146-154, 2014.

This study used a group comparison on self-report questionnaires to examine the multidimensional self-concept, global self-esteem, and psychological adjustment of an age- and gender-matched study sample of 41 individuals with traumatic brain injury (TBI) compared with 41 control participants. Three self-report questionnaires (Rosenberg Self-Esteem Scale, Tennessee Self-Concept Scale, and the Hospital Anxiety and Depression Scale) were administered to all study subjects.

Results: TBI clients showed significantly lower means of global self-esteem, and self-concept on the Rosenberg Self-Esteem and Tennessee Self-Concept scales. TBI subjects rated themselves lower on self-dimensions related to social, family, academic/work, and personal self-concept as compared to controls. TBI survivors also reported higher mean levels on the Hospital Anxiety and Depression Scales.

Application to Your Clinical Practice: Recognition of self-concept and self-esteem as potential issues for TBI clients, with negative emotional consequences may be an important underlying dynamic with these clients. Strategies to enhance self-esteem, and strengthen self-concept should be components of effective care for TBI clients.

APPLICATIONS

SELF-CONCEPT

The "Applications" section identifies strategies to strengthen self-concept, self-efficacy, and self-esteem in health care relationships and communication. It is

TABLE 9-1 Erikson's Stages of Psychosocial Development, Clinical Behavior Guidelines, and Stressors

Stage of Personality Guidelines	Ego Strength or Virtue	Clinical Behavior Guidelines	Stressors
Trust vs. mistrust	Hope	Appropriate attachment behaviors Ability to ask for assistance with an expectation of receiving it Ability to give and receive information related to self and health Ability to share opinions and experiences easily Ability to differentiate between how much one can trust and how much one must distrust	Unfamiliar environment or routines Inconsistency in care Pain Lack of information Unmet needs (e.g., having to wait 20 minutes for a bedpan or pain injection) Losses at critical times or accumulated loss Significant or sudden loss of physical function (e.g., a client with a broken hip being afraid to walk)
Autonomy vs. shame and doubt	Willpower	Ability to express opinions freely and to disagree tactfully Ability to delay gratification Ability to accept reasonable treatment plans and hospital regulations Ability to regulate one's behaviors (overcompliance, noncompliance, suggest disruptions) Ability to make age-appropriate decisions	Overemphasis on unfair or rigid regulation (e.g., putting clients in nursing homes to bed at 7 p.m.) Cultural emphasis on guilt and shaming as a way of controlling behavior Limited opportunity to make choices in a hospital setting Limited allowance made for individuality
Initiative vs. guilt	Purpose	Ability to develop realistic goals and to initiate actions to meet them Ability to make mistakes without undue embarrassment Ability to have curiosity about health care Ability to work for goals Ability to develop constructive fantasies and plans	Significant or sudden change in life pattern that interferes with role Loss of a mentor, particularly in adolescence or with a new job Lack of opportunity to participate in planning of care Overinvolved parenting that does not allow for experimentation Hypercritical authority figures No opportunity for play
Industry vs. inferiority	Competence	Work is perceived as meaningful and satisfying Appropriate satisfaction with balance in lifestyle pattern, including leisure activities Ability to work with others, including staff Ability to complete tasks and self-care activities in line with capabilities Ability to express personal strengths and limitations realistically	Limited opportunity to learn and master tasks Illness, circumstance, or condition that compromises or obliterates one's usual activities Lack of cultural support or opportunity for training

Stage	Virtue	Positive Indicators	Threats
Identity vs. identity diffusion	Fidelity	Ability to establish friendships with peers Realistic assertion of independence and dependence needs Demonstration of overall satisfaction with self-image, including physical characteristics, personality, and role in life	Lack of opportunity Overprotective, neglectful, or inconsistent parenting Sudden or significant change in appearance, health, or status Lack of same-sex role models
Identity vs. isolation	Fidelity	Ability to express and act on personal values Congruence of self-perception with nurse's observation and perception of significant others	
Intimacy vs. isolation	Love	Ability to enter into strong reciprocal interpersonal relationships Ability to identify a readily available support system Ability to feel the caring of others Ability to act harmoniously with family and friends	Competition Communication that includes a hidden agenda Projection of images and expectations onto another person Lack of privacy Loss of significant others at critical points of development
Generativity vs. stagnation and self-absorption	Caring	Demonstration of age-appropriate activities Development of a realistic assessment of personal contributions to society Development of ways to maximize productivity Appropriate care of whatever one has created Demonstration of a concern for others and a willingness to share ideas and knowledge Evidence of a healthy balance among work, family, and self-demands	Aging parents, separately or concurrently with adolescent children Obsolescence or layoff in career "Me generation" attitude Inability or lack of opportunity to function in a previous manner Children leaving home Forced retirement
Integrity vs. despair	Wisdom	Expression of satisfaction with personal lifestyle Acceptance of growing limitations while maintaining maximum productivity Expression of acceptance of certitude of death, as well as satisfaction with one's contributions to life Lack of opportunity	Rigid lifestyle Loss of significant other Loss of physical, intellectual, and emotional faculties Loss of previously satisfying work and family roles

EXERCISE 9-2	Erikson's Stages of Psychosocial Development

Purpose: To help students apply Erikson's stages of psychosocial development to client situations.

Procedure

This exercise may be done as a homework exercise with the results shared in class.

To set your knowledge of Erikson's stages of psychosocial development, identify the psychosocial crisis or crises each of the following clients might be experiencing:

1. A 16-year-old unwed mother having her first child
2. A 50-year-old executive "let go" from his job after 18 years of employment
3. A stroke victim paralyzed on the left side
4. A middle-aged woman caring for her mother, who has Alzheimer disease

Discussion

1. What criteria did you use to determine the most relevant psychosocial stage for each client situation?
2. What conclusions can you draw from doing this exercise that would influence how you would respond to each of these clients?

important to start care relationships with the premise that each client is a unique person with both obvious and hidden strengths, values, cultural beliefs and experiential life concerns. What health providers say, how they say it, and what they do matters in establishing relationships supportive of client personhood and client centered care (Drench, et. al. 2011).Self-concept variables can act as facilitators or create barriers to a client's efforts to engage in healthier lifestyle behaviors and self-management of chronic disorders. Self-concept is an essential starting point for understanding client behaviors related to coping, engagement in meaningful activities, and improved mood (van Tuyl et al., 2014).

PATTERNS AND NURSING DIAGNOSIS RELATED TO SELF-CONCEPTS

Gordon (2007) identifies related functional health patterns as self-perception, self-concept, and value-belief patterns. Injury, illness, and treatment can challenge these functional health patterns, regardless of specific medical diagnosis. As a person's perception of self-concept is disturbed, perception of the future becomes uncertain and unpredictable (Ellis-Hill and Horn, 2000). The importance of self-concept in nursing practice is further underscored by NANDA International (2014), which characterizes self-concept pattern disturbances as valid nursing diagnoses. Included in the spectrum of nursing diagnoses related to self-concept and self-esteem are

- *Body Image disturbance* (physical)
- *Personal Identity disturbance* (cognitive and perceptual awareness)

- *Altered Role Performance* (functional capacity and self-efficacy)
- *Self-Esteem* disturbance (emotional valuing)
- *Spiritual Distress* (connectivity with a higher purpose or God)

BODY IMAGE DISTURBANCE

Body image involves people's perceptions, thoughts and behaviors associated with their appearance Bolton et al. (2010) Perception of one's body image changes throughout life, influenced by the process of aging, appraisals of others, cultural and social factors, and physical changes resulting from illness, injury, and even treatment effects. For example, the potential for impotence and incontinence with prostate surgery can create a body image issue for men, secondary to treatment (Harrington, 2011).

Body image refers to how people *perceive* their physical characteristics, not how they realistically appear to others. A critical dimension of body image is the value people place on their appearance, biological or functional intactness (Slatman, 2011). For example, individuals with an eating disorder may see themselves as "fat" people despite being dangerously underweight. Ideal body image reflects sociocultural norms and popular media portrayals. Different cultures characterize similar physical characteristics as positive and others as negative. In the United States, a trim figure for women and a lean, muscular body for men are admired (Vartanian, 2009). In other cultures, obesity may be viewed as a sign of prosperity, fertility, or the ability to survive (Boston Women's Health Book Collective, 1998).

Body image is closely linked to self-concept such that any change in physical appearance or function can challenge it (Dropkin, 1999).

Permanent and even temporary changes in appearance influence how others respond to us, in words and actions. Discrimination can be subtle or overt, and the experience of a distorted body image can be long lasting. In a study of overweight adolescents, a primary theme that emerged was "a forever knowing of self as overweight" (Smith and Perkins, 2008, p. 391).

Some body images disturbances are not visible to others, for example, infertility, loss of bladder function, and loss of energy from radiation treatments. Chronic pain can undermine a person's self-identity and self-confidence creating a sense of vulnerability about oneself. People having these issues or conditions with fluctuating symptoms, such as epilepsy, can experience similar feelings of insecurity and uncertainty related to body image.

NURSING STRATEGIES

The *meaning* of body image differs from person to person. Some, such as Helen Keller or Andrea Bocelli frame a potentially negative body image as a positive feature of who they are. Others let a physical deviation become their defining feature. Clients with the same medical condition can have different body image issues (Bolton et al., 2010). Assessment should take into account

- Verbal expression of negative feelings about the body
- No mention of changes in body structure and function or preoccupation with changed body structure or function following medical interventions
- Reluctance to look at or touch a changed body structure
- Social isolation and loss of interest in friends after a change in body structure, appearance, or function
- Expressed concerns about psychosocial and role performance adjustment

Client-centered assessment includes the client's strengths, expressed needs and goals, the nature and accessibility of the client's support system, and the impact of body image change on lifestyle. Frequently there is so much focus on a client's deficits that potential compensatory personal resources are overlooked. Personal strengths can include religious beliefs, supportive family and friends, being able to care for oneself, persistence, life skills and talents, and hope. A simple query, "tell me about yourself" can start a conversation, which broadens client perspective.

Case Example

"My basic attitude toward life . . . people, things, life circumstances, has always been a positive one. The change I experience in the fifties is that it is a free and sincere reaction to life, not an expected response that I must produce" (Arnold, 2005, p. 644)

Modeling acceptance starts with the nurse. Acceptance is a process, and clients need time to resolve body image issues. Open-ended questions about what the client expects, providing coaching, and helping clients identify social supports can facilitate acceptance. Talking with others with similar changes provides credible, practical advice, for example, a Reach to Recovery volunteer visit with a mastectomy client and referrals to support groups.

PERSONAL IDENTITY

Identity is described as an intrapersonal psychological process consisting of a person's perceptions or images of personal abilities, characteristics, and potential growth potential (Karademas et al., 2008). Personal identity develops and changes over time related to stage of life, situational factors, and diverse life experiences. There are multiple dimensions to personal identity: gender and sexual identity, role identity as parent, student, widow, worker, retiree, cultural and ethnic identity, economic contextual identity and so forth. Each facet impacts a person's "worldview," sense of self and communication with others.

Normally we pass sequentially through each life stage as outlined by Erikson; our perceptions of self-identity changing to reflect who we are in the present moment physically, psychologically contextually and spiritually. Jung (1960) contends, "The afternoon of life is just as full of meaning as the morning; only its meaning and purpose are different (p. 138). Prior to midlife the energy focus is outward; in midlife the focus changes to a more selective inner reflection, thoughtful choices and a more authentic reordering of priorities.

When a major and/or sudden change in health status forces a reappraisal of personal identity, its impact on a client can be swift and compelling.

Case Example

"When I got up at last…and had learned to walk again, one day I took a hand glass and went to a long mirror to look at myself, and I went alone. I didn't want anyone… to know how I felt when I saw myself for the first time. But here was no noise, no outcry; I didn't scream with rage when I saw myself. I just felt numb. That person in the mirror couldn't be me. I felt inside like a healthy, ordinary, lucky person—oh, not like the ONE in the mirror! Yet when I turned my face to the mirror there were my own eyes looking back, hot with shame…when I did not cry or make any sound, it became impossible that I should speak of it to anyone, and the confusion and the panic of my discovery were locked inside me then and there, to be faced alone, for a very long time to come" (Goffman, 1963).

Case Example

Linda is an RN working in a busy surgery center. Returning to work after a hospitalization for major depression, she finds she has been relieved of her position as charge nurse. Other staff are highly protective of her. She is carefully watched to ensure that she is not going to relapse and she is given simpler tasks to avoid stressing her out. Linda can't understand why her coworkers don't see her as the same person she was before. Her depression is in remission. But in the eyes of her coworkers, Linda has been "reclassified" as a mentally ill person. Her colleagues' efforts are well intentioned, but they negatively affect Linda's sense of personal identity.

Individuals with cognitive impairment experience major issues with maintaining personal identity. Sensory images enter the psyche, but the brain's normal cognitive connections people use to interpret their meaning cannot make sense of them. Lake (2014) speaks of dementia as a disorder that "slowly diminishes personhood and devastates the relationships that personhood enables" (p. 5). People with dementia lose their ability to set realistic goals, implement coherent patterns of behavior, and control basic elements of their lives. As the disease progresses, they can no longer recognize significant others or retain a sense of personal identity. As one caregiver described it, "there are two deaths with Alzheimers disease—the death of self and the actual death (Nolan, 1984). Interestingly however, in a study of adults with dementia, Fazio and Mitchell (2009) found that these clients could identify themselves in photographs taken with an instant camera despite forgetting the photo had been taken minutes earlier. This finding suggests a persistence of self even when memory is significantly impaired.

NURSING STRATEGIES

Any health change challenges a person's sense of personal identity. Heijmans et al (2004) suggest that in addition to accepting an illness and learning new self-management skills, many people have to adapt to an altered social identity and renegotiate social relationships. This activity requires an emotional appraisal and adjustment, because things are not the same either for the client or for those with whom the person interacts. Renegotiating relationships can be awkward, and clients often need the nurse's help in how to respond.

Blazer (2008) suggests developing self-perceptions of achieving personal health and well-being may be as important as objective data for predicting health outcomes over time. Nurses can help clients reestablish a more positive self-identity by carefully listening to the client and family and asking open-ended questions in a spirit of mutual discovery related to

- What is this client coping with, related to self-identity?
- What is this client able to do in his or her current circumstances?
- What is needed to support this client in reconnecting with the person that he or she is capable of being?

Including a significant family member at some point in the discussion can be helpful. Family sometimes identify a behavior or personal characteristic that the client overlooks. Benner (2003) advocates exploring what matters to the client, and emphasizing a person's strengths as a basis for developing and enhancing creative meaning. Believing that clients *can* improve their situation creates new possibilities for enhancing personal identity in serious illness. Even the smallest positive movement toward change can make a difference in a client's self-image.

Box 9-1 describes client-centered interventions to enhance personal identity.

PERCEPTION

Perception is referred to as the gatekeeper of personal identity. It is the cognitive process through which a person transforms sensory data into connected personalized image patterns. Consider the image in Figure 9-3. Depending on where your eyes focus, you could draw different conclusions. Which image do you see—a vase or two figures looking at

BOX 9-1	Patient-Centered Interventions to Enhance Personal Identity: Perceptions and Cognition

- Take time to orient newly admitted clients to the unit, patient rights, and the normal care routine.
- Pay close attention to the client's "story" of the present health care experience, including concerns about coping, impact on self and others, and hopes for the future.
- Remember that each client is unique. Respect and tailor responses to support individual differences in personality, personal responses, intellect, values, and understanding of medical processes.
- Encourage as much client input as is realistically possible into diagnostic and therapeutic regimens.
- Provide information as it emerges about changes in treatment, personnel, discharge, and after care. Include family members whenever possible, particularly when giving difficult news.
- Explain treatment procedures including rationale and allow ample time for questions and discussion.
- Encourage family members to bring in familiar objects or pictures, particularly if the client is in the hospital or care facility for an extended period.
- Encourage as much independence and self-direction as possible.
- Avoid sensory overload and repeat instructions if the client appears anxious.
- Use perceptual checks to ensure you and the client have the same understanding of important material.
- Encourage older adults to maintain an active, engaged lifestyle in line with their interests and values.

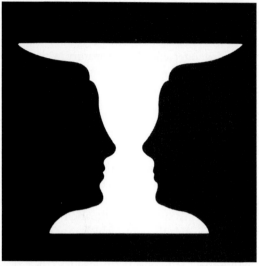

Figure 9-3 The figure-ground phenomenon. Where you focus your attention makes a difference in your perception of the figures. (*From the Westinghouse Learning Corporation:* Self-instructional unit 12: perception, 1970. *Reprinted with permission.*)

Case Example

Grace Ann Hummer is a 65-year-old widow with arthritis, a weight problem, and failing eyesight. Admitted for a minor surgical procedure, Ms. Hummer tells the nurse she does not know why she came. Nothing can be done for her because she is too old and decrepit.

Nurse: As I understand it, you came in today for removal of your bunions. Can you tell me more about your problem as you see it? (*Asking for this information separates the current situation from an overall assessment of ill health.*)

Client: Well, I've been having trouble walking, and I can't do some of the things I like to do that require extensive walking. I also have to buy "clunky" shoes that make me look like an old woman.

Nurse: So you are not willing to be an old woman yet? (*Taking the client's statement and challenging the cognitive distortion presented in her initial comments with humor allows the client to view her statement differently.*)

Client (laughing): Right, there are a lot of things I want to do before I'm ready for a nursing home.

each other? A deliberate shift of focus can transform what you see as a perceptual image.

The same phenomena is true in life situations. Reality lies in the eye of the beholder. Helping clients refocus attention on difficult circumstances from a new perspective can alter meaning and suggest different options. Perceptions differ because people develop mindsets that automatically alter sensory data in personal ways. Clients with delirium or psychoactive drug reactions experience global perceptual distortions, whereas those with mental illness can experience personalized perceptual distortions. Distorted perceptions influence communication in sending, receiving, and interpreting verbal messages and nonverbal behaviors. Simple perceptual distortions can be challenged with compassionate questioning and sometimes targeted humor. Validation of perceptual data is needed because the nurse and the client may not be processing the same reality.

Perceptual checks and active listening help clients make sense of perceptual data in a more conscious way, and the client feels heard. A constructive reframing of personal identity in the face of serious illness can contribute to treatment adherence and a stronger sense of well-being. Keeping communication simple, delivering straightforward messages with compassion, and making interactions participatory with a back-and-forth dialogue reduces the potential for acting on perceptual distortions.

COGNITION

Cognition represents the thinking processes people use to make sense of their perceptions. What people *think* about their perceptions is the throughput, which connects perceptions with associated feelings and directly influences clinical outcomes. According to Aron Beck (2011), faulty perceptions of a situation can stimulate automatic negative thoughts, which may not be realistic. Referred to as cognitive distortions, automatic thoughts about self-constructed realities create negative feelings, which can have a powerful impact on communication and behavior. As clients become more open to examining their cognitive distortions and the erroneous beliefs supporting them, they are better able to develop realistic solutions to difficult health problems. Conscious reality based thought processes are essential to acquiring and sustaining an accurate interpretation of self. Nurses can use to supportive strategies as outlined in the following paragraphs to help clients rebalance thinking operations conducive to effective functioning. Figure 9-4 demonstrates the link between perceptions and behaviors.

SUPPORTIVE NURSING STRATEGIES

Cognitive behavioral approaches, originally developed by Aaron Beck, focus on encouraging clients to reflect on difficult situations from a broader respective. Beck refers to cognitive distortions as "thinking errors." Reflecting on different potential explanations provide clients with more options to realistically interpret the meaning of their perceptions. A sudden mood change suggests an automatic thought. Cognitive approaches help clients identify, reflect on, and challenge negative automatic thinking processes instead of accepting them as reality. Common cognitive distortions are identified in Box 9-2.

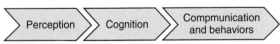

Figure 9-4 Cognitive reappraisal should be the process focus for changing negative automatic thoughts.

Other strategies to help clients reframe negative thinking patterns include providing additional alternative information, and Socratic questioning. Modeling cues to behavior, and coaching clients to challenge cognitive distortions with positive self-talk and mindfulness is helpful too. Feedback and social support are powerful antidotes to cognitive distortions. Exercise 9-3 provides practice with recognizing and responding to cognitive distortions.

SELF-ESTEEM

Self-esteem is defined as the *emotional* value a person places on his or her self-concept, expressed as either a positive or negative evaluation. People who view themselves as worthwhile and as being valuable members of society have high self-esteem. They are able to challenge negative beliefs that are unproductive or interfere with successful functioning. With a positive attitude about self, an individual is more likely to view life as a glass half full rather than half empty. People with low self-esteem do not value themselves and do not feel valued by others. Self-esteem can be related to either a specific dimension of self, "I am a good writer," or it may have a more global meaning, "I am a good person who is worth knowing."

BOX 9-2	Examples of Cognitive Distortions

- "All or nothing" thinking—the situation is all good or all bad; a person is trustworthy or untrustworthy.
- Overgeneralizing—one incident is treated as if it happens all the time; picking out a single detail and dwelling on it.
- Mind reading and fortune telling—deciding a person does not like you without checking it out; assuming a bad outcome with no evidence to support it.
- Personalizing—seeing yourself as flawed, instead of separating the situation as something you played a role in but did not cause.
- Acting on "should" and "ought to"—deciding in your mind what is someone else's responsibility without perceptual checks; trying to meet another's expectations without regard for whether it makes sense to do so.
- "Awfulizing"—assuming the worst; every situation has a catastrophic interpretation and anticipated outcome.

High self-esteem is associated with self-concept clarity (Stopa et al., 2010). People with high self-esteem respect and like who they are. They are generally satisfied with their looks, personality, skills, and ability to successfully negotiate their lives. They accept responsibility for their success *and* failures and take calculated risks to achieve important personal goals. They are more likely to be motivated to make changes. Life's inevitable problems are viewed as challenges that one can learn and grow from. Table 9-2 identifies behaviors associated with high versus low self-esteem.

Self-esteem is closely linked to our emotions, particularly those of pride or shame (Brown and Marshall, 2001). Verbal and nonverbal behaviors presenting as powerlessness, frustration, inadequacy, anxiety, anger,

or apathy suggest low self-esteem. They tend to be defensive in relationships and seek constant reassurance from others because of self-doubt. Instead of taking constructive actions that could raise self-esteem, they worry about issues they cannot control and see life challenges as problems rather than as opportunities. People with low self-esteem are less likely to correctly identify the informational value of their feelings (Harden, 2005). This is important as they are easily influenced by what is referred to at an affective margin of distortion that can color communication (displayed in figure 9-4).

The experience of success or failure can cause fluctuations in self-esteem (Crocker et al., 2006). Sources of situational challenges include loss of a job; loss of

TABLE 9-2	Behaviors Associated with High vs. Low Self-Esteem	
People with High Self-Esteem	**People with Low Self-Esteem**
Expect people to value them	Expect people to be critical of them
Are active self-agents	Are passive or obstructive self-agents
Have positive perceptions of their skills, appearance	Have negative perceptions of their skills, appearance, sexuality, and behaviors
Perform equally well when being observed as when not being observed	Perform less well when being observed
Are nondefensive and assertive in response to criticism	Are defensive and passive in response to criticism
Can accept compliments easily	Have difficulty accepting compliments
Evaluate their performance realistically	Have unrealistic expectations about their performance
Are relatively comfortable relating to authority figures	Are uncomfortable relating to authority figures
Express general satisfaction with life	Are dissatisfied with their lot in life
Have a strong social support system	Have a weak social support system
Have a primary internal locus of control	Rely on an external locus of control

EXERCISE 9-3	What Matters to Me?

Purpose: To help students understand the relationship between self-concepts and what is valued.

Procedure
This exercise may be done as a homework exercise and shared with your small group.
1. Spend 10 to 15 minutes reflecting about the three things you value most in your life. (There are no right or wrong answers.)
2. Now prioritize them and identify the one that you value the most.
3. In one to two paragraphs, explain why the top contender is most important to you.

4. In small groups of four to six students, share your results.

Discussion
1. Were you surprised by any of your choices, or what you perceived as being most important to you?
2. In what ways do your choices affirm self-concept and self-esteem?
3. What are the implications of doing this exercise for your helping clients understand what they value and how this reflects self-esteem?

an important relationship; and negative change in appearance, role, or status. Long-standing issues of verbal or physical abuse, neglect, chronic illness, codependency, and criticism by significant others can result in lowered self-esteem. Illness, injury, and other health issues also challenge a person's self-esteem. Findings from a sizable number of research studies demonstrate an association in changes in health status, functional abilities, and emotional dysfunction, and lowering of self-esteem (Vartanian, 2009; Vickery et al., 2008).

Case Example

Jenna was a professor at a major university when she was diagnosed with advanced metastatic breast cancer. All her life, Jenna had been a take-charge person and relished her capacity to run her life effectively and efficiently. People respond to her with high regard and respect because of her position and her personality. Admitted to the hospital, Jenna brought her pre-illness self-image of being treated with deference to the hospital. She expected similar responsiveness from hospital staff. Her health care providers, unfamiliar with her background and personal identity issues, expected compliance with no challenges to their authority. Angry at being unable to control her medical situation, she was demanding and angry. The staff considered her a difficult, obstinate client. Viewed from being a "patient" context, Jenna's behavior seemed irrational; understood from the perspective of a having a sudden challenge to a lifelong self-concept of independence and deference, her seemingly "irrational" behavior made sense. Once the connection was made to Jenna's personal identity issues, a different dialogue emerged between staff and client, with a deeper respect for Jenna's set of expectations and interpersonal needs. Provision of needed support for information and collaborative interpersonal responses resulted in a positive change in Jenna's attitude, and full participation in her treatment.

Reed's (2014) middle range theory of self-transcendence (has the capacity to help clients expand self-boundaries in several ways as a human resource in difficult times. The theory encompasses the four components below related to achieving a deeper sense of human potential through self-awareness of the human potential present in every life situation.

- "Intrapersonally (toward greater awareness of one's philosophy, values and dreams
- Interpersonally (to relate to others and one's environment
- Temporally (to integrate one's past and future in a way that has meaning for the present) and
- Transpersonally (to connect with dimensions beyond the typically discernible world)" p. 111)

Self-esteem also can be enhanced through trying new things and learning new skills. Rebuilding relationships with family, friends, teachers, and successful participation in social activities and clubs promote the process of achieving self-esteem. Exercise 9-4 introduces the role of social support in building self-esteem.

Nurses can help clients sort out and clarify the facts and emotions that get in the way of a person's awareness of his or her intrinsic value. Note how the client describes achievements. Does the client devalue accomplishments, project blame for problems on others, minimize personal failures, or make self-deprecating remarks? Does the client express shame or guilt? Does the client seem hesitant to try new things or situations, or express concern about ability to cope with events? Observe defensive behaviors. Lack of culturally appropriate eye contact, poor hygiene, self-destructive behaviors, hypersensitivity to criticism, need for constant reassurance, and an inability to accept compliments are behaviors associated with low self-esteem. Table 9-2 identifies characteristic behaviors related to self-esteem.

EXERCISE 9-4	Social Support

Purpose: To help students understand the role of social support in significant encounters.

Procedure
1. Describe a "special" interpersonal situation that had deep meaning for you.
2. Identify the person or people who helped make the situation meaningful for you.
3. Describe the actions taken by the people or person just identified that made the situation memorable.

Discussion
1. What did you learn about yourself from doing this exercise?
2. What do you see as the role of social support in making memories?
3. How might you use this information in your practice?

THERAPEUTIC STRATEGIES

When people have low self-esteem, they feel they have little worth, and that no one really cares enough to bother with them. Armed with an understanding of the underlying feelings as a threat to self-esteem, (e.g., intense fear, anguish about an anticipated loss, and lack of power in an unfamiliar situation), nurses can provide an opening for the client to tell his or her story. The nurse might identify a legitimate feeling by saying, "It must be frustrating to feel that your questions go unanswered," and then saying, "How can I help you?"

The nurse also helps clients increase self-esteem by being psychologically present as a sounding board. Just the process of engaging with another human being who offers a different perspective can have the effect of enhancing self-esteem. The implicit message the nurse conveys with personal presence and interest, information, and a guided exploration of the problem is twofold. The first is confirmation of the client: "You are unique, you are important, and I will stay with you through this uncomfortable period." The second is the introduction of the possibility of hope: "There may be some alternatives you haven't thought of that can help you cope with this problem. "Would you ever consider…?" Once a person starts to take charge of his or her life, a higher level of well-being can result.

Focused questions calling attention to client strengths help clients see a fuller picture. It is helpful to say… "The thing that impresses me about you is…" or "What I notice is that although your body is weaker, it seems as if your spirit is stronger. Would you say this is true?" Such questions help the client focus on positive strengths. Behaviors suggestive of enhanced self-esteem include the following:

- Taking an active role in planning and implementing self-care
- Verbalizing personal psychosocial strengths
- Expressing feelings of satisfaction with self and ways of handling life

SELF-EFFICACY

Self-efficacy is a term originally developed by Albert Bandura (2007), which refers to a person's perceptual belief that he or she has the capability to perform general or specific life tasks successfully. Self-efficacy is strongly associated with self-concept, self-esteem

and the nursing diagnosis of Powerlessness. People who believe that they can handle threatening situations value their competence and ability to succeed. They are less likely to harbor self-doubts or dwell on personal deficiencies when difficulties arise. Successful self-management depends on developing self-efficacy (Marks et al., 2005; Simpson and Jones, 2013).

Support of self-efficacy is critical to helping people with mental illness live successfully in the community (Suzuki, et. al., 2011). Self-efficacy improves motivation and helps clients sustain their efforts in the face of temporary setbacks.

Self-management support should extend beyond traditional knowledge-based client education to include specific problem-solving skills and processes clients need to cope with chronic health care issues. Start small. Breaking difficult tasks down into achievable steps and completing them constructs a resilient sense of self-efficacy. Explain why each step is important to the next one and remind clients of progress toward a successful outcome.

Look for client strengths. Skills training in areas where clients have deficits and commending clients on effort and persistence encourage clients to take the next step. Work with the client to use solutions and resources within their means. For example, exercise may become an acceptable option if clients know of free or low-cost exercise programs for seniors living in the community. Encourage parents and significant others in the client's life world to give support and approval. Families appreciate having specific suggestions and opportunities to give appropriate positive reinforcement.

Self-help and support groups can be helpful adjuncts to treatment for clients having trouble with self-efficacy in managing their illness or injury. Discovering that others with similar issues have found ways to successfully cope with problem situations encourages clients and reinforces a sense of self-efficacy and hope that they too can achieve similar success. The understanding, social support, and reciprocal learning found in these groups provide opportunities for valuable information sharing and role modeling (Humphreys, 2004).

ROLE PERFORMANCE

Role performance requires self-efficacy with links to self-concept. Johnson and colleagues (2012) suggest that professional identity can be conceptualized as a "logical consequence of self-identity," (p. 562). Quality of life, a priority goal in *Healthy People 2020*, and role performance are also interrelated. How effectively a person is able to function within expected roles influences his or her reputation within society and affects personal self-esteem.

Role performance, and associated role relationships matter to people as evidenced in depression symptoms, feelings of emptiness, and even suicide when a significant personal or professional role ceases to exist.

Case Example

My values in life have changed completely. It was incredibly difficult to realize that as a 45-year-old man I was "good for nothing." I was the rock that everybody relied on. Suddenly, it was I who had to ask others for help. I'm prone to this disease and I know that one day I will fall ill again (Raholm, 2008, p. 62).

Nurses need to be sensitive to the changes in role relationships that illness and injury produce for self, family, and work relationships. An individual's social role can change in a short time span from one of independent self-sufficiency, to one of vulnerability and dependence on others. New role behaviors may be unfamiliar, and at odds with previously held self-concepts. Asking open-ended and focused questions about the client's family relationships, work, and social roles is a useful strategy. Box 9-3 presents suggestions, which can be integrated into client assessments.

Preconceived notions of role disruption for an ill or disabled person occur more commonly when the illness is protracted, recurrent, or seriously role disruptive. Walker (2010) notes that when clients have to leave paid employment because of a chronic illness, it impact self concept because many people's social identity is tied to work roles. Nurses can coach clients about how to present themselves when they return to work. They can help clients learn how to respond to subtle and not-so-subtle discriminatory actions associated with people's lack of understanding of the client's health situation.

SPIRITUAL ASPECTS OF PERSONAL IDENTITY

The findings of Blazek and Besta (2012) suggest that self-concept clarity can be a significant predictor of meaning and purpose in life. Spiritual self-concepts, found in the innermost core of an individual,

---

| BOX 9-3 | Sample Assessment Questions Related to Role Relationships |

Family
- "What changes do you anticipate as a result of your illness (condition) in the way you function in your family?"
- "Who do you see in your family as being most affected by your illness (condition)?"
- "Who do you see in your family as being supportive of you?"

Work
- "What are some of the concerns you have about your job at this time?"
- "Who do you see in your work situation as being supportive of you?"

Social
- "How has your illness affected the way people who are important to you treat you?"
- "To whom do you turn for support?"
- "If (name)_____ is not available to you, who else might you be able to call on for support?"

---

are concerned with a person's relationship with God or a higher power, and the vital life forces that support wholeness. When a person's body fails, or circumstances seem beyond one's control, it is often the spirit that sustains a person's sense of self-integrity and helps them maintain a more balanced equilibrium. Baldacchino and Draper (2001) note the presence of a spiritual force in a client's strong will to live, positive outlook, and sense of peace.

Spirituality is a unified concept, closely linked to a person's worldview, providing a foundation for a personal belief system about the nature of God or a Higher Power, moral-ethical conduct, and reality. Spirituality is a term often used synonymously with religion, but it is a much broader concept (Baldacchino and Draper, 2001). A key difference is that religion involves a formal acceptance of beliefs and values within an organized faith community, whereas spirituality describes self-chosen beliefs and values that give meaning to a person's life. It may or may not be associated with a particular faith (Tanyi, 2006).

Spirituality is associated with meaning and purpose in life (Sessana et al., 2007; Tanyi, 2006). A number of research studies link spirituality to health, quality of life, and well-being (Molzahn and Sheilds, 2008,

Sapp, 2010). Spirituality helps people answer vital questions about what it is to be human, which human events have depth and value, and what are imaginative possibilities of being. Steger and Frazier (2005) suggest that people derive a strong sense of well-being related to the experience of religious feelings and activities. Over the course of a lifetime, spiritual beliefs change, deepen, or are challenged by circumstances that are beyond a person's control. Spiritual strength allows nurses and other health care professionals to willingly stand with others in darkness, and yet remain whole—to deal with the everyday challenges and stresses of nursing in a spirit of peace and hope.

Spiritual aspects of self-concept can be expressed through

- Membership in a specific religious faith community with a set of formal, organized beliefs
- Nature, meditation, or other personalized lifeways and practices linked with a higher purpose in life
- Cultural and family beliefs about forgiveness, justice, human rights, right and wrong learned in early childhood
- Crisis, or existential situations that stimulate a search for purpose, meaning, and values lying outside the self

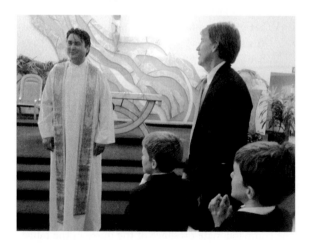

Assessment

The Joint Commission (2004) mandates that health care agencies, including long-term hospice and home care services, assess spiritual needs, provide for the spiritual care of clients and their families, and supply appropriate documentation of that care. Health crises can be a time of spiritual renewal, when one discovers new inner resources, strengths, and capacities never before tested. Alternatively, it can signal a period of spiritual desolation, leaving the individual feeling abandoned, and powerless to control or change important life circumstances.

Spiritual dimensions encompass people's spiritual beliefs, religious affiliation and level of participation, personal spiritual practices such as prayer or meditation, feeling connected to a Higher Power, and the subjective importance of these variables in a person's life (Blazer, 2012). Carson and Stoll (2008) refer to three areas of spiritual concern as a framework for nursing assessment: spiritual distress, spiritual needs, and spiritual well-being. Spiritual distress wears many faces: a lack of purpose and meaning in life, inability to forgive, loss of hope, and spirit of alienation. NANDA (2014) nursing diagnoses present specific nursing interventions for providing spiritual support: Risk for Spiritual Distress, Spiritual Distress, Readiness for Enhanced Hope, and Readiness for Enhanced Spiritual Well-being.

Assessment of spiritual needs should be approached with respect and sensitivity for the client's beliefs and values. Assessment should take account of the client's

- Willingness to talk about personal spirituality or beliefs
- Belief in a personal God or Higher Power
- Relevance of specific religious practices to the individual
- Changes in religious practices or beliefs
- Areas of specific spiritual concern activated by the illness, for example, Is there an afterlife?
- Extent to which illness, injury, or disability has had an effect on spiritual beliefs
- Sources of hope and support
- Desire for visitation from clergy or pastoral chaplain

A client's spiritual needs may be obvious and firmly anchored in positive relationships with clergy and a personal God, with a defined philosophical understanding of life and one's place in it. Alternatively, a spiritual sense of self can be expressed as a disavowal of a spiritual sense of self or allegiance to religious beliefs. Spiritual needs can reveal evidence of conflict or anger toward a Higher Power, who is held responsible for a negative health situation. For example, the noted author C. S. Lewis (1976) called his God "the cosmic sadist" as he experienced his personal grief following the death of his wife. Spiritual pain can be as severe as physical pain and often is closely accompanied by emotional pain.

Identifying a client's current religious affiliations and practices is important, as is inquiry about religious rituals. Josephson and Peteet (2007) suggest that the client's words can be an entry into a discussion of spirituality; for example, if the client uses a phrase such as "By the grace of God, I passed the final examination," you might ask something like, "It sounds like God plays a role in your life, is that true?" (p. 186).

Spiritual rituals and practices can be used to promote hope, support, and peace for a client experiencing spiritual pain. Inquire about current spiritual practices and preferences by asking, "Are there any spiritual practices that are particularly important to you now?" When assessing the client's current spiritual preferences, you should also consider past religious affiliations. It is not unusual for the religion listed on the client's chart to be different from the religious practices the client currently follows. In addition, people who have never committed to a strong sense of religion previously will seek religious support in times of crisis (Baldacchino and Draper, 2001). Spiritual assessment information should be documented in the client's record.

Miller (2007) suggests, "Hope is central to life and specifically is an essential dimension for successfully dealing with illness and for preparing for death" (p. 12). Spiritual well-being can be demonstrated through hopefulness in the face of adversity, compassion for self and others, and a sense of inner peace. Hope is critical in maintaining the "spirit" of a person in health care settings. How else can one explain the will to live or the complete serenity of some individuals in the face of life's most adverse circumstances? Hope does not guarantee a positive outcome. It simply helps a person stay connected with life. Lack of hope is expressed in feelings of powerlessness, hopelessness, and frustration. Useful assessment questions might consist of "What do you see as your primary sources of strength at the present time?" and "In the past, what have been sources of strength for you in difficult times?" Miller (2007) identified several hope-inspiring strategies found in the literature, for example, helping clients and families to develop achievable aims, realize a sense of interpersonal connectedness, live in the present, and find meaning in their illness or situation. Sharing uplifting memories, affirmation of worth, and unconditional caring presence can stimulate a sense of hopefulness.

Case Example

At age 16, Robert became a double amputee as a result of a skiing accident. One morning, Mrs. Johnson walked into Robert's room and found him crying. Her first response was to leave the room as she thought, "I can't handle this today." But she managed to stop herself, and she went over to Robert and touched his shoulder. He continued to sob and said, "What am I going to do? I wish I were dead. My whole life is sports. I would have qualified for an athletic scholarship if this hadn't happened. I feel like my life is over at 16."

Mrs. Johnson recognized the feelings of despair that Robert was expressing and said to him, "It doesn't seem like life has any meaning at all. You are feeling that this is such an unfair thing to have happened to you. I agree with you, it is. But let's talk about it" (Carson and Koenig, 2008, pp. 140-141).

Exercise 9-5 focuses on spiritual responses to distress. Spirituality can be a powerful resource for families and it is important to incorporate questions about the family's spirituality if they are involved with the client. Each family's expression of spirituality and use of spiritual resources is unique. Tanyi (2006) suggests nurses can incorporate spiritual assessment with the family, using questions such as

> What gives the family meaning in their daily routines?
>
> What gives the family strength to deal with stress or crisis?
>
> How does the family describe their relationship with God/Higher Power or the universe?
>
> What spiritual rituals, practices, or resources do the family use for support?
>
> Are there any conflicts between family members related to spiritual views, and if so, what might be the impact on the current health situation?

Nursing Strategies

The compassionate presence of the nurse in the nurse-client relationship is the most important tool the nurse has in helping the client explore spiritual and existential concerns (Carson and Koenig, 2008). Providing opportunities for clients to be self-reflective about their spirituality helps people sustain their beliefs, values, and spiritual sense of self in the face of tragedy. Gordon and Mitchell (2004) wrote, "Spiritual care is usually provided in a one-to-one relationship, is

EXERCISE 9-5	**Responding to Issues of Spiritual Distress**

Purpose: To help students understand responses in times of spiritual distress.

Procedure

Review the following case situations and develop an appropriate response to each.

1. Mary Trachter is unmarried and has just found out she is pregnant. She belongs to a fundamentalist church in which sex before marriage is not permitted. Mary feels guilty about her current status and sees it as "God punishing me for fooling around."
2. Linda Carter is married to an abusive, alcoholic husband. Linda reads the Bible daily and prays for her husband's redemption. She feels that God will turn the marriage around if she continues to pray for changes in her husband's attitude. "My trust is in the Lord," she says.
3. Bill Compton tells the nurse, "I feel that God has let me down. I was taught that if I was faithful to God, He would be there for me. Now the doctors tell me I'm going to die. That doesn't seem fair to me."

Discussion

1. Share your answers with others in your group.
2. Give and get feedback on the usefulness of your responses.
3. In what ways can you use this new knowledge in your nursing care?

---

completely person centered and makes no assumptions about personal conviction or life orientation" (p. 646).

Providing privacy and quiet times for spiritual activities is important. The support of "nursing presence" and unstructured time for helping clients cope with spiritual issues, combined with referrals to chaplains, is an important component of nursing intervention. Nurses can help individuals and families contact spiritual advisors or clergy and act as advocates in ensuring appropriate spiritual rituals are followed related to dietary restrictions, Sabbath activities, meditating or praying, and at end of life. For example, in some forms of the Jewish religion, turning lights on or off or adjusting the position on an electric bed is not permitted on the Sabbath. There is no rule against these tasks being accomplished by the nurse.

Philosophical discussion may not be necessary. Spiritual connections can provide comfort for the dying and their families through prayer or hymns. Informal family presence, coupled with a loving touch can be a spiritual act with profound meaning for all at end of life.

Prayer and Meditation

Praying with a client, even when the client is of a different faith, can be soothing for some clients. Nurses need to distinguish between their own spiritual orientation and needs and those of their clients. It is not appropriate to impose a spiritual ritual on a client that would be at odds with his or her spiritual beliefs. There should be some evidence from the client's conversation that praying or reading the Bible with a client would be a desired support. According to some researchers (Daaleman et al., 2008; Sulmasy, 2006), spiritual support can be effectively provided through *indirect* means such as protecting client dignity, helping clients find meaning in their suffering, offering presence (sitting with clients and families), and talking about what is important to them.

Client outcomes associated with successful resolution of spiritual distress, and/or spiritual well-being include connecting or reconnecting with God or a higher power, decreased guilt, forgiveness of others, expressions of hope, and evidence that the client finds meaning in his or her current situation. Even in death, there are blessings as well as pain that have meaning for the person and enrich self-concept. Thomas (2011) describes his spiritual process of being "introduced, enticed, and sometimes dragged into the magnificent life of the soul" by the two soul mates he lost through death as follows:

> Twice I have walked into the Valley of the Shadow of Death, lost my cherished mate, collapsed into the Canyon of Grief, and with their guidance managed to struggle out as a confident, spiritually embraced person. I live with a deep understanding of, and appreciation for, the meaning of God's Grace and blessings" p. 8.

The self-concept is a dynamic construct, capable of developing new paths to help answer the questions, "Who am I?' and what is important to me in this situation or phase of life? As a professional nurse you will have many opportunities to help clients answer these questions.

SUMMARY

Chapter 9 focuses on the self-concept as a key variable in the nurse-client relationship. Self-concept refers to an acquired constellation of thoughts, feelings, attitudes, and beliefs that individuals have about the nature and organization of their personality. Self-concepts are created through experiences with the environment and personal characteristics.

Aspects of self-concept patterns discussed in the chapter included body image, personal identity, role performance, self-esteem, and spirituality. Disturbances in body image refer to issues related to changes in appearance and physical functions, both overt and hidden. Personal identity is constructed through cognitive processes of perception and cognition. Serious illnesses such as dementia and psychotic disorders threaten or crush a person's sense of personal identity. Self-esteem is associated with the emotional aspect of self-concept and reflects the value a person puts on the personal self-concept and its place in the world. Assessment of spiritual needs and corresponding spiritual care is a Joint Commission requirement for quality care.

Understanding the dimensions of self-concept and the critical role it plays in directing behavior is key to working effectively with clients and families. It is always a core variable to consider in communication and supportive nurse-client relationships. Nurses play an important role in providing support and guidance for clients related to self-concept.

ETHICAL DILEMMA What Would You Do?

Sarah Best, a 22-year-old ice-skater, is brought into the emergency department after being in a car accident. The physician examines Sarah and determines that her right leg needs to be amputated below the knee. Sarah's parents are traveling in Europe and cannot immediately be located. Sarah refuses surgery. The physician asks Sarah's nurse, Ann, to get Sarah's consent. If you were in Ann's position, what would you do?

DISCUSSION QUESTIONS

1. What role does social media play in the development, and/or validation of a person's self-concept?
2. In what ways are spirituality and worldview connected with each other in defining self-concept?
3. Drawing on your experience, what are some specific ways you can help another person develop a stronger sense of self?
4. Describe a personal exchange with a client or an observed clinical encounter with another provider in which you felt that you learned something important about the value of presence in promoting self worth.

REFERENCES

Adler R, Rosenfeld L, Proctor R: *Interplay: The Process of Interpersonal Communication*, New York, 2012, Oxford University Press.

Arnold E: A voice of their own: women moving into their fifties, *Health Care Women Int* 26(8):630–651, 2005.

Bailey J: Self-image, self-concept, and self-identity revisited, *J Natl Med Assoc.* 95(5):383–386, 2003.

Baldacchino D, Draper P: Spiritual coping strategies: a review of the literature, *J Adv Nurs* 34(6):833–841, 2001.

Bandura A: Self-efficacy in health functioning. In Ayers S, editor: *Cambridge handbook of psychology, health and medicine*, ed 2, New York, 2007, Cambridge University Press, pp 191–193.

Beck J, Beck A: Chapter 3: Cognitive conceptualization. In 2nd ed, *Cognitive Behavior Therapy* New York, NY, 2011, Guilford Press, pp 29–46.

Benner P: Reflecting on what we care about, *Am J Crit Care* 12(2):165–166, 2003.

Blazek M, Besta T: Self-concept clarity and religious orientations: Prediction of purpose in life and self-esteem, *J Relig Health* 51(3):947–960, 2012.

Blazer D: Religon/spirituality and depression: What can we learn from empirical studies? *Am J Psychiatry* 169:10–12, 2012.

Blazer D: How do you feel about…? Health outcomes late in life and self-perceptions of health and well-being, *Gerontologist* 48(4):415–422, 2008.

Boston Women's Health Book Collective: *Our bodies, ourselves for the new century*, New York, 1998, Touchstone Simon & Schuster.

Brown J, Marshall M: Self-esteem and emotion: some thoughts about feelings, *Pers Soc Psychol Bull* 27(5):575–584, 2001.

Carson V, Koenig H: *Spiritual dimensions of nursing practice Revised ed*, West Conshohocken, PA, 2008, Templeton Press.

Carson V Stoll R: Spirituality: Defining the indefinable and reviewing its place in nursing. In Carson V, Koenig H, editors: *Spiritual dimensions of nursing practice*, West Conshohocken, PA, 2008, Revised ed. Templeton Press.

Crocker J, Brook AT, Niiya Y: The pursuit of self-esteem: contingencies of self-worth and self-regulation, *J Pers* 74(6):1749–1771, 2006.

Cunha C, Goncalves M: Commentary: Accessing the experience of a dialogical self: Some needs and concerns, *Cult Psychol* 15(3):120–133, 2009.

Daaleman T, B.M.Usher BM, Williams S, et al.: An exploratory study of spiritual care at the end of life, *Ann Fam Med* 6(5):406–411, 2008.

Diehl M, Hay E: Contextualized self-representations in adulthood, *J Pers* 75(6):1255–1283, 2007.

Drench M, Noonan A, Sharby N, et al.: *Psychosocial Aspects of Health Care*, 3rd edition, Englewood Cliffs, NJ, 2011, Prentice Hall.

Dropkin MJ: Body image and quality of life after head and neck cancer surgery, *Cancer Pract* 7:309–313, 1999.

Elliott A: *Concepts of the self*, Malden, 2008, MA Polity Press.

Ellis-Hill C, Horn S: Change in identity and self-concept: a new theoretical approach to recovery following a stroke, *Clin Rehabil* 14(3):279–287, 2000.

Erikson E: *Identity and the life cycle: Selected papers*, Oxford, UK, 1959, International Universities Press. Also: Published as a Norton Paperback (1980).

Erikson E: *Identity: youth and crisis*, New York, 1968, Norton.

Erikson E: *The life cycle completed: a review*, New York, 1982, Norton.

Fazio S, Mitchell D: Persistence of self in individuals with Alzheimer's disease, *Dementia* 8:39–59, 2009.

Goffman E: *Stigma and social identity. (1963). Stigma: Notes on the Management of Spoiled Identity*, Englewood Cliffs, NJ, 1963, Prentice Hall.

Gordon M: Self-perception-self-concept pattern, *Manual of nursing diagnoses*, ed 11, Chestnut Hill, MA, 2007, Bartlett Jones.

Gordon T, Mitchell D: A competency model for the assessment and delivery of spiritual care, *Palliat Med* 18(7):646–651, 2004.

Guerrero L, Anderson P, Afifi W: *Close Encounters: Communication in Relationships*, 4th ed. Thousand Oaks, CA, 2014, Sage Publications.

Harden K: Self-esteem and affect as information, *Pers Soc Psychol Bull* 31(2):276–288, 2005.

Harrington J: Implications of treatment on body image and quality of life, *Semin Oncol Nurs* 27(4):290–299, 2011.

Heijmans M, Rijken M, Foets M, et al.: The stress of being chronically ill: from disease-specific to task-specific aspects, *J Behav Med* 27:255–271, 2004.

Humphreys K: *Circles of recovery: self-help organizations for addictions*, Cambridge, 2004, Cambridge University Press.

Hunter E: Beyond death: inheriting the past and giving to the future, transmitting the legacy of one's self, *Omega* 56(40):313–329, 2008.

Jackson J: *Introducing language and intercultural communication*, New York, 2014, Routledge.

Johnson M, Cowin LS, Wilson I, Young H: Professional identity and nursing. Contemporary theoretical developments and future research challenges, *Int Nurs Rev* 59(4):562–569, 2012.

Josephson A, Peteet J: Talking with patients about spirituality and worldview: practical interviewing techniques and strategies, *Psychiatr Clin North Am* 30:181–197, 2007.

Karademas E, Bakouli A, Bastouonis A, et al.: Illness perceptions, illness-related problems, subjective health and the role of perceived primal threat: Preliminary findings, *J Health Psychol* 13(8):1021–1029, 2008.

Konig J: Moving experience: dialogues between personal cultural positions, *Cult Psychol* 15(1):97–119, 2009.

Lake N: *The Caregivers: A Support Group's Stories of Slow Loss, Courage, and Love*, New York, NY, 2014, Simon & Schuster, Inc.

Leerdam L, Rietveld L, Teunissen D, Lagro –Janseen A: Gender-based education during clerkships: A focus group study, *Adv Med Educ Pract* 26(5):53–60, 2014.

Lewis CS: *A grief observed*, New York, 1976, Bantam Books.

Lodi-Smith J, Roberts B: Getting to know me: Social role experiences and age differences in self-concept clarity during adulthood, *J Pers* 78(5):1383–1410, 2010.

Luft J, Ingham H: *The Johari window, a graphic model of interpersonal awareness. Proceedings of the western training laboratory in group development*, Los Angeles, 1955, University of California.

Marks R, Allegrante J, Lorig K: A review and synthesis of research evidence for self-efficacy-enhancing interventions for reducing chronic disability. Implications for health education practice (Part II), *Health Promot Pract* (6)148–156, 2005.

Markus H, Nurius P: Possible selves, *Am Psychol* 41:954–969, 1986.

Martin C, Ruble D: Patterns of gender development, *Annu Rev Psychol* 61:353–381, 2010.

McCormick M, Hardy M: *Re-visioning family therapy: race, culture and gender in clinical practice*, ed 2, New York NY, 2008, The Guilford Press.

Myers D: *Chapter 3: Developing through the life span. Psychology in Every Day Life*, New York, NY, 2012, Worth Publishers.

Miller J: Hope: A construct central to nursing, *Nurs Forum* 42(1):12–19, 2007.

Molzahn A, Sheilds L: Why is it so hard to talk about spirituality? *Can Nurse* 10(4):25–29, 2008.

NANDA International: *Nursing Diagnoses: Definitions and Classification 2012–2014*, Oxford UK, 2014, Wiley Blackwell.

Oyserman D, Markus H: Self as social representation. In Flick U, editor: *The psychology of the social*, Cambridge, United Kingdom, 1998, Cambridge University Press, pp 107–125.

Raholm MB: Uncovering the ethics of suffering using a narrative approach, *Nurs Ethics* 15(1):62–72, 2008.

Reed PG: Chapter 6 Theory of self-transcendence. In Smith MJ, Liehr PR, editors: *Middle range theory for nursing*, 3rd ed, New York, 2014, Springer, pp 109–140.

Rogers C: *Client centered therapy*, New York, 1951, Houghton Mifflin.

Sapp S: What have religion and spirituality to do with aging? Three approaches, *Gerontologist* 50(2):271–275, 2010.

Sessana L, Finnell D, Jezewski MA: Spirituality in nursing and health related literature: a concept analysis, *J Holist Nurs* 25(4):252–262, 2007.

Simpson E, Jones MC: An exploration of self-efficacy and self-management in COPD patients, *Br J Nurs* 13(2219):1105–1109, 2013.

Slatman J: The meaning of body experience evaluation in oncology, *Health Care Anal.* 19:295–311, 2011.

Smith MJ, Perkins K: Attending to the voices of adolescents who are overweight to promote mental health, *Arch Psychiatr Nurs* 22(6): 391–393, 2008.

Steger M, Frazier P: Meaning in life: one link in the chain from religion to well-being, *J Counsel Psychol* 52:574–582, 2005.

Stewart AJ, Ostrove JM, Helson R: Middle aging in women: Patterns of personality change from the 30s to the 50s, *J Adult Dev.* 8:23–37, 2001.

Stopa L, Brown M, Luke MA, Hirsch CR: Constructing a self: The role of self-structure and self-certainty in social anxiety, *Behav Res Ther* 48(10):955–965, 2010.

Sulmasy DP: Spiritual issues in the care of dying patients, *JAMA* 296(11):1385–1392, 2006.

Suzuki M, Amagai M, Shibata F, Tsai J. Participation related to self-efficacy for social participation of people with mental illness, *Arch Psychiatr Nurs* 25(5):359–65, 2011.

Tanyi R: Spirituality and family nursing: spiritual assessment and interventions for families, *J Adv Nurs* 53(3):287–294, 2006.

Thomas J: *My Saints Alive:Reflections on a Journey of Love*, Loss and Life Charlottesville VA, 2011, CreateSpace Independent Publishing Platform.

Usborne E, Taylor D: The role of cultural identity clarity for self-concept, clarity, self-esteem, and subjective well-being, *Pers Soc Psychol Bull* 36(7):883–897, 2010.

Vartanian L: When the body defines the self: Self-concept clarity, internalization, and body image, *J Soc Clin Psychol* 28(1):94–126, 2009.

Vickery C, Sepehri A, Evans C: Self-esteem in an acute stroke rehabilitation sample: a control group comparison, *Clin Rehabil* 22:179–187, 2008.

Walker C: Ruptured identities: Leaving work because chronic illness, *Int J Health Serv* 40(4):629–643, 2010.

CHAPTER 10

Developing Therapeutic Relationships

Elizabeth C. Arnold

OBJECTIVES

At the end of the chapter, the reader will be able to:
1. Define the therapeutic relationship in health care.
2. Describe fundamental differences between a therapeutic and a social relationship.
3. Discuss key characteristics of therapeutic nurse-client relationships.
4. Discuss therapeutic use of self in nurse-client relationships.
5. Discuss tasks in each of the four phases of the relationship.
6. Apply concepts of therapeutic relationships to contemporary practice.

Carter (2009) describes the therapeutic relationship as the cornerstone of professional nursing practice, while The Joint Commission (2001) observes, "Nearly every person's every health care experience involves the contribution of a registered nurse. Birth and death, and all the various forms of care in between, are attended by the knowledge, support and comforting of nurses" (p. 5). Understanding the nature of therapeutic relationships is essential as nursing moves into the community with shorter term, less structured therapeutic alliances between nurse and client and family. Chapter 10 explores key characteristics of the helping relationship related to authenticity, presence and positive regard, empathy, boundaries, and self-awareness. The chapter addresses developmental stages of nurse-client relationships and describes communication strategies nurses can apply to long- and short-term relationships to meet identified health care goals.

BASIC CONCEPTS

Lazenby (2013) notes that while nursing is built on a scientific evidenced based foundation, the nature of nursing, and its natural home lies in understanding the lived human experience of individuals in need of professional nursing care. Half a century later, Virginia Henderson's (1964) proposal that:

"The nurse is temporarily the consciousness of the unconscious, the love of life of the suicidal, the leg of the amputee, the eyes of the newly blind, a means of locomotion for the newborn, knowledge and confidence for the young mother, a voice for those too weak to speak, and so on" (p. 63) acts as an accurate descriptor of the professional nurse's role in client centered relationships. Finally, Porter et al. (2011) assert: "a core value of nursing is that the people we serve are uniquely valuable as human beings" (p. 107). This tenet forms the context in which nurse/client-centered relationships are implemented.

DEFINITIONS

A **therapeutic relationship** is defined as a professional, interpersonal alliance in which the nurse and client join together for a defined period to achieve health-related treatment goals. The interactions within each relationship are unique, because each nurse and client has a distinctive personality, and the health circumstances and context differs (Chauhan and Long, 2000). The time spent in a therapeutic relationship may be short, spanning up to an 8-hour shift in a hospital. It can be longer term, lasting weeks or months in a rehabilitation center, or it can consist of short episodic encounters in a primary care setting. Regardless of the time spent, each nurse-client encounter can be meaningful.

Empathetic communication in therapeutic relationships facilitates its direction and focus. To be effective, nurses need to think through and organize their ideas, actively listen and question, and choose their messages carefully for maximum impact. This integrated planning strategy allows the client and nurse to jointly and authentically construct the meaning of a health experience. Without a shared understanding and appreciation for the diversity of ideas, that create the common ground for constructive problem solving and high quality decision-making, effective decision making is limited.

The goals of therapeutic relationships are associated with one or more of the following:

- Supporting clients and families to accurately understand the client's personalized experience of an illness
- Helping clients and their families learn practical strategies to effectively self-manage chronic health conditions
- Providing emotional and informational support to help clients and their families make informed and better decisions about their health care
- Assisting clients to cope and find meaning in difficult health circumstances
- Helping clients discover new directions in line with their interests and capabilities
- Connecting clients and families with other members of the collaborative health care team
- Empowering clients with the knowledge and tools they need to be successful negotiators in their health care

THEORETICAL ORIENTATIONS

Hildegarde Peplau's interpersonal relationship nursing theory (1952, 1997) offers a way to conceptualize therapeutic relationships and lays the groundwork for crafting strategies based on those understandings. Peplau describes four sequential phases of a nurse-client relationship, each characterized by specific tasks and interpersonal skills: *preinteraction, orientation, working phase* (problem identification and exploitation), and *termination*. The phases are overlapping and serve to broaden as well as deepen the emotional connection between nurses and their clients (Reynolds,

1997). Although Peplau's model is more applicable to long-term relationships, the concepts hold true for short therapeutic alliances. Peplau (1952) identified six professional roles the nurse can assume during the course of the nurse-client relationship (Box 10-1).

Other relevant perspectives to the study of therapeutic relationships are those of Martin Buber (1958) and Carl Rogers (1958). Buber (1958) described an "I-thou" relationship as an equal relationship marked by respect, mutuality, and reciprocity. In an I-thou relationship, each person is aware of and respects the other. Together they engage in building a shared reality based on their interactions. Neither person in the relationship is an "object" of study. Instead there is a process of mutual discovery and each person feels free to be authentic. An I-thou relationship allows each person to be who he or she is, as a unique human being worthy of respect even when the person is being difficult.

Buber's work forms a theoretical foundation for using confirming responses in which the helping person identifies an observable strength of another person and comments on it. He described this way of responding as follows: "Man wishes to be confirmed in his being by man and wishes to have a presence in the being of the other. Secretly and bashfully, he watches for a yes which allows him to be" (Buber, 1957, p. 104).

PRINCIPLES OF CLIENT-CENTERED CARE

The client-centered model developed by Carl Rogers provides a theoretical construct for the focus of

| **BOX 10-1** | **Peplau's Six Nursing Roles** |

1. *Stranger* role: Receives the client the same way one meets a stranger in other life situations; provides an accepting climate that builds trust.
2. *Resource* role: Answers questions, interprets clinical treatment data, and gives information.
3. *Teaching* role: Gives instructions and provides training; involves analysis and synthesis of the learner experience.
4. *Counseling* role: Helps client understand and integrate the meaning of current life circumstances; provides guidance and encouragement to make changes.
5. *Surrogate* role: Helps client clarify domains of dependence, interdependence, and independence; acts on client's behalf as advocate.
6. *Leadership* role: Helps client assume maximum responsibility for meeting treatment goals in a mutually satisfying way.

therapeutic relationships. The terms *client* or *patient* can refer to any individual, family, group, or community with an identified health need requiring nursing intervention. McCormack and McCance (2010) define client-centered care as "an approach to practice established through the formation and fostering of therapeutic relationships between all care providers... patients and others significant to them in their lives" (p. 13). Client-centered approaches are based on the belief that each person has within him or herself the capacity to heal, if given support with respect and unconditional regard in a caring, authentic therapeutic relationship. Client-centered care focuses on each person's individual preferences, values, beliefs, and needs as a fundamental consideration in all nursing interventions.

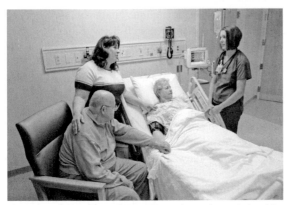

The nurse-client relationship is an interdependent relationship.

Patient/client-centered care is conceptualized as a core value in health service delivery. Its relevance as an essential component of quality health care measures was strongly stated in the Institute of Medicine (2001) published report *Crossing the Quality Chasm: A New Health System for the 21st Century*. This document charges health care systems to:

- Respect clients' values, preferences, and expressed needs.
- Coordinate and integrate care across boundaries of the system.
- Provide the information, communication, and education that people need and want.
- Guarantee physical comfort, emotional support, and the involvement of family and friends (pp. 52-53).

Nurses enter therapeutic relationships with a specialized body of knowledge, a genuine desire to help others, and openness to each client's experience.

Guiding principles (e.g., presence, purpose, positive regard, mutuality, authenticity, empathy, active listening, confidentiality, and respect for the dignity of the client) strengthen the healing influence of a therapeutic relationship (McGrath, 2005). Box 10-2 identifies strategies to facilitate empathy.

Clients are personal experts on their life experiences. The nurse's expertise derives from integrated empirical, personal, aesthetic, and ethical ways of knowing. This knowledge helps nurses guide clients to reflect on and clarify what is important about their experiences, and offers professional insights that the client may not have considered previously. From a functional perspective, client-centered relationships require nurses to step back and compassionately listen to each individual client or family concerns. Working with the client's values and beliefs is as relevant as treating the client's clinical symptoms. Each person's experience of a health-related situation is unique, despite similarities in diagnosis or personal characteristics (McCance, 2010). Relevant questions relate to: "What is this person's human experience of living with this illness, or injury" and "How can I as a health care professional help you at this point in time?" Empathy acts as a human echo in acknowledging the helper's understanding and interest in a client's perspectives and concerns (Egan, 2014).

BOX 10-2	Suggestions for Integrating Empathy into Listening Responses

- Actively listen carefully to your client's concerns. (Use open-ended questions; avoid closed-ended questions.)
- Tune in to physical and psychological behaviors that express the client's point of view.
- Do self-checks often for stereotypes or premature understanding of the client's issues.
- Set aside judgments or personal biases.
- Be tentative in your listening responses and ask for validation frequently.
- Mentally picture the client's situation and ask appropriate questions to secure information about areas or issues you are not clear about.
- Give yourself time to think about what the client has said before responding or before asking the next question.
- Mirror the client's level of energy and language.
- Be authentic in your responses.

Modified from Egan G: *The skilled helper*, ed 7, Pacific Grove, CA, 2002, Brooks Cole, by permission.

COLLABORATIVE PARTNERSHIP

The concept of collaborative patient-centered treatment planning has been strengthened to include active involvement in shared decision making (Mead and Bower, 2000; Elwyn et al, 2012). New models of client-centered care include shift reports at the bedside, reviewing care plans for the day early in the shift with clients, asking about their priorities, and working closely with other health team members to deliver quality care (Jasovsky et al., 2010).

Clients are expected to act as active team partners in their own health care (McGrath, 2005; McQueen, 2000). Nurse-client relationships are designed to empower clients and families to assume as much responsibility as possible in self-management of chronic illness. Both nurse and client have responsibilities to work toward agreed-on goals. Shared knowledge, negotiation, mutual decision-making power, and respect for the capacity of clients to actively contribute to their health care to whatever extent is possible are active components of the partnership required of client-centered care (Gallant et al., 2002). Exercise 10-1 looks at shared decision making.

A client-centered partnership honors the client's right to self-determination and gives the client and family maximum control over health care decisions. The client always has the right to choose personal goals and courses of action, even when they are at odds with the nurse's ideas. A collaborative partnership between nurse and client results in enhanced self-management, better health care utilization, and improved health outcomes (Hook, 2006).

Client Rights and Responsibilities

The American Hospital Association (AHA, 2003) has developed a brochure outlining the rights and responsibilities of client care partnership to replace its former Client's Bill of Rights. It is accessible in multiple languages on the AHA web site. Hospitals today have copies of comprehensive client rights posted on their web sites. Written copies are given to clients on admission. A sample listing of common client rights and responsibilities is provided in Box 10-3.

PROFESSIONAL BOUNDARIES

Emotional integrity in the nurse-client relationship is "reliant on maintaining relational boundaries" (LaSala, 2009, p. 424). **Professional boundaries** represent invisible structures imposed by legal, ethical, and professional standards of nursing that respect nurse and client rights, and protect the functional integrity of the alliance between nurse and client. Bruner and Yonge (2006) suggest that "rather than a line, boundaries represent a continuum with issues related to boundaries ranging from a lack of involvement to overinvolvement" (p. 39). Examples of relationship boundaries involve the setting, time, purpose, and length of contact, maintaining confidentiality, and use of appropriate professional behaviors.

Professional boundaries define how nurses should relate to clients as a helping person, that is, not as a friend, not as a judge, but as a skilled professional companion committed to helping the client achieve mutually defined health care goals (Briant and Freshwater, 1998). Maintaining appropriate professional behavior is a clear interpersonal boundary that

---

EXERCISE 10-1	Shared Decision Making

Purpose: To develop awareness of shared decision making in treatment planning.

Procedure
1. Read the following clinical situation.
   Mr. Singer, age 48 years, is a white, middle-class professional recovering from his second myocardial infarction. After his initial attack, Mr. Singer resumed his 10-hour workday, high-stress lifestyle, and usual high-calorie, high-cholesterol diet of favorite fast foods, alcohol, and coffee. He smokes two packs of cigarettes a day and exercises once a week by playing golf.
   Mr. Singer is to be discharged in 2 days. He expresses impatience to return to work, but also indicates that he would like to "get his blood pressure down and maybe drop 10 pounds."
2. Role-play this situation in dyads, with one student taking the role of the nurse, and another student taking the role of the client.
3. Develop treatment goals that seem realistic and achievable, taking into account Mr. Singer's preferences and values, and health condition.
4. After the role-playing is completed, discuss some of the issues that would be relevant to Mr. Singer's situation and how they might be handled. For example, what are some of the ways in which you could engage Mr. Singer's interest in changing his behavior to facilitate a healthier lifestyle?

makes the relationship safe for the client in much the same way as guardrails protect the public from falling into danger when observing a tourist attraction. Professional boundaries spell out the parameters of the health care relationship (Fronek et al., 2009). Nurses are ethically bound to observe the boundaries needed

BOX 10-3	Client Rights and Responsibilities

All clients have the following rights:
- Impartial access to the most appropriate treatment regardless of race, age, sexual preference, national origin, religion, handicap, or source of payment for care
- To be treated with respect, dignity, and personal privacy in a safe, secure environment
- Confidential treatment of all communication and other records related to care or payment, except as required by law or signed insurance contractual arrangements (all clients should receive Notice of Privacy Practices)
- Active participation in all aspects of decision making regarding personal health care
- To know the identity and professional status of each health care provider
- To have treatments and procedures explained to them in ways they can understand
- To receive competent interpreter services, if required to understand care or treatment
- To refuse treatment, including life-saving treatment, after being told of the potential risks associated with such refusal
- To receive appropriate pain management
- To express grievances regarding any violation of client rights internally and/or to the appropriate agency

All clients have the following responsibilities:
- To treat their care providers with respect and courtesy, including timely notification for appointment cancellations
- To provide accurate, complete information about all personal health matters
- To follow recommended treatment plans
- To assume responsibility for personal actions, if choosing to refuse treatment
- To follow hospital regulations regarding safety and conduct

Sources: American Hospital Association (AHA): *The patient care partnership: understanding expectations, rights and responsibilities.* 2003. Available online: http://www.aha.org/content/00-10/pcp_en glish_030730.pdf; U.S. Department of Health and Human Services, Agency for Healthcare Research and Quality (AHRQ): *President's advisory commission on consumer protection and quality in the health care industry.* 1997. Available online: http://www.hcqualityco mmission.gov/final/append_a.html.

to make a relationship therapeutic (Sheets, 2001). When clients seek health care, they are in a vulnerable position and look to their health care providers as responsive guides to help them achieve optimum health and well-being.

BOUNDARY VIOLATIONS AND CROSSINGS

The National Council of State Boards of Nursing (NCSBN, 2009) describes professional boundaries as the spaces between the nurse's position power and client vulnerability. The nurse, not the client, is responsible for maintaining professional boundaries. **Boundary violations** take advantage of the client's vulnerability and represent a conflict of interest that usually is harmful to the goals of the therapeutic relationship. Examples of boundary violations include sexual encounters with clients, excessive personal disclosures, personal or business relationships, and requests for or acceptance of special favors or expensive gifts. Extensive following of a client after discharge is a common boundary violation. Boundary violations are ethically wrong.

Boundary crossings are less serious infractions. They give the appearance of impropriety but do not actually violate prevailing ethical standards. Hartley (2002) suggests, "With boundary crossings, context is everything. What is appropriate behavior in one context may not be in another" (p. 7). Examples of boundary crossings include meetings outside of the relationship or disclosing personal intimate details about aspects of the nurse's life that would not be common knowledge (Bruner and Yonge, 2006). Repeated boundary crossings such as continuing a biased, rather than an impartial, relationship with a client should be avoided.

Nurses need to carefully examine their behaviors, look for possible misinterpretations or unintended consequences, and seek supervision when boundary crossings occur. For example, suppose the client perceives your extra involvement as more than a responsive gesture. How will other clients or family members view the extra attention? Is reliance on the extra time or effort spent with a client likely to jeopardize that client's journey to independence (Hartley, 2002)?

LEVEL OF INVOLVEMENT

An important feature of a therapeutic relationship is the helping person's level of involvement. The term *involvement* relates to the degree of the nurse's attachment and active participation in the client's care. The level of involvement may fluctuate, depending on the needs of the client, but it should never exceed the boundaries of professional behavior (Figure 10-1). It becomes problematic when the nurse limits the level of involvement to perfunctory tasks or becomes emotionally overinvolved in the client's care. To be effective, nurses must maintain emotional objectivity while remaining human and present to clients. Heinrich (1992) notes that nurses constantly walk a thin line between having compassion for a client and developing a relationship that is too close, resulting in a friendship with potential serious complications for the client, as well as the nurse.

Overinvolvement (also avoidance) can be associated with **countertransference**, which occurs when something in the client activates a nurse's unconscious unresolved feelings from previous relationships or life events (Scheick, 2011). It often occurs when the client is particularly needy or feeds the nurse's ego by considering him or her as special or the only one who understands. Overinvolvement results in the nurse's loss of an essential objectivity needed to support the client in meeting health goals (Kines, 1999). In addition to its effect on the nurse-client relationship, overinvolvement can compromise the nurse's obligation to the service agency, a professional commitment to the treatment regimen, collegial relationships with other health team members, and professional responsibilities to other clients (Morse, 1991).

Warning signs that the nurse is becoming overinvolved include the following:
- Giving extra time and attention to certain clients
- Visiting clients in off hours
- Doing things for clients that the clients could do for themselves
- Discounting the actions of other professionals
- Keeping secrets with the client
- Believing that the nurse is the only one who understands the client's needs

The opposite of overinvolvement is *disengagement*, which occurs when nurses find themselves withdrawing from clients because of a client's behavior or the intensity of client suffering. Deaths and high stress levels on a unit can create compassion fatigue, which can lead to disengagement as a self-protective mechanism (Hofmann, 2009). Nurses tend to disengage from clients who are sexually provocative, complaining, hostile, or extremely anxious or depressed. Physical characteristics such as poor hygiene, marked physical disability, socially stigmatized illness, or an unusual or altered appearance can negatively affect the nurse's willingness to engage with a client.

Signs of disengagement include withdrawal, limited perfunctory contacts, minimizing the client's suffering, and defensive or judgmental communication. Regardless of the reason, the outcome of disengagement is that the client feels isolated and sometimes abandoned when care is mechanically delivered with limited human connection.

Maintaining a helpful level of involvement is always the responsibility of the professional nurse (see Figure 10-1). Carmack (1997) suggests that nurses can take the following actions to regain perspective:
- Assume full responsibility for the process of care while acknowledging that the outcome usually is not within your control.
- Focus on the things that you can change while acknowledging that there are things over which you have no control.
- Be aware and accepting of your professional limits and boundaries.
- Monitor your reactions and seek assistance when you feel uncomfortable about any aspect of the relationship.
- Balance giving care to a client with taking care of yourself, without feeling guilty.

Debriefing after a highly emotional event helps nurses resolve and put strong feelings into perspective.

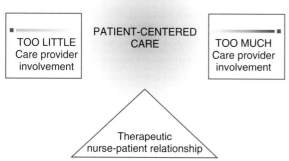

Figure 10-1 Levels of involvement: a continuum of professional behavior. *(Source: National Council of State Boards of Nursing (NCSBN): A nurse's guide to professional boundaries. Chicago: NCSBN, 2009. Available online:* https://www.ncsbn.org/ProfessionalBoundaries_Complete.pdf.)

Support groups for nurses working in high-acuity nursing situations and mentoring of new nurses are recommended.

THERAPEUTIC USE OF SELF

The therapeutic relationship is not simply about what the nurse does, but who the nurse *is* in relation to clients and families. One of the most important tools nurses have at their disposal is the use of self. LaSala (2009) uses the words of Florence Nightingale in that a nurse achieves "the moral ideal" whenever he or she uses "the whole self" to form relationships with "the whole of the person receiving care" (p. 423) to explain the optimum involvement of self in the nurse-client relationship. The relationships that nurses establish with clients and their families and other practitioners in which "the whole self" is drawn into the process serves as the primary means for putting into action health treatments and healing interventions needed for client support and self-care.

AUTHENTICITY

Authenticity is a precondition for the therapeutic use of self in the nurse-client relationship. Authenticity or genuineness requires self-awareness. It means recognizing and acknowledging your personal vulnerabilities, strengths, and limitations (Daniels, 1998). Once recognized, nurses can incorporate their personal strengths in the service of the client and can seek help to offset limitations in ways that further relationship goals. For example, Levigne and Kautz (2010) describe a situation in which the nurse realized that the respiratory therapist would be better equipped to explain the process of weaning the client from a ventilator. She arranged for the therapist to provide the explanation while providing her support by staying with the client during the explanation and the weaning process.

SELF-AWARENESS

Self-awareness allows you to fully engage with a client, knowing that parts of the relationship may be painful, distasteful, or uncomfortable. Nurses need to be clear about their personal values, beliefs, stereotypes, and personal perspectives because of their potential influence on client decisions (McCormack and McCance, 2006; Morse et al., 1997). There are some clients whom nurses simply do not like working with (Erlen and Jones, 1999). It is up to the nurse, not the client,

to resolve interpersonal issues that get in the way of a productive relationship. Nurses need to acknowledge overinvolvement, avoidance, anger, frustration, or detachment from a client when it occurs. A useful strategy in such situations is to seek further understanding of the client as a person by acknowledging your knowledge deficit and seeking to correct it.

Case Example

Brian Haggerty is a homeless individual who tells the nurse, "I know you want to help me, but you can't understand my situation. You have money and a husband to support you. You don't know what it is like out on the streets." Instead of feeling defensive, his nurse responds, "You are right, I don't know what it is like to be homeless, but I would like to know more about your experiences. Can you tell me what it has been like for you?" With this listening response, the nurse invites the client to share his experience. The data might allow the nurse to appreciate and address the loneliness, fear, and helplessness the client is experiencing, which are universal feelings.

Authenticity requires admitting mistakes. For example, a nurse might promise a client to return immediately with a pain medication and then forget to do so because of other pressing demands. When the nurse brings the medication, the client might accuse the nurse of being uncaring and incompetent. It would be appropriate for the nurse to apologize for forgetting the medication and for the extra discomfort suffered by the client.

PRESENCE

Bridges\ and colleagues (2013) define **presence** as the "nurse's ability to be 'present' in the relationship (rather than adopting a work persona), to expose themselves to the client's and their own experiences, to be open and truthful in their dealings and to be generous in committing to the client's best interests" (p. 764). Being present requires the full attention of the nurse, attuned to every nuance of the client's experience.

Presence involves the nurse's capacity to know when to provide help and when to stand back, when to speak frankly and when to withhold comments because the client is not ready to hear them. McDonough-Means and colleagues (2004) describe presence as having two dimensions: "being there" and "being with" (p. S25). The sense of connectivity is simultaneously experienced by those involved in the process: nurse, client, family.

Nursing presence is evidenced through active listening; relevant caring communication; and sharing of skills, knowledge, and competencies related to client-specific problems (McCormack and McCance, 2006; Morse et al., 1997). The gift of presence enriches the sense of self, and life of both client and nurse, in ways that are unique to each person and situation (Covington, 2003; Easter, 2000; Hawley and Jensen, 2007).

SELF-AWARENESS

Peplau (1997) notes that nurses must observe their own behavior, as well as the client's, with "unflinching self-scrutiny and total honesty in assessment of their behavior in interactions with clients" (p. 162). Self-awareness requires a reflective process that seeks to understand one's personal values, feelings, attitudes, motivations, strengths, and limitations—and how these affect practice and client relationships. By critically and simultaneously examining the behaviors of the client and the nurse and what is going on in the relationship, nurses can create a safe, trustworthy, and caring relational structure (Lowry, 2005).

Developing an Evidence-Based Practice

Haugan G. The relationship between nurse-patient interaction and meaning-in-life in cognitively intact nursing home patients. *J of Adv Nurs* 70(1):107-120, 2013.

The purpose of this cross-sectional descriptive research study was to investigate relationships between nurse-patient interaction and meaning-in-life in a nursing home population. A total of 202 clients participated in the study. Using structural equation modeling, the hypothesized relationship between nurse-client and interaction and meaning was assessed with LISREL 8.8.

Results: Study results revealed a significant direct relationship between nurse-client interaction and enhanced meaning in life for cognitively intact nursing home clients.

Application to Your Clinical Practice: Having meaning and purpose in life influences a person's sense of well-being. This need becomes increasing important as many older adults, particularly in long term settings, have fewer opportunities for consistent dialogue and a sense of connectedness. As our nation's population increasingly embraces an older adult population, finding ways to help clients develop new meaning and purpose seems highly relevant.

APPLICATIONS

Although therapeutic helping relationships share many characteristics of a social relationship, there are distinct structural and functional distinctions. Table 10-1 presents the differences between a therapeutic helping relationship and a social relationship. The goal of a therapeutic relationship is ultimately promotion of the client's health and well-being. This is true even when the client is dying or is uncooperative.

Peplau's developmental phases (1952) parallel the nursing process. The orientation phase correlates with the assessment phase of the nursing process. The identification component of the working phase corresponds to the planning phase, whereas the exploitation phase parallels the implementation phase. The final resolution phase of the relationship corresponds to the evaluation phase of the nursing process (see Chapter 2 for details on the nursing process).

PREINTERACTION PHASE

The preinteraction phase is the only one in which the client does not directly participate. Awareness of professional goals is important. Developing professional goals helps the nurse select concrete, specific nursing actions that are purposeful and aligned with individualized client needs.

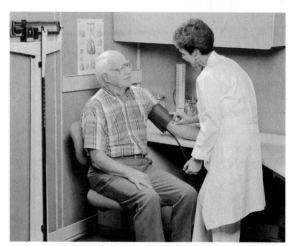

Concepts of the therapeutic relationship are present even in brief encounters.

Professional goals differ from client goals, having to do with the nurse's knowledge, competence, and control of role responsibilities in the nurse-client relationship. Although professional goals are not communicated

| TABLE 10-1 | Differences Between Helping Relationships and Social Relationships |

Helping Relationships	Social Relationships
Health care provider takes responsibility for the conduct of the relationship and for maintaining appropriate boundaries.	Both parties have equal responsibility for the conduct of the relationship.
Relationship has a specific health-related purpose and goals.	Relationship may or may not have a specific purpose or goals.
Meeting the professional health-related needs and goals of the client determine the duration of the relationship.	Relationship can last a lifetime or terminate spontaneously at any time.
Focus of the relationship is on needs of the client.	The needs of both partners can receive equal attention.
Relationship is entered into because of a client's health care need.	Relationship is entered into spontaneously for a wide variety of purposes.
Choice of who to be in relationship is not available to either helper or helpee.	Behavior for both participants is spontaneous; people choose companions.
Self-disclosure by the nurse is limited to data that facilitates the health-related relationship. Self-disclosure by the client is expected and encouraged.	Self-disclosure for both parties in the relationship is expected and encouraged.

directly to clients, they are present as professional behaviors in all aspects of nursing care.

Having an idea of potential client issues before meeting with the client is helpful. For example, a different approach is required for a client whose infant is in the neonatal intensive care unit, than for a client who is rooming in with a healthy infant.

If the relationship is to be ongoing, for example, in a subacute, rehabilitation, or psychiatric setting, it is important to share initial plans related to time, purpose, and other details with staff. This simple strategy helps avoid scheduling conflicts.

Creating the Physical Environment

Specific client needs dictate the most appropriate interpersonal setting. In hospital settings, if the door is closed, you need to knock before entering the room. When an assessment interview takes place at the client's bed in a hospital setting, the curtain should be drawn. Remember that for a limited time, this area is the client's "space."

One-on-one relationships with psychiatric clients commonly take place in a designated private space apart from the client's bedroom. In the client's home, the nurse is always the client's guest. A private space in which the nurse and client can talk without being uninterrupted is essential. Each time a nurse is sensitive to the environment in a nurse-client relationship, the nurse models thoughtfulness, respect, and empathy.

ORIENTATION PHASE

Nurses enter interpersonal relationships with clients in the "stranger" role. The client does not know you, and you do not know the client as a person. Begin the process of developing trust by providing the client with basic information about yourself (e.g., name and professional status) and essential information about the purpose, nature, and time available for the relationship (Peplau, 1997). It can be a simple introduction: "I am Susan Smith, a registered nurse, and I am going to be your nurse on this shift." Nonverbal supporting behaviors of a handshake, eye contact, and a smile reinforce spoken words. Introductions are important even with clients who are confused, aphasic, comatose, or unable to make a cogent response because of mental illness or dementia. Introductions may need to be repeated, particularly for cognitively disabled clients.

Next, you can ask the client, "How would you prefer to be addressed?" Assure the client that personal information will be treated as confidential (Heery, 2000). Explain that data will be shared with other members of the health care team as needed for making relevant clinical decisions and informing the client about the general composition of the health care team. Exercise 10-2 is designed to give you practice in making introductory statements.

Clarifying the Purpose of the Relationship

Clarity of purpose related to identifiable health needs is an essential dimension of the nurse-client relationship

EXERCISE 10-2	Introductions in the Nurse-Client Relationship

Purpose: To provide experience with initial introductions.

Procedure

The introductory statement forms the basis for the rest of the relationship. Effective contact with a client helps build an atmosphere of trust and connectedness with the nurse. The following statement is a good example of how one might engage the client in the first encounter:

"Hello, Mr. Smith. I am Sally Parks, a nursing student. I will be taking care of you on this shift. During the day, I may be asking you some questions about yourself that will help me to understand how I can best help you."

Role-play the introduction to a new client with one person taking the role of the client; another, the nurse; and a third person, an involved family number, with one or more of the following clients:

- Mrs. Dobish is a 70-year-old client admitted to the hospital with a diagnosis of diabetes and a question about cognitive impairment.

- Thomas Charles is a 19-year-old client admitted to the hospital following an auto accident in which he broke both legs and fractured his sternum.
- Barry Fisheis is a 53-year-old man who has been admitted to the hospital for tests. The physician believes he may have a renal tumor.
- Marion Beatty is a 9-year-old girl admitted to the hospital for an appendectomy.
- Barbara Tangiers is a 78-year-old woman living by herself. She has multiple health problems including chronic obstructive pulmonary disease and arthritis. This is your first visit.

Discussion

1. In what ways did you have to modify your introductions to meet the needs of the client and/or circumstances?
2. What were the easiest and hardest parts of doing this exercise?
3. How could you use this experience in your clinical practice?

(LaSala, 2009). It is difficult to fully participate in any working partnership without understanding its purpose and expectations. Clients need basic information about the purpose and nature of the interview or relationship, including what information is needed and how the information will be used, how the client can participate in the treatment process, and what the client can expect from the encounter. To understand the importance of orientation information, consider the value of having a clear syllabus for your nursing courses.

The length of the relationship dictates the depth of the orientation. An orientation given to a client by a nurse assigned for a shift would be different from that given to a client when the nurse assumes the role of primary care nurse over an extended period. When the relationship is of longer duration, the nurse should discuss the parameters of the relationship (e.g., length of sessions, frequency of meetings, and role expectations of the nurse and client).

Initial meetings should have two outcomes: First, the client should emerge from the encounter with a better idea of the most relevant health issues; second, the client should feel that the nurse is interested in him or her as a person. At the end of the contact, the nurse should thank the client for his or her participation and indicate what will happen next.

Establishing Trust

Carter (2009) defines **trust** as "a relational process, one that is dynamic and fragile, yet involving the deepest needs and vulnerabilities of individuals" (p. 404). Starting with the first encounter, clients begin to assess the trustworthiness of each nurse who cares for them. As clients experience the nurse as a person they can depend on, their sense of vulnerability decreases (Dinc and Gastmans, 2012). Kindness, competence, and a willingness to become involved are communicated through the nurse's words, tone of voice, and actions. Does the nurse seem to know what he or she is doing? Is the nurse tactful and respectful of cultural differences? Data regarding the level of the nurse's interest and knowledge base are factored into the client's decision to engage actively in a therapeutic relationship. Confidentiality, sensitivity to client needs, and honesty strengthen the relationship.

The client's level of trust fluctuates with illness, age, and the influence of past successful or unsuccessful encounters with others (Carter, 2009). Knowledge of the client's developmental level helps frame therapeutic conversations. For example, you would hold a different conversation with an adolescent client than you would with an elderly client. The acutely ill client will need short contacts that are to the point and related to providing comfort and care. The client's current health situation is a good starting place for choice of topic. The nurse's sensitivity to all aspects of the client's clinical situation and individualized needs helps clients begin to rely on the nurse as a trustworthy competent provider.

Trusting the nurse is particularly difficult for the seriously mentally ill, for whom the idea of having a professional person care about them can be incomprehensible. Having this awareness helps the nurse look beyond the bizarre behaviors that some clients present in response to their fears about helping relationships. Many mentally ill clients will respond better to shorter, frequent contacts until trust is established. Schizophrenic clients often enter and leave the space occupied by the nurse, almost circling around a space that is within visual distance of the nurse. With patience and tact, the nurse engages the client slowly with a welcoming look and brief verbal contact. Over time, brief meetings that involve an invitation and a statement as to when the nurse will return help reduce the client's anxiety, as indicated in the dialogue in the following case example.

Case Example

Nurse (with eye contact and enough interpersonal space for comfort): Good morning, Mrs. O'Connell. My name is Karen Quakenbush. I will be your nurse today.
(Client looks briefly at the nurse and looks away, then gets up and moves away.)
  Nurse: This may not be a good time to talk with you. Would you mind if I checked back later with you? (The introduction coupled with an invitation for later communication respects the client's need for interpersonal space and allows the client to set the pace of the relationship.)
  Later, the nurse notices that Mrs. O'Connell is circling around the area the nurse is occupying but does not approach the nurse. She smiles encouragingly and repeats nondemanding invitations to the client until the client is more willing to trust. (Creating an interpersonal environment that places little demand on either party initially allows the needed trust to develop in the relationship.)

Identifying Client Needs

Therapeutic relationships should directly revolve around the client's needs and preferences. Small and Small, 2011 state, the patient experience from the client's perspective should be a measurable outcome of client and family centered care (PFCC). The experience should reflect safe, effective, equitable and efficient care delivery starting with the initial nurse client encounter. Each person's experience and of the relationship will be different but all interactions need to be characterized by respect and dignity, active collaborative participation between providers and clients, and transparent information sharing regardless of length or diagnosis (IPCC, 2010). The nurse bears the responsibility for managing the conduct of the relationship and the client's experience of it as a positive one.

How clients perceive their health status, reasons for seeking treatment at this time, and expectations for health care are critical data, which you can begin to elicit by simply asking the client why he or she is seeking treatment at this time. Using questions that follow a logical sequence and asking only one question at a time help clients feel more comfortable and is likely to elicit more complete data.

Client and family expectations can facilitate or hinder the treatment process. For example, when health professionals treat elderly, adolescent, or physically handicapped clients as though they are mentally incapacitated in assessment interviews, it devalues them as a person. Conversely, family members are sometimes reluctant to challenge a client's perceptions in front of the client and may need a private interview. Nurses need to include *both* perspectives for accurate assessment.

Similarities and differences between client and family perceptions of illness and treatment are important data. If there is reason to suspect the reliability of the client as a historian, interviewing significant others assumes greater importance. Family/client agreement or disagreements about diagnosis, treatment goals, or ways to provide care are critical data. For example, if a client has one perception about personal self-care abilities and family members have a completely different awareness, these differences can become a nursing concern.

Participant Observation

Peplau describes the role of the nurse in all phases of the relationship as being a 'participant observer'. This means that the nurse simultaneously participates in and observes the progress of the relationship from the nurse and the client perspective. When validated with the client, observations about the client's behavior and words serve as guides for subsequent dialogue and actions in the relationship. According to Peplau, observation includes self-awareness and self-reflection on the part of the nurse. This is as critical to the success of the relationship as is the assessment of the client's situation (McCarthy and Aquino-Russell, 2009).

Case Example

Terminally ill client (to the nurse): It's not the dying that bothers me as much as not knowing what is going to happen to me in the process.

    Nurse: It sounds as though you can accept the fact that you are going to die, but you are concerned about what you will have to experience. Tell me more about what worries you.

By linking the emotional context with the content of the client's message, the nurse enters into the client's world and shows a desire to understand the situation from the client's perspective. Nurses need to be aware of the different physical and nonverbal cues clients give with their verbal messages. Noting facial expressions and nonverbal cues with "You look exhausted" or "You look worried" acknowledges the presence of these factors and normalizes them. Exercise 10-3 is designed to help you to critically observe a person's nonverbal cues.

Defining the Problem

Nurses act as a sounding board, asking questions about parts of the communication that are not understood and helping clients to describe their problems in concrete terms. The nurse asks for specific details to bring the client's needs into sharper focus, for example, "Could you describe for me what happened next," or "Tell me something about your reaction to (your problem)," or "How do you feel about…"? Time should be allowed between questions for the client to respond fully. Commonly, such questions are asked, but not enough time is allowed for the client to respond.

Clients usually find it easier to talk about factual data related to a problem rather than to express the feelings associated with the issue. For example, saying, "It sounds as if you feel _____ because of _____" helps the client to articulate the relationships between situational data and its emotional impact.

Once the nurse and client develop a working definition of the problem, they can begin to brainstorm the best ways to meet treatment goals. The brainstorming process occurs more easily when nurses are relaxed and willing to understand views different from their own. Brainstorming involves generating multiple ideas and suspending judgment until after all possibilities are presented. The next step is to look realistically at ideas that could work given the resources the client has available right now. Resistance can be worked through with empathetic reality testing. Peplau (1997) suggests that a general rule of thumb in working with clients is to "struggle with the problem, not with the client" (p. 164). The last part of the process relates to determining the kind of help needed and who can best provide it. Assessment of the most appropriate source of help is an important but often overlooked part of the evaluation needed in the orientation phase.

Defining Goals

Unless clients are physically or emotionally unable to participate in their care, they should be treated as active partners in developing personal goals. Goals should have meaning to the client. For example, modifying

---

EXERCISE 10-3	Nonverbal Messages

Purpose: To provide practice in validation skills in a nonthreatening environment.

Procedure
1. Each student, in turn, tries to communicate the following feelings to other members of the group without words. They may be written on a piece of paper, or the student may choose one directly from the following list.
2. The other students must guess what behaviors the student is trying to enact.

Pain	Anxiety	Shock	Disinterest
Anger	Disapproval	Disbelief	Rejection
Sadness	Relief	Disgust	Despair
Confidence	Uncertainty	Acceptance	Uptightness

Discussion
1. Which emotions were harder to guess from their nonverbal cues? Which ones were easier?
2. Was there more than one interpretation of the emotion?
3. How would you use the information you developed today in your future care of clients?

the exchange lists with a diabetic adolescent's input so that they include substitutions that follow normal adolescent eating habits can facilitate acceptance of unwelcome dietary restrictions. The nurse conveys confidence in the client's capacity to solve his or her own problems by expecting the client to provide data, to make constructive suggestions, and develop realistic goals.

WORKING (EXPLOITATION/ACTIVE INTERVENTION) PHASE

With relevant treatment goals to guide nursing interventions and client actions, the conversation in the working phase turns to active problem solving related to assessed health care needs. Clients are able to discuss deeper, more difficult issues and to experiment with new roles and actions. Corresponding to the implementation phase of the nursing process, the working phase focuses on self-direction and self-management to whatever extent is possible in promoting the client's health and well-being.

Peplau (1997) categorized the client role as dependent, interdependent, or independent, based on the amount of responsibility the client is willing or able to assume for his or her care. Nurses should provide enough structure and guidelines for clients to explore problem issues and develop realistic solutions, but no more than are needed (Ballou, 1998). Avoid taking more responsibility for actions than the client or situation requires. For example, it may seem more efficient to give a bath to a stroke victim than to watch the client struggle through the bathing process with the nurse providing coaching when the client falters. However, what happens when the client goes home if she has not learned to bathe herself?

Breaking a seemingly insoluble problem down into simpler chunks is a nursing strategy that makes doing difficult tasks more manageable. For example, a goal of eating three meals a day may seem overwhelming to a person suffering from nausea and loss of appetite associated with gastric cancer. A smaller goal of having applesauce or chicken soup and a glass of milk three times a day may sound more achievable, particularly if the client can choose the times.

In even the most difficult nursing situations, there are options, even if the choice is to die with dignity or to change one's attitude toward an illness or a family member. The client's right to make decisions, provided they do not violate self or others, needs to be accepted by the nurse, even when it runs contrary to the nurse's thinking. This protects the client's right to autonomy.

Case Example

LaSala (2009) presents a case example (courtesy of Lindsey O'Brien) in which a client with lymphoma refused a blood transfusion after her first round of chemotherapy. Her physician was upset that she would not accept this logical treatment. The nurse in this case example said, "I explained to him what her beliefs were and why she refused blood. He continued to look confused, and I said, 'We may not understand it fully, but we have to respect her decision and not let our personal opinions impede our care.' He looked at me and said I was absolutely right" (LaSala, p. 425 [quote from O'Brien]).

Tuning In to Client Response Patterns

The art of nursing requires that nurses recognize differences in client response patterns. Elderly adults may need a slower pace, and people in crisis will need a simple structured level of support. Throughout the working phase, nurses need to be sensitive about whether the client is still responding at a useful level. Looking at difficult problems and developing strategies to resolve those problems is not an easy process, especially when resolution requires significant behavioral changes. If the nurse is perceived as inquisitive rather than facilitative, communication breaks down.

It is the responsibility of the nurse, not the client, to pace interactions in ways that offer support, as well as challenge. Deciding whether to proceed is a clinical judgment that should be based on the client's response and overall body language. Examples of warning signs that the pace may need adjustment include loss of eye contact, fidgeting, abrupt changes in subject, or asking to be left alone. Conversely, strong emotion should not necessarily be interpreted as reflecting a level of interaction stretching beyond the client's tolerance. Tears or an emotional outburst may reflect honestly felt emotion. A well-placed comment, such as, "I can see that this is difficult for you," acknowledges the feeling and may stimulate further discussion.

Health disruptions create distress and usually require adaptive changes in more than one life domain. In addition to providing direct care, nurses help clients and families cope with the unique emotional and reality challenges associated with the client's health disruption. Tuning into the client's response patterns focuses on shared engagement and joint actions that connect, collaborate and create new possibilities for health and well-being. In the process of shared inquiry about the issues at hand, new possibilities can emerge even in brief encounters. Nurses are in a position to be able to discuss the unique integration of biological and social processes that can influence a successful recovery process.

If problems arise, they should be treated as temporary setbacks, which provide new information about what needs to happen next. Helping clients develop multiple strategies, and successfully cope with unexpected responses can strengthen a client's problem-solving abilities. Compelling the person to consider alternative options (i.e., a Plan B) when the original plan does not bring about the desired results is empowering.

Shared Decision Making

Barry and Edgman-Levitan (2012) identify shared decision making as the "pinnacle of patient-centered care" (p. 780). This concept requires transparent communication and active involvement of clients and families in considering the pros and cons of treatment options, and developing a decision that best fits the client's preferences and values, and the reality of the clinical situation. In addition to providing clients with information about their disease process or injury, clients need to have a clear understanding of treatment options, including side effects and consequences of each option, including what happens if no treatment is given. Elwyn (2012) outlines three key steps involved in an effective shared decision making process. He call these:

- Choice talk: Consists of finding out what information the client has, how much information the client wants, and who should be involved in the decision making process.
- Option talk: Consists of checking in with clients about potential fears, expectations, and other ideas the client may have about different options. Providing relevant information about potential treatment options, pros and cons of one option versus another, and taking into consideration what the health provider knows about the client's values and preferences, and concerns. The extent of risk for a particular client based on values, preferences, age and other health related factors, and the potential for uncertainty are relevant factors that should be discussed.

- Decision talk: Involves a more active engagement because it requires the client to make a decision. Whenever possible, clients should not forced to make a choice without being ready to make one. It is helpful to ask, "are you ready to make a decision, or do you need more time to think about it?" Some clients need not only time, but more information. It is critical that the decision be based on a client's informed preferences and that the client is comfortable with the decision.

Defusing Challenging Behaviors

Challenging behaviors can sabotage the therapeutic relationship. There is no unique way to approach a client, and no single interpersonal strategy that works equally well with every client. Some clients clearly are more emotionally accessible and attractive to work with than others. When a client seems unapproachable or uninterested in human contact, it can be quite disheartening for the nurse. It is not uncommon for the nurse to report the kind of initial contact with a client seen in the following case examples.

Case Example

"I tried, but he just wasn't interested in talking to me. I asked him some questions, but he didn't really answer me. So I tried to ask him about his hobbies and interests. It didn't matter what I asked him. He just turned away. Finally, I gave up because it was obvious that he just didn't want to talk to me."

Although, from the nurse's perspective the behavior of the client in the preceding case example may represent a lack of desire for a relationship, in many cases, the rejection is not personal. It can reflect boredom, insecurity, or physical discomfort. Anxiety expressed as anger or unresponsiveness may be the only way a client can control fear in a difficult situation. Rarely does it have much to do with the personal approach used by the nurse unless the nurse is truly insensitive to the client's feelings or the needs of the situation. In this situation, the nurse might say, "It seems to me that you just want to be alone right now. But I would like to help you, so if you don't mind, I'll check back later with you. Would that be okay with you?" Most of the time, clients appreciate the nurse's willingness to stay involved.

For novice nurses, it is important to recognize that all nurses have experienced some form of client rejection at one time or another. The nurse needs to explore whether the timing was right, whether the client was in pain, and what other circumstances might have contributed to the client's attitude. Behaviors that initially seem maladaptive may appear quite adaptive when the full circumstances of the client's situation are understood.

Before confronting a client, the nurse should anticipate possible outcomes. The nurse needs to appreciate the impact of the confrontation on a client's self-esteem. Calling a client's attention to a contradiction in behavioral response is usually threatening. Preserving the client's personal dignity is a basic human right that nurses should always keep in mind irrespective of the client's external behaviors (Stievano et al, 2013) Constructive feedback involves drawing the client's attention to the existence of unacceptable behaviors or contradictory messages while respecting the fragility of the therapeutic alliance and the client's need to protect the integrity of his/her self-concept. To be effective, constructive confrontations is best attempted when the following criteria have been met:

- The nurse has established a firm, trusting bond with the client.
- The timing and environmental circumstances are appropriate.
- The confrontation is delivered in a private setting and in a nonjudgmental and empathetic manner.
- Only those behaviors capable of being changed by the client are addressed.
- The nurse supports the client's right to self-determination.

Case Example

Mary Kiernan is 5 feet 2 inches tall and weighs 260 pounds. She has attended weekly weight management sessions for the past 6 weeks. Although she lost 8 pounds the first week, 4 pounds in week 2, and another 4 pounds by week 5, her weight loss seems to have hit a plateau. Jane Tompkins, her primary nurse, notices that Mary seems to be able to stick to the diet until she gets to dessert; then she cannot resist temptation. Mary is very discouraged about her lack of further progress.

Consider the effect of each response on the client.

Response A

Nurse: You're supposed to be on a 1200-calorie-a-day diet, but instead you're sneaking dessert. If you eat dessert when you are on a diet, you are kidding yourself that you will lose weight.

Response B:

Nurse: I can understand your discouragement, but you have done quite well in losing 16 pounds. It seems as though you can stick to the diet until you get to dessert. Do you think we need to talk a little more about what hooks you when you get to dessert? Maybe we need to find alternatives that would help you get back on track.

The first statement is direct, valid, and concise, but it is likely to be disregarded or experienced as unfeeling by the client. In the second response, the nurse reframes a behavioral inconsistency as a temporary setback. By first introducing an observed strength of the progress achieved so far, the nurse reaffirms trust in the client's resourcefulness. Both responses would require similar amounts of time and energy on the part of the nurse; however, the client is likely to accept the nurse's second comment as more supportive.

Self-disclosure

Self-disclosure by the nurse refers to an intentional revealing of relevant personal experiences or feelings used to enhance the nurse/client relationship. Limited self-disclosure can be useful if it serves the purposes of the relationship. Applications can deepen trust, and role-model self-disclosure as a beneficial mode of communicating for people who have trouble disclosing information about themselves. Deering (1999) suggests, appropriate self-disclosure can facilitate the relationship, providing the client with information that is both immediate and personalized. She suggests the following guidelines for keeping *self-disclosure* at a therapeutic level: (a) use self-disclosure to help clients open up to you, not to meet your own needs; (b) keep your disclosure brief; and (c) do not imply that your experience is exactly the same as the client's.

A nurse's self-disclosure should be solely for the clinical benefit of the client and never to meet the personal agenda of the nurse. Nurses should not share intimate details of their lives with their clients. The nurse, not the client, is responsible for regulating the amount of disclosure needed to facilitate the relationship. If the client asks a nonoffensive, superficial question, the nurse may answer briefly with a minimum of information and return to a client focus. Simple questions such as, "Where did you go to nursing school?" and "Do you have any children?" may represent the client's effort to establish common ground for conversation (Morse, 1991). Answering the client briefly and returning the focus to the client is appropriate. If the client persists with questions, the nurse may need to redirect the client by saying, "I'd like to spend this time talking about you," or simply indicate that personal questions are not relevant to understanding the client's health care needs. Exercise 10-4 provides an opportunity to explore self-disclosure in the nurse-client relationship.

TERMINATION PHASE

It is important to be clear from the beginning about how long a therapeutic relationship will last. During the course of the relationship, termination can be mentioned, and clients should be told well in advance of an impending termination date. In the termination phase, the nurse and client evaluate the client's responses to treatment and explore the meaning of the relationship and what goals have been achieved. Discussing client achievements, how the client and nurse feel about ending the relationship, and plans for the future are an important part of the termination phase.

Termination is a significant issue in long-term settings such as skilled nursing facilities, bone marrow transplant units, rehabilitation hospitals, and state psychiatric facilities. Meaningful long-term relationships can and do develop in these settings. If the relationship has been effective, real work has been accomplished. Nurses need to be sufficiently aware of their own feelings so that they may use them constructively without imposing them on the client. It is appropriate for nurses to share some of the meaning the relationship held for them, as long as such sharing fits the needs of the interpersonal situation and is not excessive or too emotionally intense.

Termination of a meaningful nurse-client relationship in long-term settings should be final. To provide the client with even a hint that the relationship will continue is unfair. It keeps the client emotionally involved in a relationship that no longer has a health-related goal. This is a difficult issue for nursing students, who either see no harm in telling the client they will continue to keep in contact or who feel they have used the client for their own learning needs and to completely close the door is unfair. However, this perception underestimates the positive things that the client received from the relationship and denies the fact that good-byes, painful as they may be, are a part of life and certainly not new for the client or for the nursing student.

Termination behaviors the nurse may encounter include avoidance, minimizing of the importance of the relationship, anger, demands, or additional reliance on the nurse. When the client is unable to express feelings about endings, the nurse may recognize them in the client's nonverbal behavior.

EXERCISE 10-4   **Recognizing Role Limitations in Self-Disclosure**

Purpose: To help students differentiate between a therapeutic use of self-disclosure and spontaneous self-revelation.

Procedure
1. Make a list of three phrases that describe your own personality or the way you relate to others, such as the following:
   I am shy.
   I get angry when criticized.
   I'm nice.
   I'm sexy.
   I find it hard to handle conflicts.
   I'm interested in helping people.
2. Mark each descriptive phase with one of the following:
   A = Too embarrassing or intimate to discuss in a group.
   B = Could discuss with a group of peers.

C = This behavior characteristic might affect my ability to function in a therapeutic manner if disclosed.
3. Share your responses with the group.

Discussion
1. What criteria were used to determine the appropriateness of self-disclosure?
2. How much variation is there in what each student would share with others in a group or clinical setting?
3. Were there any behaviors commonly agreed on that would never be shared with a client?
4. What interpersonal factors about the client would facilitate or impede self-disclosure by the nurse in the clinical setting?
5. What did you learn from doing this exercise that could be used in future encounters with clients?

Case Example

A teenager who had spent many months on a bone marrow transplant unit had developed a real attachment to her primary nurse, who had stood by her during the frightening physical assaults to her body and appearance, occasioned by the treatment. The client was unable to verbally acknowledge the meaning of the relationship with the nurse directly, despite having been given many opportunities to do so by the nurse. The client said she couldn't wait to leave this awful hospital and that she was glad she didn't have to see the nurses anymore. Yet, this same client was found sobbing in her room the day she left, and she asked the nurse whether she could write to her. The relationship obviously had meaning for the client, but she was unable to express it verbally.

Gift Giving

Clients sometimes wish to give nurses gifts at the end of a constructive relationship because they value the care nurses have given to them. Gift giving is a delicate matter that does not lend itself to absolute dictums, but instead invites reflection and professional judgment. Nurses should consider: What meaning does the gift have for the relationship, and in what ways might accepting it change the dynamics of the therapeutic alliance? Would giving or receiving a gift present issues for other clients or their families?

There is no one answer about whether gifts should or should not be exchanged. In fact, if the nurse handled every situation in the same fashion, the nurse would be denying the uniqueness of each nurse-client relationship. Each relationship has its own character and its own strengths and limitations, so what might be appropriate in one situation would be totally inappropriate in another. Token gifts such as chocolates or flowers may be acceptable. In general, nurses should not accept money or gifts of significant material value. Should this become an issue, you might suggest making the gift to the health care agency or a charity. It is always appropriate to simply thank the client for their generosity and thoughtfulness (Lambert, 2009). Exercise 10-5 is designed to help you think about the implications of gift giving in the nurse-client relationship.

Evaluation

Objective evaluation of clinical outcomes achieved in the nurse-client relationship should focus on the following:

- Was the problem definition adequate and appropriate for the client?
- Were the interventions chosen adequate and appropriate to resolve the client's problem?
- Were the interventions implemented effectively and efficiently to both the client's and the nurse's satisfaction in the allotted time frame?

EXERCISE 10-5   Gift-Giving Role-Play

Purpose: To help students develop therapeutic responses to clients who wish to give them gifts.

Procedure
Review the following situations and answer the discussion questions.

Situation
Mrs. Terrell, a hospice nurse, has taken care of Mr. Aitken during the last 3 months of his life. She has been very supportive of the family. Because of her intervention, Mr. Aitken and his son were able to resolve a longstanding and very bitter conflict before he died. The whole family, particularly his wife, is grateful to Mrs. Terrell for her special attention to Mr. Aitken.

Role-Play Directions for Mrs. Aitken
You are very grateful to Mrs. Terrell for all of her help over the past few months. Without her help, you do not know what you would have done. To show your appreciation, you would like her to have a $300 gift certificate at your favorite boutique. It is very important to you that Mrs. Terrell fully understand how meaningful her caring has been to you during this very difficult time.

Role-Play Directions for Mrs. Terrell
You have given the Aitken family high-quality care and you feel very good about it, particularly the role you played in helping Mr. Aitken and his son reconcile before Mr. Aitken's death. Respond as you think you might in this clinical situation, given the previous data.

Discussion
1. Discuss the responses made in the role-playing situation.
2. Discuss the other possible responses and evaluate the possible consequences.
3. Would you react differently if a client gave you a gift of $200 or a hand-crocheted scarf? If so, why?
4. Are there gifts clients give a nurse that are intangible? How should these gifts be acknowledged?

- Is the client progressing toward maximum health and well-being? Is the client satisfied with his or her progress and care received?
- If follow-up care is indicated, is the client satisfied and able to carry forward his or her treatment plan in the community?

ADAPTATION FOR SHORT-TERM RELATIONSHIPS

Hagerty and Patusky (2003) argue the need to reconceptualize the nurse-client relationship to one of human relatedness, given the brevity of hospital stays in today's evolving health care arena. They identify four essential qualities needed to establish relatedness in short term relationships: "sense of belonging, reciprocity, mutuality and synchrony" (Moser et al, 2010, p. 218). Driven by the economics of managed care, nurses must help clients determine what they need and how to quickly develop solutions that fit their situation. Critical to the development of autonomous responsive relationships to support self-management of chronic illness and short-term hospitalizations is a sustained collaborative engagement between nurse and client. Although nurses can and should follow the phases of the relationship, developing a therapeutic relationship in short-term care could be more accurately termed a *working alliance with active support*.

Communication is key at every stage of the relationship. The same recommendations for self-awareness, empathy, therapeutic boundaries, active listening, competence, mutual respect, partnership, and level of involvement hold true as key elements of brief therapeutic relationships.

Orientation Phase

The therapeutic alliance begins with a similar introduction and description of purpose identified for long-term relationships plus an emphasis on the nurse and client working as partners to develop a shared understanding of the client's health problems. Establishing a working alliance where time is an issue requires a "here and now" focus on problem identification, with an emphasis on quickly understanding the context in which the problem is embedded. Meaningful connections occur when nurses initially strive to view each client as a person to be engaged with rather than focusing on what needs to be done (Nicholson et al., 2010).

Eliciting the client's concerns and allowing the client to tell his or her story conveys respect and interest. Listen for what is left out and pay attention to what the client's story elicits in you. Support and empathy help build trust quickly. Acknowledge the client's feelings with a statement such as "Tell me more about..." (with a theme picked up from the client's choice of words, hesitancy, or nonverbal cues).

Anderson (2001) echoes Roger's belief that all people have potential for self constructive behaviors. As the nurse interacts with the client, there are opportunities to observe client strengths and to comment on them. Every client has healthy aspects of his or her personality, and personal strengths that can be drawn on to facilitate individual coping responses. Exercise 10-6 provides an opportunity to explore the value of acknowledging personal strengths.

An important component of brief therapeutic relationships is the rapid development of a central focus, which is developed during an initial client evaluation. A simple statement posed at the beginning of each shift, such as, "What is your most important need

---

EXERCISE 10-6	Identifying Client Strengths

Purpose: To identify personal strengths in clients with serious illness

Procedure
1. Think about a client you have had or a person you know who has a serious illness.
2. What personal strengths does this person possess that could have a healing impact? Strengths can be courage, patience, fighting spirit, family, and so on.

3. Write a one-page description of the client and the personal strengths observed, despite the client's medical or psychological condition.

Discussion
1. If you had not had to write the description, would you have been as aware of the client's strengths?
2. How could you help the client maximize his or her strengths to achieve quality of life?
3. What did you learn from this exercise that you can use in your clinical practice?

today?" or "What is the most important thing I can do for you today?" helps focus the relationship on matters important to the client (Cappabianca et al 2009). This type of question demonstrates intent to understand and meet each client's unique needs in a shortened time frame. It helps client and nurse develop a shared understanding of what is uniquely important to the client in the present moment.

Even the briefest therapeutic encounter should be client centered with an emphasis on understanding the client's personalized experience of an illness and its social context (Bardes, 2012). Client satisfaction is an identifiable outcome. Researchers consider client centered care as being "defined by a focus on outcomes that people notice and care about including, not only survival, but function, symptoms and modifiable aspects of QOL (Rodriguez et al, 2013 p. 1795; Patient-Centered Outcomes Research Insitute, 2013). Because the time frame for a therapeutic relationship may last only a few hours or days, nurses need to focus on what is absolutely essential, rather than everything that might be nice to know. Finding out how much the client already knows can save time. Planning will be smoother if the nurse and client choose problems, which are of interest to the client and offer the best return on investment. Included in the planning should be the risks and cost-benefits for each targeted clinical outcome. The more actively engaged and involved a client is taking responsibility, the stronger are the clinical outcomes. Tailoring coaching and support to a client's level of activation and encouraging small achievable steps are actions nurses can take to maximize effectiveness (Greene and Hibbarad, 2012). Looking at the client's needs from a broader contextual perspective, one that takes into consideration which problems, if treated, would also help correct other health problems, has a double benefit in terms of client success and satisfaction. Engaging the client's family early in the treatment process is helpful. Nurses must be familiar enough with the client's symptoms and behaviors so they can accurately communicate the meaning of symptoms and suffering to family members or other health care colleagues and team members. This experiential data allows nurses to advocate for their clients (Bridges et al., 2013).

As nurses increasingly move from a bedside role into a managerial coordination role, they become responsible for clarifying, integrating, and coordinating different aspects of the client's care, as part of an interprofessional team. (See chapters 8 and 22). An important component of this responsibility is ensuring that the client and family understands and is able to negotiate treatment initiatives with health care team providers. The nurse is frequently the liaison resource between the team and the client/family for follow up explanations.

Working Phase

Brief relationships should be solution-focused right from the start. Giving clients your undivided attention and using concise active listening responses is absolutely essential to being able to frame issues in a solution-focused way. A central focus, agreed on by nurse and client, promotes the small behavioral changes and related coping skills needed to meet client goals in short-term relationships. Finding ways to collaborate makes the most effective use of time, and confrontation should be avoided. Longer-term issues are not examined in depth. Support beyond what is needed to stabilize the client usually is not directly offered.

Clients respond best to nurses who appear confident and empathetic. An excellent way of helping clients discover the solutions that fit them best is by engaging the client in determining and implementing activities to meet therapeutic goals at every realistic opportunity. Conveying a realistically hopeful attitude that the goals developed with the client are likely to be achieved is important. Action plans should be as simple and specific as possible. Changes in the client's condition or other circumstances may require treatment modifications that should be expected in short-term relationships. Keeping clients and families informed and working with them on alternative solutions is essential to maintaining trust in short-term relationships.

Termination Phase

The termination phase in short-term relationships includes discharge planning, agency referrals, and arranging for follow-up appointments in the community for the client and family. Anticipatory guidance in the form of simple instructions or review of important skills is appropriate, Interpersonal relationships with other health care disciplines, families, and communities to support positive client health changes should be the norm, not the exception with short-term therapeutic relationships as these will be needed for appropriate aftercare. Check with the hospitalist or discharging physician, share the expected departure time with the staff, and ensure the client has everything in order.

The importance of the relationship, no matter how brief, should not be underestimated. Sudden illness or an exacerbation of a chronic illness can dramatically change a person's life in unexpected ways. Although the client may be one of several persons the nurse has taken care of during a shift, the relationship may represent the only interpersonal or professional contact available to a lonely and frightened person. Even if contact has been brief, the client's assigned nurse should stop by the client's room to say good-bye. The dialogue in such cases can be simple and short: "Mr. Jones, I will be going off duty in a few minutes. I enjoyed working with you. Miss Smith will be taking care of you this evening." "Is there anything I can do for you before I go?" Check to see if the client has the call button. If you will not be returning at a later date, this information should be shared with the client.

SUMMARY

The nurse-client relationship represents a purposeful use of self in all professional relations with clients and other people involved with the client. Respect for the dignity of the client and self, person-centered communication, and authenticity in conversation are process threads underlying all communication responses.

Therapeutic relationships have professional boundaries, purposes, and behaviors. Boundaries keep the relationship safe for the client. They spell out the parameters of the therapeutic relationship and nurses are ethically responsible for maintaining them throughout the relationship. Effective relationships enhance the well-being of the client and the professional growth of the nurse. The professional relationship goes through a developmental process characterized by four overlapping yet distinct stages: preinteraction, orientation, working phase, and termination phase. The preinteraction phase is the only phase of the relationship the client is not part of. During the preinteraction phase, the nurse develops the appropriate physical and interpersonal environment for an optimal relationship, in collaboration with other health professionals and significant others in the client's life.

The orientation phase of the relationship defines the purpose, roles, and rules of the process, and provides a framework for assessing client needs. The nurse builds a sense of trust through consistency of actions. Data collection forms the basis for developing relevant nursing diagnoses. The orientation phase ends with a therapeutic contract mutually defined by nurse and client.

The working phase is the problem-solving phase of the relationship, paralleling the planning and implementation phases of the nursing process. As the client begins to explore difficult problems and feelings, the nurse uses a variety of interpersonal strategies to help the client develop new insights and methods of coping.

The final phase of the nurse-client relationship occurs when the essential work of the active intervention phase is finished. The ending should be thoroughly and compassionately defined early enough in the relationship that the client can process it appropriately. Primary tasks associated with the termination phase of the relationship include summarization and evaluation of completed activities and referrals when indicated. Short-term relationships incorporate the same skills and competencies as traditional nurse-client relationships, but with a sharper focus on the here and now. The action plan needs to be as simple and specific as possible.

ETHICAL DILEMMA   What Would You Do?

Kelly, age 20 years, has been admitted with a tentative medical diagnosis: rule out acquired immunodeficiency syndrome (AIDS). John is a 21-year-old student nurse assigned to care for Kelly. He expresses concern to his instructor about the client's sexual orientation. The instructor notes that John spends the majority of his time with his only other assigned client, who is in for treatment of a minor heart irregularity. What conclusions might be drawn regarding the reason John spends so little time caring for Kelly? If you were John's clinical instructor, how would you approach this situation, and what do you see as the ethical concerns in this scenario?

DISCUSSION QUESTIONS

1. In what ways do organizational structure and expectations in your clinical setting enhance or impede development of therapeutic relationships in nursing care?
2. What does the phrase, "being present in health care relationships," mean?
3. In what specific ways do therapeutic interpersonal relationships support effective client and family decision-making processes?

REFERENCES

American Hospital Association (AHA): *The patient care partnership: understanding expectations, rights and responsibilities.* 2003. Available online: http://www.aha.org/content/00-10/pcp_english_030730.pdf

Anderson H: Postmodern collaborative and person-centered therapies: what would Carl Rogers say? *J Fam Ther* 23(4):339–360, 2001.

Bardes C: Defining "client-centered medicine." *N Engl J Med* 366:782–783, 2012.

Ballou K: A concept analysis of autonomy, *J Prof Nurs* 14(2):102–110, 1998.

Barry M, Edgman-Levitan S: Shared decision making—the pinnacle of client-centered care, *N Engl J Med* 366:780–781, 2012.

Briant S, Freshwater D: Exploring mutuality within the nurse-client relationship, *Br J Nurs* 7(4):204–206, 1998.

Bridges J, Nicholson C, Maben J, Pope C, Flatle M, Wilkinson C, Meyer J, Tziggili M: Capacity for care: meta-ethnography of acute care nurses' experiences of the nurse client relationship, *J Adv Nurs* 69(4):760–772, 2013.

Bruner B, Yonge O: Boundaries and adolescents in residential treatment centers: what clinicians need to know, *J Psychosoc Nurs* 44(9):38–44, 2006.

Buber M: *Between Man and Man*, 2nd ed (Routledge Classics) New York, NY, 2002, Routledge.

Buber M: Distance and relation, *Psychiatry* 20:97–104, 1957.

Buber M. I and Thou, New York: Charles Scribner's Sons, 1958.

Cappabianca A, Julliard K, Raso R, Ruggiero J: Strengthening the nurse-client relationship: what is the most important thing I can do for you today, *Creat Nurs* 15(3):151–156, 2009.

Carmack B: Balancing engagement and disengagement in caregiving, *Image (IN)* 29(2):139–144, 1997.

Carter M: Trust, power, and vulnerability: a discourse on helping in nursing, *Nurs Clin North Am* 44:393–405, 2009.

Chauhan G, Long A: Communication is the essence of nursing care. 2: ethical foundations, *Br J Nurs* 9(15):979–984, 2000.

Covington H: Caring presence: delineation of a concept for holistic nursing, *J Holist Nurs* 21(3):301–317, 2003.

Daniels L: Vulnerability as a key to authenticity, *Image J Nurs Sch* 30(2):191–193, 1998.

Deering CG: To speak or not to speak? Self-disclosure with clients, *Am J Nurs* 99(1 Pt 1):34–38, 1999.

Dinc L, Gastmans C: Trust and trustworthiness in nursing: An argument-based literature review, *Nursing Inq* 19(3):223–237, 2012.

Easter A: Construct analysis of four modes of being present, *J Holist Nurs* 18(4):362–377, 2000.

Egan G: *The skilled helper: A Problem-Management and Opportunity-Development Approach to Helping.* 10th ed, Brooks Cole: Belmont, CA, Cenage Learning, 2014.

Egan G: *The skilled helper*, ed 7, 2002, Brooks Cole: Pacific Grove, CA.

Elwyn G, Frosch D, Thompson R, et al.: Shared decision making: a model for clinical practice, *J Gen Intern Med* 27:1361–1367, 2012.

Erlen JA, Jones M: The client no one liked, *Orthop Nurs* 18(4):76–79, 1999.

Fronek P, Kendall M, Ungerer G, Malt J, Eugarde E, Geraghty T: Towards healthy professional-client relationships: the value of an interprofessional training course, *J Interprof Care* 23(10):16–29, 2009.

Gallant M, Beaulieu M, Carnevale F: Partnership: an analysis of the concept within the nurse-client relationship, *J Adv Nurs* 2:149–157, 2002.

Greene J, Hibbard J: Why does client activation matter? An examination of the relationships between client activation and health-related outcomes, *J Gen Inte rn Med* 27:520–526, 2012.

Hagerty B, Patusky K: Reconceptualizing the nurse-client relationship, *J Nurs Scholarsh* 35(2):145–150, 2003.

Hartley S: Drawing the lines of professional boundaries, *Renalink* 3(2):7–9, 2002.

Hawley MP, Jensen L: Making a difference in critical care nursing practice, *Qual Health Res* 17(5):663–674, 2007.

Heery K: Straight talk about the client interview, *Nursing* 30(6):66–67, 2000.

Heinrich K: When a client becomes too special, *Am J Nurs* 22(11): 62–64, 1992.

Henderson V: The nature of nursing, *Am J Nurs* 64(8):62–68, 1964.

Hofmann P: Addressing compassion fatigue. The problem is not new, but it requires more urgent attention, *Healthc Exec* (Sept/Oct). 24(5):40–42, 2009.

Hook M: Partnering with clients—A concept ready for action, *J Adv Nurs* 56(2):133–143, 2006.

Institute of Medicine: *Crossing the quality chasm: a new health system for the 21st century*, Washington, DC, 2001, National Academies Press.

Institute for Patient-and Family-Centered Care: *FAQs*. Retrieved: (July 23, 2014) www.ipfcc.org/faq.html, 2010.

Jasovsky D, Morrow M, Clementi P, et al.: Theories in action and how nursing practice changed, *Nurs Sci Q* 23(1):29–38, 2010.

The Joint Commission. (2001) *The Health care at the crossroads: strategies for addressing the evolving nursing crisis* Author: Washington, DC

Kines M: The risks of caring too much, *Can Nurs* 95(8):27–30, 1999.

Lambert K: Gifts and gratuities for the case manager, *Prof Case Manag* 14(1):53–54, 2009.

O'Brien L, Quoted in, LaSala C: Moral accountability and integrity in nursing practice, *Nurs Clin North Am* 44:423–434, 2009.

Levigne D, Kautz DD: The evidence for listening and teaching may reside in our hearts, *Medsurg Nurs* 19:194–196, 2010.

Lazenby M. On the humanities of nursing. *Nurs Outlook* 61(1) e9–14, 2013.

Lowry M: Self-awareness: is it crucial to clinical practice? Confessions of a self-aware-aholic, *Am J Nurs* 105(11):72CCC–72DDD, 2005.

McCance T, McCormack B, Dewing J: An exploration of person-centeredness in practice, *OJIN* 16, 2011. No.02, Manuscript 01.

McCarthy C, CA Aquino-Russell CA: comparison of two nursing theories in practice: Peplau and Parse, *Nurs Sci Q* 22(1):34–40, 2009.

McCormack B, McCance T: *Person-centred Nursing: Theory and Practice*, Wiley Blackwell, 2010, Oxford.

McCormack B, McCance TV: Development of a framework for person-centred nursing, *J Adv Nurs* 56(5):472–479, 2006.

McDonough-Means M, Kreitzer I, Bell: Fostering a healing presence and investigating its mediators, *J Altern Complement Med* 10(Suppl 1):S25–S41, 2004.

McGrath D: Healthy conversations: key to excellence in practice, *Holist Nurs Pract* 19(4):191–193, 2005.

McQueen A: Nurse–client relationships and partnership in hospital care, *J Clin Nurs* 9(5):723–731, 2000.

Mead N, P. Bower B: Client-centredness: a conceptual framework and review of empirical literature, *Social Science and Medicine* 51: 1087–1110, 2000.

Morse J: Negotiating commitment and involvement in the nurse-client relationship, *J Adv Nurs* 16:455–468, 1991.

Morse JM, Havens GA, Wilson S: The comforting interaction: developing a model of nurse-client relationship, *Sch Inq Nurs Pract* 11(4):321–343, 1997.

Moser A, Houtepen R, Spreeuwenberg C, Widdershoven G: Realizing autonomy in responsive relationships, *Med Health Care Philos* 13:215–223, 2010.

National Council of State Boards of Nursing (NCSBN): *A nurse's guide to professional boundaries*, Available online Chicago, 2009, NCSBN. Accessed December 15, 2009. https://www.ncsbn.org/ProfessionalBoundaries_Complete.pdf.

Nicholson C, Flatley M, Wilkinson C, Meyer J, Dale P, Wessel L: Everybody matters 2: promoting dignity in acute care through effective communication, *Nurs Times* 106(21):12–14, 2010.

Patient-Centered Outcomes Research Institute: http://www.pcori.org/about/mission-and-vision/, 2013.

Peplau HE: *Interpersonal relations in nursing*, New York, 1952, Putnam.

Peplau HE: Peplau's theory of interpersonal relations, *Nurs Sci Q* 10(4):162–167, 1997.

Porter S, O'Halloran P, Morrow E: Bringing values back into evidenced based nursing: Role of clients in resisting empiricism, *Nurs Sci Q* 34(2):106–118, 2011.

Reynolds W: Peplau's theory in practice, *Nurs Sci Q* 10(4):168–170, 1997.

Rodriguez A, Mayo N, Gagnon B: Independent contributors to overall quality of life in people with advanced cancer, *BJC* 108:1790–1800, 2013.

Rogers C: The characteristics of the helping relationship, *Person Guid J* 37(1):6–16, 1958.

Scheick D: Developing self-aware mindfulness to manage countertransference in the nurse-client relationship: An evaluation and Developmental study, *J Prof Nurs* 27(2):114–123, 2011.

Sheets V: Professional boundaries: staying in the lines, *Dimens Crit Care Nurs* 20(5):36–40, 2001.

Small D, Small R: Patients First! Engaging the Hearts and Minds of Nurses with a Patient-Centered Practice Model. *Online J Issues in Nurs* 16(2), May 31, 2011. manuscript 2.

Stievano A, Rocco G, Sabatino L, Alvaro R: Dignity in professional nursing: guaranteeing better patient care, *JRN* 32(3):120–123, 2013.

CHAPTER 11

Bridges and Barriers in Therapeutic Relationships

Kathleen Underman Boggs

OBJECTIVES

At the end of the chapter, the reader will be able to:

1. Identify concepts that enhance development of therapeutic relationships: caring, empowerment, trust, empathy, mutuality, and confidentiality.
2. Describe nursing actions designed to promote trust, empowerment, empathy, mutuality, and confidentiality.
3. Describe barriers to the development of therapeutic relationships: anxiety, stereotyping, and lack of personal space and limited time.
4. Identify nursing actions that can be used to reduce anxiety and respect personal space and confidentiality.
5. Identify research-supported relationships between communication outcomes, such as client empowerment and improvements in self-care.
6. Discuss how findings from research studies can be applied to clinical practice.

This chapter focuses on the components of the nurse-client relationship, showing how nursing communication affects client health outcomes and satisfaction. Health communication is a multidimensional process and includes aspects from both the sender and the receiver of the message. Your communication skills influence client outcomes such as anxiety, adherence to treatments, and satisfaction with care. To establish a therapeutic relationship, you need to understand and apply the concepts of respect, caring, empowerment, trust, empathy, and mutuality, as well as confidentiality and veracity (Figure 11-1). Additional bridges fostering the relationship are your ability to put into practice the ethical aspects of respecting the client's autonomy and treating your client in a just and beneficent manner. Numerous studies show a strong link between effective communication and adherence to treatment, as well as client satisfaction. In your every encounter with a client, you need to become aware of their many variations in verbal and nonverbal responses (Knoerl et al., 2011).

Understanding communication barriers in the relationship (e.g., anxiety, stereotyping, or violations of personal space or confidentiality) affects the quality of the relationship. Implementing actions that convey feelings of respect, caring, warmth, acceptance, and understanding to the client is an interpersonal skill that requires practice. Caring for others in a meaningful way improves with experience. Novice students may encounter interpersonal situations that leave them feeling helpless and inadequate. Feelings of sadness, anger, or embarrassment, although overwhelming, are common. Through discussion of these feelings in peer groups and experiential learning practice activities, you gain skill. The self-awareness strategies identified in Chapter 9 and the use of educational groups described in Chapter 8 provide useful guidelines for working through your feelings.

BASIC CONCEPTS

BRIDGES TO THE RELATIONSHIP

Nursing communication is crucial to efficient provision of quality care for your clients. Your communication skills affect client outcomes such as satisfaction with care, improved coping, adherence to treatment, adaptation to institutional care, peaceful death, and

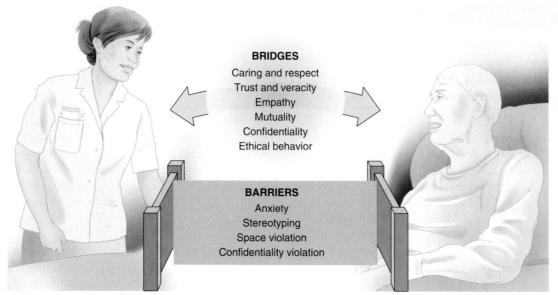

Figure 11-1   Relationships can move in a positive or negative direction. Nursing actions can be bridges or barriers to a good nurse-client interaction.

level of anxiety. Communication also affects us as providers in terms of our job satisfaction and stress levels. The following concepts will help you improve your communication. Barriers to use of each concept are described.

RESPECT

Conveying genuine respect for your client assists in building a professional relationship with him or her. Because your mutual goal is to maximize your client's health status, you convey respect for his or her values and opinions. Asking clients what they prefer to be called and always addressing them as such is a correct initial step. Of course, you avoid the sort of casual addresses portrayed in bad television shows, such as "How are you feeling, honey?" "Mom, hold your baby," or "How are we feeling today?" We try to remember that hospitalized clients feel a loss of control in relation to interpersonal relationships with staff.

BARRIER: LACK OF RESPECT

In the Williams and Irurita study (2004), clients felt devalued when they perceived that staff were avoiding talking with them or were unfriendly; they felt comforted when a little "chitchat" was exchanged. Lack of respect among members of the team has also been often cited as a cause of poor communication

leading to adverse client outcomes, especially lack of respect for the nurse by physicians. In a true collaborative model, each team member conveys respect and assumes responsibility for initiating clear communication. In establishing client-centered care, you treat your client as a respected member of the team (a QSEN competency).

Safety issues and related communication tools are discussed in Chapter 4.

CARING

Caring is an intentional human action characterized by commitment and a sufficient level of knowledge and skill to allow you to support the basic integrity of your client. You offer caring to your client by means of the therapeutic relationship. Nursing theorists, especially Watson, describe the need to develop and sustain a helping-trusting caring relationship (Lachman, 2012). Your ability to care develops from a natural response to help those in need, from the knowledge that caring is a part of nursing ethics, and from respect for self and others. As a caring nurse, you will involve clients in their struggle for health and well-being rather than simply doing things for your clients.

Provision of a caring relationship that facilitates health and healing is identified as an essential feature of contemporary nursing practice in the Social Policy

EXERCISE 11-1	Application of Caring

Purpose: To help you apply caring concepts to nursing.

Procedure
Identify some aspect of caring that might be applied to nursing practice. Work in a group to compile a list.

Discussion
Discuss examples of how this form of caring could be implemented in a nurse-client situation.

Statement of the American Nurses Association (ANA, 2010). In the professional literature, the focus of the caring relationship is clearly placed on meeting your client's needs. A formal model is even titled "patient-centered care." This is the first of the six prelicensure QSEN competencies described in Chapter 2. The behavior of "caring" is not an emotional feeling. Rather, it is a chosen response to your client's need. You willingly give of yourself to another through your compassion, concern, and interest. Caring is an ethical responsibility that guides you to advocate for your clients.

Clients want us to understand why they are suffering. Health care workers tend to speak in a medical language that values facts and events. Clients, in contrast, value associations and causes. To bridge this potential gap, you need to convey a sense that you truly care about your client's perspective. Caring has a positive influence on health status and healing. Clients can focus on accomplishing the goals of health care instead of worrying about whether care is forthcoming. The nurse gains from the caring relationship by experiencing satisfaction in meeting the client needs.

Families also need to experience a sense of caring from the nurse. Many families do not believe we have a clear understanding of the problems they are encountering while caring for their ill family member. This is especially true if the illness is not easily observable. One French study of effects of proactive communication with families of dying clients found that "caring" interventions in the form of longer conferences where family members could express emotions and talk with ethics and palliative care experts in conjunction with written materials did decrease their anxiety and depression (Lautrette et al., 2007).

BARRIER: LACK OF CARING

Although nursing has had a long-standing commitment to client-focused care, sometimes you may observe a situation in which you feel a nurse is apathetic, trying to meet his or her own needs rather than the client's needs. Some nurses develop a detachment that interferes with expressions of caring behaviors. At other times, nurses can be so rushed to meet multiple demands that they seem unable to focus on the client. Exercise 11-1 will help you focus on the concept of caring.

EMPOWERMENT

Empowerment is assisting the client to take charge of his or her own life. Our nursing care goal is to use our communication skills to build bridges to form partnership with our clients (patient-centered care, a QSEN competency). We use the interpersonal process to provide information, tools, and resources that help our clients build skills to reach their health goals. Empowerment is an important aim in every nurse-client relationship and is addressed by nursing theories such as Orem's view of the client as an agent of self-care. Studies demonstrate that the more involved clients are in their own care, the better the health outcome.

At a personal level, empowered clients feel valued, adopt successful coping methods, and think positively. Empowerment has to do with people power: In helping our clients to take control of their lives, we identify and build on their existing strengths.

BARRIERS

Empowerment is purposeful. It encourages clients to assume responsibility for their own health. This is in direct contrast with the paternalistic attitude formerly found in medicine and characterized by the attitude of "I know what is best for you or I can do it better." Lack of information about giving care, managing medicines, or recognizing approaching crises can be a major impediment to empowering family members to care for sick relatives. Failure to allow our client to assume personal responsibility, or failure to provide our client with appropriate resources and support, undermines empowerment.

TRUST

Establishing **trust** is the foundation in all relationships. The development of a sense of interpersonal trust, a sense of feeling safe, is the keystone in the nurse-client relationship. Trust provides a nonthreatening interpersonal climate in which clients feel comfortable revealing their needs. The nurse is perceived as dependable. Establishment of this trust is crucial toward enabling you to make an accurate assessment of your client's needs.

Trust is also the key to establishing workable relationships. Lack of trust in the workplace has detrimental effects for the organization and coworkers, undermining performance and commitment. According to Erikson (1963), trust is developed by experiencing consistency, sameness, and continuity during care by a familiar caregiver. Trust develops based on past experiences. In the nurse-client relationship, maintaining an open exchange of information contributes to trust. For the client, trust implies a willingness to place oneself in a position of vulnerability, relying on health providers to perform as expected. Honesty is a basic building block in establishing trust. Studies show that clients or their surrogates want "complete honesty" and most prefer complete disclosure. Box 11-1 lists interpersonal strategies that help promote a trusting relationship.

BARRIER: MISTRUST

Mistrust has an effect not only on communication but on healing process outcomes. Trust can be replaced with mistrust between nurse and client. Just as some agency managers treat employees as though they are not trustworthy, some nurses treat some clients as though they are misbehaving children. Such would be the case if a client fails to follow the treatment regimen and is labeled with the nursing diagnosis of "noncompliant." In other examples, the community health nurse who is inconsistent about keeping client appointments or the pediatric nurse who indicates falsely that an injection will not hurt are both jeopardizing client trust. It is hard to maintain trust when one person cannot depend on another. Energy that should be directed toward coping with health problems is rechanneled into assessing the nurse's commitment and trustworthiness. Having confidence in the nurse's skills, commitment, and caring allows the client to place full attention on the situation requiring

BOX 11-1	Techniques Designed to Promote Trust

- Convey respect.
- Consider the client's uniqueness.
- Show warmth and caring.
- Use the client's proper name.
- Use active listening.
- Give sufficient time to answer questions.
- Maintain confidentiality.
- Show congruence between verbal and nonverbal behaviors.
- Use a warm, friendly voice.
- Use appropriate eye contact.
- Smile.
- Be flexible.
- Provide for allowed preferences.
- Be honest and open.
- Give complete information.
- Provide consistency.
- Plan schedules.
- Follow through on commitments.
- Set limits.
- Control distractions.
- Use an attending posture: arms, legs, and body relaxed; leaning slightly forward.

resolution. Clients can also jeopardize the trust a nurse has in them. Sometimes clients "test" a nurse's trustworthiness by sending the nurse on unnecessary errands or talking endlessly on superficial topics. As long as nurses recognize testing behaviors and set clear limits on their roles and the client's role, it is possible to develop trust. Exercise 11-2 is designed to help students become more familiar with the concept of trust.

EMPATHY

Empathy is the ability to be sensitive to and communicate understanding of the client's feelings. Empathy is the ability to put yourself into your client's position. Empathy and empathetic communication are crucial to the practice of nursing (McMillan and Shannon, 2011), characteristic of a helping relationship. Empathy is an important element of a therapeutic relationship. The ability to effectively communicate empathy to your client is associated with improved client satisfaction and client adherence to treatments. A policy statement from the American Academy of Pediatrics extends this communication component to your client's family (Levetown, 2008).

EXERCISE 11-2	Techniques That Promote Trust

Purpose: To identify techniques that promote the establishment of trust and to provide practice in using these skills.

Procedure
1. Read the list of interpersonal techniques designed to promote trust (Box 11-1).
2. Individual: Describe the relationship with your most recent client. Was there a trusting relationship? How do you know? Which techniques did you use? Which ones could you have used?

3. Small group: Break class up into groups of three. Have students interview another group member to obtain a brief health history. The third member observes and records trusting behaviors. Exchange places so that everyone is an interviewer. Interviews should last 5 minutes each. At the end of 15 minutes, share findings.

Discussion
Compare techniques.

An empathetic nurse perceives and *understands* the client's emotions *accurately*. Some nurses might term this as *compassion*, which has been identified by staff nurses as being crucial to the nurse-client relationship. Communication skills are used to convey respect and empathy. Although expert nurses recognize the emotions a client feels, they hold on to their objectivity, maintaining their own separate identities. As a nurse, you should try not to overidentify with or internalize the feelings of the client. If internalization occurs, objectivity is lost, together with the ability to help the client move through his or her feelings. It is important to recognize that the client's feelings belong to the client, not to you.

Communicate your understanding of the meaning of a client's feelings by using both verbal and nonverbal communication behaviors. Maintain direct eye contact, use attending open body language, and keep a calm tone of voice. Acknowledge your clients' message about their feelings by restating what you understand them to be conveying. Then, have the clients validate that this is accurate. If you need more information about their feelings, ask them to expand on their message, perhaps asking, "Are there other things about this that are bothering you?" Now that you have full information, you can directly make interventions to address their needs. Armed with accurate data, you can communicate your clients' feelings to other providers if necessary.

BARRIER: LACK OF EMPATHY

Failure to understand the needs of clients may lead you to fail to provide essential client education or to provide needed emotional support. The literature indicates that major barriers to empathy exist in the clinical environment, including lack of time, lack of trust, lack of privacy, or lack of support. Several studies suggest that lack of empathy will affect the quality of care, result in less favorable health outcomes, and lower client satisfaction. However, we providers can consciously choose to express empathy.

MUTUALITY

Mutuality basically means that the nurse and the client agree on the client's health problems and the means for resolving them and that both parties are committed to enhancing the client's well-being. This is characterized by mutual respect for the autonomy and value system of the other. In developing mutuality, you maximize your client's involvement in all phases of the nursing process. Mutuality is collaboration in problem solving and "drives" the communication at the initial encounter. Evidence of mutuality is seen in the development of individualized client goals and nursing actions that meet a client's unique health needs. Exercise 11-3 gives practice in evaluating mutuality.

As nurses, we respect interpersonal differences. We involve clients in the decision-making process. We accept their decisions even if we do not agree with them. Effective use of values clarification as described in Chapter 3 assists clients in decision making. Clients who clearly identify their own personal values are better able to solve problems effectively. Decisions then have meaning to the client. There is a greater probability they will work to achieve success. When a mutual relationship is terminated, both parties experience a sense of shared accomplishment and satisfaction.

EXERCISE 11-3   **Evaluating Mutuality**

Purpose: To identify behaviors and feelings on the part of the nurse and the client that indicate mutuality.

Procedure
Complete the following questions by answering yes or no after terminating with a client; then bring it to class. Discuss the answers. How were you able to attain mutuality, or why were you unable to attain it?
1. Was I satisfied with the relationship?
2. Did the client express satisfaction with the relationship?

3. Did the client share feelings with me?
4. Did I make decisions for the client?
5. Did the client feel allowed to make his or her own decisions?
6. Did the client accomplish his or her goals?
7. Did I accomplish my goals?

Discussion
In a large group, discuss mutuality.

EXERCISE 11-4   **Building Communication Bridges Simulation**

Purpose: To evaluate current communication skills.

Directions
In small groups, role-play a client telling the nurse her story of some past unpleasant medical experience while another student plays the nurse conversing with the client.

Discussion
1. What aspects of the interaction demonstrated empathy, respect, caring, and so forth?

2. Listeners should give the following feedback:
   a. Comment on positive aspects observed.
   b. Offer constructive criticism only after making a positive comment.
   c. Identify any behaviors that served as barriers.
   d. Suggest alternative strategies the nurse could use.
   e. Think about times when you used bridges or barriers.

VERACITY

As described in Chapters 2 and 3, legal and ethical standards mandate specific nursing behaviors, such as confidentiality, beneficence, and respect for client autonomy. These behaviors are based on professional nursing values that stem from the ethical principles. By adhering to these "rules," nurses build their therapeutic relationships with individual clients. *Veracity* contributes to the establishment of a therapeutic relationship. When clients know they can expect the truth, the development of trust is promoted and helps build the relationship.

OTHER BARRIERS TO THE RELATIONSHIP

A few additional barriers that affect the development of the nurse-client relationship include anxiety, stereotyping, and lack of personal space. Barriers inherent in the health care system are also commonly discussed in the professional literature. Under managed care, barriers often reflect cost-containment measures. Such barriers include lack of consistent assignment of nurse to client and increased use of temporary staff such as agency nurses or "floats." Lack of time can result from low staff-to-client ratios or early discharge. The primary care literature describes agency demand for minimal appointment time with clients. Primary care providers, such as nurse practitioners, are often constrained to focus just on the chief complaint to maximize the number of clients seen, leading to "the 15-minute office visit." Other system barriers include communication conflicts with other health professionals, conflicting values, poor physical arrangements, and lack of value placed on caring by for-profit agencies. These system barriers limit the nurse's ability to develop substantial rapport with clients. Adequate time is essential to develop therapeutic communication to achieve effective care responsive to client needs. Try Exercise 11-4.

ANXIETY

Anxiety is a vague, persistent feeling of impending doom. It is a universal feeling; no one fully escapes it.

EXERCISE 11-5	Identifying Verbal and Nonverbal Behaviors Associated with Anxiety

Purpose: To broaden the learner's awareness of behavioral responses that indicate anxiety.

Procedure

List as many anxious behaviors as you can think of. Each column has a few examples to start. Discuss the lists in a group and then add new behaviors to your list.

Verbal
Quavering voice
Rapid speech
Mumbling
Defensive words

Nonverbal
Nail biting
Foot tapping
Sweating
Pacing

TABLE 11-1	Levels of Anxiety with Degree of Sensory Perceptions, Cognitive and Coping Abilities, and Manifest Behaviors

Level of Anxiety	Sensory Perceptions	Cognitive and Coping Ability	Behavior
Mild	Heightened state of alertness; increased acuity of hearing, vision, smell, touch	Enhanced learning, problem solving; increased ability to respond and adapt to changing stimuli; enhanced functioning*	Walking, singing, eating, drinking, mild restlessness, active listening, attending, questioning
Moderate	Decreased sensory perceptions; with guidance, able to expand sensory fields	Loss of concentration; decreased cognitive ability; cannot identify factors contributing to the anxiety-producing situation; with directions can cope, reduce anxiety, and solve problems; inhibited functioning	Increased muscle tone, pulse, respirations; changes in voice tone and pitch, rapid speech, incomplete verbal responses; engrossed with detail
Severe	Greatly diminished perceptions; decreased sensitivity to pain	Limited thought processes; unable to solve problems even with guidance; cannot cope with stress without help; confused mental state; limited functioning	Purposeless, aimless behaviors; rapid pulse, respirations; high blood pressure; hyperventilation; inappropriate or incongruent verbal responses
Panic	No response to sensory perceptions	No cognitive or coping abilities; without intervention, death is imminent	Immobilization

*Functioning refers to the ability to perform activities of daily living for survival purposes.

The impact on the self is always uncomfortable. It occurs when a threat (real or imagined) to one's self-concept is perceived. Lower satisfaction with communication is associated with increased client anxiety. Anxiety is usually observed through the physical and behavioral manifestations of the attempt to relieve the anxious feelings. Although individuals experiencing anxiety may not know they are anxious, specific behaviors provide clues that anxiety is present. Exercise 11-5 identifies behaviors associated with anxiety. Table 11-1 shows how an individual's sensory perceptions, cognitive abilities, coping skills, and behaviors relate to the intensity and level of anxiety experienced.

A mild level of anxiety heightens one's awareness of the surrounding environment and fosters learning and decision making. Therefore, it may be desirable to allow a mild degree of anxiety when health teaching is needed or when problem solving is necessary. It is not prudent, however, to prolong even a mild state of anxiety.

Greater levels of anxiety decrease perceptual ability. The anxious state is accompanied by verbal and nonverbal behaviors that inhibit effective individual functioning. For example, anxiety causes you to hold your breath, which can lead to even greater levels of anxiety. Moderate-to-severe anxiety on the part of either nurse or client hinders the development of the therapeutic relationship. To accomplish goals and attain mutuality, greater levels of anxiety must be reduced. Once the presence of anxiety has been identified, the nurse needs to take appropriate action. Strategies to reduce anxiety are listed in Box 11-2.

Severe anxiety requires medical and psychiatric intervention to alleviate the stress. A prolonged panic

BOX 11-2	Nursing Strategies to Reduce Client Anxiety

- Active listening to show acceptance
- Honesty; answering all questions at the client's level of understanding
- Clearly explaining procedures, surgery, and policies, and giving appropriate reassurance based on data
- Acting in a calm, unhurried manner
- Speaking clearly, firmly (but not loudly)
- Giving information regarding laboratory tests, medications, treatments, and rationale for restrictions on activity
- Setting reasonable limits and providing structure
- Encouraging clients to explore reasons for the anxiety
- Encouraging self-affirmation through positive statements such as "I will" and "I can"
- Using play therapy with dolls, puppets, and games
- Drawing for young clients
- Using therapeutic touch, giving warm baths, back rubs
- Initiating recreational activities such as physical exercise, music, card games, board games, crafts, and reading
- Teaching breathing and relaxation exercises
- Using guided imagery
- Practicing covert rehearsal

From Gerrard B, Boniface W, Love B: *Interpersonal skills for health professionals*, Reston, VA, 1980, Reston Publishing.

state is incompatible with life. It is such an extreme level of anxiety that without immediate medical and psychiatric assistance, suicide or homicide may ensue. Some of these interpersonal strategies used to reduce moderate anxiety also are used during severe anxiety and panic attacks as part of a team approach to client care.

Choosing from various strategies to reduce client anxiety can be difficult. Not all methods are appropriate or work equally well with all clients. If a nurse attempting to build trust pushes a client too fast into revealing what he or she is not yet ready to discuss, this can increase anxiety. You need to accurately identify your client's level of anxiety. You should also identify and reduce your own anxiety. Anxiety can cloud your perceptions and interfere with relationships.

STEREOTYPING AND BIAS

Stereotyping is the process of attributing characteristics to a group of people as though all persons in the identified group possessed them. People may be stereotyped according to ethnic origin, culture, religion, social class, occupation, age, and other factors. Even health issues can be the stimulus for stereotyping individuals. For example, alcoholism, mental illness, and sexually transmitted diseases are fertile grounds for the development of stereotypes. Stereotypes have been shown to be consistent across cultures and somewhat across generations, although the value placed on a stereotype changes.

Stereotypes are learned during childhood and reinforced by life experiences. They may carry positive or negative connotations. Some suggest that our culture has stereotyped an image of men as less feeling than women. We all have personal biases, usually based on unconscious past learning. As nurses, we may act on these unknowingly. Stereotypes negate empathy and erode the nurse-client relationship. As nurses, we must work to develop insight into our own expectations and prejudgments about people. Reportedly, some nurses admit to distrust in fathers' competence to provide care for ill children. If so, this is certainly an example of stereotyping. Making an intentional resolution to avoid a stereotype enables one to change.

Stereotypes are never completely accurate. No attribute applies to every member of a group. All of us like to think that our way is the correct way, and that everyone else thinks about life experiences just as we do. The reality is that there are many roads in life, and one road is not necessarily any better than another.

Emotions play a role in the value we place on negative stereotypes. Stereotypes based on strong emotions are called prejudices. Highly emotionally charged stereotypes are less amenable to change. In the extreme, this can result in discrimination. Discrimination as a legal statute refers to actions in which a person is denied a legitimate opportunity offered to others because of prejudice. In the United States, federal laws prohibit workplace discrimination based on age, creed, gender, sexual preference, disability, race, religion, or genetics.

Everyone has biases. If nurses bring their biases with them to the clinical situation, they will distort their perception, prevent client change, and disrupt the provider-client relationship. Nurses need to make it a goal to reduce bias. We do this by recognizing a client as a unique individual, both different from and similar to self. Acceptance of the other person needs to be total. This unconditional acceptance, as described

EXERCISE 11-6   Reducing Clinical Bias by Identifying Stereotypes

Purpose: To identify examples of nursing biases that need to be reduced. Practice in identifying professional stereotypes and in how to reduce them is one component of maintaining high-quality nursing care.

Procedure
Each of the following scenarios indicates a stereotype. Identify the stereotype and how it might affect nursing care. As a nurse, what would you do to reduce the bias in the situation? Are there any individuals or groups of people for whom you would not want to provide care (e.g., homeless women with foul body odor and dirty nails)?

Situation A
Mrs. Daniels, an obstetric nurse who believes in birth control, comments about her client, "Mrs. Gonzales is pregnant again. You know, the one with six kids already! It makes me sick to see these people on welfare taking away from our tax dollars. I don't know how she can continue to do this."

Situation B
Mrs. Brown, a registered nurse on a medical unit, is upset with her 52-year-old female client. "If she rings that buzzer one more time, I'm going to disconnect it. Can't she understand that I have other clients who need my attention more than she does? She just lies in bed all day long. And she's so fat; she's never going to lose any weight that way."

Situation C
Mrs. Waters, a staff nurse in a nursing home, listens to the daughter of a 93-year-old resident, who says, "My mother, who is confused most of the time, receives very little attention from you nurses, while other clients who are lucid and clear-minded have more interaction with you. It's not fair! No wonder my mother is so far out in space. Nobody talks to her. Nobody ever comes in to say hello."

---

by Carl Rogers (1961), is an essential element in the helping relationship. It does not imply agreement or approval; acceptance occurs without judgment. Mr. Fred Rogers, the children's television show host, ended his programs by telling his audience, "I like you just the way you are." How wonderful if we, as nurses, could convey this type of acceptance to our clients through our words and actions. Exercise 11-6 examines ways of reducing clinical bias.

OVERINVOLVEMENT AS A BARRIER

Objectivity is important if you are to provide competent, professional care. This may be more likely to occur in a long-term relationship. Sharing too much information about yourself, your job problems, or about your other clients can become a barrier if your clients become unclear about their role in your relationship. Many of us enjoy warm relationships with our clients, but if we are to remain effective, we need to be alert to the disadvantages of overinvolvement.

VIOLATION OF PERSONAL SPACE

Personal space is an invisible boundary around an individual. The emotional personal space boundary provides a sense of comfort and protection. It is defined by past experiences, current circumstances, and our culture.

Proxemics is the study of an individual's use of space. The optimal territorial space needed by most individuals living in Western culture is 86 to 108 square feet of personal space. Other research has found that 60 square feet is the minimum needed for each client in multiple-occupancy rooms, and 80 square feet is the minimum for private rooms in hospitals and institutions. Critical care units offer even less square footage.

Among the many factors that affect the individual's need for personal distance are cultural dictates. In some cultures, people approach each other closely, whereas in others, more personal space is required. In most cultures, men need more space than women do. People generally need less space in the morning. The elderly need more control over their space, whereas small children generally like to touch and be touched by others. Although the elderly appreciate human touch, they generally do not like it to be applied indiscriminately. Situational anxiety causes a need for more space. Persons with low self-esteem prefer more space, as well as some control over who enters their space and in what manner. Usually people will tolerate a person standing close to them at their side more readily than directly in front of them. Direct eye contact causes a need for more space. Placing oneself at the same level (e.g., sitting while the client is sitting, or standing at eye level when the client is standing) allows the nurse more access to the client's personal space because such a stance is perceived as less threatening.

Hospitals are not home. Many nursing care procedures are a direct intrusion into your client's personal space. Commonly, procedures that require tubes (e.g., nasal gastric intubation, administration of oxygen, catheterization, and intravenous initiation) restrict the mobility of the client and the client's sense of control over personal territory. When more than one health professional is involved, the impact of the intrusion on the client may be even stronger. In many instances, personal space requirements are an integral part of a person's self-image. When clients lose control over personal space, they may experience a loss of identity and self-esteem. It is recommended you maintain a social physical body distance of 4 feet when not actually giving care.

When institutionalized clients are able to incorporate parts of their rooms into their personal space, it increases their self-esteem and helps them to maintain a sense of identity. This feeling of security is evidenced when a client asks, "Close my door, please." Freedom from worry about personal space allows the client to trust the nurse and fosters a therapeutic relationship. When invasions of personal space are necessary while performing a procedure, you can minimize impact by explaining why a procedure is needed. Conversation with clients at such times reinforces their feelings that they are human beings worthy of respect and not just objects being worked on. Advocating for the client's personal space needs is an aspect of the nursing role. This is done by communicating your client's preferences to other members of the health team and including them in their care plan.

Home is not quite home when the home health nurse, infusion nurse, or other aides invade the client's personal space. Some modification of "take-charge" behavior is required when giving care in a client's home.

TIME LIMITATIONS

In our care for clients with increasingly complex health problems and heavier workloads, we may think we lack the time to spend communicating with each client (Hemsley, 2012). Developing quality communication using team rounds may be a solution. This method of reporting at the bedside includes the client as a team partner in the day's care goals. However, Rehder and associates found that becomes a barrier to communication if the nurse tries to multitask (2012).

CULTURAL BARRIERS

Cross-cultural communication is discussed extensively in Chapter 7. Every interaction encounters a basic challenge of communication when the culture of your client differs from your own. Barriers include health literacy problems or cultural definitions of the sick role. For example, in some cultures the sick role is no longer valid after symptoms disappear, so when your client's diabetes is under control, family members may no longer see the need for special diet or medication. As we move into a more multicultural society, all health care providers need to work to become culturally competent communicators.

Cultural competence requires us to become aware of the arbitrary nature of our own cultural beliefs. *Culturally competent communication* is characterized by a willingness to try to understand and respond to your client's beliefs. Knowledge of the client's cultural preferences helps you avoid stereotyping and allows you to adapt your communication.

GENDER DIFFERENCES

Gender is defined as the culture's attributions of masculine or feminine. Recently, more attention has been given to gender role, communication barriers, and health inequalities. Research results give mixed findings. Male student nurses have been reported to be less empathetic (Ouzouni, 2012), while female nurses have been disrespected (Hoglund and Holmstrom, 2008). Other studies suggest that client perceptions differ according to the nurse's gender or that females are better communicators. For example, although American culture equates female touch with caring, some individuals view male touch as sexual and therefore inappropriate.

Gender need not be a factor in developing therapeutic communication with clients. Research does support the need for communications training for all health care workers. It takes practice for you to master nurse-client communication skills such as clarification, use of open-ended questions, empathy, listening, self-disclosure, and confrontation. We need to tailor our communication to meet the needs and preferences of our clients, determining what type of communication is expected.

Developing an Evidence-Based Practice

A higher level of evidence-based practice (EBP) results from meta-analysis of multiple research findings to determine the actual "best practice." Agency for Healthcare Research and Quality (AHRQ) has published many online for you to access.

The chapter on "Promoting Engagement by Patients and Families to Reduce Adverse Events," cites more than 30 studies. Review *results*, among which are those listed below:

Application to your practice: As we engage our clients' help in reducing adverse occurrences, we use communication skills that might promote trust, caring and empowerment, such as asking clients to:

- Remind or ask every health care worker touching them and their equipment to wash their hands.
- Have the nurse give a personalized list of hospital medications and check this list each time someone gives the client a medication.

APPLICATIONS

Many nursing actions recommended here are mandated by the American Nurses Association (ANA) Code of Ethics for Nurses discussed in Chapter 2. The actions specified include confidentiality, autonomy, beneficence, veracity, and justice. Mutuality is addressed in the ANA position statement on human rights. Providers with good communication skills have greater professional satisfaction and experience less job-related stress. Studies of client perceptions generally show a correlation between good nurse communicators and good quality of care. Practice exercises provide you with opportunities to improve your skills. Part of any simulation exercise to strengthen nursing communication is the offering of feedback.

STEPS IN THE CARING PROCESS

Several articles identify four steps to help you communicate C.A.R.E. to your client:

C = First, *connect* with your client. *Offer your attention.* Here you introduce your purpose in developing a relationship with your client (i.e., meeting his or her health needs). Use the client's formal name and avoid terms of endearment such as "sweetie." Show an intent to care. Attentiveness is a part of communication skill training that is probably decreased by work-related stress, time constraints, and so forth.

A = The second step is to *appreciate* the client's situation. Although the health care environment is familiar to you, it is a strange and perhaps frightening situation for your client. Acknowledge your client's point of view and express concern.

R = The third step is to *respond* to what your client needs. What are your client's priorities? What are your client's expectations for health care?

E = The fourth step is to *empower* the client to problem-solve with you. Here your client gains strength and confidence from interactions with providers, enabling him or her to move toward achievement of goals.

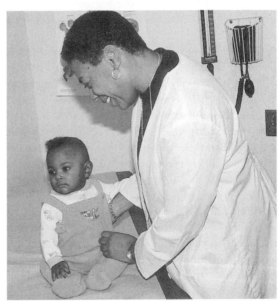

Infants lack verbal communication skills. The nurse's comforting touch and pleasant vocal tone help overcome this barrier. *(Courtesy Adam Boggs.)*

The ability to become a caring professional is influenced by your previous experiences. A person who has received caring is more likely to be able to offer it to others. Caring should not be confused with caretaking. Although caretaking is a part of caring, it may lack the necessary intentional giving of self. Self-awareness about feelings, attitudes, values, and skills is essential for developing an effective, caring relationship.

STRATEGIES FOR EMPOWERMENT

Your goal is to assist your clients to assume more responsibility for their health conditions by teaching them new roles and skills to manage their illnesses. We may never fully understand the decisions some clients make, but we support their right to do so. Your method for **empowering** should include the following key strategies:

- *Accept* your clients as they are by refraining from any negative judgments.
- Assess their level of understanding, *exploring their perceptions and feelings* about their conditions and discussing issues that may interfere with self-care.
- Establish mutual goals for client care by forming an alliance, *mutually deciding* about their care.
- Find out how much information your clients want to know.
- Reinforce client *autonomy,* for example, by allowing them to choose the content in your teaching plan.
- *Offer information* in an environment that enables them to use it.
- Make sure your clients *actively participate* in their care plan.
- Encourage clients to network with a support group.
- Clarify with your clients that they hold the major *responsibility* for both the health care decisions they make and their consequences.

APPLICATION OF EMPATHY TO LEVELS OF NURSING ACTIONS

Nursing actions that facilitate empathy can be classified into three major skills: (a) recognition and classification of requests, (b) attending behaviors, and (c) empathetic responses.

Processing requests: Two types of requests are for information and action. These requests do not involve interpersonal concerns and are easier to manage. Another form of request is for understanding involvement, which entails the client's need for empathetic understanding. This type of request requires greater interpersonal skills. It can be misinterpreted as a request for action or information. You may have to clarify whether your clients need only what they specifically ask for or whether further exploration of meaning of their needs is necessary.

Use attending behaviors: *Attending behaviors* facilitate empathy and include an attentive, open posture; responding to verbal and nonverbal cues through

appropriate gestures and facial expressions; using eye contact; and allowing client self-expression. Verbally acknowledging nonverbal cues shows you are attending. As does offering time and attention, showing interest in the client's issues, offering helpful information, and clarifying problem areas. These responses encourage clients to participate in their own healing.

Make empathetic responses: You communicate *empathy* when you show your clients that you understand how they are feeling. This helps them identify emotions that are not readily observable and connect them with the current situation. For example, observing nonverbal client cues such as worried facial expression and verbalizing this reaction with an empathetic comment, such as "I understand that this is very difficult for you," validates what your clients are feeling and tells them you understand them. Using the actions listed in Table 11-2, the nurse applies attending behaviors and nursing actions to express empathy. Verbal prompts such as "Hmm," "Uh-huh," "I see," "Tell me more," and "Go on" facilitate expression of feelings. The nurse uses open-ended questions to validate perceptions. Using

TABLE 11-2	Levels of Nursing Actions	
Level	Category	Nursing Behavior
1	Accepting	Uses client's correct name
		Maintains eye contact
		Adopts open posture
		Responds to cues
2	Listening	Nods head
		Smiles
		Encourages responses
		Uses therapeutic silence
3	Clarifying	Asks open-ended questions
		Restates the problem
		Validates perceptions
		Acknowledges confusion
	Informing	Provides honest, complete answers
		Assesses client's knowledge level
		Summarizes
4-5	Analyzing	Identifies unknown emotions
		Interprets underlying meanings
		Confronts conflict

informing behaviors listed in Table 11-2 enlarges the database by providing new information and gives feedback to your client. Remember, demonstrating empathy as a communication behavior has been shown to positively affect the outcome of your care (Rao et al., 2010). If your client's condition prevents use of familiar communication strategies to demonstrate empathy, the nurse can use alternative techniques such as touch.

REDUCTION OF BARRIERS IN NURSE-CLIENT RELATIONSHIPS

Recognition of barriers is the first step in eliminating them, and thus enhancing the therapeutic process. Practice with exercises in this chapter should increase your recognition of possible barriers. Findings from many studies emphasize the crucial importance of honesty, cultural sensitivity, and caring, especially in listening actively to suggestions and complaints from client and family. Refer to Box 11-3 for a summary of strategies to reduce barriers to the nurse-client relationship.

VERACITY AND TRUST

Trust has a strong influence on the health-related behaviors of your clients (Moore et al., 2013). Historically nurses and physicians withheld negative prognosis information, citing beneficence as a rationale. However, any deception (lies or omissions) erodes your clients' trust in their care providers. There may be a need to balance truth-telling with the need to preserve some hope, according to Pergert and Lutzen (2012). Avoiding demeaning comments about other health providers, which will damage client trust, along with some limited self-disclosure on the part of the nurse has been found to aid in establishing a trusting relationship

| BOX 11-3 | Tips to Reduce Relationship Barriers |

- Establish trust.
- Demonstrate caring and empathy.
- Empower the client.
- Recognize and reduce client anxiety.
- Maintain appropriate personal distance.
- Practice cultural sensitivity and work to be bilingual.
- Use therapeutic relationship-building activities such as active listening.
- Avoid medical jargon.

(Babatsikou and Gerogianni, 2012; Nygardh et al., 2011). When questioned by a client, you can support their desire to seek a second medical opinion.

RESPECT FOR PERSONAL SPACE

Before providing care, you need to assess your client's personal space needs. A comprehensive assessment includes cultural and developmental factors that affect perceptions of space and reactions to intrusions. To increase your client's sense of personal space, you can decrease close, direct eye contact. Instead, sit beside the client or position the chairs at angles for counseling or health teaching. Clients in intensive care units, where there are many intrusive procedures, benefit from decreased eye contact during certain times, such as when being bathed or during suction, wound care, and changing of dressings. At the same time, it is important for you to talk gently with your client during such procedures and to elicit feedback, if appropriate.

To minimize the loss of a sense of personal space, we should demonstrate regard for our client's dignity and privacy. Closed doors for private rest and periods of uninterrupted relaxation are respected. Personal belongings are arranged and treated with care, particularly with very old and very young clients, for whom personal items may be highly significant as a link with a more familiar environment. Elderly clients can become profoundly disoriented in unfamiliar environments because their internal sensory skill in processing new information is often reduced. Encouraging persons in long-term facilities to bring pictures, clothing, and favorite mementos is an important nursing intervention with such clients.

RESPECT FOR PERSONAL SPACE IN HOSPITAL SITUATIONS

Obviously, there is a discrepancy between the minimum amount of space an individual needs and the amount of space hospitals are able to provide in multiple-occupancy rooms. Actions to ensure private space and show respect include

- Providing privacy when disturbing matters are to be discussed
- Explaining procedures before implementing them
- Entering another person's personal space with warning (e.g., knocking or calling the client's name) and, preferably, waiting for permission to enter
- Providing an identified space for personal belongings

- Encouraging the inclusion of personal and familiar objects on the client's nightstand
- Decreasing direct eye contact during hands-on care
- Minimizing bodily exposure during care
- Using only the necessary number of people during any procedure
- Using touch appropriately

VIOLATION OF CONFIDENTIALITY

Discussing private information casually with others is an abuse of confidentiality. Nursing reports and interdisciplinary team case conferences are examples of acceptable forums for the discussion of privileged communication. This information is not discussed outside what is needed for nursing or medical care; to do so would undermine the basis for your therapeutic relationship with your client. Federal confidentiality regulations are discussed in Chapter 2.

AVOIDING CROSS-CULTURAL DISSONANCE

The ANA's statement on cultural diversity in nursing practice highlights the importance of recognizing intracultural variation and assessing each client as an individual (ANA, 1991). Becoming culturally sensitive includes avoiding barriers to communication that occur when generalizing about our client's beliefs based on their membership, rather than taking the time to learn personal preferences. Identify your client's health values, beliefs, health practices, or family factors that may affect their communication with you.

SUMMARY

This chapter focuses on essential concepts needed to establish and maintain a therapeutic relationship in nursing practice: caring, empowerment, trust, empathy, mutuality, and confidentiality. Respect for the client as a unique person is a basic component of each concept.

Caring is described as a commitment by the nurse that involves profound respect and concern for the unique humanity of every client and a willingness to confirm the client's personhood.

Empowerment is assisting the client to take charge of his or her own health.

Trust represents an individual's emotional reliance on the consistency and continuity of experience. The client perceives the nurse as trustworthy, a safe person

with whom to share difficult feelings about health-related needs.

Empathy is the ability to perceive accurately another person's feelings and to convey their meaning to the client. Nursing behaviors that facilitate the development of empathy are accepting, listening, clarifying and informing, and analyzing. Each of these behaviors implicitly recognizes the client as a unique individual worthy of being listened to and respected.

Mutuality includes as much shared communication and collaboration in problem solving as the client is capable of providing. To foster mutuality within the relationship, nurses need to remain aware of their own feelings, attitudes, and beliefs.

Barriers that affect the development of the nurse-client relationship, such as anxiety, stereotyping, over-familiarity, intrusion into personal space and limited time for nurse-client communication are described. High levels of anxiety decrease perceptual ability. The nurse needs to use anxiety- and stress-reduction strategies when clients demonstrate moderate anxiety levels. Stereotypes are generalizations representing an unsubstantiated belief that all individuals of a particular social group, race, or religion share the same characteristics. No allowance is made for individual differences. Developing a nonjudgmental, neutral attitude toward a client helps the nurse reduce clinical bias in nursing practice. Personal space, defined as an invisible boundary around an individual, is another conceptual variable worthy of attention in the nurse-client relationship. The emotional boundary needed for interpersonal comfort changes with different conditions. It is defined by past experiences and culture. Proxemics is the term given to the study of humans' use of space. To minimize a decreased sense of personal space, you demonstrate a regard for your client's dignity and privacy.

ETHICAL DILEMMA | What Would You Do?

There are limits to your professional responsibility to maintain confidentiality. Any information that, if withheld, might endanger the life or physical and emotional safety of the client or others needs to be communicated to the health team or appropriate people immediately.

Consider the teen who confides his plan to shoot classmates. Can you breach confidentiality in this case? How about the 5-year-old child in whom you notice genital warts (human papillomavirus) on his anus, but who shows no other signs of sexual abuse?

DISCUSSION QUESTIONS

1. What behaviors demonstrated empathy in Exercise 11-4? Could you add the phrase, "That must have been difficult," to what the nurse role-player said?

2. What stereotypes in addition to those identified in Exercise 11-6 have you heard about in health care settings?

3. What is your own preferred space distance? To what do you attribute this preference? Under what circumstances do your needs for personal space change?

REFERENCES

American Nurses Association (ANA), 1991 Cultural diversity in nursing practice [position statement] Author: Washington, DC

American Nurses Association (ANA): *Nursing's Social Policy Statement: The Essence of the Profession*, Washington, DC, 2010, Silver Spring, MD: Author. Available online http://nursingworld.org/social-policy-statement/.

Babatsikou FP, Gerogianni GK: The importance of role-play in nursing practice, *Health Sci J* 6(1):4–10, 2012. A Nursing Department Technological Educational Institute of Athens online publication. Available at www.hsj.gr.

Erikson E: *Childhood and society*, ed 2, New York, 1963, Norton.

Hemsley B, Balandin S, Worrall L: Nursing the patient with complex communication needs: time as a barrier and a facilitator to successful communication in hospital, *J Adv Nurs* 68(1):116–126, 2012.

Hoglund AT, Holmstrom I: "It's easier to talk to a woman": aspects of gender in Swedish telenursing, *J Clin Nurs* 17:2979–2986, 2008.

Knoerl AM, Esper KW, Hasenau SM: Cultural sensitivity in patient health education, *Nurs Clin North Am* 46(2011):335–340, 2011.

Lachman VD: Applying the ethics of care to your nursing practice, *Medsurg Nurs* 21(2):112–116, 2012.

Lautrette A, Darmon M, Megarbane B, et al.: A communication strategy and brochure for relatives of patients dying in the ICU, *N Engl J Med* 356(5):459–478, 2007.

Levetown M: American Academy of Pediatrics Committee on Bioethics: Communicating with children and families: from everyday interactions to skill in conveying distressing information, *Pediatrics* 121(5), 2008. e1442–e1460.

McMillan LR, Shannon D: Program evaluation of nursing school instruction in measuring students' perceived competence to empathetically communicate with patients, *Nurs Educ Perspect* 32(3):150–154, 2011.

Moore AD, Hamilton JB, Pierre-Louis BJ, Jennings BM: Increasing access to care and reducing mistrust: Important considerations when implementing the patient-centered medical home in Army health clinics, *Mil Med* 178(3):291–298, 2013.

Nygardh A, Malm D, Wikby K, Ahlstrom G: The experience of empowerment in the patient-centered encounter: the patient's perspective, *J Clin Nurs* 21:897–904, 2011.

Ouzouni C, Nakakis K: An exploratory study of student nurses' empathy, *Health Sci J* 6(3):534–552, 2012.

Pergert P, Lutzen K: Balancing truth-telling in the preservation of hope: A relational ethics approach, *Nurs Ethics* 19(1):21–29, 2012.

QSEN Institute. QSEN competencies. http://qsen.org. Accessed May 30, 2013.

Rao JK, Anderson LA, Sukumar B, Beauchesne DA, Stein T, Frankel RM: Engaging communication experts in a Delphi process to identify patient behaviors that could enhance communication in medical encounters, *BMC Health Serv Res* 10:97, 2010, http://dx.doi.org/10.1186/1472-6963-10-97. 2010 Apr 19.

Rehder KJ, Uhl TL, Meliones DA, Turner DA, Smith PB, Mistry KP: Targeted interventions improve shared agreement of daily goals in the pediatric intensive care unit, *Pediatr Crit Care Med* 13(1):6–10, 2012.

Rogers C: *On becoming a person*, Boston, 1961, Houghton-Mifflin.

Williams AM, Irurita VF: Therapeutic and non-therapeutic interpersonal interactions: the patient's perspective, *J Clin Nurs* 13(7):806–815, 2004.

CHAPTER 12

Communicating with Families

Revised by Shari Kist

OBJECTIVES

At the end of the chapter, the reader will be able to:

1. Define family and identify its components.
2. Apply family-centered concepts to the care of the family in clinical settings, using standardized family assessment tools.
3. Apply the nursing process to the care of families in clinical settings.
4. Identify nursing interventions for families in the intensive care unit (ICU).
5. Identify nursing interventions for families in the community.

The purpose of this chapter is to describe family-centered relationships and communication strategies that nurses can use to support family integrity in health care settings. The chapter identifies family theory frameworks, which provide a common language for describing family relationships. Practical assessment and intervention strategies address family issues that affect a patient's recovery, and support self-management of chronic health conditions, or peaceful death in clinical practice.

BASIC CONCEPTS

DEFINITION OF FAMILY

The term family can have several definitions, particularly in today's society. One definition is, "A group of individuals living under one roof and usually under one head" (*Merriam-Webster Online*, n.d.). The U.S. Census Bureau (2013) offers the following, "A family is a group of two people or more (one of whom is the householder) related by birth, marriage, or adoption and residing together; all such people (including related subfamily members) are considered as members of one family. A household consists of all people who occupy a housing unit regardless of relationship. A household may consist of a person living alone or multiple unrelated individuals or families living together." However, as health care providers, it is more appropriate to use the definition, "A **family** is who they say they are" (Wright and Leahey, 2009, p. 70). Identified family members may or may not be blood related. Strong emotional ties and durability of membership characterize family relationships regardless of how uniquely they are defined. Even when family members are alienated or distanced geographically, they "can never truly relinquish family membership" (Goldenberg and Goldenberg, 2013, p.3).

During times of crisis, such as a seriously ill family member, family members react to the situation and each other with a wide range of reactions. Each family member responds in unique ways. Communication, even when reactive, is designed to maintain the integrity of the family. Understanding the family as a system is relevant in today's health care environment, as the family is an essential part of the health care team. Families have a profound influence on ill family members as advisors, caretakers, supporters, and sometimes irritants. Patients who are very young, very old, and those requiring assistance with self-management of chronic illness are particularly dependent on their families.

Support from the health care team during times of stress and crisis are necessary to provide information and empowerment to successfully adapt. Both resources and supports are essential for family empowerment (Trivette et al., 2010). Resources and supports include beliefs, past experiences, help-giving and receiving practices, strengths and capabilities, and are pieces of information that help explain patient and family responses to health disruptions.

Conducting a family assessment is essential "to: (1) assure that the needs of the family are met, (2) uncover any gaps in the family plan of action, (3) offer multiple supports and resources to the family" (Kaakinen et al., 2010, p. 104).

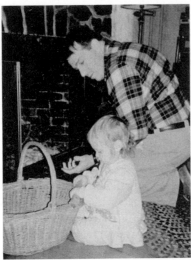

Young children learn family rules for communication from their parents.

FAMILY COMPOSITION

There is significant diversity in the composition of families, family beliefs and values, how they communicate with each other, ethnic heritage, life experiences, commitment to individual family members, and connections with the community (Goldenberg and Goldenberg, 2013, p. 2). Families today are much more complex than in past generations. Box 12-1 identifies different types of family composition.

The "typical American family" today has many variations (Goldenberg and Goldenberg, 2013, p. 3). Single-parent families must accomplish the same developmental tasks as two-parent families, but in many cases they do it without the support of the

| BOX 12-1 | Types of Family Composition |

- **Nuclear family:** a father and mother, with one or more children, living together as a single family unit
- **Extended family:** nuclear family unit's combination of second- and third-generation members related by blood or marriage but not living together
- **Three-generational family:** any combination of first-, second-, and third-generation members living within a household
- **Dyad family:** husband and wife or other couple living alone without children
- **Single-parent family:** divorced, never married, separated, or widowed male or female and at least one child; most single-parent families are headed by women
- **Stepfamily:** family in which one or both spouses are divorced or widowed with one or more children from a previous marriage who may not live with the newly reconstituted family
- **Blended or reconstituted family:** a combination of two families with children from one or both families and sometimes children of the newly married couple
- **Common law family:** an unmarried couple living together with or without children
- **No kin:** a group of at least two people sharing a nonsexual relationship and exchanging support who have no legal, blood, or strong emotional tie to each other
- **Polygamous family:** one man (or woman) with several spouses
- **Same-sex family:** a homosexual or lesbian couple living together with or without children
- **Commune:** groups of individuals (may or may not be related) living together and sharing resources
- **Group marriage:** all individuals are "married" to one another and are considered parents of all the children

other partner or sufficient financial resources. Blended families have a different life experience than those in an intact family because their family structure often is more complex. Children may be members of more than one family unit, linked biologically, physically, and emotionally to people who may or may not be part of their daily lives. Parents, step- or half-brothers and sisters, two or more sets of grandparents, and multiple aunts and uncles may make up a blended family (Kaakinen et al., 2010, p. 135). The child may spend extended periods in separate households, each with a full set of family expectations that may or may not be similar. Initially, the parents in blended families may

TABLE 12-1	Comparing Differences Between Biological and Blended Families

Biological Families	Blended Families
Family is created without loss.	Family is born of loss.
There are shared family traditions.	There are two sets of family traditions.
One set of family rules evolves.	Family rules are varied and complicated.
Children arrive one at a time.	Instant parenthood of children at different ages occurs.
Biological parents live together.	Biological parents live apart.

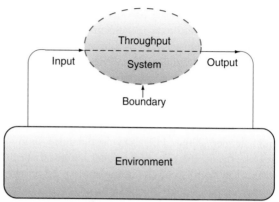

Figure 12-1 Systems model: interaction with the environment.

cohabitate, making for a sense of uncertainty for all involved (Jensen and Schafer, 2013). Blended families can offer a rich experience for everyone concerned, but they are more complex because of multiple connections. Table 12-1 displays some of the differences between biological and blended families. Issues for blended families include discipline, money, use of time, birth of an infant, death of a stepparent, inclusion at graduation, and marriage and health care decisions.

THEORETICAL FRAMEWORKS

Theoretical frameworks are used to provide a means for understanding certain processes and relationships between and among essential concepts. Numerous theoretical frameworks exist that can be used to understand family composition. Kurt von Bertalanffy's (1968) general systems theory provides a conceptual foundation for family system models (Barker, 1998). Having a systems perspective allows one to examine the interdependence among all parts of the system and see how they support the system as a functional whole. Systems' thinking maintains that the whole is greater than the sum of its parts with each part reciprocally influencing its function. If one part of the system changes or fails, it affects the functioning of the whole. A clock is a useful metaphor. It displays time correctly, but only if all parts work together. If any part of the clock breaks down, the clock no longer tells accurate time.

A system interacts with other systems in the environment. An interactional process occurs when

inputs are introduced into the system in the form of information, energy, and resources. Within each system, the information is processed internally as the system actively processes and interprets its meaning. The transformation process of raw data into desired outputs is referred to as *throughput*. The *output* refers to the result or product that leaves the system. Each system is separated from its environment by boundaries that control the exchange of information, energy, and resources into and out of the system. Evaluation of the output and feedback loops from the environment inform the system of changes needed to achieve effective outputs. Figure 12-1 identifies the relational components of a human system's interaction with the environment, using von Bertalanffy's model.

Systems theory can be applied to the human system. Individuals take in food, liquids, and oxygen to nourish the body (inputs). Within the body, a transformational process occurs through enzymes and other metabolic processes (throughputs), so that the body can use them. This interactional process results in the human organism's growth, health, and capacity to interact with the external environment (outputs). Nonusable outputs excreted from the body include urine, feces, sweat, and carbon dioxide. A person's skin represents an important boundary between the environment and the human system.

Family systems have boundaries that regulate information coming into and leaving the family system. Family systems theory helps explain how families strive for harmony and balance *(homeostasis)*, how the family is able to maintain its continuity despite challenges, *(morphostasis)*, and how the family is able to change and grow over time in response to challenges *(morphogenesis). Feedback loops* describe the patterns of interaction that facilitate movement toward morphogenesis or morphostasis. They impact goal setting in behavior systems. The systems principle of *equifinality* describes how the same outcome or end state can be reached through different pathways. This principle helps explain why some individuals at high risk for poor outcomes do not develop maladaptive behaviors (Cicchetti and Blender, 2006). Hierarchy is the term used to describe the complex layers of smaller systems that exist within a system. Communication can also be thought of as a complex system in which the message or output must be interpreted within an appropriate context.

BOWEN'S SYSTEMS THEORY

Murray Bowen (1978) family systems theory conceptualizes the family as an interactive emotional unit. He believed that family members assume reciprocal family roles, develop automatic communication patterns, and react to each other in predictable connected ways, particularly when family anxiety is high. Once anxiety heightens within the system, an emotional process gets activated (Nichols and Schwartz, 2009) and dysfunctional communication patterns can emerge. For example, if one person is overly responsible, another family member is less likely to assume normal responsibility. Until one family member is willing to challenge the dysfunction of an emotional system by refusing to play his or her reactive part, the negative emotional energy fueling a family's dysfunctional communication pattern persists.

Bowen developed eight interlocking concepts to explain his theoretical construct of the family system (Bowen Center for the Study of the Family, 2013; Gilbert, 2006).

- **Differentiation of self** refers to a person's capacity to define him- or herself within the family system as an individual having legitimate needs and wants. It requires making "I" statements based on rational thinking rather than emotional reactivity. Self-differentiation takes into consideration the views of others but is not dominated by them. Poorly differentiated people are so dependent on the approval of others that they discount their own needs (Hill et al., 2011). Individuals with a well-differentiated sense of self exhibit a balanced, realistic dependence on others and can accept conflict and criticism without an excessive emotional reaction. Self-differentiation serves as the fundamental means of reducing chronic anxiety within the family system and enhancing effective problem solving. Self-differentiation emphasizes thinking rather than feeling in communication.

- **Multigenerational transmission** refers to the emotional transmission of behavioral patterns, roles, and communication response styles from generation to generation. It explains why family patterns tend to repeat behaviors in marriages, child rearing, choice of occupation, and emotional responses across generations without understanding why it happens.

- **Nuclear family emotional system** refers to the way family members relate to one another within their immediate family when stressed. Family anxiety shows up in one of four patterns: (1) dysfunction in one spouse, (2) marital conflict, (3) dysfunctional symptoms in one or more of the children, or (4) emotional distancing.

- **Triangles** refer to a defensive way of reducing, neutralizing, or defusing heightened anxiety between two family members by drawing a third person or object into the relationship (MacKay, 2012). If the original triangle fails to contain or stabilize the anxiety, it can expand into a series of "interlocking" triangles, for example, into school issues or an extramarital affair.

- **Family projection process** refers to an unconscious casting of unresolved anxiety in the family on a particular family member, usually a child. The projection can be positive or negative, and it can become a self-fulfilling prophecy as the child incorporates the anxiety of the parent as part of his or her self-identity.

- **Sibling position**, a concept originally developed by Walter Toman (1992), refers to a belief that sibling positions shape relationships and influence a person's expression of behavioral characteristics. Each sibling position has its own strengths and weaknesses. This concept helps explain why siblings in the same family can exhibit very different characteristics. For example:
  - Oldest or only children are more serious, assume leadership roles, and like to be in control. They may experience more trouble with staying connected with others or depending on them.
  - Youngest siblings are characterized as being followers, spontaneous, and fun loving, with a stronger sense of humor. They are more likely to be interested in quality of life and relationships.
  - Middle child positions embrace characteristics of oldest and youngest; they are likely to be adventuresome and independent, but not leaders. The child in the middle position may feel neglected or take on the role of peacemaker.

TABLE 12-2	Key Features of Other Family Theories	
Theory	**Key Elements**	**References**
Structural Family Theory	Emphasizes how the family unit is structured (subsystems, hierarchies, and boundaries). Function is assessed in relation to instrumental functioning (completing tasks during times of health and illness) and expressive functioning (communication patterns, problem solving, and power structures). Families strive to maintain homeostasis.	Fivaz-Depeursinge et al.; Minuchin
Developmental Family Theory	Eight specific developmental tasks are outlined starting with a childless couple and ending with retirement. Traits that demonstrate successful family development are identified.	Antle et al.; Duvall
Family Stress Theory	Family response to and coping with stressful events are explained. Factors associated with positive resolution include family system resources, flexibility, and problem solving skills.	Frain et al.; Lavee

Antle BF, Christensen DN, van Zyl MA, Barbee AP: The impact of the Solution Based Casework (SBC) practice model on federal outcomes in public child welfare, *Child Abuse Negl* 36(4):342-353, April 2012. doi:10.1016/j.chiabu.2011.10.009; Duvall E: *Marriage and family development*. Philadelphia, 1958, JB Lippincott; Fivaz-Depeursinge E, Lopes F, Python M, Favez N: Coparenting and toddler's interactive styles in family coalitions, *Fam Process* 48(4):500-516, 2009. doi:10.1111/j.1545-5300.2009.01298.x; Frain M, Berven N, Chan F, Tschopp M: Family resiliency, uncertainty, optimism, and the quality of life of individuals with HIV/AIDS, *Rehabil Counsel Bull* 52(1):16-27, 2008; Lavee Y Stress processes in families and couples. In Peterson GW, Bush KR (eds) Handbook of Marriage and the Family. New York Springer 2013 p. 159-176; Minuchin S: *Families and family therapy*. Boston, 1974, Harvard University Press.

- Although sibling position is a factor in explaining different relational behaviors, it is not useful as a descriptor of life functioning as a person occupying any sibling position can be either successful or unsuccessful (Gilbert, 2006).
- **Emotional cutoff** refers to a person's withdrawal from other family members as a means of avoiding family issues that create anxiety. Emotional cutoffs range from total avoidance to remaining in physical contact, but in a superficial manner. All persons have unresolved emotional attachments, but the extent varies widely among individuals.
- **Societal emotional process** refers to parallels that Bowen found between the family system and the emotional system operating at the institutional level in society. As anxiety grows within a society, many of the same polarizations, lack of self-differentiation, and emotion-based thinking dominate behavior and system outcomes.

Family legacies have a powerful influence on family relationships and in shaping parenting practices. Families of one generation tend to function in a similar manner to the previous generation. Knowledge of family relationships helps explain behaviors that would not be clear without having a family context. Helping families gain clarity about how their family heritage can be used as an asset in health care and/or what areas need work strengthens the potential for effective family-centered care.

Many theoretical frameworks exist that support understanding of family structure and function. Other family theories fall into three groupings related to structure, development, and resiliency theories. Table 12-2 identifies major characteristics of family theories. Other family-related theoretical frameworks based on social sciences, family therapy, and nursing exist (Kaakinen et al., 2010, p. 9).

The challenge for health care providers is to be able to apply a theoretical understanding of family structure and function to an actual patient care situation (Segaric and Hall, 2005). In many settings, nurses have a tendency to focus care on the individual. This is important, but the nurse also must understand that the family is impacted by even minor health deviations of a family member. Thus understanding families from a theoretical perspective is necessary.

Developing an Evidence-Based Practice

Bishop SM, Walker MD, Spivak IM: Family presence in the adult burn intensive care unit during dressing changes, *Crit Care Nurse* 33(1):14-22, 2013.

This article describes a quality improvement initiative to allow family members to be present during dressing changes in the adult burn intensive care unit. The impetus for this project was a hospital-wide patient- and family-centered care (PFCC) initiative. The traditional practice of not allowing family members to be present during dressing changes was inconsistent with the aims of PFCC. Previously, family members had been excluded from dressing changes because they were considered to increase the risk for infection and because it was thought family members would not be able to tolerate viewing the procedure. It was believed that the lack of family involvement contributed to lower patient and family satisfaction scores as well as lack of preparation for care upon discharge.

Following a comprehensive literature review and discussion with members of the health care team, the decision was made to permit family presence during dressing changes. Either the patient or their designee (if unable to make decisions) had to agree to allow other family members to be present during dressing changes. Family members who wished to participate were educated on what would happen during the entire dressing change process. In addition, family members were instructed on handwashing and the use of personal protective equipment. They were also instructed on what to do in the event they became faint, weak, or nauseous. Following the dressing change, family members had the opportunity to provide their reaction to the experience, as well as to answer questions related to the procedure.

The outcome measures included patient satisfaction and rates of infection. More than 2 years of data both before and after implementation of family presence were used for comparison. Family members who were present during dressing changes reported greater satisfaction with being informed and involved, discharge planning, and perception of staff attitudes when compared with the time period without family presence. Infection rates demonstrated a decrease during the implementation of family presence during dressing changes. Limitations were identified as low response rates and the fact that multiple practice changes were simultaneously implemented.

Application to Your Clinical Practice: The results of this quality improvement initiative demonstrate the positive effects of PFCC. It was not just family members seeing the dressing change being performed, but additional benefits included an increased interaction with family members that helps to improve family members' comfort with interacting with staff members. By allowing family members to be more involved in multiple aspects of patient care, the nurse-family relationship is enhanced, which can contribute to improved patient outcomes.

APPLICATIONS

FAMILY-CENTERED CARE

Family-centered care allows health care providers to have a uniform understanding of the patient and family's knowledge, preferences, and values as the basis for shared decision-making. This provides consistent information to all involved in the patient's care and allows the family to identify any barriers that might arise with the care plan.

Health events of one family member have the potential to affect the whole family. Trotter and Martin (2007) note, "Families share genetic susceptibilities, environments, and behaviors, all of which interact to cause different levels of health and disease" (p. 561). They are instrumental in helping patients appreciate the need for diagnosis and treatment and in encouraging the patient to seek treatment. Family members are involved in a patient's health care decisions ranging from treatment options to critical decisions about end-of-life care. Families play a pivotal advocacy role in treatment by monitoring and insisting on quality care for a family member.

The challenges for the nurse in family-centered care are:

- To understand the impact of a medical crisis on family functioning and dynamics
- To appreciate and respond empathetically to the emotional intensity of the experience for the family
- To determine the appropriate level of family involvement in holistic care of the patient, based on an understanding of fundamental family system concepts (Leon and Knapp, 2008)

ASSESSMENT

As defined at the beginning of this chapter, nurses should consider that "a family is who they say they are" (Wright and Leahey, 2009, p. 70). For immediate health care purposes, family is defined as the significant people in the patient's environment who are capable and willing to provide family-type support. Regardless of how it occurs, any health disruption becomes a family event. Even when the family is not directly involved in the family member's care, they will have feelings and opinions about the situation. Negative family responses have been associated with negative patient outcomes, while supportive positive family responses are associated with positive patient outcomes (Rosland et al., 2012). Exercise 12-1 allows you to analyze positive and negative family responses. Box 12-2 provides examples of situations that could warrant family assessment and nursing intervention.

EXERCISE 12-1	Positive and Negative Family Interactions

Purpose: To examine the effects of functional versus dysfunctional communication.

Procedure

Answer the following questions in a brief essay:

1. Recall a situation in dealing with a patient's family that you felt was a positive experience. What characteristics of that interaction made you feel this way?
2. Recall a situation in dealing with a patient's family that you felt was a negative experience.

What characteristics of that interaction made you feel this way?

Discussion

Compare experiences, both positive and negative. What did you see as the most striking differences? In what ways were your responses similar or dissimilar from those of your peers? What do you see as the implications of this exercise for enhancing family communication in your nursing practice?

BOX 12-2	Indicators for Family Assessment

- Initial diagnosis of a serious physical or psychiatric illness or injury in a family member
- Family involvement and understanding needed to support recovery of patient
- Deterioration in a family member's condition
- Illness in a child, adolescent, or cognitively impaired adult
- A child, adolescent, or adult child having an adverse response to a parent's illness
- Discharge from a health care facility to the home or an extended care facility
- Death of a family member
- Health problem defined by family as a family issue
- Indication of threat to relationship (abuse), neglect, or anticipated loss of family member

ASSESSMENT TOOLS

Initially, the nurse may not have the opportunity to complete a thorough family assessment. However, throughout the initial assessment and during ongoing nurse-patient interactions, the nurse must be attentive to cues indicating potential family-related concerns. The nurse should take into consideration anticipated health needs of the individual patient upon discharge. For example, a 30-year-old patient who had major reconstructive knee surgery and cannot bear weight on the affected leg for 4 weeks will require consistent personal assistance for a period of time. Family members are often called into action in such circumstances. However, if some type of family discord previously existed, the patient may not feel comfortable requesting assistance from family members and may feel uncomfortable asking even close friends for assistance. In this case, the nurse acts as intermediary to facilitate conversations among potential caregivers.

Other situations (see Box 12-2 for example) require a more in-depth assessment of family structure and function. Wright and Leahey's (2009) 15-minute interview, consisting of the genogram, ecomap, therapeutic questions, and commendations provide a comprehensive look at family relationships. Assessment tools such as the genogram, ecomap, and family time lines are used to track family patterns. The structured format of these tools focuses on getting relational data quickly and can sensitize clinicians to systemic family issues that affect patterns of health and illness (Gerson et al., 2008).

GENOGRAMS

A **genogram** uses a standardized set of connections to graphically record basic information about family members and their relationships over three generations. Genograms can be updated and/or revised as new information emerges. A genogram can be used to identify patterns of inheritable medical conditions, but when used as part of a family psychosocial assessment, it provides information about family relationships, as well as the personal perspective of the individual providing information (Chrzastowski, 2011). Such information may be used to guide in-depth family assessment and future interventions.

There are three parts to genogram construction: mapping the family structure, recording family information, and describing the nature of family relationships. Figure 12-2 identifies the symbols used to map family structure, with different symbols representing pregnancies, miscarriages, marriages, deaths, and other family events. Male family members are noted with a square and females with a circle. The oldest sibling is placed on the left, with younger siblings following from left to right, in order of birth. In the case of multiple marriages, the

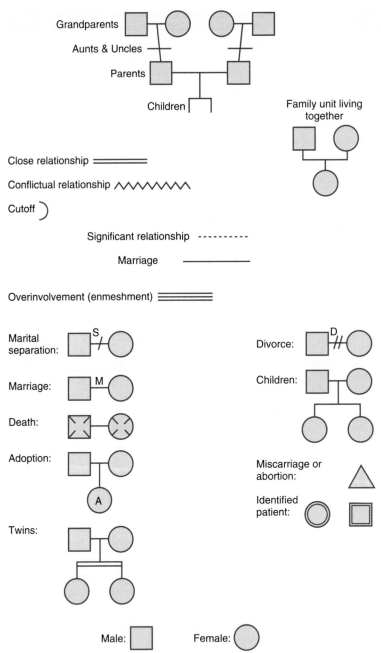

Figure 12-2 Symbols for a genogram.

earliest is placed on the left and the most recent on the right. Lines drawn between significant family members identify the strength of relational patterns that are overly close, close, distant, cut off, or conflicted. An example of a family genogram is presented in Figure 12-3.

The genogram explores the basic dynamics of a multigenerational family. Its multigenerational format, which traces family structure and relationships through three generations is based on the assumption that family relationship patterns are systemic, repetitive, and adaptive. Data about ages, birth and death dates, miscarriages, relevant illnesses, immigration, geographical location of current members, occupations and employment status, educational levels, patterns of family members entering

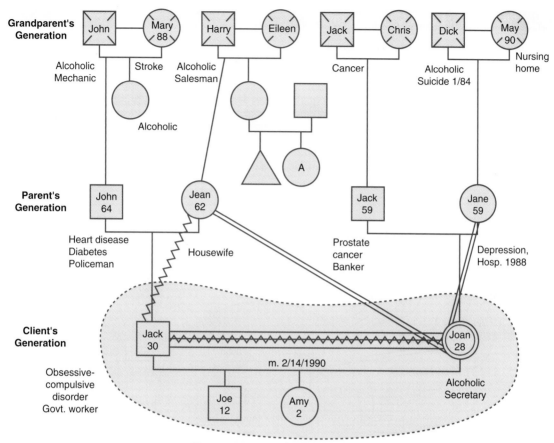

Figure 12-3 Basic family genogram.

or leaving the family unit, religious affiliation or change, and military service are written near the symbols for each person. The recorded information about family members allows families and health professionals to simultaneously analyze complex family interaction patterns in a supportive environment. The impact of multiple generations on family relationships is more readily visible.

The genogram offers much more than a simple diagram of family relationship. Formal and informal learning about appropriate social behaviors and roles takes place within the family of origin. People learn role behaviors and responsibilities expected in different life stages experientially, by way of role modeling, and through direct instruction. Exercise 12-2 provides practice with developing a family genogram.

ECOMAPS

An **ecomap** visually illustrates relationships between family members and the external environment (Kaakinen et al., 2010, p. 112). Beginning with an individual family

unit or patient, the diagram extends to include significant social and community-based systems with which they have a relationship. The diagram provides a quick visual of friends and community resource utilization. Adding the ecomap is an important dimension of family assessment, providing awareness of community supports that could be or are not being used to assist families (Rempel et. al., 2007). Ecomaps can point out resource deficiencies and conflicts in support services that can be corrected.

An ecomap starts with an inner circle representing the family unit, labeled with relevant family names. Smaller circles outside the family circle represent significant people, agencies, and social institutions with whom the family interacts on a regular basis. Examples include school, work, church, neighborhood friends, recreation activities, health care facilities or home care, and extended family. Lines are drawn from the inner family circle to outer circles indicating the strength of the contact and relationship. Straight lines indicate relation, with additional lines used to indicate the strength of

EXERCISE 12-2   Family Genograms

Purpose: To practice creating a family genogram.

Procedure
Students will break into pairs and interview one another to gain information to develop a family genogram. The genogram should include demographic information, occurrence of illness or death, and relationship patterns for three generations. Use the symbols for diagramming in Figure 12-2 to create a visual picture of the family information. Validate your genogram for accuracy with your informant.

Discussion
Each person will display the genogram they developed and discuss the process of obtaining information. Discuss strategies for obtaining information expediently yet sensitively and tactfully. Consider additional questions that could be used to gather additional information. Were you able to identify patterns that could be helpful in assisting individuals to cope with a health crisis? Discuss how genograms can be used by a nurse in a clinical setting.

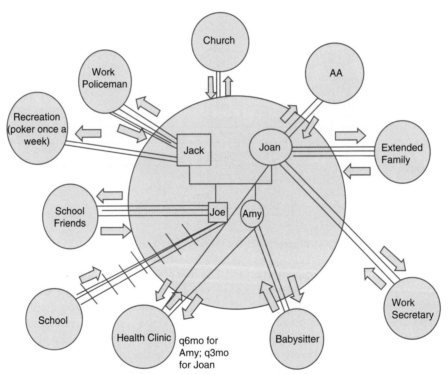

Figure 12-4   Example of an ecomap. *(Source: From Rempel GR, Neufeld A, Kushner KE: Interactive use of genograms and ecomaps in family caregiving research, J Fam Nurs 13(4):403-419, 2007.)*

the relationship. Dotted lines suggest tenuous relationships. Stressful relationships are represented with slashes placed through the relationship line. Directional arrows indicate the flow of the relational energy. Figure 12-4 shows an example of an ecomap. Exercise 12-3 provides an opportunity to construct an ecomap.

FAMILY TIME LINES
Time lines offer a visual diagram that captures significant family stressors, life events, health, and developmental

patterns through the life cycle. Family history and patterns developed through multigenerational transmission are represented as vertical lines. Horizontal lines indicate timing of life events occurring over the current life span. These include such milestones as marriages, graduations, and unexpected life events such as disasters, war, illness, death of person or pet, moves, births, and so forth (Figure 12-5). Time lines are useful in looking at how the family history, developmental stage, and concurrent life events might interact with the current health concern.

EXERCISE 12-3 | Family Ecomaps

Purpose: To practice creating a family ecomap.

Procedure
Using the interview process, students will break into pairs and interview one another to gain information to develop a family ecomap. The ecomap should include information about resources and stressors in the larger community system, such as school, church, health agencies, and interaction with extended family and friends for each student's family.

Discussion
Each person will display his or her ecomap and discuss the process of obtaining information. Discuss strategies for obtaining information expediently yet sensitively and tactfully. Explain how additional information obtained from an ecomap improves understanding of a family. Analyze the ecomap for areas that could be problematic if the informant were faced with a serious health issue. Describe how ecomaps can be used by a nurse in a clinical setting.

Note: Exercises 12-3 and 12-4 can be carried out during the same interview.

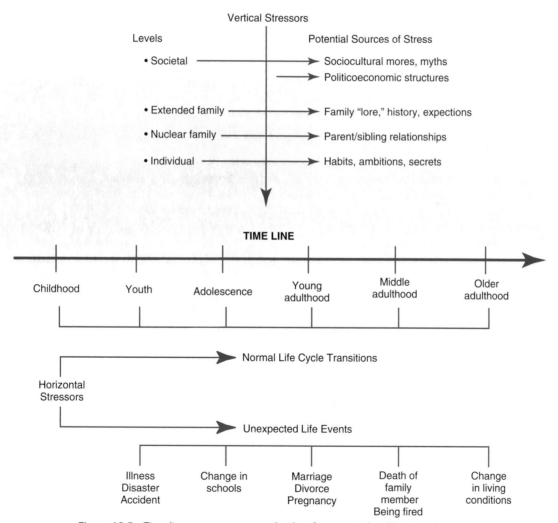

Figure 12-5   Time line assessment example identifying vertical and horizontal stressors.

By completing a family assessment, the nurse is able to develop a personalized plan of care for both the patient and family. The findings of a family assessment should be documented for use by other members of the health care team and to avoid redundant collection of data.

APPLYING THE NURSING PROCESS

ORIENTING THE FAMILY

The nurse-family relationship depends on reciprocal interactions between nurses and family members in which both are equal partners. Nurses should begin offering information to the family as soon as the patient is admitted to the hospital or service agency. Orientation to the facility, location of the cafeteria and restrooms, parking options, nearby lodging, and access to the hospitalist or physician are important points to include in early family interactions.

The initial family encounter sets the tone for the relationship. How nurses interact with each family member may be as important as what they choose to say. Begin with formal introductions and explain the purpose of gathering assessment data. Even this early in the relationship, you should listen carefully for family expectations and general anxiety that may be revealed more through behavior than through words.

When interacting with families, the nurse must ensure the patient's right to privacy. With the implementation of Health Insurance Portability and Accountability Act (HIPAA), family members may receive information regarding patient status only with the permission of either the patient or their designee (U.S. Department of Health and Human Services, 2008). This means that as a nurse, you cannot give out information regarding your patient's health status either over the phone or in person without consent. Most facilities have developed strategies to ensure that staff members do not disclose unauthorized information. For example, some facilities have adopted the use of a "code word" that is established upon admission. The code word is shared with only those family members who the patient wishes to receive information (McCullough and Schell-Chaple, 2013). If the person inquiring about the patient does not know the code word, then the nurse should politely inform the individual that for privacy reasons information cannot be provided.

GATHERING ASSESSMENT DATA

Determining the association of the family member to the patient is an initial step nurses can take in establishing a relationship. You might say, "I would like to hear what you think is the impact of your child's illness on the entire family." This statement guides your assessment, but also reminds the family that each family member is of concern to the health care team (Ylven and Granlund, 2009). Box 12-3 illustrates a framework for a family assessment with a patient entering cardiac rehabilitation. Family participation in the assessment process enhances the therapeutic relationship and completeness of the data. It is important to inquire about the family's cultural identity, rituals, values, level of family involvement, decision making, spiritual beliefs, and traditional behaviors as it relates to the health care of the patient (Leon and Knapp, 2008).

Knowledge of a family's past medical experiences, concurrent family stressors, and family expectations for treatment are essential pieces of family assessment data. Suggested questions include:

- How does the family view the current health crisis?
- What is each family member's most immediate concern?
- Has anyone else in the family experienced a similar problem?
- Are there any other recent changes or sources of stress in the family that make the current situation worse (pile up of demands?)
- How has the family handled the problem to date?
- Can you tell me what you expect from the health care team?
- As you close the session, ask, "Is there anything else I should know about your family and this experience?" Exercise 12-4 looks at assessment of family coping strengths.

PROBLEM IDENTIFICATION/NURSING DIAGNOSIS

Based on assessment data (initial and ongoing), the nurse identifies if problems related to family communication and functioning exist. Even if no problem is identified, the nurse must be alert for cues that indicate potential problems in family communication and function. Some problems related to family function may require referral to a social worker, family therapist, or other member of the health care team. In other instances, it may be appropriate for the nurse to provide

| BOX 12-3 | Family Assessment for Patient Entering Cardiac Rehabilitation |

Coping and Stress
- Who lives with you?
  _____

- How do you handle stress?
  _____

- Have you had any recent changes in your life (e.g., job change, move, change in marital status, loss)?
  _____

- On whom do you rely for emotional support?
  _____

- Who relies on you for emotional support?
  _____

- How does your illness affect your family members or significant others?
  _____

- Are there any health concerns of other family members?
  _____

- If so, how does this affect you?
  _____

Communication and Decision Making
- How would you describe the communication pattern in your family?
  _____

- How does your family address issues and concerns?
  _____

- Can you identify strengths and weaknesses within the family?
  _____

- Are family members supportive of each other?
  _____

- How are decisions that affect the entire family made?
  _____

- How are decisions implemented?
  _____

Role
- What is your role in the family?
  _____

- Can you describe the roles of other family members?
  _____

Value Beliefs
- What is your ethnic or cultural background?
  _____

- What is your religious background?
  _____

- Are there any particular cultural or religious healing practices in which you participate?
  _____

Leisure Activities
- Do you participate in any organized social activities?
  _____

- In what leisure activities do you participate?
  _____

- Do you anticipate any difficulty with continuing these activities?
  _____

- If so, how will you make the appropriate adjustments?
  _____

- Do you have a regular exercise regimen?
  _____

Environmental Characteristics
- Do you live in a rural, suburban, or urban area?
  _____

- What type of dwelling do you live in?
  _____

- Are there stairs in your home?
  _____

- Where is the bathroom?
  _____

- Are the facilities adequate to meet your needs?
  _____

- If not, what adjustments will be needed?
  _____

- How do you plan to make those adjustments?
  _____

- Are there any community services provided to you at home? (explain)
  _____

- Are there community resources available in your area?
  _____

- Do you have any other concerns at this time?
  _____

- Is there anything that we have omitted?
  _____

Signature _____ (must be completed by RN) Date/Time

Developed by Conrad J, University of Maryland School of Nursing, 1993.

EXERCISE 12-4 | Family Coping Strategies

Purpose: To broaden awareness of coping strategies among families.

Procedure

Each student is to recall a time when his or her family experienced a significant health crisis and how they coped. (Alternative strategy: Pick a health crisis you observed with a family in clinical practice.) Respond to the following questions:

1. Did the crisis cause a readjustment in roles?
2. Did it create tension and conflict or did it catalyze members, turning to one another for support? Look at the behavior of individual members.
3. What would have helped your family in this crisis? Write a descriptive summary about this experience.

Discussion

Each student shares his or her experience. Discuss the differences in how families respond to crisis. Compile a listing of coping strategies and helpful interventions on the board. Discuss the nurse's role in support to the family.

---

assistance to the family. Potential NANDA diagnoses related to communication with families might include:

- Compromised Family Coping
- Ineffective Family Therapeutic Regimen Management
- Readiness for Enhanced Family Processes
- Readiness for Enhanced Relationship (Ackley and Ladwig, 2011, p. 49)

PLANNING

The development of appropriate nursing actions should be based on mutually established goals. For the bedside nurse, these goals are often short term, focusing on improving awareness of areas to improve communication (see the following subsection regarding interventive questioning). The more the family can be involved in the planning process, the greater the likelihood of successful adaptation (Kaakinen et al., 2010, p. 116). Resources are available to help ensure family engagement.

The Agency for Healthcare Research and Quality (AHRQ) has developed the *Guide to Patient and Family Engagement in Hospital Quality and Safety*. This document has a multidisciplinary focus with four specific strategies:

Strategy 1: Working with patients and families as advisors

Strategy 2: Communicating to improve quality

Strategy 3: Nurse bedside shift report

Strategy 4: IDEAL discharge planning (AHRQ, 2013)

The preceding resources provide overall guidelines for patient- and family-centered care. As part of the overall plan of care, the nurse makes the most of communication skills to provide care to patients and families.

Interventive Questioning

Wright and Leahey (2009) identify questioning as a nursing intervention that nurses can use with families to identify family strengths; help family members sort out their personal fears, concerns, and challenges in health care situations; and provide a vehicle for exploring alternative options. Interventive questioning can be either linear or circular. **Linear questions** facilitate understanding of a situation by both the nurse and family members.

Circular questions lead to introspection, greater depth of understanding, and behavior change. Circular questions focus on family interrelationships and the effect a serious health alteration has on individual family members and the equilibrium of the family system. Examples of therapeutic questions are found in Box 12-4. Both linear and circular questioning should be used as part of effective nursing care. The nurse uses information the family provides as the basis for additional questions.

The following case example demonstrates its use when the nurse asks a family, "What has been your biggest challenge in caring for your mother at home?"

Case Example

Daughter: My biggest challenge has been finding a balance between caring for my mother and also caring for my children and husband. I have also had to learn a lot about the professional and support resources that are available in the community.

Son-in-law: For me, the biggest challenge has been convincing my wife that I can take over for a while, in order for her to get some rest. I worry that she will become exhausted.

BOX 12-4	Examples of Therapeutic Questions

- Who in the family is best encouraging your mother to comply with her diet?
- What information do you still need to understand the prognosis of your disease? Who else would benefit from this information?
- Who is suffering the most?
- What do you feel when you see your family member in pain?
- If there were one question you could have answered now, what would it be?
- How can we best help you and your family?
- If your family member's treatment does not go well, who will be most affected?

Adapted from Wright LM, Leahey M: *Nurses and families: a guide to family assessment and intervention*, ed 5, Philadelphia, 2009, FA Davis.

Mother: I have appreciated all the help that they give me. My biggest challenge is to continue to do as much as possible for myself so that I do not become too much of a burden on them. Sometimes I wonder about moving to a palliative care setting or a hospice (Leahey and Harper-Jaques, 1996, p. 135).

In this example, each family member's concern is related but different. The therapeutic circular question opens a discussion about each person's anxiety. As family members hear the concerns of other family members and as they hear themselves respond, their perspective broadens. The resulting conversation forms the basis for developing strategies that are mutually acceptable to all family members.

Family-centered interventions relate to: "(1) providing direct care, (2) removing barriers to needed services, and (3) improving the capacity of the family to act on its own behalf and assume responsibility" (Kaakinen et al., 2010, p. 117).

Meaningful involvement in the patient's care not only differs from family to family, it differs among individual family members (Ylven and Granlund, 2009). Individual family members have different perspectives. Hearing each family member's perspective helps the family and nurse develop a unified understanding of significant treatment goals and implications for family involvement.

Although treatment plans should be tailored around personal patient goals, acknowledging family needs, values, and priorities enhances compliance,

especially if they are different. Shared decision making and development of realistic achievable goals makes it easier for everyone concerned to accomplish them with a sense of ownership and self-efficacy about the process. Taking little achievable steps is preferred to attempting giant steps that misjudge what the family can realistically do. Exercise 12-5 provides practice with developing a family nursing care plan.

IMPLEMENTATION

Nurses can only *offer* interventions; it is up to the family to accept them (Wright and Leahey, 2009). Suggested nursing actions to promote positive change in family functioning include

- Encouraging the telling of illness narratives
- Commending family and individual strengths
- Offering information and opinions
- Validating or normalizing emotional responses
- Encouraging family support
- Supporting family members as caregivers
- Encouraging respite

Encouraging Family Narratives

Families need to tell their story about the experience of their loved one's illness or injury; it may be quite different from how the patient is experiencing it. The differences can lead to a more complete understanding. Such sharing can help build mutual support and empathy (Walsh, 2002). Nurses play an important role in helping families understand, negotiate, and reconcile differences in perceptions without losing face.

Case Example

Frances is a patient with a diagnosis of breast cancer. When she sees her oncologist, Frances reports that she is feeling fine, eating and able to function in much the same way as before receiving chemotherapy. Her husband's perception differs. He reports that her appetite has declined such that she only eats a few spoonfuls of food and she spends much of the day in bed. What Frances is reporting is true. When she is up, she enjoys doing what she did previously, although at a slower pace, and she does eat at every meal. Frances is communicating her need to feel normal, which is important to support. What her husband adds is also true. Her husband's input allows Frances to receive the treatment she needs to stimulate her appetite and give her more energy.

EXERCISE 12-5	Developing a Family Nursing Care Plan

Developed by Conrad J: University of Maryland School of Nursing, Baltimore, MD, 1993.

     Purpose: To practice skills needed with difficult family patterns.

Procedure

Read the case study and think of how you could interact appropriately with this family.

     Mr. Monroe, age 43 years, was chairing a board meeting of his large, successful manufacturing corporation when he developed shortness of breath, dizziness, and a crushing, viselike pain in his chest. An ambulance was called and he was taken to the medical center. Subsequently, he was admitted to the coronary unit with a diagnosis of an impending myocardial infarction (MI).

     Mr. Monroe is married with three children: Steve, age 14; Sean, age 12; and Lisa, age 10. He is the president and majority stockholder of his company. He has no history of cardiovascular problems, although his father died at the age of 38 of a massive coronary occlusion. His oldest brother died at the age of 42 from the same condition, and his other brother, still living, became a semi-invalid after suffering two heart attacks, one at the age of 44 and the other at 47.

     Mr. Monroe is tall, slim, suntanned, and very athletic. He swims daily; jogs every morning for 30 minutes; plays golf regularly; and is an avid sailor, having participated in every yacht regatta and usually winning. He is very health-conscious and has had annual physical checkups. He watches his diet and quit smoking to avoid possible damage to his heart. He has been determined to avoid dying young or becoming an invalid like his brother.

     When he was admitted to the coronary care unit, he was conscious. Although in a great deal of pain, he seemed determined to control his own fate. While in the unit, he was an exceedingly difficult patient, a trial to the nursing staff and his physician. He constantly watched and listened to everything going on around him and demanded complete explanations about any procedure, equipment, or medication he received. He would sleep in brief naps and only when he was totally exhausted. Despite his obvious tension and anxiety, his condition stabilized. The damage to his heart was considered minimal, and his prognosis was good. As the pain diminished, he began asking when he could go home and when he could go back to work. He was impatient to be moved to a private room so that he could conduct some of his business by telephone.

     When Mrs. Monroe visited, she approached the nursing staff with questions regarding Mr. Monroe's condition, usually asking the same question several times in different ways. She also asked why she was not being "told everything."

     Interactions between Mr. Monroe and Mrs. Monroe were noted by the staff as Mr. Monroe telling Mrs. Monroe all of the things she needed to do. Little intimate contact was noted.

     Mr. Monroe denied having any anxiety or concerns about his condition, although his behavior contradicted his denial. Mrs. Monroe would agree with her husband's assessment when questioned in his company.

Discussion

1. What questions would you ask the patient and family to obtain data regarding their adaptation to crisis?
2. What family nursing diagnosis would apply with this case study?
3. What nursing interventions are appropriate to interact with this patient and his family?
4. What other members of the health care team should be involved with this family situation?
5. How would you plan to transmit the information to the family?
6. What outcomes and measures would you use to determine success or failure of the nursing care plan?

Incorporating Family Strengths

Otto (1963) introduced the concept of family strengths as potential and actual resources families can use to make their life more satisfying and fulfilling to its members. When health care changes are required, and they usually are with patients suffering from serious illness or injury, working through family strengths rather than focusing on deficits is useful. Viewing the family as having strengths to cope with a problem rather than *being* a problem is a healing strategy. The intent is not that the family comes away from a stressful event or period without blemish, but instead that the existing skills and coping strategies are used in a healthy manner (Walsh, 2002). While each family's experience with illness varies, commonalities exist. The nurse should share strategies that families in similar situations have found effective.

Giving Commendations

Commendations involve "recognizing capabilities, skills and competencies" (Poor, 2013). Commendations are particularly effective when the family seems dispirited or confused about a tragic illness or accident. More than a simple compliment, commendations should reflect *patterns* of behavior existing in the

EXERCISE 12-6	Offering Commendations

Purpose: To practice with using commendation skills.

Procedure
Students will work in groups of three students. Each student will develop a commendation about the two other students in the group. The commendation should reflect a personal strength that the reflecting student has observed over a period time. Examples might include kindness, integrity, commitment, persistence, goal-directedness, tolerance, or patience. Write a brief paragraph about the trait or behavior you observe in this person. If you can, give some examples of why you have associated this particular characteristic with the person. Each student, in turn, should read his or her reflections about the other two participants, starting the conversation with good eye contact, the name of

the receiving student, and a simple orienting statement (e.g., "Kelly, this is what I have observed in knowing you...").

Discussion
Class discussion should focus on the thought process of the students in developing particular commendations, the values they focused on, and any consideration they gave to the impact of the commendation on the other students. The students can also discuss the effect of hearing the commendations about themselves and what it stimulated in them. Complete the discussion by considering how commendations can be used with families and how they can be used to counteract family resistance to working together.

family unit over time. Wright and Leahey (2009) differentiate between a commendation ("Your family is showing much courage in living with your wife's cancer for 5 years.") and a compliment ("Your son is so gentle despite feeling so ill.") (p. 270). They suggest giving at least one commendation per interview. There may be situations that seem extremely dire, but by identifying even one positive factor a family may feel empowered to push through the difficult situation. Exercise 12-6 provides practice with giving commendations.

Informational Support

Helping a family become aware of information from the environment and how to access it empowers families. By showing interest in the coping strategies that have and have not worked, the nurse can help the family recognize progress in their ability to cope with a difficult situation.

You can offer family members support related to talking with extended family, children, and others about the patient's illness. You can help family members prepare questions for meeting with physicians. Encouraging family members to write down key points to be addressed with other family members and physicians can be helpful. Written instructions should also be provided upon discharge.

The statement that discharge planning begins at admission is very true when it comes to providing families with information. The nurse should anticipate assistance that will be necessary upon discharge that will require family involvement. Because family members are not available consistently, the nurse should plan family teaching sessions prior to the time of discharge in order

to create an environment more conducive to learning (Kornburger et al., 2013). The use of the "teach-back" method can be used with families as well as individual patients. Refer to Chapter 15 regarding health teaching.

When patients and their family access the health care system, the nurse should see this as an opportunity to provide information regarding end-of-life decision making. Decisions regarding end-of-life care are best carried out when families are not in a "crisis mode." Thus you can engage with families in discussions about the cultural, ethical, and physical implications of using or discontinuing life-support systems. This is nursing's special niche, as these conversations are rarely one-time events, and nurses can provide informal opportunities for discussing them during care provision. Refer to Chapter 21 for additional information regarding advanced directives and end of life care planning.

Meeting the Needs of Families with Critically Ill Patients

Having a family member in an intensive care unit (ICU) represents a serious crisis for most families. Eggenberger and Nelms (2007) suggest, "Patients enter a critical care unit in physiological crisis, while their families enter the hospital in psychological crisis" (p. 1619). Box 12-5 identifies care needs of families of critically ill patients. Family-centered relationships are key dimensions of quality care in the ICU.

Proximity to the patient. The need to remain near the patient is a priority for many family members of patients in the ICU (Perrin, 2009). Although the family may appear to hover too closely, it is usually an

BOX 12-5	Caring for Family Needs in the Intensive Care Unit

Families of critically ill patients need to:
- Feel there is hope
- Feel that hospital personnel care about the patient
- Have a waiting room near the patient
- Be called at home about changes in the patient's condition
- Know the prognosis
- Have questions answered honestly
- Know specific facts about the patient's prognosis
- Receive information about the patient at least once a day
- Have explanations given in understandable terms
- Be allowed to see the patient frequently

Perrin K: *Understanding the essentials of critical care nursing* (pp. 40–41), Upper Saddle River, NJ, 2009, Pearson Prentice Hall.

attempt to rally around the patient in critical trouble (Leon, 2008). Viewed from this perspective, nurses can be more empathetic. As the family develops more confidence in the genuine interest and competence of staff, the hovering tends to lessen. Visitation policies may need to be adjusted based on the availability of family members (Hart et al., 2013). Staff need to be aware that family members may have obligations that prevent visits at expected times of day. When families visit loved ones in the ICU, the nurse should acknowledge them and provide any updated information that is available.

Families can be a primary support to patients, but they usually need encouragement and concrete suggestions for maximum effect and satisfaction. Family members feel helpless to reverse the course of the patient's condition and appreciate opportunities to help their loved one. Suggesting actions that family members can take at the bedside include doing range-of-motion exercises, holding the patient's hand, positioning pillows, and providing mouth care or ice chips. Talking with and reading to the patient, even if the person is unresponsive, can be meaningful for both the family and patient.

Helping families balance the need to be present with the patient's needs to conserve energy and have some alone time to rest or regroup is important. Family members also need time apart from their loved one for the same reasons. Tactfully explaining

the need of critically ill patients to have family presence without feeling pressure to interact can be supportive. Encouraging families to take respite is equally important. Providing information regarding dining and lodging can facilitate periods of rest for family members.

At the same time, nurses need to be sensitive to and respect a family member's apprehension or emotional state about their critically ill family member. Individual family members may need the nurse's support in talking about difficult feelings. Nurses can role-model communication with patients, using simple caring words and touch. Families are quick to discern the difference between nurses who are able to connect with a critically ill patient in this way, as evidenced in a family member's comment that "some seem to have a way with him and they talk to him like he is awake" (Eggenberger and Nelms, 2007, p. 1623).

Breaking Bad News to Families. The physician is the provider that most often delivers life-threatening critical information to patients and families. It is often the nurse at the bedside who ensures adequate patient and family understanding of information that has been provided. Additionally, nurses often notify patients and family members of significant changes in patient status, such as poor wound healing, transfers, need for further testing, and so forth (Edwards, 2010). Oftentimes, this occurs over the telephone, which further complicates the communication process. In each instance, well-planned communication can facilitate positive coping and adaptation.

The situation, background, assessment, recommendation (SBAR) format (see Chapter 2) can be adapted to guide communication of bad news to families. The nurse should plan for notifying patients and families of bad news in a similar manner to communicating with other health team members. Making notes of key points can assist the nurse to remember items to be addressed during a conversation. If the bad news is to be delivered in person, then the nurse should plan for a private, quiet setting (Pirie, 2012). If the news is to be delivered over the phone, the nurse should ask if it is a good time for a conversation. Present some background information and alert the person that bad news is coming. The bad news should be presented in a factual concise manner. Then the nurse should allow for a period of silence to show respect for the individual and to allow the person to process the information. In follow-up, the nurse should ask if the person understands the information that has been presented and ask for questions. The interaction should close with a summary of the treatment plan and when further communication can be expected (Pirie, 2012).

Providing Information. Families with family members in the ICU have a fundamental need for information, particularly if the patient is unresponsive. Many families have stated, "Not knowing is the worst part." Providing updated information as a clinical situation changes is critical. This information is particularly critical when family members must act as decision makers for patients who cannot make them on their own (Perrin, 2009). The use of a "Family Supportive Care Algorithm" that guided communication among family members and the health care team demonstrated improved families' sense of participation in decision making and perception of staff working as a team (Huffines et al., 2013).

Identifying one family member to act as the primary contact helps ensure continuity between staff and family. A short daily phone call when family members cannot be present maintains the family connection and reduces family stress (Leon, 2008). Families need ongoing information on the patient's progress, modifications in care requirements, and any changes in expected outcomes, with opportunities to ask questions and clarify information. Nurses in the ICU often serve as mediators between patient, family, and other health providers to ensure that data streams remain open, coordinated, and relevant.

How health care providers deliver information is important. Even if the patient's condition or prognosis leaves little room for optimism, the family needs to feel some hope and that the staff genuinely cares about what is happening with the patient and family (Perrin, 2009).

Caring for Families in the Pediatric Intensive Care Unit. Most parents of hospitalized children, particularly those in the pediatric intensive care unit (PICU) want to be with their children as often as possible (Kaakinen et al., 2010, p. 361). Parents of children in the PICU need frequent reassurance from the nurse about why things are being done for their child and about treatment-related tubes and equipment. They want to actively participate in their child's care and have their questions honestly answered.

Families act as the child's advocate during hospitalization, either informally by insisting on high-quality care or formally as the legal surrogate decision maker designated to make health care decisions on behalf of the patient. The nurse is a primary health care provider agent in working with families facing these issues. A critical intervention for the family as a whole and its individual members is to help them recognize their limitations and hidden strengths and to maintain a balance of health for all members.

Family-Centered Relationships in the Community

Nearly half of all adult U.S. citizens are affected by at least one chronic disease (CDC, 2012). Four modifiable risk factors (physical activity, obesity, smoking, and alcohol consumption) contribute substantially to the financial and emotional burden associated with chronic disease. Community-based nurses have many opportunities to educate and assist individuals to decrease risk factors and self-manage existing diseases. Many individuals are able to self-manage their disease, but an increasing number require family support with coping, self-management, and palliative care.

With the implementation of the Patient Protection and Affordable Care Act (PPACA), it is projected that the demand for health care providers will increase (Henry J. Kaiser Family Foundation, 2011). Nurses in non-acute care settings will have multiple opportunities to provide screening and health teaching to newly insured families. A major portion of these interactions should focus on encouraging families to adopt a healthy lifestyle in order to decrease the incidence of disease and illness. Concurrently, the concept of patient-centered care is becoming widely adopted throughout health care. For community-dwelling individuals the concept of patient-centered care focuses on empowering individuals to not only self-manage chronic diseases, but also to make appropriate lifestyle modifications with the intent of either preventing disease or minimizing the effects of disease. The combination of PPACA and patient-centered care will stimulate nurses to consider what constitutes effective communication when providing health teaching to families. Families need to feel empowered to take responsibility for their health state (Kaakinen et al., 2010, p. 478). Family empowerment develops when well-designed interventions are appropriate to the needs and resources of the family unit. The concepts presented in Chapters 16 can be used within the context of family health teaching.

Family caregivers are common as more people live with chronic illness on a daily basis; the level of assistance required varies on a person-by-person basis. Healthy family members have concurrent demands on their time from their own nuclear families, work, church, and community responsibilities. A significant change in health status can exacerbate previously unresolved relationship issues, which may need advanced intervention, in addition to the specific health care issues. When individual family members are experiencing a transition, for example, ending or entering a relationship, or job change, they may not be as available as support and can experience unnecessary guilt. Nurses need to consider the broader family responsibilities people have as an important part of the context of health care in providing holistic care to a family.

Meeting Family Informational Needs. Providing information to family caregivers often starts when the patient is discharged from an acute care facility. With the passage of time, the individual's needs for assistance may change, but the caregiver may lack the ability to adequately modify the care being provided. The sense of "preparedness" was identified as a factor in contributing to hope and anxiety for caregivers (Henriksson and Arestedt, 2013). As a result, nurses in clinics and community-based centers should be responsive to cues from caregivers indicating deficient knowledge. Nurses can offer suggestions about how to respond to these changes and offer support to the family caregiver as they emerge. Helping family members access services, support groups, and natural support networks at each stage of their loved one's illness empowers family members because they feel they are helping in a tangible way.

Supporting the Caregiver. Providing emotional support is crucial to helping families cope. Remaining aware of one's own values and staying calm and thoughtful can be very helpful to a family in crisis. Remember that your words can either strengthen or weaken a family's confidence in their ability to care for an ill family member. Focus initially on issues that are manageable within the context of home caregiving. This provides a sense of empowerment. The nurse can encourage the family to develop new ways of coping or can list alternatives and allow the family to choose coping styles that might be useful to them. Focus on what goes well, and ask the family to share their ideas about how to best care for the patient.

Many families will need information about additional home care services, community resources and options needed to meet the practical, and financial and emotional demands of caring for a chronically ill family member.

Encouraging families to use natural helping systems increases the network of emotional and economic support available to the family in time of crisis. Examples of natural helping systems include contact with other relatives, neighbors, friends, and churches. Promoting effective coping strategies and minimizing barriers to providing care should be implemented by community-based nurses (Leeman et al., 2008).

Validating and Normalizing Emotions. Families can experience many conflicting emotions when placed in the position of providing protracted care for a loved one. Compassion, protectiveness, and caring can be intermingled with feelings of helplessness and being trapped. Major role reversals can stimulate anger and resentment for both patient and family caregiver.

Sibling or family position or geographic proximity may put pressure on certain family members to provide a greater share of the care. Criticism or advice from less involved family members can be disconcerting and conflicts about care decisions can create rifts in family relationships. Some caregivers find themselves mourning for their loved one, even though the person is still alive, wishing it could all end and feeling guilty about having such thoughts.

These emotions are normal responses to abnormal circumstances. Listening to the family caregiver's feelings and struggles without judgment can be the most healing intervention you can provide. Nurses can normalize negative feelings by offering insights about common feelings associated with chronic illness. Family members may need guidance and permission to get respite and recharge their commitment by attending to their own needs. Support groups can provide families with emotional and practical support and a critical expressive outlet.

Psychosocial concerns for parents with chronically ill children can cover many relationship issues, for example, how to respond and discipline children with chronic illness. Parents must balance caring for their chronically ill child along with parenting other children (Kaakinen et al., 2010, p. 255). Healthy siblings may experience feelings of resentment, worry that they might contract a similar illness, or have unrealistic expectations of their part in the treatment process. Siblings need clear information about the sick child's diagnosis and care plan, as well as the opportunity to experience their own childhood as fully as possible. Exercise 12-7 provides practice with using intervention skills with families.

| EXERCISE 12-7 | Using Intervention Skills with Families |

Purpose: To practice using intervention skills with families.

Procedure

Describe a situation in which your have worked with a family. This may be from a clinical experience or other personal experience. Think about how you talked with the family related to a specific problem.

Consider the following:

- Did you talk with the family about the problem and learn how they have dealt with the problem, their perception of the problem, and its impact on their family?
- What would be some approaches identified in the text to help them explore the problem in more depth and begin to develop viable options?
- Did you feel you were too intrusive or not assertive enough?

- Did you validate all members' perceptions and perspectives? Did you clarify information and feelings? Did you remain nonjudgmental and objective?
- Did you respect the family's values and beliefs without imposing your own? Did you assist the family in clarifying and understanding the problem in a way that could lead to resolution?

Discussion

In small groups, discuss your responses to the questions above. Be attentive to the experiences of others. Did they have similar experiences? Discuss strategies to facilitate goal-directed communication and resolution of problems. How can nurses best provide support to families? How could families learn to use honest communication most of the time? How does one influence this in one's own family?

Pitfalls to Avoid

While we as nurses strive to be effective in all communication, there are times that our communication efforts are less than ideal. Wright and Leahey (2009) identified three common errors that occur in family nursing.

1. Failure to create context for change. In such instances, the nurse does not establish a therapeutic environment for open discussion of family concerns. Another example would be a plan of care that would not be effective in light of the family situation (resources, distance, health state). To avoid this pitfall, the nurse should be respectful of each family member, obtain as much information about the family and its members as possible, and acknowledge the difficulty of the situation.

2. Avoid taking sides. This can be done either inadvertently or purposively, however, the nurse is most effective when assuming the role of the investigator and mediator. To minimize the risk for taking sides, the nurse should use questioning skills that help family members develop insight into the depth and scope of the problem. The use of circular questions as discussed earlier can be helpful.

3. Giving too much advice prematurely. Nurses inherently are in a position to provide patients and families with information and advice. However, it must be well-timed and appropriate to the particular situation without sounding like a dictator.

To avoid this pitfall, obtain as much information from family members as possible before providing suggestions. Advice should be framed so that it is expressed as a suggestion, rather than a set of rules. Follow-up with family members to get their reaction to your suggestion.

Using Technology to Enhance Family Communication

The use of the Internet and wireless communication has progressed dramatically. Many community-dwelling individuals use electronic communication devices on daily basis, whether it is a cellular phone or the World Wide Web. The utilization of electronic communication with patients and families is less common but increasing rapidly. Numerous risks and hazards are associated with any type of electronic communication; however, many opportunities exist for nurses to improve family communication via technology. It is important to remember that e-mail and other text-based communication can be misconstrued and misinterpreted. Federal regulations as outlined in HIPAA apply to all modes of communication and must be considered when communicating with family members in an electronic format.

Families today are often geographically separated. Encouraging and assisting patients to send e-mail or call using a wireless phone can decrease that distance. Simply hearing the voice of a patient can help to allay fear for distant relatives. Other technologies such as Skype, FaceTime, Twitter, Facebook, and other social media can be used to enhance communication. Caring Bridge (caringbridge.org) is an organization that offers free personalized web sites for individuals undergoing serious health concerns. Online support groups are becoming more prevalent for those experiencing health issues, as well as for families and caregivers (van der Eijk et al., 2013). The nurse should assess the comfort level of family members with the use of technology. Learning to use a smart phone, e-mail, or other technology-based communication can add to the stress of an already anxious situation. Such efforts should be attempted only with caution.

EVALUATION

Evaluation should include both determining effectiveness of nursing interventions, as well as self-reflection by the nurse regarding personal effectiveness. The nurse at the bedside may not see long-term benefits from family interactions due to the episodic nature of contemporary health care. It is important that the nurse provide closure to patient interactions in any setting. This can be accomplished by summarizing the interaction, asking the family if they have questions, and providing information regarding follow-up. Bereaved families have reported that the support received from nurses played an important role in how they were able to cope (MacConnell et al., 2012). No matter how brief family interactions are, the impact may be substantial.

Referrals should include a summary of the information gained to date and should be communicated by the health team member most knowledgeable about the patient's condition. Patients and families should be provided with information related to referrals.

Self-evaluation and self-reflection by the nurse can be used to identify which communication strategies were successful in a given situation and which were not (Kaakinen et al., 2010, p. 119). By identifying effective and ineffective family communication techniques, a repertoire of skills can be developed, thus enhancing the overall effectiveness of nurses' communication and practice.

SUMMARY

This chapter provides an overview of family communication and the complex dynamics inherent in family relationships. Families have a structure, defined as the way in which members are organized. Family function refers to the roles people take in their families, and family process describes the communication that takes

place within the family. Family-centered care is developed through a combination of strategies designed to gather information in a systematic, efficient manner starting with the genogram, ecomap, and timeline. Therapeutic questions and giving commendations are interventions nurses can use with families. Families with critically ill members need continuous updated information and the freedom to be with their family member as often as possible. Involving the family in the care of the patient is important. Parents want to participate in the care of their acutely ill patient. Nursing interventions are aimed at strengthening family functioning and supporting family coping during hospitalization and in the community.

ETHICAL DILEMMA   What Would You Do?

Terry Connors is a 90-year-old woman living along in a two-story house. She has two daughters, Maria and Maggie. Maria lives 90 miles away, but works two jobs because her husband has been laid off for 9 months. Her other daughter Maggie lives in another state. So far, Terry has been able to live by herself, but within the past 2 weeks, she fell down a few stairs in her house and she has trouble hearing the telephone. Terry has very poor vision, walks with a cane, and relies on her neighbors for assistance several times a week. Maria and her husband visit every 2 weeks to bring groceries. Both Maria and Maggie worry about her and would like to see her in a nursing home. Terry will not consider this option. As the nurse working with this family, how would you address your ethical responsibilities to Terry, Maria, and Maggie?

DISCUSSION QUESTIONS

1. Identify family communication situations (e.g., end of life, family discord) that you believe would be professionally challenging. Describe strategies that you as a nurse could use to be prepared to better manage those situations.
2. How would you personally feel as a nurse delivering bad news to a family?

REFERENCES

Ackley BJ, Ladwig GB: *Nursing diagnosis handbook: an evidence-based guide to planning care*, St. Louis, MO, 2011, Mosby.

Antle BF, Christensen DN, van Zyl MA, Barbee AP: The impact of the Solution Based Casework (SBC) practice model on federal outcomes in public child welfare, *Child Abuse Negl* 36(4):342–353, April 2012. http://dx.doi.org/10.1016/j.chiabu.2011.10.009.

Barker P: Different approaches to family therapy, *Nurs Times* 94(14):60–62, 1998.

Bishop SM, Walker MD, Spivak IM: Family presence in the adult burn intensive care unit during dressing changes, *Crit Care Nurse* 33(1):14–22, 2013.

Bowen M: *Family therapy in clinical practice*, Northvale, NJ, 1978, Jason Aronson.

Centers for Disease Control and Prevention (CDC): Chronic diseases and health promotion. http://www.cdc.gov/chronicdisease/overview/index.htm, 2012. Retrieved December 19, 2013.

Cicchetti D, Blender JA: A multiple levels of analysis perspective on resilience: implications for the developing brain, neural plasticity, and preventive interventions, *Ann N Y Acad Sci* 1094:248–258, 2006.

Chrzastowski SK: A narrative perspective on genograms: revisiting classical family therapy methods, *Clin Child Psychol Psychiatry* 16(4):635–644, 2011. http://dx.doi.org/10.1177/1359104511400966.

Duvall E: *Marriage and family development*, Philadelphia, 1958, JB Lippincott.

Edwards M: How to break bad news and avoid common difficulties, *Nurs Residential Care* 12(10):495–497, 2010.

Eggenberger S, Nelms T: Being family: the family experience when an adult member is hospitalized with a critical illness, *J Clin Nurs* 16(9):1618–1628, 2007.

Fivaz-Depeursinge, Lopes F, Python M, Favez N: Coparenting and toddler's interactive styles in family coalitions, *Fam Process* 48(4):500–516, 2009. http://dx.doi.org/10.1111/j.1545-5300.2009.01298.x.

Henry J, Kaiser Family Foundation: *Focus on Health Reform: Summary of the Affordable Care Act*, Washington, DC, 2011, Author. Accessed December 2013. http://kaiserfamilyfoundation.files.wordpress.com/2011/04/8061-021.pdf.

Frain M, Berven N, Chan F, Tschopp M: Family resiliency, uncertainty, optimism, and the quality of life of individuals with HIV/AIDS, *Rehabil Counsel Bull* 52(1):16–27, 2008.

Gerson R, McGoldrick M, Petry S: *Genograms: assessment and intervention*, ed 3, New York, NY, 2008, WW Norton & Co.

Gilbert R: *The eight concepts of Bowen theory*, Falls Church, VA, 2006, Leading Systems Press.

Goldenberg H, Goldenberg I: *Family therapy: an overview*, Belmont, CA, 2013, Cenage Brooks/Cole.

Agency for Healthcare Research and Quality (AHRQ): Guide to Patient and Family Engagement in Hospital Quality and Safety. Retrieved December 28, 2013. http://www.ahrq.gov/professionals/systems/hospital/engagingfamilies/guide.html.

Hart A, Hardin SR, Townsend AP, Ramsey S, S., Mahrle-Henson A: Critical care visitation: nurse and family preference, *Dimens Crit Care Nurs* 32(6):289–299, 2013. http://dx.doi.org/10.1097/01.DCC.0000434515.58265.7d.

U.S. Department of Health and Human Services: *Health Information Privacy*, 2008. Retrieved December 28, 2013 from http://www.hhs.gov/ocr/privacy/hipaa/faq/disclosures_to_friends_and_family/523.html.

Henriksson A, Arestedt K: Exploring factors and caregiver outcomes associated with feelings of preparedness for caregiving in family caregivers in palliative care: a correlational, cross-sectional study, *Palliat Med* 27(7):639–646, 2013.

Hill WJ, Hasty C, Moore C: Differentiation of self and the process of forgiveness: a clinical perspective for couple and family therapy, *Aust New Zeal J Fam Ther* 32(1):43–57, 2011.

Huffines M, Johnson KL, Smitz Naranjo LL, Lissauer M, Fishel MA, D'Angelo Howes SM, Pannullo D, Ralls M, Smith R: Improving family satisfaction and participation in decision making in an intensive care unit, *Crit Care Nurse* 33(5):56–68, 2013.

Jensen T, Schafer K: Stepfamily functioning and closeness: children's views on second marriages and stepfather relationships, *Soc Work* 58(2):127–136, 2013.

Kaakinen JR, Gedaly-Duff V, Coehlo DP, Hanson SMH: *Family health care nursing: theory practice and research*, Philadelphia, PA, 2010, F. A. Davis.

Kornburger C, Gibson C, Sadowski S, Maletta K, Klingbeil C: Using "Teach-Back" to promote a safe transition from hospital to home: an evidence-based approach to improving the discharge process, *J Pediatr Nurs* 28:282–291, 2013.

Leahey M, Harper-Jaques S: Family-nurse relationships: core assumptions and clinical implications, *J Fam Nurs* 2(2):133–152, 1996.

Leeman J, Skelly AH, Burns D, Carlson J, Soward A: Tailoring a diabetes self-care intervention for use with older, rural African American women, *Diabetes Educat* 34(2):310–317, 2008.

Leon A: Involving family systems in critical care nursing: challenges and opportunities, *Dimens Crit Care Nurs* 27(6):255–262, 2008.

Leon A, Knapp S: Involving family systems in critical care nursing: challenges and opportunities, *Dimens Crit Care Nurs* 27(6):255–262, 2008.

Lavee Y: Chapter 8: Stress processes in families and couples. In Peterson GW, Bush KR, editors: *Handbook of Marriage and the Family*, New York, 2013, Springer, pp 159–176.

MacConnell G, Aston M, Randel P, Zwaagstra N: Nurses' experiences providing bereavement follow-up: an exploratory study using feminist poststructuralism, *J Clin Nurs* 22:1094–1102, 2012.

MacKay L: Trauma and Bowen Family Systems Theory: working with adults who were abused as children, *Aust New Zeal J Fam Ther* 33(3):232–241, 2012.

McCullough J, Schell-Chaple H: Maintaining patients' privacy and confidentiality with family communications in the intensive care unit, *Crit Care Nurse* 33(5):77–79, 2013.

Merriam-Webster OnLine: s.v. "family." Accessed November 3, 2013. www.merriam-webster.com.

Minuchin S: *Families and family therapy*, Boston, 1974, Harvard University Press.

Nichols M, Schwartz R: *Family therapy: concepts and methods*, ed 9, Upper Saddle River NJ, 2009, Prentice Hall.

Otto H: Criteria for assessing family strength, *Fam Process* 2:329–338, 1963.

Perrin K: *Understanding the essentials of critical care nursing*, Upper Saddle River, NJ, 2009, Pearson Prentice Hall.

Pirie A: July-August. Pediatric palliative care communication: resources for the clinical nurse specialist, *Clin Nurs Spec* 26(4):212–215, 2012.

Poor CJ: Important interactional strategies for everyday public health nursing practice, *Public Health Nurs* 1–7, 2013, Dec. 10. http://dx.doi.org/10.1111/phn.12097. [Epub ahead of print].

Rempel G, Neufeld A, Kushner K: Interactive use of genograms and ecomaps in family caregiving research, *J Fam Nurs* 13(4):403–419, 2007.

Rosland A, Heisler M, Piette J: The impact of family behaviors and communication patterns on chronic illness outcomes: a systematic review, *J Behav MedM* 35(2):221–239, 2012.

Segaric CA, Hall WA: The family theory-practice gap: a matter of clarity? *Nurs Inq* 12(3):210–218, 2005.

Bowen Center for the Study of the Family: Bowen theory: societal emotional process. Accessed December 9, 2013 Available online http://www.thebowencenter.org/pages/conceptsep.html. 2013.

Toman W: *Family therapy and sibling position*, New York, 1992, Jason Aronson Publishers.

Trivette CM, Dunst CJ, Hamby DW: Influences of family-systems intervention practices on patent-child interactions and child development, *Top Early Child Spec Educ* 30(1):3–19, 2010.

Trotter T, Martin HM: Family history in pediatric primary care, *Pediatrics* 120(Suppl):S60–S65, 2007.

U.S. Census Bureau: Current Population Survey: Definitions. . Retrieved November 3, 2013 from http://www.census.gov/cps/about/cpsdef.html, 2013.

van der Eijk M, Faber M, Aarts J, Kremer J, Munneke M, Bloem B: Using online health communities to deliver patient centered care to people with chronic conditions, *J Med Internet Res* 15(6):e115, 2013. http://dx.doi.org/10.2196/jmir.2476.

von Bertalanffy L: *General systems theory*, New York, 1968, George Braziller.

Walsh F: A family resilience framework: innovative practice applications, *Fam Relat* 51(2):130–136, 2002.

Wright LM, Leahey M: *Nurses and families: a guide to family assessment and intervention*, ed 5, Philadelphia, 2009, FA Davis.

Ylven R, Granlund M: Identifying and building on family strength: a thematic analysis, *Infants Young Child* 22(4):253–263, 2009.

CHAPTER 13

Resolving Conflicts between Nurse and Client

Kathleen Underman Boggs

OBJECTIVES

At the end of the chapter, the reader will be able to:

1. Describe the goal of a collaborative nurse-client relationship.
2. Define conflict and contrast the functional with the dysfunctional role of conflict in a therapeutic relationship.
3. Recognize personal style of response to conflict situations and discriminate among passive, assertive, and aggressive responses to conflict situations.
4. Specify the characteristics of assertive communications strategies to promote conflict resolution in nurse-client relationships.
5. Discuss strategies to de-escalate violence in the workplace.
6. Discuss how findings from research studies and evidenced-based practices can be applied to communicating with clients holding differing values in your clinical practice.

Patient-centered care is one of the six QSEN competencies described in Chapter 2. Our goal is to fully partner with our clients, so they are active participants in the management of their care (Rosenberg and Gallo-Silver, 2011). A QSEN desired Attitude says we will respect the centrality of our patient as a core member of the health team. However, even when nurse-client goals are mutual, our values or viewpoints may differ. Collaboration is our focus but, as in all interactions among human beings, some disagreements are inevitable.

Conflict is a natural part of human relationships. We all have times when we experience negative feelings about a situation or person. When this occurs in a nurse-client relationship, clear, direct communication is needed. This chapter emphasizes the dynamics of conflict and the problem-solving skills needed for successful resolution between you and your client. (Conflicts among health team members will be discussed in Chapter 23.) Because workplace violence is on the increase, this chapter will also present this information.

Effective nurse-client communication is critical to efficient care provision and to receiving quality care. When conflict occurs, knowing how to respond calmly allows you to use feelings as a positive force. Some clients approach their initial encounter with a nurse with verbal hostility or even physical aggression, such as when we admit an intoxicated client to the emergency department. Maintaining safety for self and client is paramount. To listen and to respond creatively to intense emotion when your first impulse is to withdraw or to retaliate demands a high level of skill, empathy, and self-control.

BASIC CONCEPTS

DEFINITION

Conflict is defined as disagreement arising from differences in attitudes, values, or needs, in which the actions of one party frustrate the ability of the other to achieve their expected goals. This results in stress or tension. Conflicts serve as warning that something in the relationship needs closer attention. Conflict is not necessarily a negative; it can become a positive force leading to growth in relationships. Conflict resolution is a learned process.

NATURE OF CONFLICT

All conflicts have certain things in common: (a) a concrete *content problem issue*; and (b) relationship or *process issues*, which involve our emotional response to the situation. It is immaterial whether the issue makes realistic sense to you. They feel real to your client and need to be dealt with. Unresolved, they will interfere with success in meeting goals. Most people experience conflict as discomfort. Previous experiences with conflict situations, the importance of the issue, and possible consequences all play a role in the intensity of our reaction. For example, a client may have great difficulty asking questions of the physician regarding treatment or prognosis, but experience no problem asking similar questions of the nurse or family. The reasons for the discrepancy in comfort level may relate to previous experiences. Alternatively, it may have little to do with the actual persons involved. Rather, the client may be responding to anticipated fears about the type of information the physician might give.

CAUSES OF CONFLICT

Lack of communication or poor communication are the main causes of misunderstanding and conflict. Other psychological causes of conflict include differences in values or personality and multiple demands or issues causing high levels of stress. Then too, if your nursing care does not fit in with your client's cultural belief system, conflict can result. Recognize that our culture has moved toward greater incivility in mainstream society. This is somewhat reflected within the health care system.

RISK FOR VIOLENCE: INCIDENCE STATISTICS

Conflict can escalate to violent threats or actions. The stressful nature of illness can aggravate factors that lead to violent behavior by clients or their family members. Society in general is becoming less civil. **Violence** against health care workers is increasing. Nurses are at greater risk because of their close contact with clients (International Council of Nurses [ICN], 2006; Waschgler et al., 2013). In fact, nurses and social workers are at three times greater risk to experience violence in their workplace than are other professionals (American Association of Critical Care Nurses [AACN], 2004;

American Nurses Association [ANA], 2002, 2012). Approximately 80% of nurses will experience violence sometime during their career (Rittenmeyer, 2012). The Joint Commission's (TJC) "Sentinel Event Alert, Issue 45," addresses prevention specifying controlling access to health care agencies and staff education. TJC notes that communication failures were inherent in 53% of reported acts of violence (2010).

Violence against health care workers ranges from threats to assaults to murder, yet it is estimated that about 80% of these occurrences remain unreported. Certain locations tend to be at higher risk for emergence of conflict. Nurses working in emergency departments, psychiatric facilities, or even in nursing homes are at even higher risk with up to half of these nurses being recipients of violent or aggressive acts (ANA, 2012; U.S. Department of Labor Occupational Safety and Health Administration [OSHA], 2004; Zeller et al., 2012). Consider the case of Mr. Dixon in the following case example.

Case Example: Mr. Dixon

Experienced staff nurse, Ms. Kaye RN, works in a busy emergency department where access to the treatment rooms is blocked by a locked security door. Staff do not wear necklaces or neck chains, nor carry implements but Ms. Kaye does wear an ID badge (per the U.S. Department of Labor Occupational Safety and Health Administration [OSHA] recommendations). While Dr. Hughes is treating Donny, age 12, who appears to be suffering from convulsions related to overdosing on methylphenidate (Ritalin), Ms. Kaye notices Mr. Dixon is becoming increasingly agitated in the waiting room.

Mr. D: "Why aren't you people doing more?"

Nurse (in a low tone of voice): "My name is Ms. Kaye and I am helping with your son. I'll be keeping you up to date with information as soon as we know anything. I know this is a stressful…"

Mr. D (interrupting in a louder voice): "I demand to know why you people won't tell me what is going on."

Nurse: "I see that you are really upset and feeling angry. Let's move over here to the conference ell for privacy."

Mr. D: "You guys are no good."

Nurse: "I want to understand your point of view. You…"

Mr. D shoves a chair.

Nurse: "This is an upsetting time for you, but violence is not acceptable. Please calm down and we will sit down. Let's both take a deep breath, then you can explain to me what you need…"

Strategies to prevent escalation of violent behavior are discussed in the "Application" section of this chapter. Physical and organizational safeguard suggestions are available from OSHA (www.osha.gov).

STAGE OF ANGER

- Mild: Feels some tension, irritability. Acts argumentative, sarcastic, or is difficult to please
- Moderate: Observably angry behaviors such as motor agitation and loud voice
- Severe: Shows acting out behaviors, cursing, using violent gestures but is not yet out of control
- Rage: Behaving in an out-of-control manner, physically aggressive toward others or self

CONFLICT OUTCOMES: WHY WORK FOR CONFLICT RESOLUTION?

Outcomes of unresolved nurse-client conflict impede the quality and safety of client care. Not only does it undermine your therapeutic relationship, it can result in your emotional exhaustion leading to **burnout** (Guidroz et al., 2012). Energy is transferred to conflict issues instead of being used to build the relationship. Conflict and exposure to violent behaviors have also been shown to result in increased stress, cynicism, somatic illnesses, while resulting in decreased job satisfaction and psychological wellbeing (Papadopoulos et al., 2012). In addition to physical harm to the worker, *Healthy People 2020* (U.S. Department of Health and Human Services, 2014) and other sources have identified problems for the health system, such as increased agency costs due to lost work days, job turnover, and occasionally litigation.

GOAL

As nurses, our goal is to collaborate with clients to maximize their health. To accomplish this goal we need to communicate clearly to prevent or reduce levels of conflict. We know that resolving some long-standing conflicts is a gradual process in which we may have to revisit the issue several times to fully resolve the conflict.

CONFLICT RESOLUTION PRINCIPLES

It goes without saying that professionals always demonstrate respect for clients. Gender and cultural factors that influence responses are described elsewhere. Figure 13-1 lists some principles of conflict resolution. These may also be applied to conflicts with colleagues.

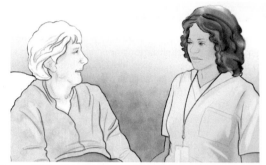

Figure 13-1 Principles of conflict resolution:
- Identify conflict issue: acknowledge you have the capacity to resolve
- Know own response: take responsibility for your response
- Separate issue from people involved: no blame approach
- Stay focused on issue: clarify
- Identify options: listen to others' alternative solutions
- Negotiate and agree on solution
- Summarize

UNDERSTAND OWN PERSONAL RESPONSES TO CONFLICT

Conflicts between nurse and client are not uncommon. First gain a clear understanding of your own personal response since conflict creates anxiety that may prevent us from behaving in an effective, assertive manner. No one is equally effective in all situations. Completing Exercise 13-1 may help you identify your personal responses.

Recognize your own "trigger" or "hot buttons." What words or client actions trigger an immediate emotional response from you? These could include having someone yelling at you or speaking to you in an angry tone of voice. Once you recognize the triggers, you can better control your own response. It is imperative that you focus on the current issue. Put aside past history. Listing prior problems will raise emotions and prevent both you and the client from reaching a solution. Identify *available options*. Rather than immediately trying to solve the problem, look at the range of possible options. Create a list of these options and work with the other party to evaluate the feasibility of each option. By working together, the expectation shifts from adversarial conflict to an expectation of a win-win outcome. After discussing possible solutions, select the best one to resolve the conflict. Evaluate the outcome based on fair, objective criteria.

KNOW THE CONTEXT

Second, understand the context or the circumstances in which the situation occurs. Most interpersonal conflicts

EXERCISE 13-1	Personal Responses to Conflict

Purpose: To increase awareness of how students respond in conflict situations and the elements in situations (e.g., people, status, age, previous experience, lack of experience, or place) that contribute to their sense of discomfort.

Procedure:
Break class into small groups of two. You may do this as homework or create an Internet discussion room. Think of a conflict situation that could be handled in different ways.

The following feelings are common correlates of interpersonal conflict situations that many people say they experienced in conflict situations that they have not handled well.

Anger	Competitiveness	Humiliation
Annoyance	Defensiveness	Inferiority
Antagonism	Devaluation	Intimidation
Anxiousness	Embarrassment	Manipulation
Bitterness	Frustration	Resentment

Although these feelings generally are not ones we are especially proud of, they are a part of the human experience. By acknowledging their existence within ourselves, we usually have more choice about how we will handle them.

Using words from the list, describe the following as concretely as possible:
1. The details of the situation: How did it develop? What were the content issues? Was the conflict expressed verbally or nonverbally? Who were the persons involved and where did the interaction take place?
2. What feelings were experienced before, during, and after the conflict?
3. Why was the situation particularly uncomfortable?

Discussion:
Suggest different ways to respond. Might these lead to differences in outcome?

---

involve some threat to one's sense of control or self-esteem. Nurses have been shown to respond to the stress of not having enough time to complete their work by imposing more controls on the client, who then often reacts by becoming more difficult. Other behaviors of nurses that may lead to anger in clients or families are listed in Box 13-1. Clients who feel listened to and respected are generally receptive. Be careful what you say and how you say it. How can you avoid acting in ways that create anger or conflict with clients?

Situations that may cause nurses to become frustrated or angry with clients include clients who dismiss what they say; clients who ask for more personal information than nurses feel comfortable sharing; clients who sexually harass or target a nurse for a personal attack; or family members who make demands nurses are unable to fulfill.

DEVELOP AN EFFECTIVE CONFLICT MANAGEMENT STYLE

Five distinct **styles of response** to conflict have been documented. In the past, nurses were found to commonly use avoidance or accommodation when faced with a conflict situation (Sayer et al., 2012). Many felt that any conflict was destructive and needed to be suppressed. Current thinking holds that conflict can be healthy and can lead to growth when with conflict resolution training, we develop a collaborative problem-solving approach.

BOX 13-1	Behaviors of a Nurse That Create Anger in Others

- Violating client's personal space
- Speaking in a threatening tone
- Providing unsolicited advice
- Judging, blaming, criticizing, or conveying ideas that try to create guilt
- Offering reassurances that are not realistic
- Communicating using "gloss it over" positive comments
- Speaking in a way that shows you do not understand your client's point of view
- Exerting too much pressure to make a person change their unhealthy behavior
- Portraying self as an infallible "I know best" expert
- Using an authoritarian, sarcastic, or accusing tone
- Using "hot button" words that have heavy emotional connotations
- Failing to provide health information in a timely manner to stressed individuals

Avoidance is a common response to conflict. Nurses using avoidance distance themselves from their client or provide less support. Sometimes an experience makes you so uncomfortable that you want to avoid the situation or person at all costs, so you withdraw. This style is appropriate when the cost of addressing the conflict is higher than the benefit of resolution. Sometimes you just have to "pick your battles," focusing your energy on the most important issues. However, use of avoidance postpones the conflict, leads to future problems, and damages your relationship with your client, making it an *I lose-You lose situation*.

Accommodation is another common response. We surrender our own needs in a desire to smooth over the conflict. This response is cooperative but nonassertive. Sometimes this involves a quick compromise or giving false reassurance. By giving into others, we maintain peace but do not actually deal with the issue, so it will likely resurface in the future. It is appropriate only when the issue is more important to the other person. This is an *I lose-You win situation*. Harmony results. Good will may be earned that can be used in the future (McElhaney, 1996).

Competition is a response style characterized by domination. You exercise power to gain your own goals at the expense of the other person. It is characterized by aggression and lack of compromise. Authority may be used to suppress the conflict in a dictatorial manner. This leads to increased stress. It is an effective style only when there is a need for a quick decision, but leads to problems in the long term, making it an *I win now, but then lose-You lose situation*.

Compromise is a solution still commonly found to be employed by nurses (Iglesias and Vallejo, 2012). By compromising, each party gives a little and gains a little. It is only effective when both parties hold equal power. Depending on the specific work environment and the issue in dispute, it can be a good solution, but since neither party is completely satisfied, it eventually can become an *I lose-You lose situation*.

Collaboration is a solution-oriented response in which we work together cooperatively to problem solve. To manage the conflict, we commit to finding a mutually agreeable solution. This involves directly confronting the issue, acknowledging feelings, and using open communication to solve the problem. Steps for productive confrontation include identifying concerns of each party; clarifying assumptions; communicating honestly to identify the real issue; and working collaboratively to find a solution that satisfies everyone. Collaboration is considered to be the most effective style for genuine resolution. This is an *I win-You win situation*.

STRUCTURE YOUR RESPONSE

In mastering assertive responses, it may be helpful initially to use these steps in an assertive response.

1. Express empathy: "I understand that_____"; "I hear you saying _____." *Example:* "I understand that things are difficult at home."

2. Describe your feelings or the situation: "I feel that _____"; "This situation seems to me to _____." *Example:* "But your 8-year-old daughter has expressed a lot of anxiety, saying, 'I can't learn to give my own insulin shots.'"

3. State expectations: "I want _____"; "What is required by the situation is _____." *Example:* "It is necessary for you to be here tomorrow when the diabetic teaching nurse comes so you can learn how to give injections and your daughter can, too, with your support."

4. List consequences: "If you do this, then _____ will happen" (state positive outcome); "If you don't do this, then _____ will happen" (state negative outcome). *Example:* "If you get here on time, we can be finished and get her discharged in time for her birthday on Friday."

FOCUS ON THE PRESENT

- The focus should always be on the present. Focus only on the present issue. The past cannot be changed.

Limiting your discussion to one topic issue at a time enhances the chance of success. Usually it is impossible to resolve a conflict that is multidimensional in nature with one solution. By breaking the problem down into simple steps, enough time is allowed for a clear understanding. You might paraphrase the client's words, reflecting the meaning back to the client to validate accuracy. Once the issues have been delineated clearly, the steps needed for resolution may appear quite simple.

Because it is impossible to do anything about the past except learn from it, and because the future is never completely predictable, the present is the only reality in which we have much decision-making power as to how we act. To be assertive in the face of an emotionally charged situation demands thought, energy, and commitment. Assertiveness also requires the use of common sense, self-awareness, knowledge, tact, humor, respect, and a sense of perspective. Although there is no guarantee that the use of assertive behaviors will produce desired interpersonal goals, the chances of a successful outcome are increased because the information flow is optimally honest, direct, and firm. Often the use of assertiveness brings about changes in ways that could not have been anticipated. Changes occur because the nurse offers a new resource in the form of objective feedback with no strings attached.

USE "I" STATEMENTS

Statements that begin with "You..." sound accusatory. When statements point a finger or imply judgment, most people respond defensively. "We" statements should only be used when you actually mean to look at an issue collaboratively. Use of "I" statements are one of the most effective conflict management strategies you can use. Assertive statements that begin with "I" suggest that the person speaking accepts full responsibility for his or her own feelings and position in relation to the conflict. "I" statements feel clumsy at first and take a little practice to use. The following is one suggested format:

"I feel_____ (use a name to claim the emotion you feel)

when_____ (describe the behavior non-judgmentally)

because_____ (describe the tangible effects of the behavior)."

Example: "I feel uncomfortable when a client's personal problems are discussed in the cafeteria because someone might overhear confidential information."

MAKE CLEAR STATEMENTS

Statements rather than questions set the stage for assertive responses to conflict. When you do use a question, "how" questions are best because they are neutral in nature, seek more information, and imply a collaborative effort. Avoid "why" questions as they put other people on the defensive, asking them to explain their behavior. Use a strong, firm tactful manner and state the situation clearly. Consider the following case example of Mr. Gow.

Case Example: Mr. Gow

Mr. Gow is a 35-year-old executive who has been hospitalized with a myocardial infarction. He has been acting seductively toward some of the young nurses, but he seems to be giving Miss O'Hara an especially hard time.

Client: Come on in, honey, I've been waiting for you.

Nurse (using appropriate facial expression and eye contact, and replying in a firm, clear voice): Mr. Gow, I would rather you called me Miss O'Hara.

Client: Aw, come on now, honey. I don't get to have much fun around here. What's the difference what I call you?

Nurse: I feel that it does make a difference, and I would like you to call me Miss O'Hara.

Client: Oh, you're no fun at all. Why do you have to be so serious?

Nurse: Mr. Gow, you're right. I am serious about some things, and being called by my name and title is one of them. I would prefer that you call me Miss O'Hara. I would like to work with you, however, and it might be important to explore the ways in which this hospitalization is hampering your natural desire to have fun.

In this interaction the nurse's position is defined several times, using successively stronger statements before the shift is made to refocus on the client's needs. Notice that the nurse labeled the behavior, not the client, as unacceptable. Persistence is essential when initial attempts at assertiveness appear too limited.

USE MODERATE PITCH AND VOCAL TONE

The strength of a forceful assertive statement depends on the nature of the conflict situation, as well as the degree of confrontation needed to resolve the conflict successfully. Starting with the least amount of assertiveness required to meet the demands of the situation conserves energy and does not place you in an "overkill" bind. It is not necessary to use all your resources at one time or to express your ideas too strongly. We sometimes loose effectiveness by becoming too long-winded. Long explanations detract from the spoken message. Get to the main point quickly, saying what is necessary in the simplest, most concrete way possible. This cuts down on the possibility of misinterpretation.

Pitch and tone of voice contribute to another person's interpretation of the meaning of your assertive message. A soft, hesitant, passive presentation can undermine an assertive message. The same is true if a harsh, hostile, aggressive tone is used. Try a firm but moderate presentation to effectively convey your message when you practice Exercise 13-2.

EXERCISE 13-2	Pitching the Assertive Message

Purpose: To increase awareness of how the meaning of a verbal message can be significantly altered by changing one's tone of voice.

Procedure:
Break class up into groups of five. Write on a slip of paper one of the five vocal pitches: whisper, soft tone with hesitant delivery, moderate tone and firm delivery, loud tone with agitated delivery, or screaming.

Pick one of five pieces of paper and demonstrate that tone while the others in the group try to identify correctly in which tone the person is giving the assertive message.

Discussion:
How does tone affect perceptions of a message's content?

OUTCOME: POSITIVE GROWTH

Traditionally conflict was viewed as a destructive force to be eliminated. Actually conflicts that are successfully resolved lead to stronger relationships. The critical factor is the willingness to explore and resolve it mutually. Appropriately handled, conflict can provide an important opportunity for growth. Training courses and even short practice sessions have been shown to help nurses develop needed skills (Sargeant et al., 2011). Practice of conflict management skills is essential.

OUTCOME: DYSFUNCTION, SUCH AS UNRESOLVED CONFLICT

As mentioned, unresolved conflicts tend to resurface later, impeding your ability to give quality care. If the emotional aspect of the conflict is expressed too strongly, the nurse can feel attacked.

NATURE OF ASSERTIVE BEHAVIOR

Assertive behavior is defined as setting goals, acting on those goals in a clear, consistent manner, and taking responsibility for the consequences of those actions. Assertive communication is conveying this objective in a direct manner, without anger or frustration (Rosenberg and Gallo-Silver, 2011). The assertive nurse is able to stand up for personal rights and the rights of others. Practice with Exercise 13-2.

Components of assertion communication include the following four abilities: (1) to say no; (2) to ask for what you want; (3) to appropriately express both positive and negative thoughts and feelings; and (4) to initiate, continue, and terminate the interaction. This honest expression of yourself does not violate the needs of others but

BOX 13-2	Characteristics Associated with the Development of Assertive Behavior

- Express your own position, using "I" statements.
- Make clear statements.
- Speak in a firm tone, using moderate pitch.
- Assume responsibility for personal feelings and wants.
- Make sure verbal and nonverbal messages are congruent.
- Address only issues related to the present conflict.
- Structure responses so as to be tactful and show awareness of the client's frame of reference.
- Understand that undesired behaviors, not feelings, attitudes, and motivations, are the focus for change.

does demonstrate self-respect rather than deference to the demands of others. Conflict creates anxiety that may prevent us from behaving assertively. Assertive behaviors range from making a direct, honest statement about your beliefs to taking a very strong, confrontational stand about what will and will not be tolerated. Assertive responses contain "I" statements that take responsibility. This behavior is in contrast with **aggressive behavior**, which has a goal of dominating while suppressing the other person's rights. Aggressive responses often consist of "you" statements that fix blame on the other person. Box 13-2 lists characteristics of assertive behavior. Remember assertiveness is a learned behavior and assertive responses need to be practiced!

Nonassertive behavior in a professional nurse is related to lower levels of autonomy. Continued patterns of nonassertive responses have a negative influence on you and on the standard of care you provide. Evaluate your own assertiveness with Exercise 13-3.

| EXERCISE 13-3 | Assertive Responses |

Purpose: To increase awareness of assertiveness.

Procedure:
Respond to the following scenario:
   You are working full time, raising a family, and taking 12 credits of nursing classes. The teacher asks you to be a student representative on a faculty committee. You say the following:
   1. "I don't think I'm the best one. Why don't you ask Karen? If she can't, I guess I can."

2. "Gee, I'd like to, but I don't know. I probably could if it doesn't take too much time."
3. "I do want students to have some input to this committee, but I am not sure I have enough time. Let me think about it and let you know in class tomorrow."

Discussion:
Choose the most assertive answer and comment about how other options could be altered.

SAFETY

It is your responsibility to maintain your own safety and that of clients. Note, when you are confronted by an angry client or family member, use your skills to defuse the situation, addressing their concerns. If anger enters the RAGE-STAGE, leave, get help. Do not stay in a dangerous situation. It cannot be overemphasized that if you feel in danger→ LEAVE! Each agency should have a resource team to call for intervention assistance. CALL!

| Developing an Evidence-Based Practice |

Zeller A, Dassen T, Kok G, Needham I, Halfens RJ: Factors associated with resident aggression, *J Nurs Scholarsh* 44(3):249-257, 2012.

A retrospective cross-sectional survey of 814 Swiss caregivers in nursing homes was done to identify environmental factors related to aggression. This study also identified caregiver and resident characteristics. A regression analysis was completed on items measured on the standardized tool: Survey of Violence Experienced by Staff (SOVES-G-R).

Results: Staff were found to be at high risk for aggressive behaviors. Reported aggression was very prevalent, reported by 81.6% of nurses in the prior 12-month period subcategorized as verbal aggression (76.5%), threats (27.6%), and physical aggression (54%). Feeling confident one could handle aggression was a predictor for being at higher risk for aggression, especially during basic care activities.

Application to Your Clinical Practice: The authors suggest that nursing home personnel receive training in prevention and handling of aggression from their clients.
   Nursing interventions that are effective in defusing aggression certainly need more research. An extensive review of recent literature identified scant research into managing the behavior of clients, although there is a plethora of articles on interacting with disruptive colleagues.

APPLICATIONS

Practicing the following strategies helps improve conflict resolution skills. By doing so we demonstrate that we are developing the **QSEN Attitude** of continuously improving our own communication and conflict resolution skills.

PREVENTING CONFLICT

In addition to managing your own responses to client provocations by adopting a professional, "calm" demeanor and low tone of voice, other conflict prevention strategies may be useful. Signal your readiness to listen with attending behaviors such as good body position, eye contact, and receptive facial expression. Give your undivided extra attention to a client or a visitor whom you identify as potentially becoming aggressive. The review by Finke and colleagues (2008) of 12 nurse-client communication studies showed that nurses' anticommunication attitudes were cited in half the studies as a barrier to communication. Increasing your positive appreciation of your client does facilitate communication. As nurses, we hold the belief that all clients have worth as human beings. Remind yourself of this basic belief whenever you are in a conflict situation with your client. Try some of the strategies described in this chapter to help prevent or resolve conflict.

ASSESSING THE PRESENCE OF CONFLICT IN THE NURSE-CLIENT RELATIONSHIP

To get resolution, you need to acknowledge the presence of conflict. Often the awareness of our own feelings of discomfort is an initial clue. Evidence of the presence of conflict may be *overt*, that is, observable in

| EXERCISE 13-4 | Defining Conflict Issues |

Purpose: To help begin to organize information and define the problem in interpersonal conflict situations.

Procedure:

In each conflict situation, look for specific behaviors (including words, tone, posture, and facial expression); feeling impressions (including words, tone, intensity, and facial expression); and need (expressed verbally or through actions).

Identify the behaviors, your impressions of the behaviors, and needs that the client is expressing in the following situations. Suggest an appropriate nursing action. Situation 1 is completed as a guide.

Situation 1

Mrs. Patel, an Indian client, does not speak much English. Her baby was just delivered by cesarean section, and it is expected that Mrs. Patel will remain in the hospital for at least 4 days. Her husband tells the nurse that Mrs. Patel wants to breast-feed, but she has decided to wait until she goes home to begin because she will be more comfortable there and she wants privacy. The nurse knows that breast-feeding will be more successful if it is initiated soon after birth.

Behaviors: The client's husband states that his wife wants to breast-feed but does not wish to start before going home. Mrs. Patel is not initiating breast-feeding in the hospital.

Your impression of behaviors: Indirectly, the client is expressing physical discomfort, possible insecurity, and awkwardness about breast-feeding. She may also be acting in accordance with cultural norms of her country or family.

Underlying needs: Safety and security. Mrs. Patel probably will not be motivated to attempt breast-feeding until she feels safe and secure in her home environment.

Suggested nursing action: Provide family support and guarantee total privacy for feeding.

Situation 2

Mrs. Moore is returned to the unit from surgery after a radical mastectomy. The doctor's orders call for her to ambulate, cough, and deep breathe, and to use her arm as much as possible in self-care activities. Mrs. Moore asks the nurse in a very annoyed tone, "Why do I have to do this? You can see that it is difficult for me. Why can't you help me?"

---

the client's behavior and expressed verbally. For example, the client may criticize you. No one likes to be criticized and a natural response might be anger, rationalization, or blaming others. But as a professional nurse, you recognize your response, recognize the conflict, and work toward resolution so that constructive changes may take place.

More often, conflict is *covert* and not so clear-cut. The conflict issues are hidden. Your client talks about one issue, but talking does not seem to help and the issue does not get resolved. The client continues to be angry or anxious. Subtle behavioral manifestations of covert conflict might include a reduced effort by your client to engage in self-care; frequent misinterpretation of your words; behaviors that are out of character for the client, such as excessive anger. For example, when your client seems unusually demanding, has a seemingly insatiable need for your attention, or is unable to tolerate reasonable delays in having needs met, the problem may be anxiety stemming from conflictive feelings. Client behaviors are often negatively affected by feelings of pain, loss, helplessness, frustration, or fear. As nurses, we affect the behavior of our clients through our actions. This can lead to positive or negative outcomes. See Exercise 13-4 for practice in defining conflict issues.

Sometimes the feelings themselves become the major issue, so that valid parts of the original conflict issue are hidden; consequently, conflict escalates. Consider how you would deal with Ms. Dentoni in the following situation.

Case Example: Ms. Dentoni

Ms. Dentoni is scheduled for surgery at 8 a.m. tomorrow. As the student nurse assigned to care for her, you have been told that she was admitted to the hospital 3 hours ago and that she has been examined by the house resident. The anesthesia department has been notified of the client's arrival. Her blood work and urine have been sent to the laboratory. As you enter her room and introduce yourself, you notice that Ms. Dentoni is sitting on the edge of the bed and appears tense and angry.

Client: I wish people would just leave me alone. Nobody has come in and told me about my surgery tomorrow. I don't know what I'm supposed to do—just lay around here and rot, I guess.

At this point, you probably can sense the presence of conflictive feelings, but it is unclear whether the emotions being expressed relate to anxiety over the surgery or to anger over some real or imagined invasion of privacy because of the necessary laboratory tests and physical examination. Your client might also be annoyed by you or by a lack of information from her surgeon. She may feel the need to know that hospital personnel see her as a person and care about her feelings. Before you can respond empathetically to the client's feelings, they will have to be decoded.

> *Nurse* (in a concerned tone of voice): You seem really upset. It's rough being in the hospital, isn't it?

Notice that the reply is nonjudgmental and tentative and does not suggest specific feelings beyond those the client has shared. There is an implicit request for her to validate your perception of her feelings and to link the feelings with a concrete issue. You process verbal as well as nonverbal cues. Concern is expressed through your tone of voice and words. The content focus relates to the client's predominant feeling tone, because this is the part of the conflict that she has chosen to share with you. It is important to maintain a nonanxious, relaxed presence.

TECHNIQUES FOR CONFLICT RESOLUTION

Remember your goal is to *de-escalate* the conflict. Use the strategies for conflict resolution described in this section. Mastery takes practice. Although this seems like a lot of information, an incident can occur in only a few minutes.

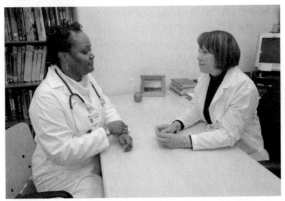

Reaching a common understanding of the problem in a direct, tactful manner is the first step in conflict resolution.

PREPARE FOR THE ENCOUNTER

Careful preparation often makes the difference between being successful or failing to assert yourself when necessary. Clearly identify the issue in conflict.

For communication to be effective, it must be carefully thought out in terms of certain basic questions:

- *Purpose.* What is the purpose or objective of this information? What is the central idea, the one most important statement to be made?
- *Organization.* What are the major points to be shared, and in what order?
- *Content.* Is the information to be shared complete? Does it convey who, what, where, when, why, and how?
- *Word choice.* Has careful consideration been given to the choice of words?
- If you wish to be successful, you must consider not only what is important to you in the discussion but what is important to the other person. Bear in mind the other person's viewpoint. The following case about Mr. Pyle illustrates this idea.

Case Example: Mr. Pyle

Mr. Pyle is an 80-year-old bachelor who lives alone. He has always been considered a proud and stately gentleman. He has a sister, 84 years old, who lives in Florida. His only other living relatives, a nephew and his wife, also live in another state. He recently changed his will so that it excludes his relatives, and he refuses to eat. When his neighbor brings in food, he eats it, but he won't fix anything for himself. He tells his neighbor that he wants to die and that he read in the paper about a man who was able to die in 60 days by not eating. As the visiting nurse assigned to his area, you have been asked to make a home visit and assess the situation.

The issue in this case example is not one of food intake alone. Any attempt to talk about why it is important for him to eat or expressing your point of view in this conflict immediately on arriving is not likely to be successful. Mr. Pyle's behavior suggests that he feels there is little to be gained by living any longer. His actions suggest further that he feels lonely and may be angry with his relatives. Once you correctly ascertain his needs and identify the specific issues, you may be able to help Mr. Pyle resolve his intrapersonal conflict. His wish to die may not be absolute or final, because he eats when food is prepared by his neighbor and he has not yet taken a deliberate, aggressive move to end his life. Each of these factors needs to be assessed and validated with him before an accurate nursing diagnosis can be made.

ORGANIZE INFORMATION

Plan your approach for a time and place conducive to collaborative discussion. Do not respond in the heat of the moment. Organizing your information and validating the appropriateness of your intervention with another knowledgeable person who is not directly involved in the process is useful. Sometimes it is wise to rehearse out loud what you are going to say. Remember to adhere to the principle of focusing on the conflict issue. Avoid bringing up the past.

MANAGE YOUR OWN ANXIETY OR ANGER

Recognizing and controlling your own natural emotional response to your client's upsetting behavior may be one key factor in managing conflict. Conflict produces anxiety **and creates** feelings of helplessness. This discomfort should signal you that you need to deal with the situation. As mentioned earlier, part of an initial assessment of an interpersonal conflict situation includes recognition of the nurse's intrapersonal contribution to the conflict, as well as that of the client. It is not wrong to have ambivalent feelings about taking care of clients with different lifestyles and values; however, this needs to be acknowledged to yourself.

Confronting the client's behavior now should keep you from losing control later as the problem escalates. Most people experience some variation of a physical response when taking interpersonal risks. A useful strategy for managing your own anger is to vent to a friend using "I" statements, as long as this does not become a complaining, whining session. Another strategy to manage your own anger is to "take a break." A cooling-off period, doing something else for a few minutes or hours until your anger subsides, is acceptable. Take care that you reengage, however, so that this does not become just an avoidance response style. Communicate with the correct person; do not take out your frustration on someone else. Focus on the one issue with the client involved. Try saying, "I would like to talk something over with you before the end of shift/before I go." Before you actually enter the client's room, do the following:

- Cool off. Wait until you can speak in a calm, friendly tone.
- Take a few deep breaths. Inhale deeply and count "1-2-3" to yourself. Hold your breath for a count of 2 and exhale, counting again to 3 slowly.
- Fortify yourself with positive statements (e.g., "I have a right to respect."). Anticipation is usually far worse than the reality.
- Defuse your own anger before confronting the patient.
- Focus on one issue.

TIME THE ENCOUNTER

Timing is a determinant of success. Know specifically the behavior you wish to have the client change. Make sure that the client is capable physically and emotionally of changing the behavior. Select a time when you both can discuss the matter privately and use neutral ground, if possible. Select a time when the client is most likely to be receptive.

Timing is also important if an individual is very angry. The key to assertive behavior is choice. Sometimes it is better to allow your client to let off some "emotional steam" before engaging in conversation. In this case, the assertive thing to do is to choose silence accompanied by a calm, relaxed body posture. These nonverbal actions convey acceptance of feeling and a desire to understand. Validating the anger and reframing are useful. Comments such as, "I'm sorry you are feeling so upset" recognize the significance of the emotion being expressed without getting into the cause.

PUT SITUATION INTO PERSPECTIVE

Do not play the blame game. Put the issue into perspective. How urgent is it to resolve this issue? How important is the issue? Will the issue be significant in a year? In 10 years? Will there be a significant situational change with resolution? This is another way of saying to pick your battles. Not every situation is worth using up your time and energy. Remind yourself that anger may be caused by a problem communicating; clients who are frustrated may become angry when they cannot make staff understand.

USE THERAPEUTIC COMMUNICATION SKILLS

Refer to the discussion on therapeutic communication in Chapter 10. Particularly useful is *active listening*. Really trying to understand what the client is upset about requires more skill than just listening to his or her words. Listening closely to what the client is saying may help you understand his or her point of view. This understanding may decrease the stress. Repeat what the client said to make sure communication is crystal clear.

	BOX 13-3	Nursing Communication Interventions: Following the C.A.R.E. Steps
C	Clarify the behavior that is a problem	Use communication skills, especially active-listening skills, to identify issues of concern to the client. • Use a calm tone and avoid conveying irritation. • Paraphrase client's message to be sure you understand. • Ask for clarification if needed. • Suggest simple interventions to decrease anxiety (deep breathing relaxation and guided imagery). • Factually state the problem, focusing only on the current issue.
A	Articulate why the behavior is a problem	Explain the institution policies. • Explain the limits of your role. • Set limits firmly.
R	Request a change in the problem behavior	Work with the entire health team so all use the same uniform approach to the client's demands. • Develop a mutual health care plan: involve patient in care and set goals. • Review and reevaluate whether you and client have same goals.
E	Evaluate progress	Provide education; explain all options, with outcomes. • Verbalize incentives and withdrawal of privileges to modify unacceptable behavior. • Promote trust by providing immediate feedback.

NURSING COMMUNICATION INTERVENTIONS: FOLLOWING THE C.A.R.E. STEPS

Riley (2012) adapted a C.A.R.E. acronym to help nurses confront conflict situations. Refer to Box 13-3. Use your therapeutic nursing communication skills described in Chapter 10. Particularly useful in dealing with conflict situations is use of active listening and paraphrasing.

C = Clarify.

Choose direct, declarative sentences. Use objective words and avoid mixed messages. Make sure verbal and nonverbal communication is congruent. Maintain an open stance and omit any gestures that might be interpreted as criticism, such as rolling your eyes or sighing heavily. Avoid mixed messages. One example of inappropriate communication might be found in the case of Larry, a staff nurse who works the 11 p.m. to 7 a.m. shift. Larry needs to get home to make sure his children get on the bus to school. A geriatric client routinely asks for a breathing treatment while Larry is reporting off. Instead of setting limits, Larry uses a soft voice and smiles as he tells her he can be late to begin the report. Another example is Mr. Carl, the 29-year-old client in Room 122 who constantly makes sexual comments to a young student nurse. She laughs as she tells him to cut it out. Directly state the behavior that is a problem.

A = Articulate why the behavior is a problem.

Acknowledge the feelings associated with conflict, because it is emotions that escalate conflict.

R = Request a behavior change.

Avoid blaming. This would only make your client feel defensive or angry. Clearly *request that the individual change* the behavior. Rather than just stating your position, try to use some objective criteria to examine the situation. Saying, "I understand your need to…, but the hospital has a policy intended to protect all our clients" might help you talk about the situation without escalating into anger. Psychiatric units have known rules against verbal abuse, violence such as throwing objects, violence against others, and so on. You can restate these "rules" together with their known violation outcomes (medication, seclusion, manual restraint), in a calm but firm voice.

There obviously will be situations in which such a thorough assessment is not possible, but each of these variables affects the success of the confrontation. For example, a client with dementia who makes a pass at a nurse may simply be expressing a need for affection in much the same way that a small child does; this behavior needs a caring response rather than a reprimand. A 30-year-old client with all his cognitive faculties who makes a similar pass needs a more confrontational response.

Mutually generate some options for resolution. Focus on ways to resolve the problem by listing possible options. You are familiar with the "fight-or-flight" response to stress: Many people can respond to conflict only by either fighting or avoiding the problem. But brainstorming possible options and discussing pros and cons can turn the "fight" response into a more mutual "seeking a solution" mode of operations. Set mutual goals between staff and client. Every one of the health care team needs to be together, presenting a similar approach to this client.

Client readiness is vital. The behavior may need to be confronted, but the manner in which the confrontation is approached and the amount of preparation or groundwork that has been done beforehand may affect the outcome.

E = Evaluate the conflict resolution.

Encourage the client to change by stating the outcomes, the positive consequences of changing, or the negative implications for failing to change. Evaluate the degree to which the interpersonal conflict has been resolved. This depends somewhat on the nature of the conflict. Sometimes a conflict cannot be resolved in a short time, but the willingness to persevere is a good indicator of a potentially successful outcome. Accepting small goals is useful when large goal attainment is not possible. Your goal is open communication with frequent feedback leading to successful problem solving.

For a client, perhaps the strongest indicator of conflict resolution is the degree to which the client is actively engaged in activities aimed at accomplishing tasks associated with treatment goals. As the nurse, there are two questions you might want to address if modifications are necessary:

- What is the best way to establish an environment that is conducive to conflict resolution? What else needs to be considered?
- What self-care behaviors can be expected of the client if these changes are made? These need to be stated in ways that are measurable.
- Consider how to manage the case of Mr. Plotsky.

Case Example: Mr. Plotsky

Mr. Plotsky, age 29, has been employed for 6 years as a construction worker. About 4 weeks ago, while operating a forklift, he was struck by a train, leaving him paraplegic. After 2 weeks in intensive care, he was transferred to a neurologic unit. When staff members attempt to provide physical care, such as changing his position or getting him up in a chair, Mr. Plotsky throws things, curses angrily, and sometimes spits at the nurses. Staff members become very upset; several nurses have requested assignment changes. Some staff members try bribing him with food to encourage good behavior; others threaten to apply restraints. The manager schedules a behavioral consultation meeting with a psychiatric nurse or clinical specialist. The immediate goal of this staff conference is to bring staff feelings out into the open and to facilitate increased awareness of the staff's behavioral responses when confronted with this client's behavior. The outcome goal is to use a problem-solving approach to develop a behavioral care plan, so that all staff members respond to Mr. Plotsky in a consistent manner.

THE ANGER MANAGEMENT PROCESS: NURSING BEHAVIORS TO AVOID VIOLENT CLIENT BEHAVIOR

Table 13-1 details nursing behaviors to avoid violence when dealing with an angry client or family member.

MAINTAIN SELF-CONTROL

Once you identify that a client in a conflict situation may be so angry he or she could be at risk for acting out behavior or violent behavior, your initial step is to maintain your own self-control.

Early recognition is the key to preventing escalation. Illness generates feelings of powerlessness where your client may feel he or she has little control. Anger is more powerful so by focusing on their anger, clients can feel they are able to regain some control. This coping mechanism may work temporarily for the client but when you are the target of anxious or angry clients, it can be difficult. Understanding this dynamic may help you to not take their behavior personally (Rittenmeyer, 2012).

To maintain the situation you attempt to help clients reduce strong emotion to a workable level by providing a neutral, accepting, interpersonal environment. Within this context, you can acknowledge your client's emotion as a necessary component of adaptation to life. You convey acceptance of the individual's legitimate right

TABLE 13-1	Five Steps for Nursing Behaviors When Dealing with an Angry Client to Avoid Violence	
Step	**Nurse**	**Angry Client or Family Member**
1. Control self	Appear calm, relax, and take two deep breaths. Remember to talk in low tone, monotone. Focus only on defusing anger or potential for violence. Remove any necklaces, cords around neck (risk of being strangled). Do not respond to insults to self or team; do not become defensive. Avoid arguing, saying no, or hurrying.	Assess for unusually stressed individual and potential for violence. Does client appear out of control? If so, *leave!* Remember, showing your anxiety will increase the client's anxiety and anger. Reasoning with an enraged individual is impossible, *focus on de-escalation.* Devote only 3-5 minutes in attempt to de-escalate! (If it takes longer, it is not working.) Skip to last step!
2. Nonverbal body posture	Never touch an angry person. Relax facial muscles; do not smile. Assume neutral position, hands down by your side, one foot in front of the other in a relaxed posture. Stay at same eye level; try to get client to sit. If standing, do not position yourself face to face; be at an angle (so you can sidestep). Never turn your back. If standing, stay four times farther away than usual: Do not "crowd" the client; maintain space (a safe distance). Do not gesture; never point finger. Always be closest to door (so you can escape if needed).	Allow client to move around, pace (movement can help control stress). Allow client to break eye contact; avoid constant stare. Monitor client's body position; watch for escalation in gestures.
3. Verbal de-escalation discussion	Use communication skills in Box 13-3 and therapeutic skills such as active listening and paraphrasing. Introduce yourself; call the client by name while making occasional eye contact. Communicate clearly and simply. Respond in a low, calm, gentle tone of voice; do not raise voice. Avoid being defensive. Do not argue. Always be respectful. Do not dismiss any client concern but always answer request for information. Appeal to cognitive rather than emotional; help client verbalize anger. Offer to work with client to help deal with the issue. Answer selectively, ignore generalized ranting comments, and focus on just giving information requested. Set limits (empathize with underlying feeling, not with client's behavior). State clearly that violence is *not* acceptable. Give options for alternative behavior, e.g., "Let's take a break, have a [paper] cup of water."	Allow client to ventilate some of his or her anger and discuss problem. Help client identify his or her own anger, e.g., "I notice you are clenching your fists and talking more loudly than usual. These are things people do when angry. Help me understand." Help client identify the source of his anger. Have client use some relaxation technique such as deep breathing. Give permission to feel angry, but set limits on acting out and violent behavior: "It's okay to feel angry about...but not okay to act on it" or "It's natural to feel angry about...but throwing isn't okay..." Support client's attempts to control his or her feelings. Client needs to hear the consequences of his or her continued acting out behavior.

Continued

TABLE 13-1	Five Steps for Nursing Behaviors When Dealing with an Angry Client to Avoid Violence—cont'd	
Step	**Nurse**	**Angry Client or Family Member**
4. Containment	Be aware of backup resources (orderlies, call to security, etc.). You can choose to leave. Use physical restraints if necessary. Place client in seclusion or locked isolation room in psychiatric setting. Use enforced chemical restraint (medication).	Implement agency violence code. Allow or ask client to leave. Represent containment as a policy of the institution, not "I will restrain you." For some clients with brain damage or mental illness, it is appropriate to remove them from the source of their irritation to a calm environment, such as a lock room, to give them a sort of a time-out.
5. Debrief immediately: analyze and report	Reflect on incident. What can be done to prevent recurrence? Can you identify the trigger? Sometimes too long a wait, too little information, or even an insensitive or hostile comment from staff was the trigger.	After calming down, client needs assistance to reflect on alternative ways of behaving and a plan for the future.

to have feelings. Telling a client, "I'm not surprised that you are angry about…" or simply stating, "I'm sorry you are hurting so much," acknowledges the presence of an uncomfortable emotion in the client, conveys an attitude of acceptance, and encourages the client to express himself or herself. Once a feeling can be put into words, it becomes manageable because it has concrete boundaries. Remember there is a continuum:

$$\text{Anxiety} \rightarrow \text{Anger} \rightarrow \text{Aggression}$$

TALK ABOUT IT

The second strategy in defusing the strength of an emotion is to talk the emotion through with someone. For the client, this someone is often the nurse. For the nurse, this might be a nursing supervisor or a trusted colleague. Unlike complaining, the purpose of talking the emotion through is to help the person bring the feeling up to a verbal level, which helps him or her gain control. Verbalization connects him or her to connect with personal feelings surrounding the incident. If one client seems to produce certain negative emotional reactions on a nursing unit, the emotional responses may need the direct attention of all staff on the unit.

USE TENSION-REDUCING ACTIONS AND THERAPEUTIC COMMUNICATION SKILLS

The third strategy is intervention. The specific needs expressed by the emotion suggest actions that might help the client deal with his or her emotion. Convey mutual respect and avoid any "put-down" type of comment about yourself or the client. Sometimes the most effective action is simply to listen. Active listening in a conflict situation involves concentrating on what the other person is upset about. Listening can be so powerful that it alone may reduce the client's feelings of anxiety and frustration.

Physical activity can also reduce tension. For example, taking a walk can help your client control anxiety behaviors and can defuse an emotionally tense situation. If your client is so upset that he or she constitutes a danger to him- or herself or others, talk softly in a calm tone; face the client but allow maximum space and an exit for yourself should it become necessary. Many hospitals and psychiatric units have a "code word" that is used to summon trained help.

Relaxation techniques may help your client regain control. Some can be quickly taught, such as deep breathing. Humor is frequently used by nurses to engage a client or to initiate the interaction. Humor can also be used as a means of reducing tension. To paraphrase a famous advice columnist, two of the most important words in a relationship are "I apologize." And she recommended making amends immediately when you have made a mistake, because it is easier to eat crow while it is still warm. Is this advice easier to take (we will not say *swallow*) because it comes with a chuckle? Humor serves as an immediate tension reliever.

CONTAINMENT

A priority is to maintain a safe environment for yourself and all agency clients. Isolation in a locked room is standard in many psychiatric facilities, as is use of restraints and chemical mood soothers. Sometimes, maintaining safety necessitates summoning agency resources such as a critical incident response team, or security, or community police.

EVALUATION: IMMEDIATE DEBRIEFING

The final strategy is to do an evaluation of the effectiveness of responses. What was the trigger? Sometimes it is simple, such as having had to wait too long to get information or hearing an insensitive or even hostile comment from a staff person. Your goal is to apply insight toward preventing future occurrences. It is not the responsibility of any nurse to help a client resolve all conflict. Long-standing conflicts require more expertise to resolve. In such cases, refer your client to the appropriate resource.

Each step in the process may need to be taken more than once and refined or revised as circumstances dictate.

CONFLICT COMMUNICATION SKILLS

BE ASSERTIVE

Assertive communication means you convey objectives with directness, not conveying anger or frustration (Rosenberg and Gallo-Silver, 2011).

DEMONSTRATE RESPECT

Responsible, assertive statements are made in ways that do not violate the rights of others or diminish their standing. They are conveyed by a relaxed, attentive posture and a calm, friendly tone of voice. Statements should be accompanied by the use of appropriate eye contact.

USE "I" STATEMENTS

Statements that begin with "You" sound accusatory and always represent an assumption because it is impossible to know exactly, without validation, why someone acts in a certain way. Because such statements usually point a finger and imply a judgment, most people respond defensively to them.

"We" statements should be used only when you actually mean to look at an issue collaboratively. Thus the statement "Perhaps we both need to look at this issue a little closer" may be appropriate in certain situations. However, the statement, "Perhaps we shouldn't get so angry when things don't work out the way we think they should" is a condescending statement thinly disguised as a collaborative statement. What is actually being expressed is the expectation that both parties should handle the conflict in one way—the nurse's way.

Use of "I" statements are one of the most effective conflict management strategies you can use. Assertive statements that begin with "I" suggest that the person making the statement accepts full personal responsibility for his or her own feelings and position in relation to the presence of conflict. It is not necessary to justify your position unless the added message clarifies or adds essential information. "I" statements seem a little clumsy at first and take some practice. The traditional format is this:

"I feel _____ (use a name to claim the emotion you feel) when _____; (describe the behavior nonjudgmentally) because _____; (describe the tangible effects of the behavior)."

Example: "I feel uncomfortable when a client's personal problems are discussed in the cafeteria because someone might overhear confidential information."

MAKE CLEAR STATEMENTS

Statements, rather than questions, set the stage for assertive responses to conflict. When questions are used, "how" questions are best because they are neutral in nature, they seek more information, and they imply a collaborative effort. "Why" questions ask for an explanation or an evaluation of behavior and often put the other person on the defensive. It is always important to state the situation clearly; describe events or expectations objectively; and use a strong, firm, yet tactful manner. The Mr. Dixon Case shows how a nurse can use the three levels of assertive behaviors to meet the client's needs in a hospital situation without compromising the nurse's own needs for respect and dignity.

In this interaction, the nurse's position is defined several times using successively stronger statements before the shift can be made to refocus on underlying client needs. Notice that even in the final encounter, however, the nurse labels the behavior, not the client, as unacceptable. Persistence is an essential feature when first attempts at assertiveness appear too limited. After careful analysis, if you find that a client's behavior is infringing on your rights, it is essential that the issues be addressed directly in a tactful manner. If they are not, it is quite likely that the undesirable behavior will continue until you are no longer willing to tolerate it.

USE PROPER PITCH AND TONE

The amount of force used in delivery of an assertive statement depends on the nature of the conflict situation, as well as on the amount of confrontation needed to resolve the conflict successfully. Starting with the least amount of assertiveness required to meet the demands of the situation conserves energy and does not place the nurse into the bind of overkill. It is not necessary to use all of one's resources at one time or to express ideas strongly when this type of response is not needed. You can sometimes lose your effectiveness by becoming long-winded in your explanation when only a simple statement of rights or intent is needed. Long explanations detract from the true impact of the spoken message. Getting to the main point quickly and saying what is necessary in the simplest, most concrete way cuts down on the possibility of misinterpretation. This approach increases the probability that the communication will be constructively received.

Pitch and tone of voice contribute to another person's interpretation of the meaning of your assertive message. A firm but moderate presentation often is as effective as content in conveying the message. (Revisit responses to Exercise 13-2, this time analyze the tone of the verbal responses.)

CLINICAL ENCOUNTERS WITH DEMANDING, DIFFICULT CLIENTS

Every nurse encounters clients who seem overly demanding of your limited time and resources. Although this may reflect a personality characteristic, most often it is a sign of their anxiety. Box 13-1 describes behaviors that increase anger in others. Reflect on how to avoid these triggers. Conversely, ignoring inappropriate behavior does not make it go away. For example in the Mr. Gow Case, discussed earlier, the nurse's client displays inappropriate sexual suggestiveness. She could have ineffectively responded by ignoring his verbal comments, or physically avoiding him. Instead she responded assertively in a "no-nonsense" professional behavior. How would you handle it? Try out some of the more therapeutic approaches in Box 13-3 and Table 13-1. Usually we have labeled people as "difficult to deal with" when our normal way

of dealing with them has failed. So remember, we cannot change another's personality but we can change the way we react to them.

CLINICAL ENCOUNTERS WITH ANGRY CLIENTS

RECOGNIZE SIGNS OF ANGER

You can expect to encounter clients who express anger. This may take the form of refusal to comply with the treatment plan, withdrawal from any positive interaction with you, or exhibition of hostile behaviors. Hostility may be verbalized or even violent physical actions. When dealing with a difficult client, ask yourself what the client is gaining from such behavior. Some people have not learned successful communication, so they revert to behavior that has gained them something in the past. For example, as children they may have only gotten needed attention when they acted out in a negative way or when they pouted or sulked. Ask yourself if the client behaving in a difficult way is getting rewarded by becoming the focus of staff attention. Does he or she just need to learn a more effective way of communicating? Remind yourself that usually clients' feelings center on their disease or treatment and are not a reflection of their feeling about you. Nurses cited by Servodidio (2008) comment, "One of the hardest things to learn as a nurse is not to take a patient's frustration or anger personally" (p. 17).

Nonverbal clues to anger include grimacing, clenching jaws or fists, turning away, and refusing to maintain eye contact. Verbal cues by a client may, of course, include use of an angry tone of voice, but they may also be disguised as witty sarcasm or as condescending or insulting remarks. To become comfortable in dealing with client anger, the nurse must first become aware of his or her own reactions to anger so that the nurse does not threaten or reject the individual expressing anger, or respond in anger. Interventions include those listed in Table 13-1.

HELP THE CLIENT EXPRESS ANGER IN AN ACCEPTABLE MANNER

Help the client own the angry feelings by getting the client to verbalize things that make him or her angry. Acknowledging a client's anger may prevent an expression of abusive ranting. It is essential that you use empathetic statements or active listening to acknowledge the client's anger and maintain a nonthreatening demeanor *before* moving on to try to discuss the issue. Remember your goal is to maintain *safety* while helping your client.

DEFUSE HOSTILITY

Avoid responding to a client's anger by getting angry yourself. Verbal attacks follow certain rules, in that the abusive person expects you to react in specific ways. Usually people will respond by becoming aggressive and attacking back or by becoming defensive and intimidated. Keep your cool using strategies discussed earlier. Take a deep breath! Remember, if you lose control, you lose! If you become defensive, you lose! Abusive people want to provoke confrontations as a means of controlling you.

- Use empathy in your communication. An angry client needs to have you acknowledge both the issue and their feelings about that issue. Only then can the client begin to interact in a meaningful way. Deliberately begin to lower your voice and speak more slowly. When we get upset, we tend to speak quickly and use a higher tone of voice. If you do the opposite, the client may begin to mimic you and thus calm down.

REALISTICALLY ANALYZE THE CURRENT SITUATION THAT IS DISTURBING THE CLIENT

- Be assertive in setting limits. If the client persists, you need to assert limits, saying, for example, "Jim, I want to help you sort this out, but if you continue to raise your voice, I'm going to have to leave. Which do you want?" or, "Yelling at me isn't going to get this worked out. I will not argue with you. Come back when you can talk calmly and I will try to help you."
- Assist the client in developing a plan to deal with the situation (e.g., use techniques such as role-playing to help the client express anger appropriately, using "I" statements such as, "I feel angry" rather than "You make me angry"). Bringing behavior up to a verbal level should help alleviate the need for other acting out of destructive behaviors.

PREVENT ESCALATION OF CONFLICT

Depending on the type of feedback received, an intrapersonal conflict can take on interpersonal dimensions. In nurse-client confrontations, recognizing "trigger" factors, which often lead to escalation, may help in prevention. Do assess whether the client is intoxicated, disoriented, or whether there may be substance abuse.

Using respectful client-centered care approaches help prevent any escalation in interpersonal conflict. Hurt feelings or misunderstandings can quickly escalate a conflict. Keep the focus on the individual's behavior rather than on the client personally. In talking to an angry client, as the client's voice rises, lower yours. If eye contact seems confrontational, then break eye contact. If the client is acting out by throwing or hitting, set limits: "No hitting (spitting, or other physical behavior) is allowed here. Such behavior is unacceptable." If you set limits, be sure to follow through. Ask the client to verbalize his or her anger (e.g., "Talk about how you feel, instead of throwing things"). Studies show that talking will dramatically reduce aggressive behavior. Use strategies described in Table 13-1 for defusing conflict situations. Engaging in active listening (i.e., really listening to your client's viewpoint), using attentive body language, and summarizing the client's viewpoint can defuse some of the tension of the conflict.

STRATEGIES USEFUL DURING CLINICAL ENCOUNTERS WITH VIOLENT CLIENTS

Your only goal is to decrease the individual's level of rage and to protect your client and yourself.

- *Approach.* In an acute situation you **de-escalate** and **contain.** If you are in danger of mortal harm, leave! Deliberately using "calming interventions" is recommended if there is no weapon.
- *Actions.* Table 13-1 list some useful strategies for coping with angry, potentially violent individuals. Remember, your goal is to defuse the threat of violence if possible and to protect yourself and others from harm. Do not try for a rational discussion, just focus on calming interactions.
- *Reporting.* It has been estimated that a significant number of incidents go unreported, some say up to 80%. This is an international problem for nurses, and ICN urges you to report all incidents of abuse or violence.
- *Analysis.* Postincident analysis may give insight into how to prevent the next situation. Some clients have mental problems, are truly confused, or have cognitive deterioration. The Agency for Healthcare Research and Quality (AHRQ, 2014) recommends clinicians assess the client's

level of cognitive functioning when this is suspected, using the Mini-Mental State Examination (MMSE). It helps you to respond more positively if you perceive that their behavior is not "evil" but a result of their illness. *Be aware that escalating conflict can be a threat not only to your client, but to your own safety. In no case is violence acceptable.* Limits must be set. Failing this, *you need to remove yourself from a potentially harmful situation.* Starcher (1999) describes the behavior of an emotionally disturbed client admitted to a geriatric unit. Sam's behavior ranged from bullying or pushing other clients to noncompliance with his treatment. Staff tried setting clear limits and identifying specific negative outcomes, including restraints and medication, without success. Eventual successful interventions included consistent response by all staff members and using written patient contracts for each of his unacceptable behaviors. Outcomes were specifically stated for both negative behaviors (restrictions) and positive acceptable behaviors (rewards with his favorite activities).

An additional strategy for helping nurse-client problem interactions is the **staff-focused consultation**. Consider the following situation. Students are particularly prone to feeling rebuffed when they first encounter negative feedback from a client. Support from staff, instructors, and peers, coupled with efforts to understand the underlying reasons for the client's feelings, help you resist the trap of avoiding the relationship. To develop these ideas further, practice.

DEFUSING POTENTIAL CONFLICTS WHEN PROVIDING HOME HEALTH CARE

Recognizing potential situations lending themselves to conflict is, of course, an important initial step. Caregivers have been shown to experience conflict through incompatible pressures suffered between caregiver demands and demands from their other roles, such as parenting their children or maintaining employment. In addition to this inter-role conflict, caregivers suffer pressures when a nurse comes into their home to participate in the care of an ill relative. A Canadian study of home health nurses and family caregivers of elderly relatives identified four evolving stages in the nurse-caregiver relationship. The initial stage is "worker-helper," with the nurse providing care

to the ill client and the family helping. Next comes "worker-worker," when the nurse begins teaching the needed care skills to family members. Third is "nurse as manager; family as worker," as the family members learn needed care skills. The final stage, "nurse as nurse for family caregiver," occurs as the family member becomes exhausted (Butt, 2000). A source of conflict for nurses was the dual expectation of the family that the nurse would provide care not only for the identified client but also provide relief for the exhausted primary caregiver. When the nurse operated as manager and treated the caregiver as worker, the discrepancy in expectations and values resulted in increased tension in the relationship. Discussion of role expectations is essential. Because of the high cost of providing direct care to chronically ill clients, home health nurses may be expected to quickly shift to teaching the necessary skills to the family members. You can clarify that this shift in responsibility results in a reduction of expensive professional time but not in your commitment to the family.

SUMMARY

Conflict represents a struggle between two opposing thoughts, feelings, or needs. It can be intrapersonal in nature, deriving from within a particular individual; or interpersonal, when it represents a clash between two or more people. This chapter focused on conflict between nurse and client or client's family.

All conflicts have certain things in common: a concrete content problem issue and relationship issues arising from the process of expressing the conflict. Generally, intrapersonal conflicts stimulate feelings of emotional discomfort. Strategies to defuse strong emotion were highlighted. Most interpersonal conflicts involve some threat, either to one's sense of power to control an interpersonal situation or to ways of thinking about the self. Giving up ineffective behavior patterns in conflict situations is difficult; such patterns are generally perceived to be safer because they are familiar.

Behavioral responses to conflict situations fall into five styles. In the past, nurses most commonly choose avoidance. However, this chapter describes other strategies (e.g., assertion) that have been more successfully used by nurses to manage client-nurse conflicts. Assertive behaviors range from making a simple statement, directly and honestly, about one's beliefs, to taking a very strong, confrontational stand about what will and will not be tolerated.

The principles of conflict management were described. To apply conflict management principles, you need to identify your own conflictive feelings or reactions. For internal conflict, feelings usually have to be put into words and related to the issue at hand before the meaning of the conflict becomes understandable. In conflict between nurse and client, you need to think through the possible causes of the conflict, as well as your own feelings, before making a response. To resolve these kinds of conflict, you need to use "I" statements and respond assertively. Chapter 13 also discussed workplace violence and strategies to maintain or restore a safe environment.

ETHICAL DILEMMA | What Would You Do?

You are caring for Kim, born at the gestational age of 24 weeks in a rural hospital and transferred this morning to your neonatal intensive care unit. Today her father arrives on the unit. Seeing you taking a blood sample from one of the many intravenous lines attached to Kim, he yells at you to "Stop poking at her! What are you trying to prove by keeping her alive? Turn off those machines." This is both a communication problem and an ethics problem. How do you respond to his anger?

DISCUSSION QUESTIONS

1. Pick a tone and pitch listed in Exercise 13-2 and describe its effect on a conflict situation.
2. How would you de-escalate a conflict resulting from a behavior listed in Box 13-1?

REFERENCES

American Association of Critical Care Nurses (AACN): *Position Statement: Workplace Violence Prevention.* http://www.aacn.org/wd/practice/docs/publicpolicy/workplace_violence.pdf, 2004.

American Nurses Association (ANA): *House of Delegates Resolution of Workplace Violence.* www.nursingworld.org, 2012.

American Nurses Association (ANA): *Preventing workplace violence,* Washington D.C., 2002, Author.

Butt G: Nurses and family caregivers of elderly relatives engaged in 4 evolving types of relationships, *Evid Based Nurs* 3:134, 2000.

Finke EH, Light J, Kitko L, et al.: A systematic review of the effectiveness of nurse communication with patients with complex communication needs with a focus on the use of argumentative and alternative communication, *J Clin Nurs* 17(16):2102–2115, 2008.

Guidroz AM, Wang M, Perez LM: Developing a model of source-specific interpersonal conflict in health care, *Stress Health* 28:69–79, 2012.

U.S. Department of Health and Human Services: *Healthy People 2020: Injury and Violence Prevention.* www.healthypeople.gov/2020/topicsobjectives2020/overview.aspx?topicid=24, 2014.

International Council of Nurses (ICN): Violence: A Worldwide Epidemic. www.icn.ch/images/stories/documents/publication/position_statements/CO1_Abuse_Violence_Nsg_Personnel.pdf.

Iglesias ME, Vallejo R: Conflict resolution styles in the nursing profession, *Contemp Nurs* 43(1):73–80, 2012.

The Joint Commission (TJC): *Sentinel Event Alert, Issue 45: Preventing Violence in the health care setting.* or www.jointcommission.org/sentinel_event_alert_issue_45_preventing_violence_in_the_healthcaresetting/, 2010. http://www.jointcommission.org/assets/1/18/SEA_45.PDF, 2010. Accessed 7/13/14.

McElhaney R: Conflict management in nursing administration, *Nurs Manag* 27(3):49–50, 1996.

U.S Department of Labor Occupational Safety and Health Administration (OSHA): *Guidelines for preventing workplace violence for health care and social service workers,* OSHA 3148-01R 2004. https://www.osha.gov/OshDoc/data_General_Facts/factsheet-workplace-violence.pdf/, 2004. Accessed 7/11/14.

Papadopoulos C, Bowers L, Quirk A, Khanom H: Events preceding changes in conflict and containment rates on acute psychiatric wards, *Psychiatr Serv* 63(1):40–47, 2012. http://dx.doi.org/10.1176/appi.ps.201000480.

QSEN International. www.qsen.org.

Riley JB: *Communication in nursing,* ed 7, St. Louis, MO, 2012, Mosby/Elsevier Inc.

Rittenmeyer L: Assessment of risk for in-hospital suicide and aggression in high-dependency care environments, *Crit Care Nurs Clin North Am* 24(1):41–51, 2012. http://dx.doi.org/10.1016/j.ccell.2012.01.002.

Rosenberg S, Gallo-Silver L: Therapeutic communication skills and student nurses in the clinical setting, *Teach Learn Nurs* 6:2–8, 2011.

Sargeant J, MacLeod T, Murray A: An interprofessional approach to teaching communication skills, *J Contin Educ Health Prof* 31(4):265–267, 2011.

Sayer MM, McNeese-Smith D, Leach LS, Phillips LR: An educational intervention to increase 'speaking-up' behaviors in nurses and improve patient safety, *J Nurs Care Qual* 27(2):154–160, 2012.

Servodidio CA: Nurses discuss working with challenging patients, *ONS Connect* 23(3):17, 2008.

Starcher S: Sam was an emotional terrorist, *Nursing* 99(2):40–41, 1999.

Agency for Healthcare Research and Quality (AHRQ): Guide to Clinical Preventive Services, 2014: Recommendations of the U.S. Preventive Services Task Force. http://www.ahrq.gov/professionals/clinicians-providers/guidelines-recommendations/guide/index.html.

Waschgler K, Ruiz-Hernandez JA, Llor-Esteban B, Garcia-Izquierdo M: Patients' aggressive behaviours towards nurses: Development and psychometric properties of the hospital aggressive behaviour scale-users, *J Adv Nurs* 69(6):1418–1427, 2013.

Zeller A, Dassen T, Kok G, Needham I, Halfens RJ: Factors associated with resident aggression, *J Nurs Scholarsh* 44(3):249–257, 2012.

Communicating to Encourage Health Literacy, Health Promotion, and Prevention of Disease

Elizabeth C. Arnold

OBJECTIVES

At the end of the chapter, the reader will be able to:

1. Define concepts related to health promotion and disease prevention.
2. Identify national agendas for health promotion and disease prevention.
3. Specify relevant conceptual frameworks for health promotion actions.
4. Apply health promotion and disease prevention strategies for individuals.
5. Apply health promotion and disease prevention strategies at the community level.
6. Explain the role of health literacy in health promotion and disease prevention strategies.

Chapter 14 focuses on the role of health promotion and disease prevention in quality health care. Included are conceptual frameworks related to health promotion at individual and community levels. The chapter addresses social determinants of health and health literacy as underlying challenges to health promotion and disease prevention efforts. Applications of communication strategies designed to help clients and targeted populations achieve a better health quality of life through education and lifestyle changes are presented.

BASIC CONCEPTS

Health care reform is creating rapid and profound changes that dramatically impact how care is delivered, where it is delivered, and what its focus should be. Litchfield and Jonsdottir (2008) note the nation's new health care focus "is about changing the culture of health systems from a curative/reactive to a preventive/responsive orientation" (p. 81). Health promotion and disease prevention with special attention paid to the underlying causes of health problems is increasingly recognized as a legitimate, reimbursable, *and* essential component of comprehensive health care.

DEFINITIONS

From a health promotion perspective, health includes "being able to function normally, experiencing well-being, and having a healthy lifestyle" (Fagerlind et al., 2010, p. 104). It is considered a fundamental human right, intimately tied to a nation's social and economic development (*Jakarta Declaration*; World Health Organization [WHO], 1997). Factors such as genetics, environment, and social circumstances influence health (IOM, 2012). Other issues, for example, availability of health services, new research findings, even opportunity and luck also influence health.

Health promotion activities empower clients, families and communities with the knowledge, skills, and confidence needed to engage in healthy behaviors. ***Health promotion*** is defined as "the process of enabling individuals to take control over their health" (WHO, 1986). Health promotion encompasses a wide range of activities provided in a variety of community-based settings:

- Health education
- Preventive health services
- Advocacy and public policies

- Safeguarding environmental health
- Community-based education, for example schools, work sites, vulnerable populations, media

In practice, health promotion and disease prevention strategies complement and reinforce each other's effectiveness. Nurses are in a unique position to help clients understand the importance of consistent health habits, such as a balanced diet, regular exercise, preventive health screening, and a strong support system to living a longer healthier life.

Disease prevention focuses on actions that reduce or eliminate the onset, progression, complications, or recurrence of disease. ***Disease prevention*** is concerned with identifying modifiable risk and protective factors associated with diseases and disorders, and using this knowledge as a basis for corrective action. The goal of disease prevention is to help individuals "avoid the occurrence of a disease, disorder, or injury, to slow the progression of detectable disease and/or reduce its consequences" (WHO, 1997).

Risk and protective factors represent personal or environmental characteristics, which increase the probability of having a health problem (risk factor), or decrease the probability of its occurrence or progression (protective factor). For example, if a person is obese, eats many carbohydrates, and leads a sedentary life, these risk factors increase the probability of having a heart attack. Causal risk factors and social determinants of health play a major role in the onset and progression of emergent chronic disorders (Zubialde et al., 2009).

Many risk factors are modifiable. Clients at risk for diabetes can adjust their diet, maintain regular exercise, and monitor carbohydrate intake. Smoking, overeating and excessive alcohol consumption are associated with a range of chronic disorders, including cancer. Regular screenings can catch treatable health problems such as osteoporosis, high blood pressure and glaucoma. Those that cannot be modified may have less impact with regular screenings to catch potential treatable client problems early and encouragement of healthy lifestyles. For example, those with a genetic predisposition to chronic diseases, such as obesity, heart disease, or diabetes can reduce the impact of inherited risk factors by actively embracing habits of healthy eating patterns, adequate sleep and an active lifestyle.

Protective factors are defined as behavioral activities that have been shown to delay the emergence of chronic disease or lessen its impact. While protective factors do not guarantee a life without serious illness or early death, they play a significant role in helping clients improve their quality of life. Protective factors include developing healthy lifestyle habits, daily exercise, healthy diet, annual checkups, available support systems, health insurance etc. Health education, social marketing, and screening services help people recognize health risk factors.

Lifestyle

Milio (1976) defines **lifestyle** as "patterns of choices made from the alternatives that are available to people according to their socioeconomic circumstances and the ease with which they are able to choose certain ones over others" (quoted in Cody, 2006, p. 186). Components of a healthy lifestyle include: eating healthy meals, staying active with adequate exercise, getting adequate sleep, managing stress, building supportive relationships, and nurturing one's spirit.

Ideally, building a healthy lifestyle begins in childhood. As Frederick Douglass (BrainyQuote.com, n.d.) noted years ago, "It is easier to build strong children than to repair broken men." Nurses also serve as role models. And, they have more credibility in advocating for healthy lifestyles if they practice what they preach.

Social Determinants of Health

Social, economic, and political factors, embedded at community and larger society levels, have a significant effect on health and well-being (DHHS, 2010b). ***Social determinants of health*** is a term used to identify a wide range of contextual factors influencing the health and well-being of individuals, and communities. Although each person enters the world with a distinct set of constitutional factors, size, gender, intellect, and personality, they grow up within social and community networks and absorb community social values. A person's environment interacts with individual variables to influence, enhance, or limit health behaviors. Larger social community systems create roles and expectations that shape and modify personal health behaviors. Not everyone has the same opportunities or protective factors to encourage and safeguard their health and well-being. People living in poverty may lack the opportunity to make healthy behavior choices or to pay for medical care even if they desire to do so. ***Health disparities*** is the term used to describe causal preventable differences in adverse health outcomes and lost opportunities to achieve optimal health and well-being.

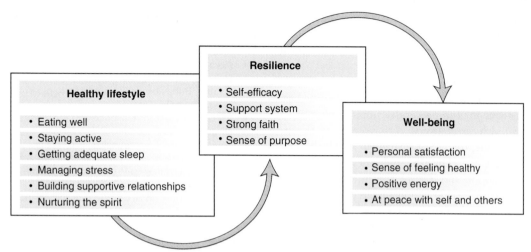

Figure 14-1   Critical elements for maintaining health and well-being.

They are related to **health equity**, defined as environmental circumstances offering all community members equal health resources to achieve their full health potential (CCLHO-CHEAC, 2013). Nationally, disparities account for significant variances in life expectancy, positive health outcomes, and the incidence of chronic disease and disability. Social determinants associated with health disparities include social isolation, cultural factors, access and availability of services, finances, lack of knowledge or education, food or job security, language barriers, health literacy, and poverty. Social determinants critically impact health, morbidity, and mortality, as "treatment alone is unlikely to have marked effects on health inequities or health status" (Frankish et al., 2006, p. 271). *Healthy People 2020*, and the Centers for Disease Control and Prevention (CDC) (2006) identify health disparities as a fundamental health concern, requiring immediate concentrated attention.

Well-being

Health promotion activities incorporate the WHO concept of an inseparable construct of health and well-being. **Well-being** is defined as a person's subjective experience of satisfaction about his or her life related to six personal dimensions: intellectual, physical, emotional, social, occupational, and spiritual (Edlin and Golanty, 2009). People experience well-being as being at peace with themselves and others even with a serious health problem or terminal diagnosis if they have hope and appropriate support (Saylor, 2004).

A challenge in contemporary health care is helping people understand the close connection between *consistent* positive lifestyle behaviors and habits and overall health and well-being. Fundamental changes in health habits and modifications in lifestyle typically improve health and well-being. Figure 14-1 displays critical elements for maintaining health and well-being.

GLOBAL AND NATIONAL HEALTH PROMOTION AGENDAS

Improving the quality of health promotion and disease prevention is a national and global health care reform initiative (Hogg et al., 2009). As you read through this section, note the similar themes in virtually all national and global agenda goals. Individually and collectively, these reports bear strong testament to the need for effective health preventive services. Strong recommendations appear about the need to explore the close interaction between personal, environmental, and social determinants of health and well-being and provide equal opportunity for quality health care. In 1986 the WHO *Ottawa Charter for Health Promotion* documented essential prerequisites and resources needed for health promotion as "peace, shelter, education, food, income, a stable ecosystem, sustainable resources, social justice, and equity" (WHO, 1986). The Charter outlined principles and functions of health promotion and identified prerequisites for improving health as:

1. Advocacy for health
2. Enabling equal opportunities and resources for people to achieve health

3. Mediation and coordinated action shared by community groups, health service agencies, and governments targeted toward the pursuit of health

In 2001 the Institute of Medicine (IOM)'s landmark report on the health of the nation identified six areas of focus for comprehensive improvement at all levels of health care delivery.

Each decade, the U.S. Department of Health and Human Services (DHHS) publishes an updated health promotion and disease prevention agenda for the nation with specific national goals and objectives. The fourth document of its kind, *Healthy People 2020* offers a natural continuation of earlier *Healthy People* initiatives, with a distinct focus on the social determinants and environmental factors contributing to the health status of individuals and populations. Its vision is to have "a society in which all people live long, healthy lives" (DHHS, 2010a). Proposed goals include:

- Eliminate preventable disease, disability, injury, and premature death.
- Achieve health equity, eliminate disparities, and improve the health of all groups.
- Create social and physical environments that promote good health for all.
- Promote healthy development and healthy behaviors across every stage of life.

Topic areas proposed to achieve these goals (Box 14-1) provide direction for what needs to be done, with focused strategies for each topic area. Objectives are organized in three categories—interventions, determinants, and outcomes. *Healthy People 2020* reinforces the importance of social determinants as critical antecedents that influence health and well-being. There is a specific goal related to "ideas of health equity that address social determinants of health and promote health across all stages of life. More information about specific recommendations is available at (www.healthy people.gov/HP2020).

The *Jakarta Declaration on Health Promotion* (WHO, 1997) is a global initiative, which recommended the following to enhance health and well-being:

- Building healthy public policy
- Creating supportive environments for health
- Strengthening community action for health
- Developing personal skills
- Reorienting health services

Passage of the Patient Protection and Affordable Care Act (2010) provides for specific coverage of preventive

---

| BOX 14-1 | *Healthy People 2020:* Topic Areas with Health Indicators |

- **Access to Care:** Proportion of people with access to health care services
- **Healthy Behavior:** Proportion of people engaged in healthy behaviors
- **Chronic Disease:** Prevalence and mortality of chronic disease
- **Environmental Determinants;** Proportion of people with a healthy physical environment
- **Social Determinants:** Proportion of people with a healthy social environment
- **Injury:** Proportion of people that experiences injury
- **Mental Health:** Proportion of people experiencing positive mental health
- **Maternal and Infant Health:** Proportion of healthy births
- **Responsible Sexual Behavior:** Proportion of people engaged in responsible sexual behavior
- **Substance Abuse:** Proportion of people engaged in substance abuse
- **Tobacco:** Proportion of people using tobacco
- **Quality of Care:** Proportion of people receiving quality health care services.

Adapted from: U.S. Department of Health and Human Services: *Leading health indicators for Healthy People 2020: letter report.* 2011. Available online: http://iom.edu/Reports/2011/Leading-Health-Indicators-for-Healthy-People-2020.aspx. Accessed September 7, 2013.

---

care. Mandatory health risk assessment requirements during subsidized annual comprehensive physical examinations for medicare recipients reinforce the primacy of health promotion and disease prevention as an essential component of contemporary health care. Kushner and Sorenson (2013) suggest that *"lifestyle medicine"* may represent a new disciplinary approach for the management of chronic illness and disease prevention.

THEORY-BASED FRAMEWORKS

Theory frameworks for health promotion examine how people make choices and decisions about their health. Pender's health promotion model, Prochaska's transtheoretical model, and Bandura's social learning theory are useful frameworks to guide health promotion strategies.

Pender's Health Promotion Model

A person's capacity to absorb and use health promotion information depends to a large degree on what

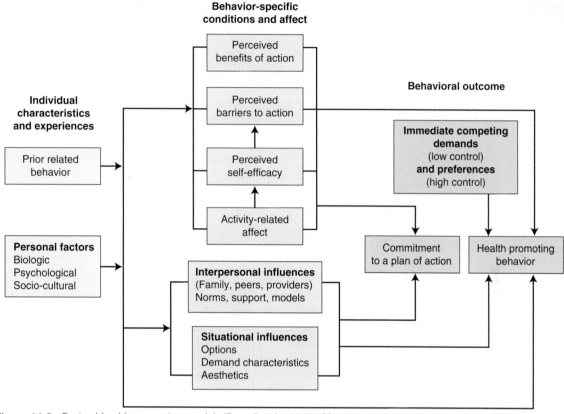

Figure 14-2   Revised health promotion model. *(From Pender N: Health promotion in nursing practice, ed 6, Upper Saddle River, NJ, 2011, Prentice Hall, p. 45.)*

people believe about their health and the extent to which their personal actions (self-efficacy) will produce positive outcomes. Health promotion interventions target behavioral change. Nurses use Nola Pender's revised health belief model to understand what motivates people to engage in personal health behaviors. The model expands on an earlier health belief model developed by Rosenstock and his associates in the 1950s. The model (Figure 14-2) proposes that a person's willingness to engage in health promotion behaviors is best understood through examining personal beliefs about the nature and seriousness of a health condition and the person's capacity to influence its outcome.

Pender's model identifies perceived benefits, barriers, and ability to take action related to health and well-being as important components of people's health decision making. The dynamics act as internal or external "cues to action," which influence a person's decision to seek health care and engage in health-promoting

activities. Cues to action include required school immunizations, interpersonal reminders, past experiences with the health care system, the mass media, and ethnic approval.

Case Example

Mary Nolan knows that walking will help diminish her risk for developing osteoporosis, but the threat of potentially having this problem in her 60s is not sufficient to motivate her to take action in her 40s. Mary does not feel any signs or symptoms of the disorder, and it is easier to maintain a sedentary lifestyle. The nurse will have to understand the client's internal value system and other factors that influence readiness to learn to create the most appropriate learning conditions and types of teaching strategies Mary will need to effect positive change in health habits.

Exercise 14-1, Pender's Health Promotion Model, provides practice with applying this model to common health problems.

EXERCISE 14-1   Pender's Health Promotion Model

Purpose: To help students understand the value of the health promotion model in assessing and promoting healthy lifestyles.

Procedure
1. Using the health promotion model as a guide, interview a person in the community about his or her perception of a common health problem (e.g., heart disease, high cholesterol, osteoporosis, breast or prostate cancer, obesity, or diabetes).
2. Record the person's answers in written diagram form following Pender's model of health promotion. Identify the behavior-specific cognitions and affect action that would best fit the person's situation.

3. Share your findings with your classmates, either in a small group of four to six students with a scribe to share common themes with the larger class or in the general class.

Discussion
1. Were you surprised by anything the client said, his or her perception of the problem, or interpretation of its meaning?
2. As you compare your findings with other classmates, do common themes emerge?
3. How could you use the information you obtained from this exercise in future health care situations?

TRANSTHEORETICAL MODEL OF CHANGE

Prochaska's transtheoretical model is an evidence-based model used to explore a person's motivational readiness to intentionally change health habits (Daley et al., 2009; Prochaska and Norcross, 2013). The model identifies stages of readiness ranging from lack of awareness or acknowledgement of a problem, to taking and maintaining constructive actions to correct unhealthy behaviors. Table 14-1 presents Prochaska's stage model with suggested approaches for each stage and corresponding sample statements.

In the *precontemplation* stage, a person either does not see a health problem, (even though it may be obvious to others), or does not have any intention of modifying it in the foreseeable future. The *contemplation* stage is characterized by an awareness of a problem. The person is thinking of change, but is still ambivalent and lacks a strong commitment to take action. Prochaska and Norcross (2013) refer to contemplation as "knowing where you want to go, but not being quite ready to go there" (p. 460). In the *preparation* stage, a person begins to take small tentative steps toward changing difficult health habits, but is not fully committed to consistent action. An important component in the preparation stage is goal and priority setting. The *action* stage is marked by a strong commitment to change and taking consistent definitive actions to make behavioral changes a reality. A *maintenance* stage in which clients stabilize and consolidate gains achieved during the action stage follows. This is an important stage. It is not easy to maintain behaviors once the newness has worn off. Clients can

easily relapse and may need to recycle through previous stages several times before a new health behavior is firmly established. Relapses are treated as temporary setbacks, which can be used to identify triggers and high-risk situations.

The transtheoretical model does not represent a linear paradigm. Long-standing habits are hard to break. Clients may cycle through one or more stages several times before a permanent change takes place. Setbacks and relapse with return to old behaviors can be expected; they should be treated as an opportunity to learn from the experience, rather than as a failure. Exercise 14-2, Assessing Readiness Using Prochaska's Model, provides an opportunity to work with the transtheoretical model.

Social Learning Theory

Bandura's (1997) contribution to the study of health promotion is his concept of self-efficacy. He believed that *self-efficacy*, described as a personal belief in one's ability to execute the actions required to achieve a goal, is a powerful mediator of behavior and behavioral change.

Self-efficacy has particular relevance when people are contemplating change, but have not yet taken needed actions. If people know they have the capacity to complete a health-promoting behavior and/or have support, they are more likely to try. Self-efficacy and **motivation** are reciprocal processes; increased self-efficacy strengthens motivation, which, in turn increases the client's capacity to complete the learning task. Providing support at critical junctions can improve

TABLE 14-1	Prochaska's Stages of Change with Suggested Approaches and Sample Statements Applied to Alcoholism		
Stage	**Characteristic Behaviors**	**Suggested Approach**	**Sample Statement**
Precontemplation	Client does not think there is a problem; not considering the possibility of change.	Raise doubt; give informational feedback to raise awareness of a problem and health risks.	"Your lab tests show liver damage. These tests can be predictive of serious health problems and premature death."
Contemplation	Client thinks there may be a problem; thinking about change; goes back and forth between concern and unconcern.	Tip the balance; allow open discussion of pros and cons of changing behavior; build motivation for change; help client justify a positive commitment.	"It sounds as though you think you may have a drinking problem, but are not sure you are an alcoholic. What would your life be like without alcohol?"
Preparation	Client decides there is a problem and is willing to make a change: "I guess I do need to stop drinking."	Help the client choose the best course of action to take in resolving the problem.	"What kinds of changes will you need to make to stop drinking? Most people find Alcoholics Anonymous (AA) helpful as a support. Have you heard of them?"
Action	Client engages in concrete actions to effect needed change.	Help the client take active steps to resolve health problem; review progress; give feedback.	"I am impressed that you went to two AA meetings this week and have not had a drink either. What has this been like for you?"
Maintenance	Client perseveres with positive behavioral change.	Help client identify and use strategies to sustain progress; point out positive changes; accept temporary setbacks and use steps in preparation phase, if needed.	"It's hard to let go of old habits, but you have been abstinent for 3 months now, and your liver tests are significantly improved."

EXERCISE 14-2   **Assessing Readiness Using Prochaska's Model**

Purpose: To identify elements in teaching that can promote readiness using Prochaska's Model.

Procedure
Identify as many specific answers as possible to the following questions:
1. Patrick drinks four to six beers every evening. Last year he lost his job. He has a troubled marriage and few friends. Patrick does not consider himself an alcoholic and blames his chaotic marriage for his need to drink. There is a strong family history of alcoholism. What kinds of information might help Patrick want to learn more about his condition?

2. Lily has just learned she has breast cancer. Although there is a good chance that surgery and chemotherapy will help her, she is scared to commit to the process and has even talked about taking her life. What kinds of health-teaching strategies and information might help Lily become ready to learn about her condition?
3. Shawn has just been diagnosed as having epilepsy. He is ashamed to tell his friends and teachers about his condition. Shawn is considering breaking up with his girlfriend because of his newly diagnosed illness. How would you use health teaching to help Shawn cope more effectively with his illness?

motivation and beliefs in one's ability to master essential tasks. Mastery is considered to be the strongest outcome of self-efficacy (Srof and Velsor-Friedrich, 2006).

Bandura considers learning to be a social process. He identifies three sets of motivating factors that promote the learning necessary to achieve a predetermined goal: physical motivators, social incentives, and cognitive motivators. *Physical motivators* can be internal, such as memory of previous discomfort or a symptom that the client cannot ignore. *Social incentives*, such as praise and encouragement, increase self-esteem and give the client reason to continue learning. Bandura refers to a third set of motivators as *cognitive motivators*, describing them as internal thought processes associated with change.

In the following case example, the nurse combines the concept of a physical motivator with a social incentive related to something the client values (his grandson), and relates the process to the desired outcome. The intervention is designed to help Francis recognize how changes in his health behavior can not only improve his health and well-being but give him a social outlet that could be important to him.

Case Example

Nurse: I'm worried that you are continuing to smoke, because it affects your breathing. There is nothing you can do about the damage to your lungs that is already there, but if you stop smoking it can help preserve the healthy tissue you still have (*physical motivator*) and you won't have as much trouble breathing. I bet your grandson would appreciate it if you could breathe better and be able to play with him (*social incentive*). As Francis notices that he is coughing less when he gives up smoking, this new perceptual knowledge can act as an internal *cognitive motivator* to remain abstinent.

DISEASE PREVENTION

Disease prevention frameworks are concerned with identifying modifiable risk and protective factors associated with specific diseases and mental disorders. Nurses use case finding strategies to identify individuals and families with risk factors in health care situations. Once specific risk factors are identified, you informally can help client identify behaviors, such as regular physical exercise, proper nutrition, balanced lifestyle, and regular checkups. Three tiers of prevention—primary, secondary, and tertiary—represent a continuum of disease prevention focus.

- *Primary prevention* strategies emphasize taking proactive actions that can prevent targeted conditions. They target modifiable risk factors with health education to promote a healthy lifestyle, for example, promoting exercise and diet as ways to prevent obesity and diabetes. Other examples include immunizations; low-cost flu shots; safe sex counseling; smoking cessation; use of car seats, seat belts, and motorcycle helmets; and bans on texting while driving. Advocacy for these health protections is easily incorporated into ordinary nursing care.
- *Secondary prevention* strategies focus on early disease detection through regular health screenings for prostate cancer, osteoporosis, and diabetes; regular mammograms and pap smears for women; periodic colonoscopies; and blood pressure screenings. Individuals with known risk factors such as family history, high cholesterol, elevated blood sugar, high blood pressure, and age should be screened periodically. With early case finding, the emergence, or course of a chronic disease can be modified to allow a stronger quality of life. Screening for mental health problems during the course of primary care visits can detect undiagnosed depression, anxiety, and substance abuse.
- *Tertiary prevention* strategies focus on minimizing the damaging effects of a disease or injury once it occurs. Preventing complications and helping people achieve their highest quality of life regardless of their health circumstances is the goal of tertiary health promotion strategies.

Exercise 14-3, Developing a Health Profile, provides an opportunity to look at your own risk factors.

Developing an Evidence-Based Practice

Rothpletz-Puglia P, Jones VM, Storm DS, Parrott JS, O'Brien, KA: Building social networks for health promotion: Shout-out Health, New Jersey, 2011, *Prev Chronic Dis.* 10:E147, 2013.

Background: This exploratory study examined the impact of preventive health information developed by community members and disseminated through informal social networks to community members living in poverty areas. Preparation of the group was based on empowerment education principles. Included was discussion about how the participants would provide health promotion in the community, development of personal action plans, and tracking plans for health promotion community member encounters.

Method: Inclusion criteria for the project study included English-speaking adult woman recruited from the community agency client data base of women at risk for, or living with, human immunodeficiency virus (HIV) infection. Sixty-five women from the two cities agreed to participate, with 87% completing pre- and post-test questionnaires. Participants provided health promotion activities for 6 weeks. Descriptive statistics, t tests, and nonparametric tests were used to examine changes and group differences in pre- and posttest scores.

Results: The health promotion strategy reached 5861 people in two cities. Health promotion activities developed and delivered through informal social networks had the advantage of meeting people where they lived and congregated. The project empowered the participants' self-awareness and increased their self-efficacy. However, no significant changes were noted between pre- and postprogram scores.

Application to your clinical practice: Nurses need to be intimately involved in the development of relevant creative public health approaches. This study shows that at-risk community members can successfully provide relevant health promotion materials through informal social networks. They also can personally benefit from the process of developing relevant information.

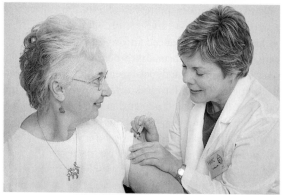

Figure 14-4   Immunizations are an important component of disease prevention. *(From James Gathany, Centers for Disease Control and Prevention [CDC], 2006.)*

APPLICATIONS

The American Association of Colleges of Nursing (AACN, 2008) declares that "Health promotion, disease, and injury prevention across the lifespan are essential elements of baccalaureate nursing practice at the individual and population levels" (p 23). The goal of health promotion and disease prevention strategies is to improve individual health and prevent disease. Health promotion interventions involve an interactive process designed to enable people to have greater control over the determinants of personal health and well-being. Interventions should demonstrate a sensitive appraisal and choice of targeted strategies.

EXERCISE 14-3	Developing a Health Profile

Purpose: To help students understand the relationship between lifestyle health assessment factors and related health goals from a personal perspective.

Procedure

Out-of-class assignment:
1. Assess your own personal risk factors related to each of the following:
   a. Family risk factors (diabetes, cardiac, cancer, osteoporosis)
   b. Diet and nutrition
   c. Exercise habits
   d. Weight
   e. Alcohol and drug use
   f. Safe sex practices
   g. Perceived level of stress
   h. Health screening tests: cholesterol, blood pressure, blood sugar

2. Identify unhealthy behaviors or risk factors
3. Develop a personalized action plan to identify strategies to address areas that need strengthening.
4. Identify any barriers that might prevent you from achieving your personal goals.

Discussion
1. In small groups, discuss findings that you feel comfortable sharing with others.
2. Get input from others about ways to achieve health-related goals.
3. In the larger group, discuss how doing this exercise can inform your practice related to lifestyle changes and health promotion.

Health promotion strategies should be a part of everyday nursing care (Beckford-Ball, 2006). Education can be introduced informally as you provide care, or presented formally through client education, screening programs, and social media. A person-centered health promotion education format considers personal values and beliefs and perceptions of personal ability to achieve health behavior changes (self-efficacy) as part of client assessment. Socioeconomic factors, level of education, age, and social networks are important considerations in understanding client preferences and working with clients to enable them to make the changes needed for a healthy lifestyle (Ochieng, 2006). Nurses need to be public advocates as well as care agents of health promotion. They can be influential in helping communities create supportive health environments. Nurses are perceived as trustworthy informants about health matters because of their close links to clients and families. They can serve on health-related community advisory committees and encourage agencies to include greater input from caregivers and clients in care and funding discussions (Hawranik and Strain, 2007).

HEALTH EDUCATION FOR HEALTH PROMOTION

Health education is an essential component of effective health promotion and disease prevention strategies (Hoving et al., 2010). Mol and colleagues (2010) note that good care involves "persistent tinkering in a world full of complex ambivalence and shifting tensions" (p. 14). Clients requiring the same educational information can demonstrate a wide range of learning, cognitive, experiential, and communication diversity. They differ in intellectual curiosity, learning preferences, motivation for learning, learning styles, and rate of learning, each of which will require adaptations to maximize learning. This is where the art of nursing comes in, to guide nurses in selecting strategies with meaning for their clients.

Health promotion learner activities need to be safe, timely, effective, patient-centered, equitable, and efficient. Programs should be designed to empower clients through an emphasis on the active role of the client as a stakeholder and a collaborative partner in all aspects of the health promotion process. Common examples of general health promotion education topics include developing a healthy lifestyle, good nutrition, regular

physical activity, adequate sleep patterns, and stress reduction.

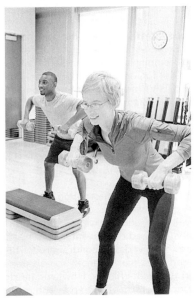

Regular health habits of balanced diet, consistent exercise, preventive health screening, and a strong support system can contribute to a longer healthier life. *(From Amanda Mills, Centers for Disease Control and Prevention [CDC], 2011.)*

Formal and informal instruction can focus on condition-specific topics. A wide variety of topics lend themselves to a health promotion focus. A sampling includes

- Alcohol, nicotine, and other drug abuse prevention
- Anger management
- Prevention and early detection of common chronic diseases such as human immunodeficiency virus (HIV), diabetes, cancer, heart disease, osteoporosis, co-occurring disorders
- Safe sex practices
- Stress reduction for informal caregivers and organizational work sites
- Healthy dietary practices
- Need for regular exercise habits
- Value of available support systems

HEALTH PROMOTION STRATEGIES FOR INDIVIDUALS

An overarching goal of health promotion for individuals is to develop a better health-related quality of life. To achieve this goal, people must want to change behaviors that compromise their health. Health promotion thinking must be responsive to particular situations, as universal applications may not be appropriately sensitive to social or economic factors, which are important to an individual or target population (Carter et al., 2011). For example, attempts to help clients modify food choices and engage in physical activity have different meanings for various cultural and socioeconomic groups. Incorporating client preferences and cultural understandings is an essential component of effective health promotion strategies. Miller and Rollnick (2013) assert "when you understand what people value you have a key to what motivates them" (p 75). People put energy into actions they believe are critical to their wellbeing. Clinical approaches to promote healthy behaviors with individuals include motivational interviewing,(MI), empowerment, social support, and education.

Motivational Interviewing

Motivational interviewing (MI) represents an evidence-based clinical application originally developed by Miller and Rollnick, (2013). A motivational framework to change unhealthy behaviors is based on a person's values, beliefs, and preferences, and fits well with concepts of client-centered care (Sandelowski et al., 2008). It is based on, and is "theoretically congruent" with the transtheoretical model of behavior change (Goodwin et al., 2009, p. 204). Originally conceptualized for use in the treatment of alcoholism, the MI framework is used with a growing range of chronic health conditions, such as diabetes or obesity, exacerbated by unhealthy lifestyle behaviors (Carels et al., 2007; Kirk et al., 2004).

Because making positive changes in health behaviors are basically the client's responsibility, motivation is important. Motivation is considered a state of readiness, rather than a personality trait (Dart, 2011). MI emphasizes an individual's capacity to take charge of his or her personal health and to control lifestyle factors that interfere with optimal health and well-being. Although initially an MI approach takes longer, it is likely to be more effective because the client chooses actions having personal meaning and will be more committed to it.

The underlying premise of motivational learning is that learning takes root from within a person. It occurs when the learner is ready and "wants" to learn because s/he believes it will make a positive difference. The decision to change, choice of goals, and commitment to trying new behaviors is always under the client's control.

Readiness to change can be influenced. Nurses can better understand and influence a client's deeper perception of a problem through Socratic questioning. Socratic questioning allows nurses to develop discrepancies between client goals or values and current behaviors without argument or direct confrontation. MI helps clients address resistance and ambivalence about making health-related lifestyle changes in a nonjudgmental environment (Hall, et al., 2012). Therapeutic strategies center on resolving problem behaviors, increasing committed collaboration, and joint decision-making (Miller and Rollnick, 2013)

Case Example

Client: "I'm ready to go home now. I know once I get home, that I'll be able to get along without help. I've lived there all my life and I know my way around."

Nurse: "I know that you think you can manage yourself at home. But most people need some rehabilitation after a stroke to help them regain their strength. If you go home now without the rehabilitation, you may be shortchanging yourself by not taking the time to develop the skills you need to be independent at home. Is that something important to you?" (*precontemplation approach to raise awareness of the problem*).

MI is designed as a client-centered participatory interaction process. Negotiating behavior change is conceptualized as a "shared endeavor" in which client and provider examine the potential and willingness to change obstructive health behaviors (Martin and McNeil, 2009, p 284). When motivational strategies match an individual's readiness to change, it increases the likelihood of positive intentional behavioral lifestyle changes. MI strategies are used with habitual health behaviors that sabotage optimal health and well-being such as alcohol or drug abuse, poor dietary control and obesity, smoking, lack of physical activity, risky sexual behaviors, even taking medications, etc. Determining a client's level of readiness to change unhealthy behaviors helps nurses engage clients in a tailored dialogue to challenge and overcome ambivalence to making desired healthy changes (Baumann, 2012).

Miller and Rollnick, (2013) describe two phases of MI. The first phase focuses on mutually exploring and resolving ambivalence to change as a collaborative endeavor. This is accomplished through weighing the pros and cons of the current situations and the actions one would have to take to make change possible. With the client in charge of determining change activities, the second phase emphasizes strengthening and supporting the client's commitment to change based on client choice and capacity for change. The process starts to clarify a collaborative relationship with a client and family in clarifying the nature of the issues. A good starting point is a simple introductory question, such as, "I wonder if you could tell me what you do to keep yourself healthy? This type of question helps you to see what the client values. As the client begins to tell you about personal health habits, you can reflect on relevant details and ask for clarification. The purpose of the dialogue is to deepen the client's thought process. Use empathy in your responses, for example, "It sounds like you have been having a tough time, without a lot of support."

Open-ended questions allow clients the greatest freedom to respond. Asking a client if he regularly exercises may yield a one-sentence answer. Asking the same client to describe his activity and exercise during a typical day, and what makes it easier or harder for him to exercise provides stronger data. Potential concerns, inconsistent with values, preferences, or goals are more readily identified. Client and family perspectives on disease and treatment are not necessarily the same as those of their health care providers. For example, you may think that an emaciated or an obese woman is worried about her weight and wants to return to a normal weight. She may value the way she looks. Likewise, her culture or family values or traditions may be in conflict with making significant behavioral changes. Until the client can understand a health-related value for making a weight change, she will not put serious efforts into making a change. This level of data allows nurses to tailor interventions based on the client's readiness to change and the availability of a support system.

As clients progress to the contemplative stage, nurses provide coaching guidance, information and practical support to help clients consider different choices and potential solutions. The pros and cons of each client choice are explored. Empathy for the challenges faced by the client and affirming the client's reflection process encourage clients to consider alternative options and to choose the most viable among them (Levensky et al., 2007). A critical component of MI is an acceptance of the client's right to make the final decision and the need for the clinician to honor each client's right to do so.

In the preparation stage, your role is to help clients establish realistic goals and develop a plan for achieving them. Goals should be realistic, client centered, and achievable. For example, having a goal to lose 10 pounds in 3 months sounds more doable than a goal to simply lose weight (too vague) or to lose 75 pounds (potentially overwhelming goal). Incremental goals build a sense of confidence, as the client sequentially meets them.

The action stage is where the most difficult work takes place. The importance of personalizing goals and treatment plans for your clients cannot be stressed enough. Each client has unique life situations, different support systems, and different ways of coping with problems. Unhealthy health habits are cumulative and hard to break. Work with clients to monitor their progress, offering suggestions, revising goals or plans when needed, and reminding clients of progress made. It is useful to help clients proactively identify potential obstacles, and anticipate next steps. You can offer additional suggestions, empathize or commend client efforts, and revisit actions from the preparation stage if goals need revision. For example, you could say, "you have really worked hard to master your exercises" or "I'm really impressed that you were able to avoid eating sweets this week." Availability to help clients problem solve or rethink plans, if needed, is also key.

EMPOWERMENT STRATEGIES

Tengland (2008) distinguishes between empowerment as a *goal* in having control over the determinants of one's quality of life and as a *process* in which one has control over problem formulation, decision making, and the actions one takes to achieve relevant health goals. Client empowerment takes place through clinician-initiated patient-centered care approaches *and* through actions clients take on their own initiative (Holmstrom and Roing, 2010).

As a process strategy, empowering people to take the initiative with their own health and well-being support a person's ability to maintain his or her role as a functioning adult and facilitates self-management of chronic disorders (Zubialde et al., 2009).

Case Example

Soon Mrs. Hixon began learning how to dress herself. At first she took an hour to complete this task. But with guidance and practice, she eventually dressed herself in 25 minutes. Even so, I practically had to sit on my hands as I watched her struggle. I could have done it so much faster for her, but she had to learn, and I had to let her (Collier, 1992, p. 63).

Other enabling strategies include a focus on knowledge and skills, tailored education and training, previous successful conquering of problems, social supports they can lean on, and reexamining existing supportive assets (Green, 2008). Learning as much as possible about healthy lifestyles and how they support self-management of chronic conditions is empowering (Coward, 2006).

Helping people use technology to find information and resources is a form of empowering clients to take charge of their health and well-being. Online support groups, chat rooms, and shared experiences provide additional support for people who live in areas that are not geographically convenient to person-to-person contact. Clients can connect with others coping with issues such as weight control and exercise and can share practical strategies through the Internet.

The Internet is a powerful resource for knowledge. Clients and families can find specific information, regardless of the stage of their illness on the Web. Nurses can augment understanding by helping clients select and critically evaluate personal relevance of web data. Not all data is completely accurate, or relevant to a particular client situation. If the client or family does not use technology, then flyers, fact sheets, and direct dialogue with opportunity for questions and follow-up can be used to reinforce information.

Most people learn best when they engage more than one sense in the learning process and have an opportunity to practice essential skills. A participatory learning format that encourages different ways of thinking and opportunities to try out new behaviors is more effective than giving simple instructions to a client or family or demonstration without teach-back feedback (Willison et al., 2005). When time is short, focus on topics that address the most pressing lifestyle need changes. Teaching strategies presented in Chapter 15 can be used or modified for health promotion teaching.

Empowerment through Social Support

Andam (2011) suggests, "empowerment implies a gathering of power, in a dynamic way, over a period of time" (p. 50). Social support from friends and family is an important empowerment resource in health promotion activities. *Social support* describes a person's "integration within a social network," and "the perceived availability of support" when it is needed (MacGeorge et al.,, 2011), p. 320). The interested support of significant others can strengthen a person's resolve, provide

input for innovative solutions, and nurture development of self-efficacy.

Health-related support groups in the community are available for a wide variety of diagnoses, providing relevant information, direct assistance, referral to appropriate resources, and being available to simply interact with others experiencing similar challenges. For example, the Alzheimer's Association (for Alzheimer disease and related disorders) holds regularly scheduled support groups to assist family members in most major locations. Community-based cancer support groups provide valuable information and support for many common cancer diagnoses. Educational and referral supports enable clients and families to learn the skills they need to effectively manage chronic conditions and to live a healthy lifestyle.

HEALTH PROMOTION AS A POPULATION CONCEPT

Community is defined as "any group of citizens that have either a geographic, population-based, or self-defined relationship and whose health may be improved by a health promotion approach" (Frankish et al., 2006, p. 174). The community offers a natural social system with special significance for facilitating health promotion activities, particularly for people who are economically or socially disadvantaged. It is difficult to change attitudes and lifestyles to promote health when a client's social or economic environment does not support prevention efforts.

Major advances in health promotion and prevention have not benefited all segments of nation's population equally (Kline and Huff, 2008). *Health disparities* is the term used to describe cohort differences in health status across ethnic groups, gender, education, or income. The term also is associated with inequalities in access, service use, and health outcomes. People with the greatest health burdens often have inadequate financial resources, and the least access to information, communication technologies, health care, and supporting social services. Individuals living in extreme poverty do not have access to preventive care, adequate nutrition, or the opportunity to live in a healthy environment. When they are at the survival level, most people are not in a position to think about health promotion techniques to acquire a better quality of life. Being mindful of the client's environment helps nurses proactively tailor interventions to engage and meet their health promotion and disease prevention client needs.

Equity and empowerment related to health care are the expected outcome of health promotion activities at the community level. Equity corresponds to the WHO directive that all people should have an equal opportunity to enjoy good health and well-being. Key health issues in economically disadvantaged communities often are those with social roots such as violence or abuse, substance abuse, teen pregnancies, and acquired immunodeficiency syndrome (AIDS) (Blumenthal, 2009).

Community empowerment "seeks to enhance a community's ability to identify, mobilize, and address the issues that it faces to improve the overall health of the community (Yoo et al., 2004, p. 256). Empowerment is fueled by *both* public policy and targeted education. Unless the community as a whole can collectively challenge and eradicate inequities in health care access and treatment provision, health promotion activities will fall short of their targeted goals (Messias et al., 2005).

Successful health promotion programs require individuals, groups, and organizations to act as active agents in shaping health practices and policies that have meaning to a target population. Specific interventions are designed to engage those people who are most involved with a common environmental concern related to health as active participants. A proactive approach to capture the attention of people who otherwise might not be predisposed to taking charge of their health and/or may not know that they are at risk is a first step. Social and political action to enhance health services can augment educational efforts to ensure program viability.

COMMUNITY VOICES IN HEALTH PROMOTION ACTIVITIES

Health promotion activities recognize the community as its principal voice in assuming control of and improving health and well-being. Health promotion represents a multidisciplinary approach, also inclusive of health education, public health, and environmental health (Corcoran, 2013). Health promotion strategies are offered in clinics, schools, communities, parishes, and during routine care in hospitals.

The Patient Protection and Affordable Care Act created the National Prevention Council to ensure that lifelong prevention services are available to all individuals, families, and communities. The council developed a prevention model with four strategic directions as identified in Figure 14-3, with seven priority action areas.

- Developing healthy and safe community environments to promote health and wellness through prevention
- Ensuring the availability of integrated clinical and community preventive services for all
- Empowering people to make healthy choices
- Eliminating disparities as a way to improve the quality of all Americans (National Prevention Council, 2011).

Successful community-based health promotion activities start with a community analysis of health issues identified by the community. Consciousness raising is critical, as engagement and buy-in of the community in which the activity is to take place is essential. WHO notes that health promotion activities should be "carried out by and with people, not on, or to people" (WHO 1997). Active participation of individuals, communities, and systems means a stronger and more authentic commitment to the establishment of the realistic regulatory, organizational, and sociopolitical supports, which will be needed to achieve targeted health outcomes (Kline and Huff, 2008).

PRECEDE-PROCEED MODEL

The PRECEDE-PROCEED community education model offers a roadmap and a structural framework for designing, implementing, and evaluating community-based health promotion programs for effective health promotion planning, intervention, and evaluation. Developed by Green and Kreuter (2005), this model is based on two fundamental assumptions: (1) health and health risks are multi-determined, and (2) health promotion interventions must be multidimensional and participatory to be effective.

The PRECEDE component refers to the assessment and planning components of program planning. It takes place as a part of the planning process *before* the educational program is offered and provides direction for each program's focus and implementation strategies. The acronym PRECEDE stands for predisposing, reinforcing, enabling causes in educational diagnosis, and identifies evaluation factors associated with the targeted problem area. Examples of diagnostic behavioral factors are presented in Table 14-2.

Careful assessment of these factors provides direction for the type of program and content most likely

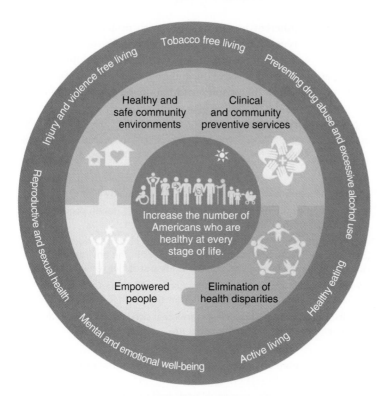

Figure 14-3 National Prevention Strategy *(From National Prevention Council: National Prevention Strategy, Washington, DC, 2011, U.S. Department of Health and Human Services, Office of the Surgeon General.)*

TABLE 14-2	PRECEDE-PROCEED Model: Examples of PRECEDE Diagnostic Behavioral Factors

Factors	Examples
Predisposing factors	Previous experience, knowledge, beliefs, and values that can affect the teaching process (e.g., culture and prior learning)
Enabling factors	Environmental factors that facilitate or present obstacles to change (e.g., transportation, scheduling, and availability of follow-up)
Reinforcing factors	Perceived positive or negative effects of adopting the new learned behaviors, including social support (e.g., family support, risk for recurrence, and avoidance of a health risk)

to engage the interest of diverse learners in community-based settings. Nurses also determine population needs and establish evaluation methods before implementation. Evaluation is a continuous process that begins when the program is implemented and is exercised throughout the educational experience.

Sufficient resources, knowledge about target populations, and leadership training are part of an essential infrastructure needed to support health promotion approaches in the community. A sustainable educational model needs political, managerial, and administrative supports for full implementation of a community-based approach to health promotion and disease prevention. The PROCEED component (policy, regulatory, organizational constructs in educational and environmental development) was added to the model by Green in the late 1980s. This component explicitly considers critical environmental and cost variables such as budget, personnel, and critical organizational relationships as part of the planning process. Having the resources in place and assessing their sustainability is important in health promotion planning, though it is not always thought through in the planning phase. Prevention activities do not generate the same level of revenue; they may not be as sustainable when resources become tight (Bernard, 2006). Nurses can play an important role in advocating for public policies supporting sustainable access to appropriate health resources on citizen advisory committees.

The PRECEDE-PROCEED model is presented in Table 14-3.

Exercise 14-4, Analyzing Community Health Problems for health promotion interventions provides an opportunity to think about the complex factors inherent in community health problems. As with all types of education and counseling, learners need to be actively engaged in goal setting and developing action plans that have meaning to them. The health care system is complex and requires a new level of client

TABLE 14-3	PRECEDE-PROCEED Model Definitions
Phase	**Definition**
PRECEDE Components	
1. Social diagnosis	People's perceptions of their own health needs, quality of life
2. Epidemiologic diagnosis	Determination of the extent, distribution, causes of health problem in target population
3. Behavioral and environmental diagnosis	Determination of specific health-related actions likely to affect problem (behavioral); systematic assessment of factors in the environment likely to influence health and quality-of-life outcomes (environmental)
4. Educational and organizational diagnosis	Assessment of all factors that must be changed to initiate or sustain desired behavioral changes and outcomes
5. Administrative and policy diagnosis	Analysis of organizational policies, resources, circumstances relevant to the development of the health program
PROCEED Components	
6. Implementation	Converting program objectives into actions taken at the organizational level
7. Process evaluation	Assessment of materials, personnel performance, quality of practice or services offered, and activity experiences
8. Impact evaluation	Assessment of program effects of intermediate objectives inclusive of all changes as a result of the training
9. Outcome evaluation	Assessment of the teaching program on the ultimate objectives related to changes in health, well-being, and quality of life

Adapted from Green L, Kreuter M: *Health program planning: an educational and ecological approach*, ed 4, New York, 2005, McGraw Hill.

EXERCISE 14-4	**Analyzing Community Health Problems for Health Promotion Interventions**

Purpose: To develop an appreciation for the multidimensional elements of a community health problem.

Procedure
In small groups of four to six students, brainstorm about health problems you believe exist in your community and develop a consensus about one public health problem that the group would prioritize as being most important.

Use the following questions to direct your thinking about developing health promotion activities for a health-related problem in your community.

- What are the most pressing health problems in your community?
- What are the underlying causes or contributing factors to this problem?
- In what ways does the selected problem impact the health and well-being of the larger community?
- What is the population of interest you would need to target for intervention?
- What types of additional information would you need to have to propose a solution?
- Who are the stakeholders, and how should they be involved?
- What step would you recommend as an initial response to this health problem?
- What is one step the nurse could take to increase awareness of this problem as a health promotion issue?

Discussion
How hard was it for your group to arrive at a consensus about the most pressing problem? Were you surprised with any of the discussion that took place about this health problem? How could you use what you learned in doing this exercise in your nursing practice?

decision-making. Shared decision making and working with personal and community-based values and beliefs provide a more holistic framework for health promotion strategies at the macro as well as micro levels (McBrien, 2009). Choosing the right strategies requires special attention to the learner's readiness, capabilities, and skills. Box 14-2 presents health promotion educational strategies.

Evaluation of health promotion activities is essential. In addition to evaluating immediate program effects, longitudinal evaluation of the impact of health promotion activities on morbidity, mortality, and quality of life is desirable. Keep in mind that what constitutes quality of life is a subjective reality for each client and may differ from person to person (Fagerlind et al., 2010).

HEALTH PROMOTION MODELS FOR COMMUNITY EMPOWERMENT

Community empowerment strategies are used to help identify and address environmental and social issues needed to improve the overall health of the community. This strategy is sometimes referred to as "capacity building." Community-focused empowerment strategies build on the personal strengths, community resources, and problem-solving capabilities already existing in individuals and communities that can be used to address potential and actual health problems. The exploratory study presented in this chapter is an example of capacity building through community mobilization of women at risk for HIV to plan, carry out, and evaluate a health promotion strategy in a poverty-stricken area. Capacity building requires the inclusion of informal and formal community leaders as valued stakeholders. Networking, partnering, and creating joint ventures with indigenous and local religious infrastructures is a powerful consensus-building strategy communities can use for effective health promotional education planning and implementation. Box 14-3 outlines a process for engaging the community in health promotion activities.

HEALTH LITERACY IN HEALTH PROMOTION AND DISEASE PREVENTION

Parker and colleagues (2003) define **health literacy** as "the degree to which people have the capacity to obtain, process, and understand basic health information and services needed to make appropriate health decisions" (p. 194). Health literacy is central to achieving good health and well-being (DHHS, 2010b). Approximately 21% of U.S. adults would be classified as functionally illiterate, which means they read below a ninth-grade level and would have trouble comprehending written instructions on medication bottles, negotiating the health care system, and fully understanding consent forms (Davis et al., 1998). This has disastrous implications for self-management, as indicated in the following case example.

BOX 14-2	Strategies in Health Education and Counseling: Recommendations of the U.S. Preventive Services Task Force

- Frame the teaching to match the client's perceptions. Consider and incorporate the clients preferences, beliefs and concerns.
- Fully inform clients of the purposes and expected outcomes of interventions and when to expect these effects.
- Suggest small changes and baby steps rather than large ones.
- Be specific.
- Add new behaviors rather than eliminating established behaviors whenever possible.
- Link new behaviors to old behaviors.
- Obtain explicit commitments from the client; Ask clients to state exactly how they plan to achieve goals (what, when, and how often---start with how will you begin?
- Refer clients to appropriate community resources that are accessible and convenient.
- Use a combination of strategies to achieve outcomes tailored to individual needs.
- Monitor progress through follow-up contact.

Adapted from Agency for Healthcare Research and Quality (AHRQ). 2002. *Guide to Clinical Preventive Services: Report of the U.S. Preventive Services Task Force*, 2nd ed. New York: International Medical Publishing, p. lxxvii-lxxx.

Case Example

Jonathan is a 14-year-old adolescent recently discharged from a mental health unit. This was his fourth admission over an 18-month period. His mother assumed responsibility for seeing that he took his medications as directed. His mother knew the names of his medications and faithfully monitored his taking of them. But Jonathan's behavior began to deteriorate again. At one of Jonathan's follow-up visits, the nurse asked him to show her the meds he was on, and how he was taking them. It turned out that Jonathan's mother couldn't read, got the meds mixed up, and was administering the daily med three times a day, and the TID medication once daily.

| BOX 14-3 | Guiding Principles for Community Engagement |

Before starting a community engagement effort:
- Be clear about the purposes or goals of the engagement effort and the populations and/or communities you want to engage.
- Become knowledgeable about the community's culture, economic conditions, political and power structures, norms and values, demographic trends, history, and experience with the efforts by outside groups to engage it in various programs. Learn about the community's perceptions of those initiating the engagement activities.

For engagement to occur, it is necessary to:
- Go to the community, establish relationships, build trust, work with the formal and informal leadership, and seek commitment from community organizations and leaders to create processes for mobilizing the community.
- Remember and accept that collective self-determination is the responsibility and right of all people who are in a community. No external entity should assume it can bestow to a community the power to act in its own self-interest.

For engagement to succeed:
- Partnering with the community is necessary to create change and improve health.
- All aspects of community engagement must recognize and respect the diversity of the community. Awareness of the various cultures of a community and other factors of diversity must be paramount in designing and implementing community engagement approaches.
- Community engagement can only be sustained by identifying and mobilizing community assets and strengths, and by developing the community's capacity and resources to make decisions and take action.
- Organizations that wish to engage a community as well as individuals seeking to effect change must be prepared to release control of actions or interventions to the community, and be flexible enough to meet the changing needs of the community.
- Community collaboration requires long-term commitment by the engaging organization and its partners.

From Clinical and Translational Science Awards (CTSA) Consortium and Community Engagement Key Function Committee Task Force on the Principles of Community Engagement: *Principles of community engagement*, ed 2. NIH Publication No. 11-7782. Washington, DC, 2011, National Academies Press, pp. 46-52. Available online: http://www.atsdr.cdc.gov/communityengagement/pdf/PCE_Report_508_FINAL.pdf. Accessed September 28, 2013.

Responsibility for health literacy is a collaborative initiative that lies with both providers and clients. Special attention needs to be given to disadvantaged A more proactive approach needs to be extended to lower socioeconomic groups and minority populations as health literacy disproportionately affects these population groups. Clients need to be encouraged to ask questions about anything they do not understand. You can normalize this circumstance for clients, for example, by saying something such as, "many people find it confusing to fully understand what is going on with them. They ask a lot of questions, and I am hoping you will too." Teach-back, (see Chapter 15) in addition to written instructions, also helps anchor instructions.

Literacy is not just about reading and writing. It also is about speaking, listening for understanding, asking questions about anything that is not understood, and checking to see that the messages sent are the same as those received.

Luckily the mother in the preceding case example responded with enough information that the nurse was able to correct her misinterpretation. When clients have left the health care setting, understanding unfamiliar complex information can be daunting. The combination of client perception of locus of control, cultural prioritization of health needs and level of health literacy skills can influence client health compliance with lifestyle self-management recommendations and medication adherence (Singleton and Krause, 2009; Ownby, 2006).

Health literacy can be compromised by visual and/or auditory impairment, diminished mental alertness, fatigue and acute illness. For example, a hard-of-hearing client may not hear the words correctly and assign meanings, which are incorrect. A client with poor vision can misread a medication label or misinterpret individual words on a consent form. Helping clients use more than one sense to interpret instructions and asking questions to validate impressions is important.

Health literacy differs from overall literacy and IQ. People with inadequate health literacy may be highly intelligent, but functionally unable to fully grasp medical terminology because of education or language differences. Many of the words and meanings associated with medical terminology are complex and not easily understood by the lay public.

The American Medical Association (AMA) defines **functional health literacy** as "the ability to read and comprehend prescription bottles, appointment slips, and the other essential health related materials to successfully function as a patient" (AMA, 1999, p. 552) Health literacy involves more than the capacity to read. It can include inability to understand the complexity and implications of medical treatments or essential system navigation skills (Dewalt and Pignone, 2005). A few well-placed questions can reveal this problem. People with inadequate health literacy skills often do not know what to do about their health, how to self-manage a chronic condition, or why it is important, especially if they have not been exposed previously to medical settings. Even when they comprehend the words, their level of understanding may be too limited to weigh possible alternate meanings or to know what questions to ask for a better interpretation. Table 14-4 presents core constructs of health literacy.

A less common, but related literacy skill is numeracy. *Numeracy* is defined as "the ability to understand and use numbers in daily life" (Rothman et al., 2008, p. 583). Lack of numeracy skills can affect the client's ability to understand dates and timing related to medications, dosage measurement of oral medications, the importance of time intervals between medications, and so forth, and why this is important. Inadequate numeracy skill is particularly relevant for clients who rely on prescribed medications given at different times and as-needed meds to cope with their illness (Rothman et al., 2008). Some try to hide the fact that they cannot read or understand the meaning of complex words or make sense of numbers. They feel ashamed, so they fake their inability to understand by appearing to agree with the nurse, by saying they will read the instructions later, or by not asking questions.

Here are some issues clients or significant others may have related to poor health literacy:

- Inability to adequately describe symptoms or health problems
- Taking instructions too literally
- Having a limited ability to generalize information to new situations
- Decoding one word at a time rather than reading a passage as a whole
- Skipping over uncommon or hard words
- Thinking in individual rather than categorical terms (Doak et al., 1996)

Partial understanding or lack of full step-by-step instructions can result in unintentional non-compliance.

Case Example

A two-year-old is diagnosed with an inner ear infection and prescribed an antibiotic. Her mother understands that her daughter should take the prescribed medication twice a day. After carefully studying the label on the bottle and deciding that it doesn't tell how to take the medicine, she fills a teaspoon and pours the antibiotic into her daughter's painful ear (Parker et al., 2003, p. 150).

Educationally disadvantaged or functionally illiterate people are interested in learning, but nurses need to adapt teaching situations to accommodate literacy learning differences. Marks (2009) suggests having written materials modified to six- to eighth-grade reading levels and providing lists of key instructions for use after visits. Using symbols and images with which the client is familiar helps overcome the barriers of low literacy. Taking the time to understand the client's use of words and phrases provides the nurse with concrete words and ideas that can be used as building blocks in helping the client understand difficult health-related concepts. Otherwise the client may misunderstand what the nurse is saying. It is also important to check

TABLE 14-4	Core Constructs of Health Literacy with Application Examples
Core Construct	**Application Examples**
I. Basic literacy or comprehension	Reading information, appointment cards
	Interpreting medical tests, dosages, and instructions, side effects, contraindications
	Understanding brochures, medication labels, informed consent, insurance documents
II. Interactive and participatory literacy (able to engage in two-way interactions)	Provision of appropriate and usable information
	Comprehension and ability to carry out information
	Mutual decision making
	Remembering and carrying out information
III. Critical literacy	Ability to weigh critical scientific facts Capacity to assess competing treatment options

Adapted from Marks R: Ethics and patient education: health literacy and cultural dilemmas, *Health Promot Pract* 10(3):328-332, 2009.

with the client about the environmental infrastructure needed to implement self-management strategies. Do not assume that the client understands the implications of a clinical recommendation.

Case Example

Michelle is a nurse practitioner in an inner city pediatric clinic. After examining a child with strep throat, she prescribed an antibiotic for her. She instructed the mother to give the child the medication four times a day and to store it in the refrigerator between doses. She asked the mother if she had any questions or concerns, and the mother indicated she did not have any. But as the mother and child were leaving the exam room, the mother turned to the nurse practitioner and said, "You know, we don't have a refrigerator. Will anything happen if I don't refrigerate the antibiotic?" If you were the nurse in this situation, how would you respond to this client? What supports would you suggest?

Use common concrete words as descriptors rather than abstract or medical terminology, for example, "Call the doctor on Monday if you still have pain or swelling in your knee." Use the same words to describe the same thing. If you use "insulin" in one instance and "medicine" or "drug" later to describe the same medication, the client may become confused. The same instructions, written exactly as they were spoken, act as a reminder once the person leaves the actual teaching situation.

Sequence the content logically beginning with a core concept. Remember that the client with low health literacy may not be able to read or interpret the label instructions on the bottle. You can use the following question sequence to teach a client about taking a new medication.

- What do I take?
- How much do I take?
- When do I take it?
- What will it do for me?
- What do I do if I get a side effect?

If there are multiple oral medications, it is useful to describe each pill's appearance. Provide a written copy of the questions and answers as a reminder.

Apply common simple concrete words such as "You should take your medicine with your meals," instead of "take this medication on an empty stomach." Sophisticated terminology, while accurate, may not be understood.

Whenever possible, *link new information and tasks with what the client already knows.* This strategy builds on previous knowledge and reinforces self-efficacy in mastering new concepts. Keeping sentences short and precise and using active verbs helps clients understand what is being taught. When technical words are necessary for clients to communicate about their condition with other health professionals, clients may need direct instruction or coaching about appropriate words to use.

DEVELOPMENTAL LEVEL

Developmental level affects both teaching strategies and subject content. You will have clients at all levels of the learning spectrum with regard to their social, emotional, and cognitive development. Developmental learning capability is not always age related; it is easily influenced by culture and stress. Social and emotional development does not always parallel cognitive

---

EXERCISE 14-5   **Developing Relevant Teaching Aids**

Purpose: To develop skill in adapting learning materials for clients with limited literacy.

Procedure
1. Develop a one-paragraph case study preferably from a client experience.
2. Choose a health promotion topic such as exercise, diet, stress reduction, or medication adherence.
3. Use the topic to develop a simple poster or teaching aid for a client with limited literacy skills.
4. Use clear plain language consistent with a fifth-to-sixth grade reading level to develop your project.
5. Check your content for accuracy

6. Use your teaching aid with your client and ask for feedback about the client understanding of your message, and reaction to the teaching aid.

Discussion:
How difficult was it to develop the teaching aid? What factors did you have to take into consideration to make it interesting and informative for your client? Were you surprised at any of the feedback you received from the client? Would you do anything differently as a result of the feedback?

maturity or literacy. Mirroring the client's communication style and framing messages to reflect developmental characteristics helps improve comprehension and understanding. Parents can provide useful information about their child's immediate life experiences and commonly used words to incorporate in health teaching.

CULTURE

Cultural understandings add to the complexity of health promotion strategies in health care. Chiu et al (2006) suggest that "empowering ethnocultural communities through informal care may be the most culturally appropriate approach for improving the health status of ethnocultural populations" (p. 3). Values, norms, and beliefs are an integral part of a person, which influence individual and community lifestyles and health perceptions (see Chapter 7). Culture helps explain assumptions about health and illness, the causes of and treatments for different types of illnesses, and traditionally accepted health actions or practices to prevent or treat illness. Cultural values affect expectations and trust of health care providers. Eliciting explanatory information regarding health and illness, and incorporating relevant material in health teaching promotes better acceptance of health promotion and disease prevention recommendations.

Cultural sensitivity includes knowledge of the preferred communication style of different cultural groups, which can be appropriately used when choosing teaching strategies. For example, Native Americans are known for learning through stories. The tradition of oral stories is a primary means of teaching that the nurse can use as a teaching methodology for health promotion purposes. In many cultures, the family assumes a primary role in care of the client even when the client is physically and emotionally capable of self-care. Including them, and especially those expected to support the learning process of the client from the outset in all aspects of health teaching for health promotion, is important. Client motivation and participation can also increase with the use of indigenous teachers and counselors. If health literacy is related to language, qualified interpreters should be used for translation and preparation of written materials.

Nurses participate routinely in community health promotion and disease prevention activities. They have an ethical and legal responsibility in health teaching to maintain the appropriate expertise and interpersonal sensitivity to client needs required for effective learning.

SUMMARY

Chapter 14 focuses on communication strategies nurses can use, which are designed to help people increase control over harmful social determinants of health. National and global agendas over the last decade reinforce the importance of developing public health policies to create supportive health environments. Specific attention to reducing health disparities, negative social determinants through strengthened community action for health, and increased access for all is advocated. Optimal health and well-being are considered the desired outcomes of health promotion activities.

Three individual health promotion frameworks are presented. Pender's health belief model identifies perceptions of benefits, barriers, and ability to take action related to health and well-being as components of peoples' willingness to engage in health promotion activities.

Prochaska's transtheoretical model is used to explore a person's motivational readiness to intentionally change health habits. This theory serves as foundation for motivational interviewing developed by Miller and Rollineck. Bandura's social learning theory explores the role of self-efficacy in empowering clients to use health promotion and disease prevention recommendations to better take care of their health.

Community-based interventions are critical in addressing broader causal influences on health, referred to as social determinants. The PRECEDE-PROCEED model is used to plan, implement, and evaluate community-based health promotion interventions. Chapter 14 also describes the important role of health literacy. Lack of health literacy, culture, and developmental status are described as factors that can compromise a client's ability to fully engage in healthy lifestyle behaviors.

ETHICAL DILEMMA   What Would You Do?

Jack Marks is a 16-year-old adolescent who comes to the clinic complaining of symptoms of a sexually transmitted disease (STD). He receives antibiotics and you give him information about safe sex and preventing STDs. Two months later he returns to the clinic with similar symptoms. It is clear that he has not followed instructions and has no intention of doing so. He tells you he's a regular jock and just can't get used to the idea of condoms. He says he can't tell you the names of his partners—there are just too many of them. What are your ethical responsibilities as his nurse in caring for Jack?

DISCUSSION QUESTIONS

1. In what ways are concepts of health literacy, and functional health literacy different, and similar to each other, and why is this important data?
2. Why are health promotion and disease prevention strategies receiving so much emphasis in contemporary health care?
3. How would you implement Pender's model to enhance personal responsibility for health promotion and disease prevention practices?

REFERENCES

American Medical Association Ad Hoc Committee on Health Literacy for the Council on Scientific Affairs. Health literacy: Report of the council on scientific affairs. *Journal of the American Medical Association*, 281, 552–557, 1999.

American Association of Colleges of Nursing: *The essentials of baccalaureate education for professional nursing practice*. Washington DC, Author, 2008.

Andam R: *Planning in Health Promotion Work*, An Empowerment Model. NY, 2011, Routledge.

Bandura A, 1997 Self-efficacy: the exercise of control WH Freeman: New York.

Baumann S: Motivational interviewing for emergency nurses, *J Emerg Nurs* 38:254–257, 2012.

Beckford-Ball J: The essence of care benchmark for patient health promotion, *Nurs Times* 102(14):23–24, 2006.

Bernard M: Health promotion/disease prevention: tempering the giant geriatric tsunami, *Geriatrics* 61(2):5–7, 2006.

Blumenthal DS: Clinical community health: revisiting "the community as patient, *Educ Health* 22(2):1–8, 2009. Available online http://www.educationforhealth.net.

Carter S, Rychetnik L, Lloyd B, et al.: Evidence, ethics, and values: A framework for health promotion, *Am J Public Health* 101:465–472, 2011.

Chiu L, Balneaves L, Barroetavena M, Doll R, Leis A. Use of complementary and alternative medicine by Chinese individuals living with cancer in British Columbia. Journal of Complementary and Integrative Medicine. 3(1): 1-19.

Davis T, Michiellurrw E, Askov E, et al.: Practical assessment of adult literacy in health care, *Health Educ Behav* 22(5):613–624, 1998.

Douglass F. (n.d.) BrainyQuote.com: Frederick Douglass. Available online http://www.brainyquote.com/quotes/quotes/f/frederickd201574.html. Accessed August 2, 2010.

Carels R, Darby L, Cacciapaglia H, et al.: Using motivational interviewing as a supplement to obesity treatment: a stepped-care approach, *Health Psychol* 26(3):369–374, 2007.

California Conference of Local Health Officers-County Health Executives Association of California (CCLHO-CHEAC): *Chronic Disease Prevention Leadership Project. Chronic Disease Prevention Framework*, Sacramento, CA, 2013, Author.

Cody W: *Philosophical and theoretical perspectives for advanced practice nursing*, ed 4, Sudbury MA, 2006, Jones and Bartlett. 183–190.

Collier S: Mrs. Hixon was more than the "CVA" in 251, *Nursing* 22(5):62–62, 1992.

Corcoran N: *Communicating Health: Strategies for Health Promotion*, 2nd ed., Thousand Oaks, CA, 2013, Sage Publications.

Coward D: Supporting health promotion in adults with cancer, *Fam Community Health* 29(Suppl 1):S52–S60, 2006.

Daley L, Fish A, Frid D, Mitchell L: Stage specific education/counseling intervention in women with elevated blood pressure, *Prog Cardiovasc Nurs* 24(2):45–52, 2009.

Dart M: *Motivational Interviewing in Nursing Practice*, Salisbury MA, 2011, Jones & Bartlett.

Dewalt DK, Pignone M: The role of literacy in health and health care, *Am Fam Physician* 72(3):387–388, 2005.

Doak CC, Doak LG, Root JH: *Teaching patients with low literacy skills*, ed 2, Philadelphia, 1996, JB Lippincott.

Edlin G, Golanty E: *Health and wellness*, ed 10, Sudbury, MA, 2009, Jones & Bartlett.

Fagerlind H, Ring L, Brulde B, Feltelius N, Lindblad A: Patients' understanding of the concepts of health and quality of life, *Patient Educ Couns* 78:104–110, 2010.

Frankish CJ, Moulton G, Rootman I, et al.: Setting a foundation: underlying values and structures of health promotion in primary health care settings, *Prim Health Care Res Dev* 7:172–182, 2006.

Goodwin A, Bar B, Reid G, Ashford S: Knowledge of motivational interviewing, *J Holist Nurs* 27(3):203–209, 2009.

Green J: Health education—the case for rehabilitation, *Crit Public Health* 18(4):447–456, 2008.

Green L, Kreuter M: *Health program planning: an educational and ecological approach*, ed 4, New York, 2005, McGraw Hill.

Hall K, Gibbie T, Lubman D: Motivational interviewing techniques: facilitating behavior change in the general practice setting, *Aust Fam Physician* 42:660–667, 2012.

Hawranik P, Strain S: Giving voice to informal caregivers of older adults, *Can J Nurs Res* 39(1):156–172, 2007.

Holmstrom I, Roing M: The relation between patient-centeredness and patient empowerment: a discussion on concepts, *Patient Educ Couns* 72(2):167–172, 2010.

Hogg W, Dahrouge S, Russell G, Tuna M, Geneau R, et al.: Health promotion activity in primary care: performance of models and associated factors, *Open Med* 3(3):e165–e173, 2009.

Hoving C, Visser A, Mullen PD, van den Borne B: A history of patient education by health professionals in Europe and North America, *Patient Educ Couns* 78(3):275–281, 2010.

Institute of Medicine (IOM): *Crossing the quality chasm: A new health system for the 21st century*, Washington DC, 2001, National Academies Press.

Institute of Medicine (IOM): *The future of the public's health in the 21st century*, Washington, DC, 2002, National Academies Press.

Institute of Medicine (IOM): *Primary care and public health: Exploring integration to improve population health*, Washington DC, 2012, National Academies Press.

Kirk A, Mutrie N, Macintyre P, Fisher M: Promoting and maintaining physical activity in people with type 2 diabetes, *Am J Prev Med* 27:289–296, 2004.

Kline M, Huff R: *Health promotion in multicultural populations: a handbook for practitioners and students*, ed 2, Thousand Oaks, CA, 2008, Sage.

Kushner RF, Sorensen KW: Lifestyle medicine: the future of chronic disease management, *Curr Opin Endocrinol Diabetes Obes* 20(5):389–395, 2013.

Levensky E, Forcehimes A, O'Donohue W, Beitz K: Motivational interviewing: an evidence-based approach to counseling helps patients follow treatment recommendations, *Am J Nurs* 107(10):50–58, 2007.

Litchfield M, Jonsdottir H: A practice discipline that is here and now, *Adv Nurs Sci* 31(1):79–91, 2008.

Marks R: Ethics and patient education: health literacy and cultural dilemmas, *Health Promot Pract* 10(3):328–332, 2009.

MacGeorge E, Feng B, Burleson B: Chapter 10 Supportive Communication. In Knapp M, Daly J, editors: *The Sage handbook of interpersonal communication*, Thousand Oaks, CA, 2011, Sage, pp 317–354.

Martins R, McNeil D: Review of motivational interviewing in promoting health behaviors, *Clin Psychol Rev* 29:283–293, 2009.

McBrien B: Translating change: the development of a person-centered triage training programme for emergency nurses, *Int Emerg Nurs* 17(1):31–37, 2009.

Messias D, De Jong M, McLoughlin K: Being involved and making a difference: empowerment and well-being among women living in poverty, *J Holist Nurs* 23(1):70–88, 2005.

Miller W, Rollnick S: *Motivational interviewing: preparing people for change*, ed 3, New York, 2013, Guilford Press.

Milio N: A framework for prevention: changing health-damaging to health-generating life patterns, *Am J Public Health* 66:435–439, 1976.

Mol A, Moser I, Pols J. (eds) 2010 Care in Practice: On Tinkering in Clinics, Homes and Farms. www.transcript-verlag.de/ts1447/ts1447.php.

National Prevention Council: *National Prevention Strategy*, Washington, DC, 2011, U.S. Department of Health and Human Services, Office of the Surgeon General.

Ochieng B: Factors affecting choice of a healthy lifestyle: implications for nurses, *Br J Community Nurs* 11(2):78–81, 2006.

Ownby L: Medication adherence and cognition: medical, personal and economic factors influence level of adherence in older adults, *Geriatrics* 61(2):30–35, 2006.

Parker R, Ratzan S, Lurie N: Health illiteracy: a policy challenge for advancing high-quality health care, *Health Aff (Millwood)* 22(4):147–153, 2003.

Pender N, Murdaugh C, Parsons M: *Health promotion in nursing practice*, ed 6, Upper Saddle River, NJ, 2011, Prentice Hall.

Prochaska J, Norcross J: *The transtheoretical model in Systems of psychotherapy: a transtheoretical analysis*, 8th ed., Stamford CT, 2013, Cengage Learning.

Rothman R, Montori V, Pignone M: Perspective: The role of numeracy in health care, *J Health Commun* 13(6):583–595, 2008.

Sandelowski M, DeVellis B, Campbell M: Variations in meanings of the personal core value "health." *Patient Educ Couns* 73(2):347–353, 2008.

Saylor C: The circle of health: a health definition model, *J Holist Nurs* 22(2):98–115, 2004.

Singleton K, Krause E: Understanding Cultural and Linguistic Barriers to Health Literacy, *OJIN: The Online Journal of Issues in Nursing* Vol. 14, Sept. 30, 2009. No. 3, Manuscript 4.

Srof B, Velsor-Friedrich B: Health promotion in adolescents: a review of Pender's health promotion model, *Nurs Sci Q* 19(4):366–373, 2006.

Tengland P-A: Empowerment: A conceptual discussion, *Health Care Anal* 16(2):77–96, 2008.

U.S. Department of Health and Human Services (DHHS): *Healthy People 2020*, Available at . Accessed May 9, 2013 www.healthypeople.gov/HP2020, 2010a.

U.S. Department of Health and Human Services (DHHS): *National Action plan to improve health literacy. Washington DC*, Author, 2010b.

Willison K, Mitmaker L, Andrews G: Integrating complementary and alternative medicine with primary health care through public health to improve chronic disease management, *J Complement Integr Med* 2(1):1–24, 2005.

World Health Organization (WHO): Jakarta declaration on leading health promotion into the 21st century. Available online www.who.int/hpr/NPH/docs/jakarta_declaration_en.pdf, 1997.

World Health Organization (WHO): Ottawa Charter for Health Promotion: First International Conference on Health Promotion, Ottawa, November 21. . Available online http://www.who.int/healthpromotion/conferences/previous/ottawa/en/, 1986. Accessed September 21, 2009.

Yoo S, Weed N, Lempa M, et al.: Collaborative community empowerment: an illustration of a six-step process, *Health Promotion Pract* 5(3):256–265, 2004.

Zubialde J, Mold J, Eubank D: Outcomes that matter in chronic illness: a taxonomy informed by self-determination and adult-learning theory, *Fam Syst Health* 27(30):193–200, 2009.

WEB RESOURCES

Harvard School of Public Health: Health Literacy Studies www.hsph.harvard.edu/healthliteracy.

Health and Literacy Special Collection http://healthliteracy.worlded.org/.

Joint Commission Report: What Did the Doctor Say?: Improving Health Literacy to Protect Patient Safety www.jointcommission.org/NR/rdonlyres/D5248B2E-E7E6-4121-8874-99C7B4888301/0/improving_health_literacy.pdf.

National Institute for Literacy Health Literacy Discussion List www.nifl.gov/mailman/listinfo/Healthliteracy.

Office of disease prevention and health promotion: Health literacy outline http://www.health.gov/healthliteracyonline/.

Health Teaching and Coaching

Elizabeth C. Arnold

OBJECTIVES

At the end of the chapter, the reader will be able to:

1. Define client (patient)-centered health education.
2. Identify the domains of learning.
3. Discuss theoretical frameworks used in client-centered health teaching.
4. Apply the nursing process in health teaching.
5. Discuss health teaching applications in different settings.
6. Describe coaching strategies for self-management of chronic conditions.

Health teaching is considered a core nursing competency used to promote quality and safety in health care across clinical settings. Chapter 15 identifies selected theories of teaching and learning as the basis for effective health teaching and client education. The chapter describes instructional principles and strategies that nurses can use to help clients learn the essential skills they need to self-manage chronic illness, make effective decisions, and work effectively with community resources to maximize health and well-being.

BASIC CONCEPTS

DEFINITIONS

Masters (2008) describes *client (patient) education* as a set of planned educational activities, resulting in changes in knowledge, health-related behaviors, and attitudes. The goal of client education is to empower clients to obtain, understand, and act on information needed for optimal health (Speros, 2011). *Health teaching* is a focused form of instructional dialogue used in client-centered relationships. The purpose of health teaching is to provide clients and families with the knowledge and life skills needed to make good decisions, slow or prevent disease progression

and mortality, and promote the highest possible quality of life. Contemporary health teaching embraces a broader context related to physical, social, and lifestyle modifications needed for self-managed health promotion, as well as treatment compliance (Farin et al., 2013; Figure 15-1).

Most definitions of client education do not address the complexity of the health teaching process (Wellard et al., 1998). The "learner" in a health care setting can be a client, a family or caregiver, a group, or a community. Individual learning characteristics of clients and families from different socioeconomic, educational, and experiential backgrounds vary greatly. A highly educated client, a noncompliant client, and a low-literacy client with similar medical conditions may present equivalent requirements for health teaching, but each requires an individualized teaching approach to ensure successful outcomes. Teaching partnerships with clients and families form the cornerstone of client education (Hudon et al, 2013). The goal is to help clients assume as much responsibility as possible with personal self-management of their chronic illness and its related life roles and changes. Problem-solving strategies, resource utilization, and health teaching across clinical settings are emphasized in contemporary health care focused on self-management of chronic disorders (Lorig and Holman, 2003). Including an

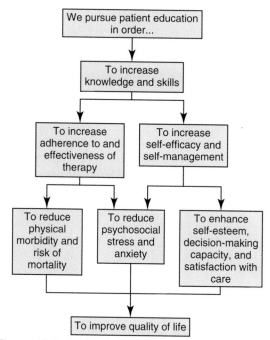

Figure 15-1 Goals of client education. *(From Feudtner C: What are the goals of patient education? West J Med 174(3):174, 2001).*

evaluation of health teaching through teach-back and return demonstrations help ensure client understanding and skill mastery.

PROFESSIONAL, LEGAL, AND ETHICAL MANDATES FOR PATIENT EDUCATION

Health teaching is *not* an option. It is a legal and ethical responsibility. The Joint Commission directives mandate tailoring health teaching to each client's needs, and health care requirements, including accommodations for developmental stage (Bastable, 2013). The Joint Commission has established standards *requiring* health care agencies to provide systematic health education and training for clients *and* families that is:

- Sufficient for clients to make informed decisions and to take responsibility for self-management activities related to their needs
- Provided to clients and families in an understandable manner and designed to accommodate various learning styles
- Reflected in documented evidence of the client's and family's understanding and response to appropriate medical information (The Joint Commission, 2014).

Similarly, nursing standards, developed by the American Nurses Association (ANA), reinforce the importance of health teaching as an essential nursing intervention. Standard 5B specifically relates to health teaching and health promotion (ANA, 2004). State Nurse Practice Acts mandate health teaching as an independent professional nursing function. Medicare requirements identify health teaching as a skilled nursing intervention for reimbursement purposes.

Documentation of client-specific education about health conditions and treatment options in language the client can fully understand is required for informed consent. Whereas the informed consent process itself is the physician's responsibility, nurses play an important role in providing appropriate follow-up health teaching, particularly with clients having limited mental capacity, and with surrogate decision makers (Menendez, 2013).

THEORETICAL FRAMEWORKS

Theory constructs discussed in Chapter 14 (the health belief model, motivational interviewing, PRECEDE/PROCEED community framework, and social cognitive theory) also contribute as a theory base for this chapter. Other noteworthy frameworks are identified in the following sections.

CLIENT-CENTERED HEALTH TEACHING

Carl Rogers' (1983) client-centered theoretical approach is applicable to client education. Emphasizing the primacy of the teacher-learner relationship, a learner-centered approach involves engaging clients as active partners in the learning process and coaching them in achieving meaningful health goals, to whatever extent is possible. Health teaching interventions are client-centered and empathetically supportive of client preferences and values. Rogers insists that the teacher must start where the learner is, and the learning process should support the learner's natural desire to learn. Relationship conditions of unconditional positive regard, empathy, and authenticity, described in earlier chapters are conceptual threads. Participatory strategies, which build on personal strengths, help clients achieve clinical outcomes. When information is provided in a meaningful context it has greater impact (Benner et al., 2010; Su et al., 2011). A collaborative learning environment allows nurses to offer sufficient information, specific instructions, and emotional support—but no more than is required—to allow each client to take as much charge of his or her health care as possible. The following case example illustrates the impact of a client-centered teaching encounter on a client.

Case Example

There was Nadine, who was an excellent preoperative teacher. She was the first person who clearly explained what a bladder augmentation entailed. She described different tubes I'd have and the purpose of each. When I returned from surgery, she helped me cope with my body image by teaching me how to use my bladder and by being a compassionate listener (Manning, 1992, p. 47).

DEVELOPMENTAL FRAMEWORK ORIENTATIONS

Andragogy refers to the "art and science of helping adults learn" (Knowles et al., 2011). Adult learners are self-directed, action oriented, and practical. They want to see the practicality of what they are learning. Generally, adults favor a problem-focused approach to learning and want to be directly engaged in developing skills needed to master immediate life problems. The adult learner expects the nurse to inquire about previous life experience and to incorporate this knowledge into the teaching plan. Figure 15-2 shows Knowles' model of adult learning.

Pedagogy refers to the processes used to help children learn. A key difference between pedagogy and andragogy is the need to provide the child learner with additional direct guidance and structure in learning content. Children come to the learning experience with far less life experience that can be tapped as resources for learning. They pass through cognitive and psychosocial stages, which dictate different teaching formats for successful participation (see Chapters 9 and 18). Kelo et al. (2013) advise that parent participation is critical to successful client education) with school-age children as a way to provide management guidance with essential emotional support.

Bastable (2013) describes a third developmental orientation to learning in older adulthood as **gerogogy**. Nurses should have a broad understanding of normal aging changes and the life experience of older adults. Accommodations for older adults can facilitate the learning process. Mobility or sensory losses and multiple comorbid chronic conditions are an unpleasant fact for many older adults, which can make learning or performing self-management more challenging. They may need a gentler or slower pace, as many are likely to be more cautious in trying new self-management strategies. Simple accommodations such as cueing, brighter lighting, and enlarged print facilitate learning. Encouragement and positive reinforcement improve motivation, self-efficacy, and performance.

THEORY OF PLANNED BEHAVIOR

Ajzen's (1991) theory of planned behavior emphasizes a person's *choice* (motivation) to perform a new behavior based on personal preference, self-efficacy (ability, and perceptions of others' favorable assessment). This theory perspective argues that a person's social nature and perception of ability to perform the behavior strongly influence learning targeted behaviors. A person's intention to perform a behavior offers one of the best predictors of whether the behavior will occur. A client is more likely to engage in a behavior when he or she has a positive view of it and thinks that others in the immediate environment hold a similar viewpoint.

BANDURA'S SOCIAL COGNITIVE MODEL

Living effectively with chronic illness requires constant adjustments as new challenges arise. Clients need a self-management response framework that goes beyond disease-specific interventions. Bandura's social cognitive model links successful behavioral changes to a person's perception that he or she has the capability to carry out the actions (self-efficacy) required to meet identified goals (outcome expectancy) within each person's unique social context, as discussed in Chapter 9. If people think they have the skills or can easily learn them, they are more likely to be successful. Bandura's use of incentive motivators is consistent with Pender's propositions that perceived competence (self-efficacy) strengthens commitment to action (see Chapter 14).

DOMAINS OF LEARNING

Health teaching is a dynamic interactive process, which involves making relevant connections to meaning within three domains: *cognitive* (understanding content), *affective* (changing attitudes and promoting acceptance), and *psychomotor* (hands-on skill development). Originally described by Bloom and associates, the utility of Bloom's taxonomy is that it provides "a common language about learning goals to facilitate communication across persons and subject matter" (Krau, 2011, p. 305).

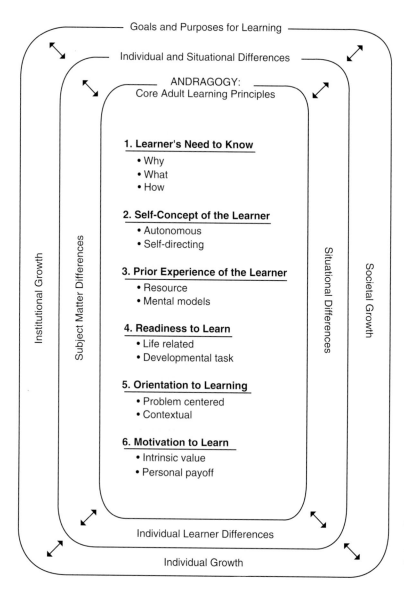

Goals and Purposes for Learning

Individual and Situational Differences

ANDRAGOGY:
Core Adult Learning Principles

1. Learner's Need to Know
- Why
- What
- How

2. Self-Concept of the Learner
- Autonomous
- Self-directing

3. Prior Experience of the Learner
- Resource
- Mental models

4. Readiness to Learn
- Life related
- Developmental task

5. Orientation to Learning
- Problem centered
- Contextual

6. Motivation to Learn
- Intrinsic value
- Personal payoff

Institutional Growth

Subject Matter Differences

Situational Differences

Societal Growth

Individual Learner Differences

Individual Growth

Figure 15-2 Andragogy model: a core set of adult learning principles. *(From Knowles M, Holton E, Swanson R: The adult learner: the definitive classic on adult education and training, Terre Haute, IL, 1998, Butterworth-Heinemann, p. 182.)*

Learning domains are interrelated. Cognitive knowledge is a prerequisite for changing attitudes (affective) and developing mastery of psychomotor skills (psychomotor) domain. When people learn about and practice a skill, they also develop "cognitive knowledge" about the reasons for using the skill and a blueprint for how it works. For example, objectives in the cognitive domain for a client with a recent diagnosis of diabetes would include knowledge of the disease; the roles of diet, exercise, and insulin in diabetic control; and personal judgments about how to identify trouble signs requiring immediate attention. Concrete cognitive information, provided through verbal discussions, images and line drawings, written instructions, and Web data, would be used to explain the steps needed to achieve client negotiated health goals.

BLOOM'S TAXONOMY

Nurses use Bloom's taxonomy as a guide to writing behavioral objectives in health care. This taxonomy identifies a hierarchy of learning objectives ranging from the least to the most complex. Bloom's leveled objectives were revised in the twenty-first century

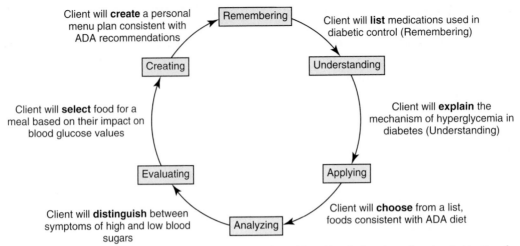

Figure 15-3   Leveled objectives using Bloom's taxonomy. *(Text adapted from Krau S: Creating educational objectives for patient education using the new Bloom's taxonomy, Nurs Clin North Am 46(3):302, 2011.)*

(bolded, in ascending order) to represent *verbs* rather than nouns. In the new hierarchy, the levels of evaluation and synthesis are reversed (Su et al., 2004). The revised Bloom's taxonomy consists of:

- Knowledge → **Remembering**: recognizing, recalling information and facts
- Comprehension → **Understanding**: interpreting, explaining, or constructing meaning
- Application → **Applying**: carrying out or executing a procedure; using information in a new way
- Analysis → **Analyzing**: considering constituent parts and how they relate to each other and the whole
- Evaluation → **Evaluating**: making judgments, critiquing, prioritizing, selecting, verifying
- Synthesis → **Creating**: putting material together in a coherent whole, reorganizing material into a new pattern, creating something new (Anderson et al., 2000). Figure 15-3 shows leveled objectives using Bloom's taxonomy.

Jointly developed objectives should have meaning to the client. Written behavioral objectives should begin with the phrase "the client will," followed by expected step-by-step achievable, measurable client behavioral progression toward treatment goals. Ideally, there should be an objective for each significant component of the teaching session. Exercise 15-1 provides practice with developing behavioral objectives.

Learning in the **affective domain** focuses on emotional attitudes related to acceptance, compliance,

valuing, and taking personal responsibility. It is more complex because of its association with values and beliefs. Objectives focusing on affective understanding are useful when clients demonstrate compliance issues or seem stalled in moving forward. The following case example illustrates learning blocks in the affective domain.

Case Example

Jack cognitively understands that adhering to his diabetic diet is essential to control his diabetes. He can tell you everything there is to know about the relationship of diet to diabetic control. Although he follows his diet at home, he eats snack foods at work and insists on extra helpings at dinner. He says he doesn't mind taking extra insulin and that it is his choice to do so. His problem with compliance lies in the affective domain; he resents having a lifelong condition that limits his food selections. The nurse will need to allow him time to vent his frustration, and then help him figure out ways to cope with a chronic illness in less self-destructive ways. If you were Jack's nurse, what health teaching strategies would you use to help him?

Skill requirements for effective self-care management usually include psychomotor learning. The **psychomotor domain** refers to skill development through *hands-on practice*. Performance learning promotes greater understanding than reading or hearing about a skill. It is more likely to be remembered. Think of the first time you road a bike. Chances are it was not until you actually got on the bike and made it move

EXERCISE 15-1	Developing Behavioral Goals

Purpose: To provide practical experience with developing teaching goals.

Procedure
Establish a nursing diagnosis related to health teaching and a teaching goal that supports the diagnosis in each of the following situations:

1. Jimmy is a 15-year-old adolescent who has been admitted to a mental health unit with disorders associated with impulse control and conduct. He wants to lie on his bed and read Stephen King novels. He refuses to attend unit therapy activities.
2. Maria, a 19-year-old single woman, is in the clinic for the first time because of cramping. She is 7 months pregnant and has had no prenatal care.
3. Jennifer is overweight and desperately wants to lose weight. However, she cannot walk past the refrigerator without stopping and she finds it difficult to resist the snack machines at work. She wants a plan to help her lose weight and resist her impulses to eat.

Discussion
1. What factors did you have to consider in developing the most appropriate diagnosis and teaching goals for each client?
2. In considering the diagnosis and teaching goals for each situation, what common themes did you find?
3. What differences in each situation contributed to variations in diagnosis and teaching goals? What contributed to these differences?
4. In what ways can you use the information in this exercise in your future nursing practice?

through your own efforts that you really "owned" the skill of bike riding. Usually psychomotor learning begins with the nurse's demonstration of a skill, followed by the client's return demonstration. Desired outcomes relate to proficiency in performing the required psychomotor skill and developing personal confidence and coping skills to adjust the performance of the skill when challenged with altered health situations.

CORE DIMENSIONS OF CLIENT EDUCATION

CLIENT CENTERED

Client-centered education starts with and respects the client's perspective. McCormack and McCance (2006) note that client-centered care approaches build on give-and-take relationships between health care professionals and clients, which in turn are based on "mutual trust, understanding and sharing collective knowledge" (p. 473). Clients are expected to participate as fully as possible in working with professionals to make realistic value-based decisions about their care, and treatment.

The teaching-learning process in health care strives to empower clients with the conceptual understandings and skills to self-manage their health and quality of life. Rather than a standalone nursing intervention, health teaching is considered a basic element of quality care integrated with other aspects of human interaction and healing partnerships with health team members, family, and significant others. Freda (2004) notes, "the goal of patient education has changed

from telling the client the best actions to take, to now assisting clients in learning about their health care to improve their own health," (p. 203). Clients are considered autonomous agents with final decision-making authority. Nurses, using a client-centered teaching framework, are expected to engage, empower, and support clients and families in developing effective self-management skills related to improved health status. Effective competency-based health teaching include tailoring the interventions to work with the client's lifestyle, providing coaching cues and behavioral counseling, and promoting the concept of social support as an essential component of chronic disease self-management.

COMPETENCY BASED

New models of client education related to self-management skill development are competency based. They include coaching and providing self-management support to strengthen a client's capability and confidence in managing his or her health condition(s). Self-management skill-enhancement strategies are designed to optimize chronic disease management in the home and community. Strategies involve obtaining an active provider/client collaborative commitment to setting realistic, achievable health goals, developing specific action plans to meet them, and evaluating their effectiveness. Competency-based health teaching begins with identifying specific learning outcomes (Su et al., 2011).

TAILORED INTERVENTIONS

What is taught and how it is taught are critical elements of competency-based health teaching. Behavioral objectives should reflect higher order cognition activities beyond remembering. Applications are grounded in evidence-based and nursing practice guidelines, tailored to each client's presenting needs, preferences, and available resources. The linkage between assessment needs and tailored actions should be transparent to everyone involved with the client's care.

Tailoring interventions requires listening for hidden emotional cues and accommodating individual differences into teaching plans. For example, a client with normal cognitive functioning might respond well to a suggestion to shower, while a client with mental issues or mild dementia may respond poorly if accommodations are not built into the teaching process. When self-management tactics fit within a client's daily routine, they are more likely to be followed. Scheduled times for exercising and taking medications helps new habits assume a regular place in the client's life.

COLLABORATIVE PARTICIPATORY PROCESS

Contemporary client education is conceptualized as a collaborative participatory process involving multilevel interventions, linked to a common purpose of maximizing a client's health and well-being. Clients are expected to be active participants and take responsibility for their health care, with collaborative support from their health care team. Nurses should use evidence-based knowledge and guidelines to facilitate and support individualized client and family decision making (Inott and Kennedy, 2011). Meaningful client-centered teaching does more than supply a basis for action: The process can improve client self-esteem and reduce health anxiety (Feudtner, 2001).

VARIED OPPORTUNITIES FOR HEALTH TEACHING

Client-centered education should be evidenced as a continuous thread, extending across health care settings and systems. Opportunities for health teaching occur in the community, schools, parish nursing, the home, hospitals, and clinics (Dreeben, 2010). Teaching formats range from informal one-to-one health relationships to formal structured group sessions, family conferences, and scheduled presentations in the care setting or community. Even emergency departments provide opportunities for "teachable moments" for clients (Szpiro et al., 2008). Health teaching can occur spontaneously during home visits as the nurse observes clients having specific difficulties with aspects of health care. Referred to as *guided care*, this type of on-the-spot health teaching is targeted to respond to specific health issues as they appear (Doherty, 2009). The media provides mass health-related client information related to primary prevention (e.g., safe sex and drug abuse prevention commercials) to targeted community groups. Health fairs for children and preventive screenings for adults provide natural health teaching spot opportunities in the community.

TECHNOLOGY INTEGRATION

Technology advances have expanded the depth and breadth of health information available to the health consumer. In addition to basic tailored health information, decision support systems can assist clients in making better health care decisions (Lewis, 2003). The Internet provides instant health information, with a wide range of learning resources to accommodate different levels of knowledge and learning styles. For example, *MedlinePlus* from the National Library of Medicine provides accurate current information about most common health conditions, palliative care, and drug information (Smith, 2013). Clients can type in a layperson's description of their problem and quickly receive links to tutorials and appropriate web sites. Web-based information on the Internet is searchable, up to date, inexpensive to obtain, and accessible at any time of day. Search engines such as Google and Bing allow clients to type in a few key words with immediate access to web sites related to their diagnosis (Gordon, 2011). National organizations, such as the American Diabetes Association and the American Cancer Society, have online tools to help clients understand their disease and treatment options. These and other web sites offer specific ideas for self-management, with a wide range of learning tools. Clients have free access to computers in public libraries and selected community centers (Bastable, 2013).

Although a powerful learning resource, the Internet has human and resource limitations. Many clients do not have easy accessibility to computers or know how to use them. Not all health information is equally relevant or directly applicable. Nurses can educate clients on how to begin searches and how to access information, as well as evaluate their quality (Gordon, 2011).

Clients and families find online sharing with others coping with similar health conditions helpful.

Recently, Holt, et al. (2011) described using cell phone technology as a health teaching aid for clients. They created an app consisting of personalized step-by-step photos beginning with essential equipment and accompanied by voice memo directions for complicated self-management of wound care.

Developing an Evidence-Based Practice

White M, Garbez R, Carroll M, Brinker E, Howie-Esquival J: Is "teach-back" associated with knowledge retention and hospital readmission in hospitalized heart failure patients? *J Cardiovasc Nurs* 28(2):137-146, 2013.

The goal of this study was to determine if the teach-back method would help hospitalized heart failure (HF) clients better retain self-care information, and whether it is associated with less readmissions. The study used a prospective design to study 276 clients hospitalized with HF. Recall of information was evaluated approximately 7 days after discharge, and readmissions were evaluated through phone calls and medical records.

Results: Study results revealed that inclusion of the teach-back method showed a significantly higher rate of correctly answered questions. There was a trend toward significance in recall for clients readmitted for HF.

Application to Your Clinical Practice: The extra step of using the teach-back method in client education holds promise for improving information retention for clients with heart failure.

APPLICATIONS

DEVELOPING INDIVIDUALIZED TEACHING PLANS

PREPARATION

Health Teaching Responsibilities

Individualized teaching plans follow the nursing process, beginning with an assessment of client learning needs, strengths, and limitations, and ending with evaluation of clinical outcomes. Common categories of health teaching responsibilities are featured in Figure 15-4.

Health teaching is a complex nursing intervention, consisting of many interlocking parts. Research demonstrates that structured client-specific teaching is more effective than generalized approaches (Friedman et al., 2011). As a health professional, you are responsible for the quality of health teaching, even though only the client can assure the outcome. Prior to beginning the teaching process, you should review evidence-based care guidelines for the client's condition (Bonaldi-Moore, 2009). Taking time to look over *key concepts and verifiable bottom-line information* needed to achieve designated client health goals facilitates later content discussion. Effective teaching plans provide clients and families with new or reorganized knowledge, skills, and attitudes based on scientific evidence—and personally tailored to client needs, resources, preferences, and values.

Nursing Roles in Health Teaching

Nurses assume several roles in health teaching. The nurse can act as a guide, an information provider, a resource, a knowledgeable emotional support, or all of these. As *guide,* nurses coach clients on actions they can take to improve their health and offer suggestions on modifications as their condition changes. As *information provider,* you help clients become more aware of why, what, and how they can learn to take better care of themselves. As *resource support,* nurses help clients connect with appropriate community social and health supports. Nurses act as a *knowledge source and emotional support provider* to encourage positive learning efforts by helping clients minimize the impact of temporary setbacks and never giving up on them. For example, helping clients to anticipate actual and potential effects of a medication or treatment reduces anxiety and the incidence of errors.

Self-Awareness

It is easier to remain engaged with self-directed, motivated client learners. It takes energy and imagination to stimulate interest in learning when a client sees little reason to participate in making essential lifestyle changes. Health teaching is a two-way process. This means rising above personal stereotypes to fully understand and appreciate each client's unique worldview. Incorporating a discovery approach to health teaching in which you encourage questions and use the client's life experiences whenever possible to help clients apply knowledge with familiar meaning to them enhances health teaching. Try to imagine yourself in the client or client's family's health situation. Empathy and understanding

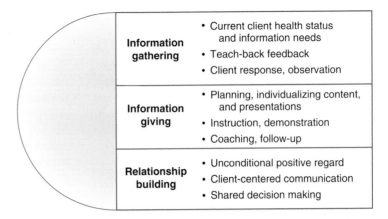

Figure 15-4 Health teaching categories.

of motivational commitment broaden health-teaching perspectives and convey respect for the client and family.

ASSESSMENT

To the extent that clients are cognitively able, they should be key informants about their personal health situations. Client education begins with a comprehensive assessment of each client's needs, issues, and concerns, including what clients already know about their health condition, and treatment. When what a client "already knows" is inaccurate, a different set of evidence-based data can be shared with the client, as another source of data.

Each learning situation has a past and a present reality, and each client's unique story model of his or her illness or disability is different. Pender's health belief model proposes that past experience and beliefs about illness, medications and treatments, cultural values, and the reactions of others produce assumptions, which directly impact motivation and the acceptance of health teaching. Physical symptoms have an emotional, relational, and social context that need to be taken into account in individualizing teaching care plans. Finding out what the client feels is his or her primary health concern is important as this may differ from the reason that the client is seeking treatment. Apart from a client's symptom history, contextual factors such as impact on work or social relationships are often of considerable concern to clients. Open-ended questions help nurses understand the unique learning needs of individual clients and families in a practical way, for example, "Can you tell me what this illness has been like for you so far?." Box 15-1 provides examples of questions nurses can use to assess client learning needs.

BOX 15-1   Characteristics of Different Learning Styles

Visual
- Learns best by seeing
- Likes to watch demonstrations
- Organizes thoughts by writing them down
- Needs detail
- Looks around; examines situation

Auditory
- Learns best with verbal instructions
- Likes to talk things through
- Detail is not as important
- Talks about situation and pros and cons

Kinetic
- Learns best by doing
- Hands-on involvement
- Needs action and likes to touch, feel
- Loses interest with detailed instructions
- Tries things out

Assessing Personal Learning Characteristics

Personal learning characteristics have a significant influence on achieving positive clinical outcomes. Preferred learning style, developmental stage, learning readiness and motivation, and low health literacy affect successful learning (Bastable, 2013).

Preferred Learning Style. There are three major types of learning styles: *visual, auditory,* and *kinesthetic*. A visual learner learns best with reading or Web-based material and graphic images, rather than explanations. Auditory learners need to hear the information and appreciate discussion rather than

---

BOX 15-2	Questions to Assess Learning Needs

- What does the client already know about his or her condition and treatment?
- In what ways is the client affected by it?
- In what ways are those persons intimately involved with the client affected by the client's condition or treatment?
- What does the client identify as his or her most important learning need?
- To what extent is the client willing to take personal responsibility for seeking solutions?
- What goals would the client like to achieve?
- What will the client need to do to achieve those goals?
- What resources are available to the client and family that might affect the learning process?
- What barriers to learning exist?

---

strictly visual material. Kinesthetic learners learn best with demonstration and hands-on practice. Beagley (2011) notes that while most clients can learn with any of these learning styles, they have a preference and respond best when their preference is incorporated in teaching plans. Box 15-2 presents characteristics of different learning styles.

Learning Readiness. Learning readiness refers to a person's mind-set and openness to engaging in a learning or counseling process for the purpose of adopting new behaviors. Motivational interviewing is a widely used strategy designed to assess and enhance the potential for client learning readiness when internal motivation seems to be lacking. Nurses use empathy, acceptance, and respect for the client's autonomy to help clients choose and commit to positive health behavior changes. Rather than challenging a client's resistance directly, nurses guide clients from wherever they are in the continuum of assuming responsibility for health promotion enhancements to a better place. Four stages of change applicable to current behaviors and client investment in making positive behavioral change (precontemplation, contemplation, action, maintenance) direct the teaching learning process.

Emotional issues can increase, as well as interfere, with learning readiness. Crisis anxiety (if it is not extreme) can create an immediate need to learn (Mezirow, 1990). Uninsured and medically underserved clients, who may lack the resources or inclination to engage in health care otherwise, also seek crisis intervention services (Gravely et al., 2011). Health teaching for these clients should be practical and carefully orchestrated to meet client immediate needs. If clients experience professional support as a helpful relationship, they may be more receptive to less crisis-oriented health teaching interventions related to chronic conditions.

Ability to Learn. Some clients are ready to learn but are unable to do so with traditional learning formats. Assessing the client's ability to learn and adapting the learning format to the learner's unique characteristics makes a difference. For example, a client's physical condition or emotional state can temporarily preclude teaching. Clients in pain can focus on little else. Nausea or weakness makes it difficult for clients to sustain attention. Medications, or a temporary period of disorientation after a diagnostic test or surgical procedure, can inhibit concentration.

Accurately assessing and managing a client's level of anxiety before health teaching is essential, as is choosing a time when the client energy wise is most likely to be receptive (Stephenson, 2006). The shock of a difficult diagnosis may require teaching in small segments or postponement of serious teaching sessions until the client has understood the diagnosis. Clients with significant thought disorders have difficulty processing information. They may need simple concrete instructions and frequent prompts to perform adequately. Comorbid health problems can interfere with the goals of client education if not recognized. For example, an exercise program might be useful for an overweight person, but if the client also has asthma or another activity-limiting issue, the intervention might require modification. Elevated stress and anxiety affects a client's ability to focus attention and process material.

Health Literacy. If the client cannot understand what is being taught, learning does not take place.

The World Health Organization (WHO, 2009) definition of health literacy is expressed as "the cognitive and social skills, which determine the motivation and ability of individuals to gain access to, understand, and use information in ways that promote and maintain good health." This broader definition heightens awareness of the social aspects of health literacy that are sometimes overlooked in immediate hectic health teaching situations. Low literacy is related to, but is not the same as low health literacy; medical vocabulary can be daunting for many people (Schwartzberg et al., 2007).

Case Example

"Everything was happening so fast and everybody was so busy," and that is why Mitch Winston, 66 years old and suffering from atrial fibrillation, did not ask his doctor to clarify the complex and potentially dangerous medication regimen that had been prescribed for him on leaving the hospital emergency department. When he returned to the emergency department via ambulance, bleeding internally from an overdose of warfarin (Coumadin), his doctor was surprised to learn that Mitch had not understood the verbal instructions he had received, and that he had ignored the written instructions and orders for follow-up visits that the doctor had provided. In fact, these had never been retrieved from Mitch's wallet. Despite their importance, they were useless pieces of paper. Mitch cannot read (The Joint Commission, 2007, p. 5).

In addition to being able to accurately read and understand words and numbers, literacy includes being able to "orally express oneself, understand and recall spoken instructions, make inferences, utilize technology, critically weigh options and make decisions, and sustain often complex behaviors" (Wolf et al., 2012, p. 1302). Since nurses are identified as key providers of client education across clinical settings, it is especially important for us to incorporate health literacy strategies in all aspects of care. (Baker and colleagues, (2011)) suggest using a limited set of essential learning goals related to:

- Explaining the outcome behavior
- Essential background information to understand the recommended behavior
- Explanation of how the behavior change will help the client feel better
- What barriers exist and how they can be overcome to produce the desired result (p. 11)

Clients with limited literacy struggle harder to understand the material and usually need more time to process information. They tend to decode messages one word at a time and may not grasp the whole message. To facilitate understanding, use fewer, rather than more words to explain a concept, and allow extra time to practice psychomotor skills with ongoing feedback. Learning goals should be simple and delivered with words familiar to the learner. Provide only essential basic information in a sequential format and avoid information overload. Using open-ended questions and other listening responses can help you clarify what the client understands.

Some clients have adequate literacy skills, but a limited background or lack of interest in medical matters makes it difficult for them to understand medical terminology and complex medical explanations. The adage, keep information simple and straightforward, applies to all health education explanations.

Developmental Factors. The client's developmental learning factors significantly influence ability to learn (Bastable, 2013). Children at different levels of cognitive development need health teaching that is specifically tailored to match their developmental level. For example, children who developmentally cannot think abstractly will not understand a conceptual explanation of what is happening to them. Instead they need simple concrete explanations and examples. Recommended teaching strategies for client learners at different developmental levels are presented in Table 15-1.

Socioenvironmental Variables. Socioenvironmental factors can impact the effectiveness of health teaching *and* even produce dangerous outcomes. Commonly overlooked assessments are potential environmental barriers, such as limited health insurance, transportation difficulties, lack of follow-up facilities, accessible food markets and health facilities, cultural considerations, and choice of priorities due to poverty. Clients may not have the money for medication. A visit to the pediatrician for an ear infection may have a co-pay that the mother cannot afford. Health illiteracy can be a product of poverty, as well as culture (Lowenstein et al., 2009). Nurses need to explore the level and types of situational support available to clients and families as part of any teaching plan.

PLANNING

Family Involvement

Constructive family involvement is an *essential* component of successful self-management. The Joint Commission standards (2014) require evidence of direct education provided to the family as well as the client. Health teaching, similar to that provided to fully functional clients is required for anyone actively involved in the client's care as a primary caregiver or reliable supportive influence. Information and anticipatory guidance about what to expect when the client goes home, and early warning signs of complications or potential problems, should also be given to family members. Knowing when to seek professional

TABLE 15-1	Recommended Teaching Strategies at Different Development Levels
Developmental Level	**Recommended Teaching Strategies**
Preschool	Allow child to touch and play with safe equipment.
	Relate teaching to child's immediate experience.
	Use child's vocabulary whenever possible.
	Involve parents in teaching.
School-age	Give factual information in simple, concrete terms.
	Focus teaching on developing competency.
	Use simple drawings and models to emphasize points.
	Answer questions honestly and factually.
Adolescent	Use metaphors and analogies in teaching.
	Give choices and multiple perspectives.
	Incorporate the client's norm group values and personal identity issues in teaching strategies.
Adult	Involve client as an active partner in learning process.
	Encourage self-directed learning.
	Keep content and strategies relevant and practical.
	Incorporate previous life experience into teaching.
Older adult	Explain why the information should be important to the client.
	Incorporate previous life experience into teaching.
	Accommodate for sensory and dexterity deficits.
	Use short, frequent learning sessions (<30 minutes).

assistance and resource support is critical information. Examples of appropriate goals for family teaching relate to empowerment of family members in using equipment, understanding what is happening to their loved one, and promoting direct therapeutic care involvement.

Any change in the level of support from primary caregivers can affect a client's willingness or ability to learn. When these supports are no longer available through death, incapacity, or other reasons, the client may lack not only motivation but also the skills to cope with complex health problems.

Case Example

Edward Flanigan, an 82-year-old recently widowed man, has severe diabetes. There is no evidence of memory problems, but there are significant emotional components to his current health care needs. All his life, his wife pampered him and did everything for him, from meal preparation to monitoring his diabetes. Since her death, Edward takes no interest in controlling his diabetes. He doesn't follow his prescribed diabetic diet and is not consistent in taking his medication. Predictably, his diabetes has become increasingly unstable. His family worries about him, but he is unwilling to consider leaving his home of 42 years. To enhance Edward's learning readiness, how could Edward's teaching plan related to diabetic self-care management skills be individualized?

Considering Special Learning Needs

Cultural Diversity. Clients interpret health care messages within the context of culturally bound traditions, beliefs, and values. Tailoring teaching interventions to meet the specific cultural needs and resources of clients is key to improving outcomes through client education (Peek et al., 2012). Explanatory models for why symptoms develop and cultural attitudes toward common treatment protocols are important information as they are not always harmless. Inquire about home remedies and applicable spiritual influences. Differences should be treated with the utmost respect. When working with culturally diverse clients, it is important to simplify self-care management strategies and to put information in a culturally familiar context.

Culturally unique perspectives and preferences for treatment can be incorporated in many situations, if it is part of the assessment. Inquiry about use of folk medicine and indigenous health informants or providers is critically important. Culturally diverse clients are more likely to trust tradition-bound health care solutions than modern medical approaches. Clients prefer a teaching plan that integrates cultural practices with mainstream biomedical approaches. Recognition and acceptance of differences as long as they are not harmful is a component of participatory decision making.

Focusing on accurate information without destroying the credibility of influential cultural health advisors is part of the art of health teaching. Nothing is gained by injuring the reputation of the person who gave the client the information, and only those behaviors with potentially adverse health consequences should be addressed. For example, you might say: "There have been some new findings that I think you might be interested in. Current thinking suggests that (*give concrete example*) works well in situations like this." With this type of statement you can expand the client's thinking without challenging the status of the person a client considers as expert. (See Chapters 7 and 14 for more ideas tailoring communication and teaching strategies to use in teaching culturally diverse clients.) It is best to use simple concrete words and images in explaining options and to ask frequently for validation of understanding.

Culturally diverse clients are not deaf. Sometimes there is a tendency for people to speak louder when instructing someone from a different culture. Instead, speak *slowly* in a normal conversational tone. When teaching a client for whom English is a second language, keep in mind that words from one language do not necessarily translate with the same meaning in another. Certain concepts do not exist, or the phrases used for expressing and describing them differs significantly. Lorig (2001) suggests that when preparing teaching materials for translation, the following are important:

- Use nouns rather than pronouns and simple unambiguous language.
- Use short simple sentences of less than 16 words each.
- Avoid the use of metaphors and informal slang.
- Avoid verb forms that have more than one meaning or include would or could (p. 181).

If a client still is unable to understand important concepts with accommodations, enlisting the services of a trained medical interpreter becomes an essential intervention.

Cognitive-Processing Deficits. Learners with memory deficits, lack of insight, poor judgment, and limited problem-solving abilities require accommodations. Special needs learners respond best when the content is presented in a consistent, concrete, and patient manner, with clear and frequent cues to action. Patience and repetition of key ideas

---

Box 15-3	Suggested Format for Teaching Care Plans

- Briefly identify client's needs and preferences.
- Write summary statement of what is to be taught (three to four main points).
- Identify realistic goal(s) or outcome(s) you want the client to achieve with your teaching in one or two sentences.
- State two to three specific measurable behavioral objectives related to goal achievement.
- Specify content (relate to objectives) in bulleted outline form.
- Describe teaching methodology (e.g., discussion, demonstration, diagrams).
- Identify materials, handouts, and resources needed to achieve client success.
- Stipulate specific evaluation measures such as teach-back or return demonstration.

---

is essential. Illustrated materials can result in greater comprehension and recall, but they should be simple, without distracting details (Friedman et al., 2011). Including significant others in the teaching session increase chances of follow through with instructions if the deficit is more than minimal.

Creating a Successful Teaching Plan

Teaching care plans provide a guide for choosing and sequencing content and for selecting the best approach. Box 15-3 provides a sample format for developing relevant teaching plans.

Choosing Appropriate Focus. Choosing focus in health teaching is a critical competency because you need to distinguish between essential information about the most important client concerns, and "what would be nice to know." Edwards (2013) suggests that providers should collaborate with the client in focusing learning goals and related activities around the client's perception of the most pressing problem(s), including, but not centered solely around medical facts and provider recommendations. In developing client learning goals, keep in mind the following:

- What essential *information* does the client **need** to have for self-management and treatment compliance?
- What *attitudes* does the client hold that could **enable** or **hinder** the learning process?
- What specific *skills* does this client **need** for self-management?

- What does the client **want** from this health experience to improve his or her quality of life?
- What *cultural* or *socioenvironmental* factors could **facilitate** or **sabotage** the learning process?

Periodically asking the client and primary caregivers, "Do you have any questions for me?" gives nurses a sense of what is most important to the client or may not be fully understood. Suggest that if things come up that the client has questions about later, the client should ask for further clarification. Often hours or days after health teaching takes place, clients have questions or concerns about received information. You can offer additional opportunities for discussion after the client has had time to absorb the initial information, and encourage clients to jot down questions that may develop as they occur.

Health-Teaching Goals. Setting realistic collaborative goals with clients with periodic reviews not only helps motivate clients; they serve as a benchmark for evaluating changes. Establish goals *with* your client rather than *for* your client. Clear learning goals that the client is interested in meeting and for which he or she has the necessary ability and resources to achieve, increase the chances for compliance (London, 2001). Prioritizing individualized goals and objectives important to client health and well-being helps nurses and clients focus on the most relevant specifics.

Identify outcome goals with a general statement of what the client needs to achieve as a result of the teaching (e.g., "After health teaching, the client will maintain dietary control of her diabetes"; an interim goal might be, "After health teaching, the client will develop an appropriate diet plan for 1 week"). Setting realistic goals prevents disappointment. Box 15-4 provides guidelines for developing effective health teaching goals and objectives.

Developing Measurable Objectives. Objectives help organize content and identify logical action steps. Collaboratively developed objectives should describe an immediate action step-by-step plan for goal achievement based on the client's most pressing clinical issues (Edwards, 2013). Each action step should build on the previous one for maximum effectiveness. Objectives should be achievable in the time frame allotted. To determine whether an objective is achievable, consider the client's level of experience, educational level, resources, and motivation, and define the objectives accordingly in specific measurable behavioral terms.

BOX 15-4	Guidelines for Developing Effective Goals and Objectives

- Link goals to the nursing diagnosis.
- Make goals action-oriented.
- Make goals specific and measurable.
- Define objectives as behavioral outcomes.
- Design objectives with a specific time frame for achievement.
- Show a logical progression with established priorities.
- Review periodically and modify goals as needed.

Objectives should directly relate to medical and nursing diagnoses and support the overall health outcome. For example, the nursing diagnosis for a client with newly diagnosed diabetes might read, "knowledge deficit related to diabetic diet." Examples of appropriate progressive learning objectives required for mastering diabetic control might occur as follows:

- First teaching session: The client will identify the purpose of a diabetic diet and appropriate foods.
- Second teaching session: The client will identify appropriate foods and serving sizes allowed on a diabetic diet.
- Third teaching session: The client will demonstrate the processes for urine and blood testing for glucose at home.
- Fourth teaching session: The client will identify foods to avoid on the diabetic diet and the rationale for compliance.
- Fifth teaching session: The client will describe symptoms and actions to take for hyperglycemia and hypoglycemia.

Timing. Health teaching is *not* an add-on; it is an essential nursing intervention. Teaching interventions should never be eliminated because the nurse lacks time. Even in the most limited situation, schedule a block of time for health teaching. Because time is a precious commodity in health care, choosing the most effective and efficient ways to achieve identified clinical goals is vital (Stephenson, 2006). You need to consider how much time is required to learn a particular skill or body of knowledge, and build this into the learning situation. Complicated skill development may need blocks of time for repeated practice with feedback. Pick times for teaching when energy levels are high, other things do not distract the client, it is not visiting time and the client is alert and not in pain. Careful observation of the client helps determine the most appropriate times for health teaching.

Even under the best of circumstances, people can absorb only so many details and fine points at a time (Suter and Suter, 2008). Keep the teaching session short, interesting, and to the point. Ideally, teaching sessions should last no longer than about 20 minutes, including time for questions. Otherwise, the client may tire or lose interest. Scheduling shorter sessions with time in between to process information helps prevent sensory overload and reinforces teaching points.

Nurses also have opportunities for informal teaching during the course of providing care. Simple, spontaneous health teaching takes minutes, but can have immeasurable effects. The following case example, taken from *Heartsounds* (Lear, 1980), illustrates this point.

Case Example

A nurse came in while he was eating dinner. "Dr. Lear," she said, "after angiography the patients always seem to have the same complaints, and I thought you might want to know about them. It might help." (This was a good nurse. I didn't know it then, because I didn't know how scared he was. But later I understood that this was a darned good nurse.)

"Thanks, it would help," he said.

"It's mostly two things. The first is, they say that during the test, they feel a tremendous flush. It's very sudden and it can be scary."

He responds to the nurse, "Okay, the flush. And what's the other thing?"

"It's...well, they say that at a certain point, they feel as though they are about to die. But that feeling passes quickly." He thanked her again. He was very grateful.

(Later, during the actual procedure, Dr. Lear remembered the nurse's words and found comfort.) "Easy. Easy. You're supposed to feel this way. This is precisely what the nurse described. The moment you feel you are dying" (Lear, 1980, pp. 120-121).

Implementation

Each teaching session should be a collaborative process with reciprocal exchange of information, feedback, and opportunities to ask questions.

Building a Logical Information Flow. No one teaching strategy can meet the needs of all clients (Su et al., 2011). Introductory content should build on the client's experiences, abilities, interests, motivation, and skills. Most clients learn best when there is a logical flow and building of information from simple to complex. *Begin by presenting a simple overview of what will be taught and why the information is important to learn.* Include only essential information in your overview; for example, give a brief explanation of the health care problem, risk factors, treatment, and self-care skills the client will need to manage at home. Incorporate or ask about previous related experience.

Concrete application of knowledge in a meaningful context increases learning (Benner et al., 2010). (2010). Ideally you should solicit input frequently and offer opportunities for client feedback and questions. Complex information can be delivered in smaller stepwise learning segments. For example, diabetic teaching could include the following segments:

- Introduction, including what the client does know
- Basic pathophysiology of diabetes (keep description simple and short)
- Diet and exercise
- Demonstration of insulin injection with return demonstration
- Recognizing signs and symptoms of hyperglycemia and hypoglycemia
- Care of skin and feet
- How to talk to the doctor

A strong closing statement summarizing major points reinforces the learning process. Exercise 15-2 provides practice with developing a mini teaching plan.

Using Clear Concrete Language

Use simple familiar words and limit the number of ideas in each learning segment. General or vague language leaves the learner wondering what the nurse actually meant. For example, "Call the doctor if you have any problems" has more than one meaning. "Problems" can refer to side effects of the medication, a return of symptoms, problems with family acceptance, changed relationships, and even alterations in self-concept. Instead say, "If you should develop a headache or feel dizzy in the next 24 hours, call the emergency department doctor right away."

Checking with clients to confirm a common understanding of words and concepts is critical to knowledge transfer in health teaching. Doak et al, (2001) suggest asking the client, "What does this material tell you about _____ [subject]? What does it tell you to do?" (p. 188). Concrete

EXERCISE 15-2	Developing Teaching Plans

Purpose: To provide practice with developing teaching plans.

Procedure

1. Using the teaching plan format, develop a mini teaching plan for one of your clients. Alternative: Develop a mini teaching plan for one of the following client situations:
   a. Jim Dolan feels stressed about returning to work after his accident. He is requesting health teaching on stress management and relaxation techniques.
   b. Adrienne Parker is a newly diagnosed diabetic. Her grandfather had diabetes.
   c. Marion Hill just gave birth to her first child. She wants to breast-feed her infant, but she does not think she has enough milk.
   d. Barbara Scott weighs 210 pounds and wants to lose weight.
2. Include the following data: a brief statement of client learning needs and a list of related nursing diagnoses in order of priority.
3. For one nursing diagnosis, develop a mini teaching plan outline that contains objectives, topical content outline, planned teaching strategies, time frame for planned activities, and evaluation criteria.

---

examples help clients understand abstract material. You can ask the client for relevant examples to make a point.

Written directions should demonstrate similar language clarity. From a study of client input about written care instructions, Buckley et al. (2013) suggest highlighting key words, for example: "After cleaning, you can **apply antibiotic ointment** 'Neosporin or bacitracin' to the wound and then put on a clean bandage" (p. 556).

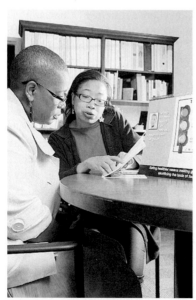

Nurses use multiple instructional aides to help clients remember essential information. *(Courtesy of Amanda Mills, Centers for Disease Control and Prevention, 2011.)*

Incorporating Visual Aids. You can use line drawings and simple diagrams of anatomical body parts or physiology related to a procedure to increase comprehension. *Simple* images and fewer words work better than complicated visual aids. For example, an illustrated chart showing how the heart pumps blood might help a client understand the anatomy and physiology of a cardiac problem better than words. Perdue and colleagues (1999) suggest that DVDs are useful in teaching clients with limited reading skills. They have the advantage of allowing clients to watch them again at their convenience. Related discussions help to correct misinterpretations and emphasize pertinent points.

Preparing Written Handouts. Written materials to which clients can refer when needed reinforce learning. Attention to the client's reading level and health care literacy helps ensure that the pamphlets will be read (CDC, 2009). Most reading materials should be geared to a sixth-grade reading level. Even people with adequate health literacy comprehend written information better when the language is simple and clear using layperson's language. Large-print pamphlets and audiotapes are helpful learning aids for those with sight problems and auditory learners. Guidelines for preparing effective written materials include the following:

- Present the most important information first.
- Use illustrations and diagrams designed to enhance clarity and appeal.
- Make sure that the content is current, accurate, objective, *and* consistent with information provided by other team members.

EXERCISE 15-3	Teach-Back

Purpose: To help students understand the teach-back process.

Procedure
Review what you learned in class about the teach-back method. Break into class groups of three students: nurse, client, and observer. Each student will take a turn being the nurse, the client, and the observer. Using one medication that your client is on, role-play the teach-back process with one person taking the role of nurse, another the client receiving the medication for the first time, and the third person an observer.

Rotate roles so each student has the opportunity to role-play the nurse role.

Discussion
After *each* teach-back role-play:
1. The nurse should reflect on what he or she did well or would have changed.
2. The observer should provide feedback on what the nurse did well and what he or she could have done better.
3. The client should add his or her perspective and anything that was not addressed by the other two participants.

- Use appropriate language at a literacy level that the reader can understand.
- Use a 12-point font and avoid using all capital letters for reading ease.
- Define technical terms in lay language and avoid medical jargon.
- Bold important points.
- Check for spelling errors and stay away from complicated sentences.
- Include resources with contact information that the client can refer to for further information or for help with problems.

Using Advance Organizers. Advance organizers, called *mnemonics*, consist of cue words, phrases, or letters related to more complex data can help clients remember difficult concepts. For example, each letter in diabetes can represent an action for diabetic control. Taken together, the client has a useful tool for remembering *all* related concepts:

D = diet
I = infections
A = administering medications
B = basic pathophysiology
E = eating schedules
T = treatment for hyperglycemia or hypoglycemia
E = exercise
S = symptom recognition

Evaluation and Documentation

Teach-Back. Teach-back or show me is a client/provider evaluation method used to confirm a client's understanding of and/or ability to execute self-management skills through demonstration or explanation of major points. It involves having the client explain relevant information and treatment instructions in his or her own words (Lorenzen et al., 2008). Teach-back offers nurses valuable data about areas of skill learning needing additional attention. To avoid having an exam-like approach, start with a statement such as, "I just want to be sure that I have explained everything you need to know. Can you tell me, in your own words, how you will determine that your blood sugar is low, and what you will do if it is?" Encourage the client to ask questions. If the content is complex, consider using teach-back after each segment, before moving on to the next concept. Redo instruction if needed. Document your use of teach-back and the client's response (Exercise 15-3).

Documenting Health Teaching. The Joint Commission (2014) *requires* written documentation of all client health teaching. Notes about the initial assessment should be succinct, but comprehensive and objective. Teaching content should be linked to assessment data, including client preferences, previous knowledge, and values. Included in the documentation are the teaching actions, the client response, and any clinical issues or barriers to compliance. If family members are involved, you should identify their role, content provided, and teaching outcomes in your documentation. Accurate documentation helps ensure continuity and prevents duplication of teaching efforts. The client's record informs other health care providers of what has been taught and what areas need further work.

Self-Management Strategies

The focus on self-management strategies in client education reflects the growth extent of chronic illness in our nation and the transformational emphasis on participatory self-management of chronic disorders as a way of reducing health costs while still providing quality care (Peeters et al., 2013). Examples of chronic illnesses requiring self-management include cancer, asthma, COPD, diabetes, multiple sclerosis, arthritis, hypertension, macular degeneration, cardiovascular disorders, and chronic mental illness. Cystic fibrosis, developmental delays or abnormalities, juvenile diabetes, sickle cell anemia, and childhood cancer are significant chronic disorders affecting children.

Skill support for clients and families requires more than informative education. Holman and Lorig (2004) research findings indicate that clients desire access to information and continuity of care as part of learning about their condition and how to self-manage their symptoms. The Center for the Advancement of Health (2002) identifies problem solving, decision making, goal setting, utilization of resources, development of client/provider partnerships, and taking action as essential self-management skills.

Essential Skill Development. Mickley et al. (2013) define self-management as "the skills and activities necessary to control symptoms of a chronic condition" (p. 323). Development of self-management skills requires a contextual, problem-based teaching approach. Key skills identified in the literature involve "monitoring, interpreting, making decisions, taking actions, making adjustments, accessing resources, providing hands-on care, working together with the ill person, and navigating the health care system" (Schumacher and Marren, 2004, p. 460). In addition to learning specific knowledge, and skills, clients need to learn how to live with a chronic illness. This usually involves special attention to the social consequences and life style changes occurring as a result of the chronic condition. A multi-strategy approach is useful, including the activation of essential resources such as social services, joining support groups, choosing different activities, and so forth (Barlow et al., 2002). Children usually require consistent parental support and encouragement to follow through with care tasks and they need reinforcement of small successes. Because of their developmental needs, children may require special adaptations to lead normal healthy lives. Nurses should be aware of school and community supports available for children with chronic disabilities.

The client's active participation is essential in the daily management of chronic medical conditions

(Udlis, 2011). Consequently, participatory decision making is a vital component of meaningful action planning and tailoring of teaching strategies for individual clients and families is a critical dimension. *Repetition is important*, as is careful inquiry with open-ended questions about new issues. Clients should understand why an action is important, what can be expected with a medication or treatment protocol, what are the risks and benefits of treatment options, and what are the warning signs of adverse reactions. Unforeseen factors affecting the self-management process such as changes in the environmental context, interactions with health professionals, and changes imposed by the chronic illness make this information essential content. Incomplete client education, resulting in clients not knowing how to self-monitor symptoms and recognize side effects is not only unsafe, it is ethically indefensible (Redman, 2011). Clients need support as they take the first steps toward autonomously assuming responsibility for self-care and whenever a health situation changes. Living with chronic illness produces unexpected transitions in care requirements associated with exacerbations. Accommodating changes is important. Self-monitoring should focus on changes in symptoms and achieving treatment goals. Client and family input, combined with professional contributions, are essential for the development of personalized self-care applications. They help incorporate specific self-management actions with a client's daily routine.

Coaching. *Coaching* is a dynamic interactive and context-based teaching strategy. It offers tailored support for self-management and problem-solving skills with clients and families experiencing unfamiliar tasks and procedures (Huffman, 2007). For example, coaching can help clients distinguish between which symptoms require immediate medical attention and which ones can be handled with self-management strategies. Nurses can assist the client or family in opening a communication with a health agency and with choosing appropriate questions to ask. A coaching intervention can be as simple as helping people seek information from several sources rather than calling only one, and waiting for a response (Lorig and Holman, 2003).

Coaching "builds on the client's strengths rather than attempting to "fix weaknesses (Dossey and Hess, 2013, p 10). It emphasizes the client's autonomy in acquiring self-management skills, because the client is always in charge of the pace and direction of the

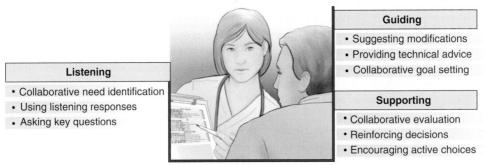

Figure 15-5   The nurse's role in coaching clients.

| **EXERCISE 15-4** | **Coaching** |

Purpose: To help students understand the process of coaching.

Procedure
Identify the steps you would use to coach a current client or a client with one of the chronic health conditions listed. Use Figure 15-1 as a guide to develop your plan.
  1. A client returning from hip replacement surgery
  2. A client recovering from a myocardial infarction
  3. A client with newly diagnosed diabetes, type II
  4. A child with partially controlled asthma
Share your suggestions with your classmates.

Discussion
1. What were the different coaching strategies you used with the client?
2. In what ways were your coaching strategies similar to or unlike those of your classmates?
3. How could you use the information you gained from this exercise to improve the quality of your coaching?

---

learning. Assessment for coaching purposes starts with an exploration of past history relevant to the client's current health situation and the client's current health issues. This dialogue provides a basis for looking at current options and taking different options based on client values and beliefs. Nurses can encourage clients to critically think about the elements of a situation, consider multiple options, consider new perspectives, and evaluate the appropriateness of choosing one option over another. Coaching involves a number of skills presented in Figure 15-5.

The coaching process involves taking the client step by step through a procedure or activities with the client taking the lead in choice of actions. The secret of successful coaching is to provide enough information and/or support to help the client take the next step without taking over. Coaching can include supervised skill practice and role-playing. For example, role-playing a potentially difficult conversation can inform the client about timing of actions, potential outcomes, areas that need special attention, and contextual issues that might not otherwise emerge in a teaching

situation. Exercise 15-4 provides practice with coaching as a teaching strategy.

Providing Transitional Cues. Clients may have difficulty with learning essential information because they do not see how information fits together, in their particular circumstances. Transitional cues linking purpose with action, for example, following the purpose of taking a medication or doing an exercise, with the actions you want the client to take. This dual approach helps fix the process in a person's mind and makes it easier to remember related instructions. When you tell a client, a medication should be taken with meals, be specific about what this means and why it is important. Ask the client (teach-back) how he or she will implement essential health management skills, such as using an inhaler or adhering to a therapeutic diet. Such discussions offer clients another opportunity to discuss any issues or concerns they have about their self-management skills. Visual cues such as a sticky note to remember to take medication or to keep an appointment are helpful too. Asking clients to keep a journal of their daily activities and responses to learning new skills so that you and the client can review these self-report logs and make changes as needed is also helpful.

Giving Feedback. Feedback is of central importance in successful health coaching. To appreciate its significance in learning new skills, consider the effect on your performance if you never received feedback from your instructor. For maximum effectiveness, give feedback as soon as possible after the learning event or observation. Consider the impact on the client. Encourage client reflection by asking open-ended questions such as, "How did you feel about doing your treatment by yourself?" "Is there anything you would do differently next time?" Indirect feedback—provided through nodding, smiling, and sharing information about the process and experiences of others—also reinforces learning. When providing feedback, keep it *participatory and simple*. Focus only on behaviors that can be changed and include strengths as well as areas needing improvement. Exercise 15-5 provides practice with giving feedback.

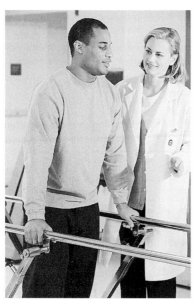

Giving immediate feedback is important with learning psychomotor tasks.

Behavioral Approaches

Behavioral approaches are based on the work of BF Skinner (1971). Behaviorists believe that reinforcement strengthens learner responses. Choice of rewards are based on the premack principle, defined as selecting positive reinforcers with meaning to the learner. This is critical because what is reinforcing to one person may not be so for another. Rewarded behaviors (positive reinforcement) tend to be repeated. Negative reinforcement (reward withdrawal) and ignoring behaviors tend to diminish their occurrence. Different types of reinforcement with examples are found in Table 15-2. Reinforcement schedules describe the timing of rewards. Schedules start with continuous reinforcement for each completed attempt. Once a new behavior is in place, interval schedules in which reinforcement is given after a certain number of successful attempts (fixed interval), or after a random number of responses (variable ratio) are introduced. Tangible rewards are gradually replaced with social reinforcement such as praise. Over time, improved health outcomes become a source of reinforcement to clients. For example, significant weight loss and the way it makes a person feel about personal appearance is a strong motivator to continue with a healthy diet.

A behavioral approach starts with a careful description of a concrete behavior requiring change. Describe each action as a single behavioral unit (e.g., failing to take a medication, cheating on a diet, or not participating in unit activities). It is important to start small so the client will experience success.

A behavioral approach requires the cooperation of the client and a shared understanding of the problem. Counting the number of times the client engages in a behavior as a baseline before implementing the behavioral approach allows the nurse and the client to monitor progress.

Behavioral objectives should be action oriented. They reframe the problem in a solution statement (e.g., "The client will lose 2 pounds"). Begin with the simplest and most likely behavior to stimulate client interest. Identify the tasks in sequential order; define specific consequences, positive and negative, for behavioral responses; and solicit the client's cooperation.

Behavioral Strategies. Modeling describes learning a behavior by observing another person performing it. Nurses model behaviors in their normal conduct of nursing activities and teaching situations. Bathing an infant, feeding an older person, and talking to a scared child in front of significant caregivers provides informal modeling.

Shaping refers to the reinforcement of successive approximations of the target behavior. The long-term goal is broken down into smaller steps. The person is

| EXERCISE 15-5 | Usable Feedback |

Purpose: To give students perspective and experience in giving usable feedback.

Procedure
1. Divide the class into working groups of three or four students.
2. Present a 3-minute sketch of some aspect of your current learning situation that you find difficult (e.g., writing a paper, speaking in class, coordinating study schedules, or studying certain material).
3. Each person, in turn, offers one piece of usable informative feedback to the presenter. In making suggestions, use the guidelines on feedback given in this chapter.

4. Place feedback suggestions on a flip chart or chalkboard.

Discussion
1. What were your thoughts and feelings about the feedback you heard in relation to resolving the problem you presented to the group?
2. What were your thoughts and feelings in giving feedback to each presenter?
3. Was it harder to give feedback in some cases than in others? In what ways?
4. What common themes emerged in your group?
5. In what ways can you use the self-exploration about feedback in this exercise in teaching conversations with clients?

| TABLE 15-2 | Types of Reinforcement |

Concept	Purpose	Example
Positive reinforcer	Increases probability of behavior through reward	Stars on a board, smiling, verbal praise, candy, tokens to "purchase" items
Negative reinforcer	Increases probability of behavior by removing aversive consequence	Restoring privileges when client performs desired behavior
Punishment	Decreases behavior by presenting a negative consequence or removing a positive one	Time-outs, denial of privileges
Ignoring	Decreases behavior by not reinforcing it	Not paying attention to whining, tantrums, or provocative behaviors

reinforced for any behavior (successive approximations) that gets him or her closer to accomplishing the desired behavior.

Learning Contracts. The learning contract with the client serves as a formal commitment to a behavioral learning process. Contracts spell out the responsibilities of each party, expected behaviors, and reinforcements. Contracts are especially useful as part of learning self-management strategies for school-aged children (Burkhart et al., 2012; Mickley, 2013). The contract should include:

- Behavioral changes that are to occur
- Conditions under which they are to occur
- Reinforcement schedule
- Time frame

Initially, each instance of expected behavior should be rewarded. If the client is noncompliant or needs to pay more attention to a particular aspect of behavior, the nurse can say, "This (*name the behavior or skill*) needs a little more work." One advantage of a behavioral approach is that it never considers the client as bad or unworthy.

Group Presentations

Group presentations offer the advantage of being able to teach a number of people at one time. The format allows people to learn from each other, as well as from the nurse educator. Health teaching topics that lend themselves to a group format include care of the newborn, diabetes, oncology, and prenatal and postnatal care (Redman, 2007).

EXERCISE 15-6	Group Health Teaching

Purpose: To provide practice with presenting a health topic in a group setting.

Procedure

1. Plan a 15- to 20-minute health presentation on a health topic of interest to you, including teaching aids and methods for evaluation. Suggested topics:

Nutrition	Weight control
Drinking and driving	Mammograms
High blood pressure	Safe sex

2. Present your topic to your class group.

Formal group teaching should occur in a space large enough to accommodate all participants. The learner should be able to hear and see the instructor and visual aids without strain. Technical equipment (if used) should be available and in working order. Should the equipment not work, it is better to eliminate the planned teaching aid completely than to spend a portion of the teaching session trying to fix it. Preparation and practice can ensure that your presentation is clear, concise, and well spoken.

Establish rapport with your audience. Extension of eye contact to all participants communicates acceptance and inclusion. Make eye contact immediately and continue to do so throughout the presentation. An initial quote capturing the meaning of the presentation or a humorous opening grabs the audience's attention. Logical organization of the material is essential. Strengthen content statements with careful use of specific examples. Citing a specific problem and the ways another person dealt with it offers a broader perspective. Repeating key points and summarizing them again at the conclusion of the session helps reinforce learning.

Use slides to identify key points. Slides help you stay on track and move through the agenda. The font should be large enough to see from a distance (32 point is recommended). Include no more than four or five items per slide. Face the audience, not the slides. Practice your presentation to ensure that you keep within the time frame and allot time for short discussion points. It is up to you as the presenter to set the pace. No matter how interesting the presentation and dialogue that it stimulates, running out of time is frustrating for the audience.

Anticipate questions and be on the alert for blank looks. No matter how good a nurse educator you are, from time to time you will experience the blank look. When this occurs, it is appropriate to ask, "Does anyone have any questions about what I just said?" Give reinforcement for comments, such as "I'm so glad you brought that up," or "That's a really interesting question (or comment)." Smiling and nodding your head are nonverbal reinforcers. If a participant has a question that you cannot answer, do not bluff. Instead, say, "That is a good question. I don't have an answer at this moment, but I will get back to you with it." Sometimes another person will have the required information and will share it. Handouts provide reinforcement. Make sure that the information is accurate, complete, easy to understand, logical, and very important, and that you have enough for all participants. Exercise 15-6 provides an opportunity to practice health teaching in a group setting.

Health Teaching in the Home. Health teaching in the home includes assessment of the home environment, family supports, and resources, as well as client needs. In many ways the home offers a teaching laboratory unparalleled in the hospital. The nurse can "see" improvisations in equipment and technique that are possible in the home environment. Family members may have ideas that the nurse would not have thought of and the nurse can see obstacles the family face. Nurses should review the basic pathophysiology and course of the client's health condition with the client and family. Everyone should understand the nature of chronic illness, the potential for exacerbation episodes. Teach-back evaluation helps reinforce learning.

The nurse is a guest in the client's home. Always call before going to the client's home. This is common courtesy; it also protects the nurse's time if the client is going to be out. Teaching in home care settings is rewarding. Often the nurse is the client's only visitor. Family members often display a curiosity and willingness to be a part of the learning group, particularly if the nurse actively uses knowledge of the home environment to make suggestions about needed modifications.

| BOX 15-5 | Medication Teaching Tips |

- Provide clients with written drug information, particularly for metered-dose inhalants and high-alert medications such as insulin.
- Include family or caregivers in the teaching sessions for clients who need extra support or reminders.
- Do not wait until discharge to begin education about complex drug regimens.
- Clearly explain directions for using each medication.
- Always require repeat demonstrations or explanations about medications to be taken at home, particularly for those requiring special drug administration techniques.
- Use the time you already spend with clients during assessments and daily care to evaluate their level of understanding about their medications.
- Keep medication administration schedule as simple and easy to follow as possible.

Adapted from Institute for Safe Medication Practices: *Patient medication teaching tips*, Huntingdon Valley, PA, 2006, Author.

Teaching in home settings should center on self-management essentials. Encourage clients or caregivers to write down their questions between visits, so critical issues can be addressed during the home visit. Start each session with an open-ended question as to how things are going. Ask if there are any new or unresolved concerns. You need to review medications with the client or caregiver on every visit. Tips for teaching clients and caregivers about medications are presented in Box 15-5. Other content should reflect specific information the client and family need to support self-care management.

An understanding of Medicare, Medicaid, and other insurance regulations, required documentation, and reimbursement schedules is important, as is knowledge of community resources *and* helping clients access them. Expert nurses know that clients often can be a source of information about resources they may not know about.

SUMMARY

This chapter describes the nurse's role in health teaching. Theoretical frameworks, client-centered teaching, developmental, and behavioral approaches guide the nurse in implementing health teaching. Teaching is designed to access one or more of the three domains of

learning: cognitive, affective, and psychomotor. Assessment for purposes of constructing a teaching plan centers on three areas: What does the client already know? What is important for the client to know? What is the client ready to learn?

No one teaching strategy can meet the needs of all clients. Essential content in all teaching plans includes information about the health care problem, risk factors, and self-care skills needed to manage at home. Client learning needs help define relevant teaching strategies. Several teaching strategies, such as coaching, use of mnemonics, and visual aids, are described. Repetition of key concepts and frequent feedback make the difference between simple instruction, and teaching that informs. Nurses use teach-back methods to confirm understanding. The Joint Commission (2014) requires documentation of client education. The client's record becomes a permanent communication tool, informing other health care workers what has been taught and what areas need to be addressed in future teaching sessions

DISCUSSION QUESTIONS

1. How can you best integrate chronic disease–related personal self-management skills with lifestyle and other aspects of the client's life?
2. Discuss what is meant by the statement: "Client education is essential to safe, ethical clinical practice."
3. What *specific* strategies would you use to help low-literacy clients learn essential health information?

ETHICAL DILEMMA   What Would You Do?

Louisa is a low literacy client at the mental health clinic who wants a refill of her medication. She states that she has reduced her medication to every other day, rather than every day because she thinks it "works better for her." She does not want to lower her dose. She also tells the nurse that she gave several of her extra pills to her brother, because he ran out of his pills. Although she listens politely to the nurse's concerns, Louisa tells her that she thinks her current regime is appropriate for her. She sees nothing wrong with sharing her meds with her brother as he is on the same medication. If you were the nurse, how would you respond to this client?

REFERENCES

American Nurses Association (ANA): *Scope and standards of practice*, Washington, DC, 2004, Author.

Anderson LW, Krathwohl DR, Airasian PW, Cruikshank KA, Mayer RE, Pintrich PR, Raths J, Wittrock MC: *A Taxonomy for Learning, Teaching, and Assessing: A revision of Bloom's Taxonomy of Educational Objectives*, New York, 2000, Pearson, Allyn & Bacon.

Ajzen I: The theory of planned behavior, *Organizational Behavior and Human Decision Processes* 50:179–211, 1991.

Baker D, DeWalt D, Schillinger D, Hawk V, et al.: Teach to goal: Theory and design Principles of an intervention to improve heart failure self-management skills of patients with low literacy, *J Health Commun 16(suppl 3)* 7:3–88, 2011.

Barlow J, Wright C, Sheasby J, Turner A, Hainsworth J: Self-management approaches for people with chronic conditions a review, *Patient Educ Couns* 48(2):177–187, 2002.

Bastable S: Nurse as educator: principles of teaching and learning for nursing practice. In *Sudbury MA: Jones & Bartlett*, 2013.

Beagley L: Educating patients: Understanding barriers, learning styles, and teaching techniques, *J Perianesthesia Nurs* 26(5):331–337, 2011.

Benner P, Sutphen M, Leonard V, et al.: *Educating nurses: a call for radical transformation*, Standford, CA, 2010, Jossey-Bass.

Bonaldi-Moore L: The nurse's role in educating postmastectomy breast cancer patients, *Plast Surg Nurs* 29(4):212–219, 2009.

Buckley B, McCarthy DM, Forth VE, Tanabe P, Schmidt MJ, Adams JG, Engel KG: Patient input into the development and enhancement of ED discharge instructions: A focus group study, *J Emerg Nurs* 39(6):553–561, 2013, http://dx.doi.org/10.1016/j.jen.2011.12.018. Epub 2012 May 9.

Burkhart P, Oakley M, Mickley K: Self-management for school-age children with asthma, *Curr Pediatr Rev* 8:45–50, 2012.

CDC 2009 *Simply Put: A Guide for Creating Easy-to-Understand Materials 3rd ed*. www.cdc.gov/healthliteracy/pdf/simply_put.pdf

Center for the Advancement of Health: *Essential elements of self-management interventions*, Washington, DC, 2002, Author.

Doherty D: Guided care nurses help chronically ill patients, *Patient Educ Manag* 16(12):139–141, 2009.

Doak C, Doak L, Gordon L, Lorig K: Selecting, preparing and using materials. In Lorig K, editor: *Patient education: a practical approach*, ed 3, Thousand Oaks, CA, 2001, Sage, pp 183–197.

Dossey B, Hess D. Professional nurse coaching: Advances in global healthcare transformation. *Global Advances in Health and Medicine*. 40(2):10–16, 2013.

Dreeben O: *Patient Education in Rehabilitation*, Sudbury MA, 2010, Jones & Bartlett Publishers.

Edwards A: Asthma action plans and self-management: Beyond the traffic light, *Nurs Clin North Am* 48:47–51, 2013.

Farin E, Gramm L, Schmidt E: Predictors of communication preferences in patients with chronic low pain, *Patient Prefer Adherence* 7:1117–1127, 2013.

Freda M: Issues in patient education, *J Midwifery Womens Health* 39(3):203–209, 2004.

Friedman AJ, Cosby R, Boyko S, et al.: Effective teaching strategies and methods of delivering for patient education: A systemic review and practice guideline recommendations, *J Cancer Educ* 26, 2011. 12-2.

Feudtner C: What are the goals of patient education? *West J Med* 174(3):173–174, 2001.

Gordon J: Educating the patient: Challenges and opportunities with current technology, *Nurs Clin North Am* 46:341–350, 2011.

Gravely S, Hensley B, Hagood-Thompson C: Comparison of three types of diabetic foot ulcer education plans to determine patient recall of education, *J Vasc Nurs* 29:113–119, 2011.

Holman H, Lorig K: Patient self-management: A key to effectiveness and efficacy in care of chronic disease, *Public Health Rep* 119:239, 2004. 239-243.

Holt JE, Flint EP, Bowers MT: Got the picture? Using mobile phone technology to reinforce discharge instructions, *Am J Nurs* 111(8)(4):6–51, 2011.

Hudon C, Tribble D, Bravo G, et al.: Family physician enabling attitudes: a study of patient perceptions, *BMC Fam Practice* 14:8–16, 2013.

Huffman M: Health coaching: A new and exciting technique to enhance patient self-management and improve outcomes, *Home Healthc Nurse* 25(4):271–274, 2007.

Inott T, Kennedy B: Assessing learning styles: practical tips for patient education, *Nurs Clin North Am* 46(3):313–320, 2011.

Kelo M, Eriksson E, Eriksson I: Pilot educational program to enhance empowering patient education of school-age children with diabetes, *J Diabetes Metab Disord* 12:18, 2014.

Knowles M, Holton E, Swanson R: *The adult learner: the definitive classic on adult education and training*, 7th ed, Oxford UK, 2011, Elsevier.

Krau S: Creating educational objectives for patient education using the new Bloom's taxonomy, *Nurs Clin North Am (46)*299–321, 2011.

Lear MW: *Heartsounds Pocket Books*, New York, 1980, Simon & Schuster.

Lewis D: Computers in patient education, *Comput Inform Nurs* 21(2):88–96, 2003.

London F: Take the frustration out of patient education, *Home Healthc Nurse* 19(3):158–160, 2001.

Lorenzen B, Melby C, Earles B: Using principles of health literacy to enhance the informed consent process, *AORN J* 88(1):23–29, 2008.

Lorig K: *Patient education: a practical approach ed 3 Sage*, Oaks, CA, 2001, Thousand.

Lorig K, Holman H: Self-management education: history, definition, outcomes and mechanisms, *Ann Behav Med* 26(1):1–7, 2003.

Lowenstein AA, Foord-May LL, Romano JJ: *Teaching strategies for health education and health promotion*, Sudbury, MA, 2009, Jones & Bartlett.

Manning S: The nurses I'll never forget, *Nursing* 22(8):47, 1992.

Masters K: *Role development in professional nursing*, Sudbury MA, 2008, Jones & Bartlett.

McCormack B, McCance T: Development of a framework for person-centred nursing, *J Adv Nurs* 56(5):472–479, 2006.

Menendez J: Informed consent: Essential legal and ethical principles for nurses, *JONA's Health Law, Ethics, and Regulations* 15(4):140–144, 2013.

Mezirow J: *Fostering critical reflection in adulthood: a guide to transformative and emancipatory learning*, San Francisco, CA, 1990, Jossey-Bass.

Mickley K, Burkhart P, Sigler A: Promoting normal development and self-efficacy in school age children managing chronic conditions, *Nurs Clin North Am* 48(2):319–328, 2013.

Peek M, Harmon S, Scott J, et al.: Culturally tailoring patient education and communication skills training to empower African Americans with diabetes, *Transl Behav Med* 2(3):296–308, 2012.

Peeters J, Wiegers T, Friele R: How technology in care at home affects patient self-care and self-management: A scoping review, *Int J Environ Res Public Health* 10(11):5541–5564, 2013.

Perdue B, Degazon C, Lunny M: Diagnoses and interventions with low literacy, *Nurs Diagn* 10(1):36–39, 1999.

Redman BK: *The practice of patient education: a case study approach*, ed 10, St. Louis, 2007, Mosby.

Redman BK: Ethics of patient education and how do we make it everyone's ethics, *Nurs Clin North Am* 46:283–289, 2011.

Rogers C: *Freedom to learn for the '80s*, Columbus, OH, 1983, Merrill.

Skinner BF: *Beyond freedom and dignity*, New York, 1971, Knopf.

Schumacher K, Marren J: Home care nursing for older adults: state of the science, *Nurs Clin North Am* 39:443–471, 2004.

Schwartzberg J, Cowett A, Vangeest J, Wolf M: Communication techniques for patients with low literacy: a survey of physicians, nurses, and pharmacists, *Am J Health Behav* 31(9):S96–S104, 2007.

Smith L: Help your patients access government health information, *Nursing* 2013:32–34, 2013.

Speros CL: Promoting health literacy: a nursing imperative, *Nurs Clin North Am* 46(3):321–333, 2011.

Stephenson P: Before the teaching begins: managing patient anxiety prior to providing education, *Clin J Oncol Nurs* 10(2):241–245, 2006.

Su WM, Osisek P, Starnes B: Applying the revised Bloom's Taxonomy to a medical–surgical nursing lesson, *Nurse Educ* 29(3):116–120, 2004.

Su WM, Herron B, Osisek P: Using a competency based approach to patient education: Achieving congruence among learning, teaching and evaluation, *Nurs Clin North Am* 46(3):291–298, 2011.

Szpiro K, Harrison M, Kerkhof Van Den, Lougheed M MD: Patient education in the emergency department, *Adv Emerg Nurs J* 30(1):34–49, 2008.

Suter PM, Suter WN: Timeless principles of learning: a solid foundation for enhancing chronic disease self-management, *Home Health Nurse* 26(2):83–88, 2008.

The Joint Commission: *Comprehensive accreditation manual for hospitals (CAMH)*, Oakbrook Terrace, IL, 2014, Author.

The Joint Commission: *What did the doctor say? Improving health literacy to promote patient safety. Health Care at the Crossroads Reports*, Oakbrook Terrace, IL, 2007, Author.

Udlis K: Self-management in chronic illness: concept and dimensional analysis, *J Nurs and Health Care in Chronic Illness* 3(2):130–139, 2011.

World Health Organization (WHO): *Health promotion. Track 2: health literacy and health behaviour 7th global conference on health promotion: track themes*, 2009. Available at http://www.who.int/healthpromotion/conferences/7gchp/track2/en/index.html. Accessed February 11, 2014.

Wellard S, Turner D, Bethune E: Nurses as patient-teachers: exploring current expressions of the role, *Contemp Nurse* 7(1):12–14, 1998.

Wolf M, Curtis L, Baker D: Literacy, cognitive function, and health: results of the LigCog study, *J Gen Intern Med* 27(100):1300–1307, 2012.

WEB RESOURCES

MedlinePlus (n.d.): Health topics. U.S. National Library of Medicine and National Institutes of Health. www.nlm.nih.gov/medlineplus/healthtopics.html

www.cdc.gov/healthliteracy/pdf/Simply_Put.pdf.

Empowerment Oriented Communication Strategies to Reduce Stress

Elizabeth C. Arnold

OBJECTIVES

At the end of the chapter, the reader will be able to:

1. Define stress and associated concepts.
2. Describe biological and psychosocial models of stress.
3. Identify concepts related to coping with stress.
4. Discuss stress assessment strategies.
5. Describe stress reduction strategies nurses can use in stressful situations.
6. Identify stress management therapies.
7. Address occupational stress in nurses.

Chapter 16 focuses on understanding the role of stress and coping in health care relationships. Included in the chapter are descriptions of biological and psychosocial models of stress reactions and models of coping with stress. The chapter identifies communication strategies nurses can use to help clients and families reduce stress levels in health care situations.

BASIC CONCEPTS

DEFINITION

Stress represents a natural physiologic, psychological, and spiritual response to the presence of a stressor. Stress is a common response to serious illness, which can affect quality of life and the client's ability to function (Haugland et al., 2013). It differs from crisis situations because it may not present the same alarm treatment intervention, and unlike crisis, it may not lessen over time. Strengthening a client's capacity to cope effectively with stress has important implications for clinical outcomes and the client's motivation and capacity to perform self-management responsibilities (Jaser et al., 2012). It also can prevent a crisis situation from emerging. Incorporating a stress assessment as part of an overall clinical assessment is part of the complex data nurses need to support a person's ability to adapt to chronic illness.

Hans Selye (1950) defines **stress** as a nonspecific response of the body to any demand made upon it, whether it is caused by the results of a pleasant, or unpleasant situation. McEwen (2012) describes stress as a state of mind, "involving both brain and body as well as their interactions" (p. 17180). Stress feelings set into motion an immediate emergency physiologic response to real or perceived threats through neuroendocrine and other body systems.

A **stressor** is defined as any demand, situation, internal stimulus, or circumstance that threatens a person's personal security or self-integrity. Internal stressors such as pregnancy, fever, menopause, or emotions originate within the body. External stressors, such as social or work stressors, accidents, debt, and exams, start outside the self. **Crisis** (detailed in Chapter 20) represents an extreme acute stressor situation for which coping mechanisms fail and the person is unable to function normally. By definition a crisis situations resolve within 6 weeks.

SOURCES OF STRESS

Stress is a universal part of life. For each person, however, stress represents a personal experience; what is stressful for one person may not be for another. Box 16-1 lists personal sources of stress. Stressors can be catastrophic (war, hurricane, earthquake), cumulative

| BOX 16-1 | Personal Sources of Stress |

Physical Stressors
- Acute or chronic illness
- Trauma or injury
- Pain
- Sleep deprivation
- Mental disorder

Psychological Stressors
- Loss of job or job security
- Loss of a significant person or pet
- Significant change in residence, relationship, work
- Personal finances
- Work relationships
- High-stress work environment
- Caretaking (frail elderly, children)
- Significant change or loss of role

Spiritual Stressors
- Loss of purpose
- Loss of hope
- Questioning of values or meaning

or continuous, or minor. Personal stressors can relate to a major life change (marriage, divorce, death, moving to a new area), or an illness or injury. A new diagnosis, loss of social ties, premature death, and potential damage from adjuvant therapy are common health-related stressors (Antoni, 2013). For family members, sources of emotional stress include watching a loved one steadily decline physically or mentally, concern about finances, uncertainty about the future, balancing family responsibilities with client care, and coping with the client's frustration. Stressors likely to stimulate an intense stress response are those in which a person has limited control over the situation, the situation is ambiguous, or aspects of the current situation resemble past unresolved stressful events.

Concurrent or cumulative stressors increase stress intensity, as does extreme or prolonged stress (Meyers, 2011). The intensity and duration of stress varies according to the circumstances, level of social support, and the emotional state of the person. The mentally ill have a double set of chronic stressors. Some stem from their mental disorder which lowers clients' threshold for stress and diminishes the capacity to act effectively on their own behalf to reduce the stress (Lavoie, 2013).

Daily hassles (traffic jam, child misbehavior, too many competing tasks, computer crashes) are mild stressors that can turn into chronic stress, especially when they are cumulative. A less commonly thought about example of daily hassle is continuing to press forward with a key unattainable life goal (Miller and Wrosch, 2007). The stress response is commonly present in all health care disruptions.

LEVELS OF STRESS

Selye used **"Eustress"** to describe a mild level of stress, which acts as a positive stress response with protective and adaptive functions. Mild stress heightens awareness and can motivate people to master challenges and develop new skills. Coping skills learned in mastering a stressful situation help people cope better in other life circumstances (Aldwin and Levenson, 2004).

Distress is identified as a negative stress level, which creates a level of anxiety, which exceeds a person's normal coping abilities. Distress diminishes performance and diminishes quality of life. *Moderate stress* occurs when people experience frustration or conflict that resists easy reduction. Moderate or chronic stress is implicated in the development and exacerbation of cardiac conditions, migraine, and digestive disorders. *High stress* levels seriously interfere with a person's ability to function. Severe, chronic stress weakens the immune system, thereby contributing to the development of stress-related illnesses (Martin et al., 2007). Stress and coping is said to account for up to 50% of the variation in psychological symptoms (Sinha and Watson, 2007). Untreated, severe mental stress reactions associated with traumatic events can develop into posttraumatic stress syndrome, a clinical disorder.

ACUTE STRESS

Acute stress requires immediate attention. Once the situation is resolved, homeostasis is reestablished. Depending on the magnitude of the stressor and/or lack of client skills in reducing the stress level, acute stress can switch into being a crisis event and lead to the development of posttraumatic stress disorder (PTSD) Yeager and Roberts, 2003). Although the PTSD diagnosis is associated with a catastrophic crisis event, the contributions of chronic stress events can tip the balance. It is important to distinguish a crisis situation, so as to secure the safety of the client and others in the immediate environment. While there is a reduction in functioning associated with stress, with a crisis the severity of the homeostatic balance disrupts normal functioning.

CHRONIC STRESS

Chronic stress manifests itself over an extended period of time as a result of repeated exposure to stressors (allostatic load). Symptoms include: fatigue, excessive anxiety, irritability, insomnia, and lack of attention to healthy lifestyle behaviors. It is important to get a picture of past trauma, quality of relationships, and family dysfunction in addition to assessing the current client presentation. These factors affect a client's ability to counteract stress-related cognitions with positive thoughts, action, and skill building.

VARIATION IN STRESS RESPONSES

Although stress is a universal occurrence, it is a highly subjective experience. People have different tolerance levels for stress. Some are extremely sensitive to any stressor. Others are laid back and less disturbed by unexpected stressful circumstances. More than mild stress reduces the efficiency of cognitive functions. Secondary stressors, such as insomnia caused by worry and financial issues, can heighten the impact of primary stressors on a person's personal life and routines (Wittenberg-Lyles et al., 2012).

Current research suggests that men and women respond to stress differently. Men respond with patterns of "fight or flight," whereas women use a "tend and befriend" approach (Taylor, 2006). Women use nurturing activities to reduce stress and promote safety for self and others. They seek social support from others, particularly from other women. Children express stress through behavior, usually corresponding to developmental stage, and family patterns. Acting out behaviors and psychosomatic illness can mask a child's distress.

STRESS FRAMEWORKS

BIOLOGICAL THEORIES

Systemic Physiological Response

Walter Cannon (1932) described stress as a systemic physiologic response to a perceived threat. The same systemic response occurs regardless of the stressor. Cannon believed that when people feel physically well, emotionally centered, and personally secure, they are in a state of dynamic equilibrium or **homeostasis**. Stress disturbs homeostasis. Physiologically, the sympathetic-adrenal medulla system in the brain sets into motion an immediate hormonal cascade designed to mobilize the body's energy resources to cope with acute stress. Cannon proposed that people attempt to adapt to stress with either a "fight or flight" response. The "fight" response refers to a person's inclination to take action against a threat if the threat appears to be resolvable. People use a flight response if they perceive that the threat cannot be overcome through personal effort.

General Adaptation Syndrome

Hans Selye (1950) described stress as a physiological whole body response to stress, evidenced primarily through the endocrine and autonomic nervous systems. He viewed it as an adaptive response that "was so general that it was like a single burglar alarm that sounds, no matter what intrudes (Meyers, 2011, p. 275). The same physiologic response occurs regardless of whether a stressor is psychological or physical.

Selye described a three-stage progressive pattern of nonspecific physiologic responses: alarm, resistance, and exhaustion. The alarm stage is similar to Cannon's acute stress response. If the stressor is not resolved in the initial alarm stage, a second adaptive phase, "resistance," occurs as the body tries to accommodate for the stressor. In the resistance stage, overt alarm symptoms subside as the immune system helps the body to adapt to the demands of the stressor. If the body fails to adapt or is unable to resist the continued stress, it leads to "exhaustion." A healthy response results in adaptation; an unhealthy response leads to exhaustion. If the body shuts down due to exhaustion, the person becomes high risk for stress-related illness or mental disorder. The longer the physiologic stress response remains elevated, the greater the negative impact on the person.

Allostasis

A recent theory of stress response, allostasis describes how the human organism achieves homeostasis through adaptation (Sterling and Eyer, 1988). The brain determines what experiences are threatening or nonthreatening and the physiologic response requirements of each situation. It serves as a "primary mediator" between the "current stressor exposure, internal regulation of bodily processes, and health outcomes" (Ganzel et al., 2010, p. 134).

Allostatic accommodation is the physiologic process through which the brain tries to find a new homeostasis, using a range of adaptive functioning. McEwen (2000) refers to this phenomenon as "stability through change" (p. 1219). The interaction between stressors and physical responses is ongoing such that individuals become more or less susceptible to the negative consequences of stress over time. Inclusion of genetic risk factors, early life events, and adaptive lifestyle behaviors offers a way to understand the interaction between stressful events and physiologic adaptation processes (McEwen, 2012). Figure 16-1 identifies relationships in the allostasis model.

Stress hormones protect the body against short-term acute stress (allostasis). Stress mediators, such as social support, can provide protective effects. When small or moderate levels of stressor exposure are encountered, and social support is available, coping with it can strengthen well-being and quality of life. According to McEwen (2007) , early life experiences with stress have implications for later biological stress experiences, and a "cumulative wear and tear of the physical and social environment on the brain and body" (p. 17180). If a stressor presents continued challenges, or coping responses are ineffective, there is "wear and tear" on the body, which can have a damaging effect. McEwen terms this phenomena *allostatic load*. The allostatic load can be negligible or severe and

protracted enough to result in significant illness or death if untreated.

PSYCHOSOCIAL FRAMEWORKS
Critical Life Events
Holmes and Rahe (1967) consider stressful life events, such as marriage, divorce, death, and losing a job, as stimuli that disrupt homeostasis and create stress. The Holmes and Rahe scale assigns each life event a weighted numerical score reflecting its potential stress impact. Stressors requiring a significant change in the person's lifestyle have greater impact, as does the number of cumulative stresses on the scale. The total score reflects a person's potential for later development of physical illness. This model has been criticized for not conveying a clear understanding of eventful changes versus indicators of ongoing strains, in creating stress (Pearlin, 1989).

Transactional Model of Stress
Lazarus and Folkman's (1984, 1991) transactional appraisal model of stress is widely used in health care. This model considers stress as a two way interactive process involving both the stressor and the individual's

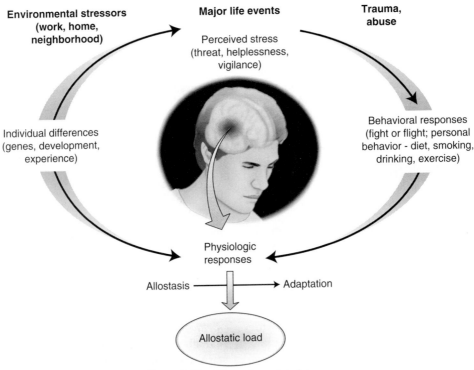

Figure 16-1 Allostasis model of stress.

response to the stressor. According to the transactional model of stress and coping when stress occurs, the stressor creates a significant adaptive demand requiring a response from the individual (Dolbier et al, 2007). It is not the objective stressor, which accounts for the stress response. Instead, the primary mediators are (1) a person's cognitive appraisal of the stressful event (primary appraisal) and (2) a (secondary) appraisal of personal coping abilities (Figure 16-2). The transactional cognitive appraisal model is as applicable to daily "hassles as it is with major events" (Neale et al., 2007).

Lazarus's transactional model helps explain individual differences in responses to stressors that objectively could be thought of as having the same stress value. A *primary appraisal* examines the strength of

a person's belief about the potential harm a stressor holds for a person; the stronger the perceived threat to self-integrity, the more severe the stress response. The **secondary appraisal** considers a person's perception of personal coping skills and availability of social and environmental resources to reduce the stressor's impact. The secondary appraisal can happen concurrently with the primary appraisal. Both appraisals are required to determine whether a stressor will be considered to be a harmful threat or challenge (Folkman, 2008). People experience stress if they appraise the stressor to be threatening and/or feel incapable of meeting the stressor's demands with available resources.

COPING

In their classic work, Pearlin and Schooler (1978) define **coping** as "any response to external life strains that serves to prevent, avoid, or control emotional distress" (p. 2). They identify three purposes of coping strategies:

- To change the stressful situation (problem focused)
- To change the meaning of the stressor (meaning focused)
- To help the person relax enough to take the stress in stride (emotion focused)

Some forms of coping, such as developing realistic goals, focused problem solving, and seeking, help yield positive results. Others are negative. Rumination, denial, use of drugs, or alcohol can increase the effects of stressors and development of distress. Culture plays a role in shaping a person's stress and coping behaviors by

1. Shaping the types of stressors a person is likely to experience
2. Influencing the client's appraisal of stress
3. Affecting the choice of coping strategies
4. Providing different resources and institutional mechanism as coping options (Aldwin, 2010, p. 564)

Skinner and colleagues (2003) suggest that a fundamental problem in defining coping is that "coping is not a specific behavior that can be unequivocally observed or a particular belief that can be reliably reported" (p. 217). People use different behaviors and actions to cope with stressful experiences. In addition to cultural differences, previous stressful experiences, financial assets and social/ self-management support

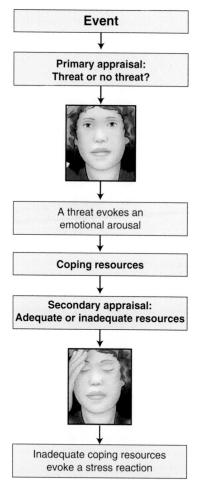

Figure 16-2 Primary and secondary appraisal in stress reactions.

influence a client's and family's ability to problem-solve and cope effectively with their health condition.

For example, in certain collective cultures (Hispanic and Asian), distress is commonly expressed through somatic symptoms (Lehrer et al., 2007). People learn coping strategies from parents, peers, and life experiences. Those with varied life opportunities and supportive people in their lives have an advantage over people who lack opportunity or support systems. People who have been overprotected or repeatedly exposed to danger without support generally lack experience with coping skills. Exercise 16-1 helps identify common coping strategies.

TYPES OF COPING

Appraisal theory describes coping as "a process by which a person makes cognitive and behavioral efforts to manage psychological stress" (Bippus and Young, 2012, p. 177). There are two types of coping: an approach problem focused style and an avoidant emotion focused style (Dolbier et al 2007). **Problem-focused coping** strategies are active, task oriented methods. Strategies use *approach* behaviors designed to change the problem or alter personal response to it. Examples include confronting a problem directly, negotiating, seeking social support, constructive problem solving, and taking action. In general, problem-focused coping strategies have been found to be the most effective in reducing stress.

Awareness of personal and external resources adds options and individuals who think they have options generally are better able to cope with stress. Common personal coping "resource options" include health, energy, problem-solving skills, the amount and availability of social supports, and other material resources

to cope effectively with the stressor. For example, Jaser and colleagues (2012) found that adolescents who used problem-solving strategies to control their diabetes demonstrated better diabetic control and higher quality of life.

By contrast, *emotion-focused coping* strategies are focused on the person and are designed to distance the person from stress. They can be helpful when clients are faced with overwhelming irreversible situations or a person needs respite from overthinking a stressful situation. Emotion-focused coping strategies, such as meditation, yoga, or spirituality, are constructive when a person deliberately chooses to "let go" of negative feelings associated with an unmanageable stressor. Most people use both types of coping strategies, with the choice of strategy dependent on the nature of the stressor and typical coping style. Meaning-focused coping strategies aim to reframe the meaning or significance of the stressor so that it loses its power as a stressor.

Defensive Coping Strategies

Ego defense mechanisms represent unconscious patterns of avoidant coping that people use to protect the self from full awareness of challenging conflict situations. They are designed to protect the ego from anxiety and loss of self-esteem by denying, avoiding, or projecting responsibility for a challenging conflict to an external source. Ego defense mechanisms can be temporarily adaptive in minimizing the threat of a potentially overwhelming stressor (Richards and Steele, 2007). Persistent use of the ego defense mechanisms presented in Table 16-1 is considered pathologic. As a primary stress reducer, defense mechanisms are ineffective because the avoidant behavior delays action and compromises trust

---

EXERCISE 16-1	**Examining Personal Coping Strategies**

Purpose: To help students identify the wide range of adaptive and maladaptive coping strategies.

Procedure
1. Identify all of the ways in which you handle stressful situations.
2. List three personal strategies that you have used successfully in coping with stress.
3. List one personal coping strategy that did not work, and identify your perceptions of the reasons it was inadequate or insufficient to reduce your stress level.

4. List on a chalkboard or flip chart the different coping strategies identified by students.

Discussion
1. What common themes did you find in the ways people handle stress?
2. Were you surprised at the number and variety of ways in which people handle stress?
3. What new coping strategy might you use to reduce your stress level?
4. Are there any circumstances that increase or decrease your automatic reactions to stress?

TABLE 16-1	Ego Defense Mechanisms
Ego Defense Mechanism	**Clinical Example**
Regression: returning to an earlier, more primitive form of behavior in the face of a threat to self-esteem	Julie was completely toilet trained by 2 years of age. When her younger brother was born, she began wetting her pants and wanting a pacifier at night.
Repression: unconscious forgetting of parts or all of an experience	Elizabeth has just lost her job. Her friends would not know from her behavior that she has any anxiety about it. She continues to spend money as if she were still getting a paycheck.
Denial: unconscious refusal to allow painful facts, feelings, or perceptions into awareness	Bill Marshall has had a massive heart attack. His physician advises him to exercise with caution. Bill continues to jog 6 miles a day.
Rationalization: offering a plausible excuse or explanation for unacceptable behavior	Ann Marie tells her friends she is not an alcoholic even though she has blackouts, because she drinks only on weekends and when she is not working.
Projection: attributing unacceptable feelings, facts, behaviors, or attitudes to others; usually expressed as blame	Ruby just received a critical performance evaluation from her supervisor. She tells her friends that her supervisor does not like her.
Displacement: redirecting feelings onto an object or person considered less of a threat than the original object or person	Mrs. Jones took Mary to the doctor for bronchitis. She is not satisfied with the doctor's explanation and feels he was condescending, but says nothing. When she gets to the receptionist's desk to make the appointment, she yells at her for not having the prescription ready and taking too much time to set the next appointment.
Intellectualization: unconscious focusing on only the intellectual and not the emotional aspects of a situation or circumstance	Johnnie has been badly hurt in a car accident. There is reason to believe he will not survive surgery. His father, waiting for his son to return to the intensive care unit, asks the nurse many questions about the equipment, and philosophizes about the meaning of life and death.
Reaction formation: unconscious assuming of traits opposite of undesirable behaviors	John has a strong family history of alcoholism on both sides. He abstains from liquor and is known in the community as an advocate of prohibition.
Sublimation: redirecting socially unacceptable unconscious thoughts and feelings into socially approved outlets	Bob has a lot of aggressive tendencies. He decided to become a butcher and thoroughly enjoys his work.
Undoing: verbal expression or actions representing one feeling, followed by expression of the direct opposite	Barbara criticizes her subordinate, Carol, before a large group of people. Later, she sees Carol on the street and tells her how important she is to the organization.

in relationships. Some defense mechanisms, humor, anticipation, affiliation (asking for help), and sublimation, can be adaptive (Reich et al., 2010).

Case Example

Lynn was diagnosed as having high cholesterol and was advised to lose weight. She sees no purpose in going on a diet because "it's all in the genes." Both her parents had high cholesterol and died of heart problems. Lynn claims there is nothing she can do about it, even though the physician has advised her differently. Her defensive interpretation prevents her from taking actions needed to reduce her risk for cardiovascular disease. Motivational interviewing (see Chapter 14) offers guidelines for gently casting doubt, providing new information, and introducing problem solving to resistant clients. Her nurse inquires about Lynn's personal health goals and provides her with information about the link between diet, exercise, and heart disease. Linking information to Lynn's stated life goals provides her with a different frame of reference.

Resilience

Resilience is a concept related to most discussions of stress. It is defined as the ability of individuals who are exposed to highly disruptive stressors to remain relatively stable and functional despite the stress (Garcia-Dia, 2013). Resilience explains why some people seem to weather stress and adversity more easily than others and are able to grow from the experience. Characteristics of resilience include empowerment and creativity (Lin et al. 2013) Resilient people develop coping mechanisms, which allow them to see a situation, as it is, to focus on what can be changed, and to accept what cannot be altered (Schieveld, 2009). Helping clients develop clear goals, shape relevant problem solving skills and take baby steps toward identified goals is a means of improving client resilience.

Resilience is associated with having a strong internal sense of control and a positive attitude (Marsiglia et al., 2011). A resilient person acquires the skills needed to move forward despite stressful life events. Resilience is advanced through self-efficacy strategies. Examples of resilience include developing an organized way of coping with stressors and cultivating a meaningful support system. A strong faith and sense of purpose are other factors associated with resilience (Freedman, 2008). A related concept is hardiness. *Hardiness* consists of three basic elements when confronted with a stressful situation: *challenge* (looking at stressors and the need for change as an opportunity for personal growth), *commitment* (consistent with a sense of purpose and a willingness to expend a strong involvement in directing one's life) and *control* (belief that one can direct one's life circumstances (Dolbier et al 2007). These variables influence a person's appraisal of global stress events as ultimately being manageable.

Developing an Evidence-Based Practice

Happel B, Dwyer T, Reid-Searl K, Caperchione C, Gaskin C: Nurses and stress: recognizing causes and seeking solutions, *J Nurs Manag* 21(4):638-647, 2013.

The purpose of this qualitative exploratory study was to describe occupational stressors and ways they could be reduced from the nurse's perspective. Thirty-eight registered nurses (RNs) participated in six focus groups to discuss sources of occupational stress and possible ways to reduce the stress.

Results: This purposive sample group of nurses identified high workloads, shift work, unsupportive management, unavailability of physicians, parking, and other human resource issues, client and client relative issues. Suggestions for modification included workload and shift hour changes, organizational development, better work conditions, and acknowledgement from management.

Application to Your Clinical Practice: All nurses have a responsibility to participate in making health care environments better and less stressful. Nurse managers should make opportunities available to discuss occupational stressors and encourage nurses to engage in stress reduction activities.

APPLICATIONS

APPLYING THE NURSING PROCESS

STRESS ASSESSMENT

Stress is an unwelcome part of most illness and injury. It is rarely a personal choice. People experience and cope with stress in different and sometimes unexpected ways. Nurses can be instrumental in helping clients cope with stress effectively so that their anxiety does not dominate their health experience and they are able to function effectively. Factors that influence the impact of stress are identified in Box 16-2.

Addressing relevant stress issues and teaching clients related coping strategies as early as possible

BOX 16-2   Factors That Influence the Impact of Stress

- Magnitude and demands of the stressor on self and others
- Multiple stressors occurring at the same time
- Suddenness or unpredictability of a stressful situation
- Accumulation of stressors and duration of the stress demand
- Level of social support available to the client and family
- Previous trauma, which can activate unresolved fears
- Presence of a co-occurring mental disorder
- Developmental level of the client
- Normal attitude and outlook
- Knowledge, expectations, and realistic picture

enhances clinical outcomes and recovery potential. With the exception of emergency treatment, reducing client stress and suffering should be an immediate focus. An initial assessment should include:

- Client's perception of current stressors
- Client's perception of the stressor causing the greatest stress
- Client's perception of stressor as a challenge or as a personal threat to self-integrity
- Client's insight about the value or meaning attached to the stressor
- Identification of usual coping strategies used to manage stressful situations
- Assessment of linked issues such as developmental stage, culture, family ways of coping, and level of support
- Cultural, religious and spiritual beliefs, and activities

This data can be integrated into the general assessment. Understanding how a stressful event relates to other life issues, including stressors from the past and current financial or family concerns, puts current stressors in context. Ask open-ended questions about changes in daily routines, new roles and responsibilities, and the client's and family's understanding of diagnosis and treatment options. Pay close attention to cultural values. What is a small stressor in one culture can be huge in another, and normal coping strategies can be quite different.

Sources of Stress in Health Care

All health disruptions create a sense of vulnerability. Health-related stressors for clients and families include fear of death, uncertainty about clinical outcomes, changes in roles, disruption of family life, and financial concerns. Hospital-related sources of stress include physical discomfort, strange noises and lights, unfamiliar people asking personal questions, and strange equipment. Clients and their families experience stress with client transfer to the intensive care unit, again when the client is transferred to a step-down or regular unit, and still again when clients are transitioning to home (Chaboyer et al., 2005). Providing immediate practical and emotional support during such transitions helps reduce excessive stress.

A client-centered approach pays attention to the type of stress a client is experiencing. For example, stress perceived as a threat provokes anxiety, whereas stress associated with loss presents as depression and grief. Strategies nurses would use to help clients reduce stress usually differ based on the source of the stress. When stress presents as anxiety, the nurse might suggest problem-solving techniques. However, if the stress is related to a significant loss, the nurse would want to focus on the loss and work with the client from a grief perspective. Box 16-3 provides an assessment and intervention tool that you can use to organize assessment data and plan interventions.

Behavioral Observations

Stress behaviors are sometimes hard to understand or accept. Distress often presents through behavior rather than through words. For example, anxiety can present in the form of heart palpations, shortness of breath, sweating, and muscle tension (Grillon, 2005). Other physical and mental symptoms of stress include

- Significant changes in eating or sleeping habits
- Headaches, gastric problems, muscular tension, aches and pains, tightness in the throat
- Restlessness and irritability
- Inability to cope with normal everyday concerns and obligations
- Inability to concentrate

Anger and Hostility. Anger and hostility are common stress emotions associated with feeling helpless or psychologically threatened. Clients (and/or families) become hostile when they feel threatened about what is happening or feel they have little control in a situation. Anxiety usually exists as the underpinning of anger. What hostile clients or families need most despite hostile behavior is understanding, comfort, and human caring.

Blame is a frequent form of hostility. Family members blame each other for undesired outcomes or the physician for operating (or not operating) on a loved one. They criticize the nurse for not responding quickly enough. Recognizing hostility as a cry for help in coping with escalating stress makes it easier to respond empathetically. Nurses can help clients stabilize an out-of-control situation by providing a calming supportive presence and working with the client to find a viable resolution of his or her anxiety.

BOX 16-3   Assessment and Intervention Tool

Assessment

A. Perception of stressors
1. Major stress area or health concern
2. Present circumstances related to usual pattern
3. Experienced similar problem? How was it handled?
4. Anticipation of future consequences
5. Expectations of self
6. Expectations of caregivers

B. Intrapersonal factors
1. Physical (mobility, body function)
2. Psychosociocultural (attitudes, values, coping patterns)
3. Developmental (age, factors related to present situation)
4. Spiritual belief system (hope and sustaining factors)

C. Interpersonal factors
1. Resources and relationship of family or significant other(s) as they relate to or influence interpersonal factors

D. Environmental factors
1. Resources and relationships of community as they relate to or influence interpersonal factors

Prevention as Intervention

A. Primary
1. Classify stressor
2. Provide information to maintain or strengthen strengths
3. Support positive coping mechanisms
4. Educate client and family

B. Secondary
1. Mobilize resources
2. Motivate, educate, involve client in health care goals
3. Facilitate appropriate interventions; refer to external resources as needed
4. Provide information on primary prevention or intervention as needed

C. Tertiary
1. Attain/maintain wellness
2. Educate or reeducate as needed
3. Coordinate resources
4. Provide information about primary and secondary interventions

Developed by J. Conrad, University of Maryland School of Nursing, Baltimore, MD, 1993.

Case Example

Client: I'm paying a lot of money, and no one wants to help me. The nursing care is terrible, and I just have to lie here in pain with no one to help me.

Nurse: I'm sorry you are feeling so bad. Can you tell me a little more what's going on with you. I'd really like to be able to help you.

Carefully listening to a client's concerns goes a long way toward neutralizing anger and hostility. The client feels heard, even if the issues cannot be fully resolved to the client's satisfaction. In the course of the conversation, both nurse and client can sort out how the client experiences a stressor. This data can serve as a basis for focusing on productive solutions. Set limits if necessary, but do so with a calm attitude and empathetic matter of fact manner. If client and/or family expectations are unrealistic, or cannot be met in the current situation, alternative explanations and suggestions can be introduced. Exercise 16-2 is designed to address the relationship between anger and anxiety.

Social Withdrawal. Stress does not always look like a "stressor response." Some people internalize stress. They withdraw or seem disengaged from an obvious stressor when stressed. Unexpressed emotions of anxiety and anger are toxic and debilitating. Nurses can help clients externalize their stress. Putting their observations into words helps clients link emotional states to specific stress reactions using words rather than behavior to express them. Words put limits on the stress experience and make it more manageable. For example, you might say, "This (*name stressor*) must be very upsetting," or "It seems like you are pretty anxious about..." Offering your presence, together with a simple statement that when people put their stress into words, they usually experience less anxiety helps normalize the feelings.

ASSESSMENT OF COPING SKILLS

Assessment of a client's coping behaviors and social support network is critical to understanding stress from a holistic perspective. Ask about coping strategies a client has used in the past and what the person is currently using to resolve stress. Relevant issues include culturally sanctioned coping approaches and

EXERCISE 16-2	**Relationships Between Anger and Anxiety**

Purpose: To help students appreciate the links between anger and anxiety and understand how anger is triggered.

Procedure
1. Think of a time when you were really angry. It need not be a significant event or one that would necessarily make anyone else angry.
2. Identify your thoughts, feelings, and behavior in separate columns of a table you construct. For example, what were the thoughts that went through your head when you were feeling this anger? What were your physical and emotional responses to this experience? Write down words or phrases to express what you were feeling at the time. How did you respond when you were angry?
3. Identify what was going on with you before experiencing the anger. Sometimes it is not the event itself, but your feelings before the incident that make the event the straw that breaks the camel's back.
4. Identify underlying threats to your self-concept in the situation (e.g., you were not treated with respect, your opinion was discounted, you lost status, you were rejected, you feared the unknown).

Discussion
1. In what ways were your answers similar to and different from those of your classmates?
2. What role did anxiety and threat to the self-concept play in the development of the anger response? What percentage of your anger related to the actual event and to self-concept?
3. In what ways did you see anger as a multidetermined behavioral response to threats to self-concept?
4. Did this exercise change any of your ideas about how you might handle your feelings and behavior in a similar situation?
5. What are the common threads in the events that made people in group angry?
6. In what ways could experiential knowledge of the close association between anger and anxiety be helpful in your nursing practice?

---

typical family coping strategies. Sample questions might include
- What do you do to relieve your stress?
- Who can you rely on when you are feeling stressed?

Discussing stress can be difficult in part because it is so uncomfortable. Clients feel more comfortable when their nurse presents an open, nonthreatening stance and a calm attitude. Use an informal conversational format. Being patient and willing to listen is important. Your client's reactions will serve as a guide as to how much and how quickly the information can be gathered.

Assessment of Immediate Social Support

Social support is an essential buffer against stress. Families can be a major support for clients in managing health-related distress (Antoni, 2013). To be sure that everyone is on the same page, nurses should inquire about the following as part of the initial assessment:
- What are the family's expectations of care?
- In what ways, if any, are family, client, and provider expectations different?
- What does the family or client need from you as the nurse? From each other?
- Is there a family spokesperson?
- What are the family's cultural, religious, and values concerning the meaning of the stressor?

- What does the family identify as sources of strength and hope? Are these similar or different from the client's list?

Community resources include support groups, social services, and other public health agencies that provide practical support, as well as social contacts. Nurses need to be aware of community support services. Exercise 16-3 is designed to help you become better acquainted with resources in your community.

Belief in a personal God or Higher Power provides interested clients with an incomparable personal resource. Multiple studies reveal that spiritual interventions can help prevent and improve physical illnesses and have helped client cope with chronic pain and death (Moeini et al, 2014). Some people rely on faith to facilitate their acceptance of a reality that cannot be changed. Assessing and providing spiritual comfort to clients is an important consideration in caring for clients experiencing stress. For example, African Americans tend to use spirituality and religious activities as preferred coping strategies (Samuel-Hodge et al., 2008).

Assessing Impact on Family Relationships

Stress Issues for Children. Health disruptions create special stress for children; they lack the words

EXERCISE 16-3	Community Resources for Stress Management

Purpose: To help students become aware of the community resources available in the community for stress management.

Procedure

1. Contact a community agency, social services group, or support group in your community that you believe can help clients cope with a particularly stressful situation. Look in the newspaper for ideas.
2. Find out how a person might access the resource, what kinds of cases are treated, what types of treatment are offered, the costs involved, and what

you as a nurse can do to help people take advantage of the resource.

Discussion

1. How did you decide which community agency to choose?
2. How difficult or easy was it to access the information about the agency?
3. What information about the community resource did you find out that surprised or perplexed you?
4. In what ways could you use this exercise in planning care for your clients?

---

and life experience to sort out the meaning of illness, either their own, or that of a significant family member (Compas et al., 2001). Children express their stress through behavior. Signs of distress, such as academic decline, gastric distress, and headaches, can alert the nurse to unvoiced stress. In the hospital, children withdraw, demonstrate clinging behaviors, or have frequent meltdowns. Uncertainty creates stress for both parents and children (Stewart and Mishel, 2000).

Parents may need help with communicating information about serious illness to children, with anticipating their child's reactions, and with advice on ways to break bad news, or set realistic limits with an ill child. Children need to have their questions answered simply and honestly, consistent with their developmental stage. Hearing information from someone they trust is important in modifying the uncertainty of a serious illness. Small children can be encouraged to express their stress feelings through drawings and manipulating puppets.

Stress Issues for Older Adults. Stress issues for older adults occur during a phase of life accompanied by multiple health challenges and increased potential for loss of important personal supports. Worry about finances and fears of not being able to live independently are common. Older adults living alone can feel vulnerable about their safety or ability to reach help should they experience a fall or sudden physical change. The loss of significant people, isolation, and loneliness can complicate treatment issues.

Nurses can help older clients develop tangible ways to promote physical and emotional safety and to maximize their health situation. Stress management

strategies for the older adult from a health promotion perspective include maintaining an active social life and a healthy lifestyle that keeps mind and body engaged and active. Sharing concerns and developing leisure or volunteer interests help older adults develop a well-balanced lifestyle that can improve quality of life and reduce stress. Sometimes all it takes is simple suggestions and well-timed questions about recreational activities or hobbies that the older adult has not considered. Most communities have low-impact exercise activities, senior centers, continuing education, and social outlets for older adults. Elderly caregivers of clients with dementia can benefit from some of the suggestions in Chapter 19 to reduce stress and balance their health and well-being with care of a family member with dementia.

STRESS REDUCTION STRATEGIES
Planning and Interventions

Offering a Safe Environment. In stressful situations, normal feelings are covered by anxiety. Your initial goal is to help clients and families feel secure. Providing emotional safety reduces anxiety and allows the space clients need to express fears, anger, and negative feelings. A calm empathetic approach helps establish a safe holding environment. Slowing the pace is essential. Name the feelings: "You seem to be really struggling right now" or "You seem to be feeling scared (stuck) right now." This can be followed by a simple question, "How can I best help you?"

Giving Information. Information is an essential stress reducer. Relevant information can range from providing basic data about visiting hours, the timing of tests and procedures, plans for discharge, contact

EXERCISE 16-4	Role-Play: Handling Stressful Situations

Purpose: To give students experience in responding to stressful situations.

Procedure

Use the following case study as the basis for this exercise.

Dave is a 66-year-old man with colon cancer. In the past, he had a colostomy. Recently, he was readmitted to your unit and had an exploratory laparotomy for small-bowel obstruction. Very little can be done for him because the cancer has spread. He is in pain and he has to have a feeding tube. His family has many questions for the nurse: "Why is he vomiting?" "How come the pain medication isn't working?" "Why isn't he feeling any better than he did before the surgery?" You have just entered the client's room; his family is sitting near him, and they want answers now.

1. Have different members of your group role-play the client, the nurse, the son, the daughter-in-law, and the wife. One person should act as observer.
2. Identify the factors that will need to be clarified in this situation to help the nurse provide the most appropriate intervention.
3. Using the strategies suggested in this chapter, intervene to help the client and the family reduce their anxiety.
4. Role-play the situation for 10 to 15 minutes.

Discussion

1. Have each player identify the interventions that were most helpful.
2. From the nurse's perspective, which parts of the client and family stress were hardest to handle?
3. How could you use what you learned from doing this exercise in your clinical practice?

---

phone numbers, to complex facts about the client's condition or treatment. Keep it simple. Information sharing should begin with orienting clients and families to the health care situation or unit and providing enough information to familiarize but not overwhelm them as to what they might expect from health care. Take time to briefly explain the following:

- What will happen during tests or surgery
- Who is likely to interview the client and why
- How the client can best cooperate or assist in his or her treatment process

In stressful situations, the perceptual field narrows. Information and directions given in the first 48 hours of an admission should be repeated, usually more than once, because this is the time of high stress. A calm approach and repetition helps clients in stressful situations relax enough to hear important instructions. Providing simple written instructions particularly about medications that can be discussed at the time, and then left with the client or family enhances understanding. Allow time to answer questions and provide the client's family with the health provider's contact numbers to call if other issues arise.

Processing Strong Feelings. When strong stress feelings get bottled up inside the client, constructive problem solving ceases. Often nurses can tell that clients are stressed from their body language, even when they deny strong feelings. Helpful statements include, "This must be very difficult for you to absorb" or "Can you tell me what you are experiencing?" Your immediate goal is to help clients step back, and relook at their situation from a balanced perspective.

A calm accepting presence and willingness to listen to the client's story allows nurses and clients to develop a shared understanding of a stressful event. Listen carefully and ask gentle, probing questions. Some clients feel they are going crazy or are out of control when experiencing stress. You can help a client normalize stressful feelings such as, "I think I'm losing my mind," with a statement such as, "What you are feeling is not unusual; although it feels that way, you are having a normal response to a sudden, overwhelming situation. Can you tell me what worries you the most?" Notice in both probes, the nurse acknowledges the legitimacy of feelings as a normal response to an abnormal situation, which helps the client reframe anxious feelings. Once the client begins to calm down, it becomes possible to look at the situation more realistically.

Exercise 16-4 provides practice in helping clients handle stressful situations.

Reappraisal of either the stress event itself (primary appraisal) or secondary appraisal of coping and personal resources is important information. For example, you can help client change the meaning of a stress event from being a failure by viewing it as a challenge or opportunity for personal growth.

Jamieson and colleagues (2011) propose that when people believe they have the resources to cope with stressors, they perceive them as a challenge rather than as a threat. Pointing out personal or community resources the client has not considered can reduce the impact of the stressor and make coping efforts more feasible. Group formats provide social support and practical education. It is important to help clients choose programs and supports that are convenient and compatible with their stage of life, regular commitments and health issues (Arnold, 1997). Concrete assistance with negotiating appropriate referral resources may be needed.

Developing Realistic Goals. Without command over controllable parts of life, most people feel helpless and stressed. Relevant goals for stress reduction should relate to assessment data, for example, client-identified needs, strengths, resources, barriers, and goal achievement priorities. Treatment goals and objectives should build on past successful coping efforts and preferences. Choosing personal responses to stress is empowering and has a ripple effect on client self-efficacy around other health issues.

Coping mechanisms such as negotiation, specific actions, seeking advice, and rearranging priorities can significantly diminish stress through direct action. Once stressors are named, nurses can use health teaching formats and coaching that help clients to

- Develop a realistic plan to offset stress.
- Deal directly with obstacles as they emerge.
- Evaluate action steps.
- Make needed modifications in the plan and essential lifestyle adjustments.

Case Example

Sam Hamilton received a diagnosis of prostate cancer on a routine physical examination. His way of coping (problem focused) included obtaining as much information on the disease as possible. He researched treatment options and sought advice from physician friends as to which surgeons had the most experience with this type of surgery. As he shared his diagnosis with friends and colleagues, he found several men who had successfully survived without a cancer recurrence. Sam used the time between diagnosis and surgery to finish projects and delegate work responsibilities. He attended a support group with his wife and was able to obtain valuable advice on handling his emotional responses to what would happen. When the time came for his surgery, Sam's actions before surgery reduced his stress.

Priority Setting. Clients do not always know where to start. Priority setting helps reduce hesitation and offers a stepwise framework for stress resolution. You can help clients determine which task elements are critical and achievable and which can be addressed later. Break objective tasks into smaller manageable progressive segments. The most important tasks should be scheduled during times when the client or family has the most energy and freedom from interruption.

The next step is to help clients identify the concrete tasks needed to achieve treatment goals, including the people involved, necessary contacts, amount of time each task will take, and specific hours or days for each task. Some tasks are more important than others in reducing stressful situations and not everything can be handled at once. A helpful suggestion might be, "Let's see what you need to do right now and what can wait a little while." The client should be the final decision maker. Tasks that someone else can do and those that are not essential to the achievement of goals should be delegated or ignored for the moment.

Intervention

Anticipatory Guidance. Fear of the unknown intensifies the impact of a stressor. **Anticipatory guidance** is a proactive strategy to help clients cope effectively with stressful situations. The term refers to the process of sharing information about a circumstance, concern, or situation *before* it occurs. Knowing what lies ahead often prevents the development of a crisis (Hoff et al., 2009). In framing a response, you might reflect on the following:

- What type of information would be most helpful to this particular client at this particular time, given what the client has told me?
- How would I feel if I was in this person's position?
- What would I want to know that might bring me comfort in this situation?

Providing anticipatory guidance can put needless worry to rest. You can prepare your clients for a procedure, beginning with a simple statement, "You've never had this procedure before. Let me explain how it works" (Keller and Baker, 2000). When providing anticipatory guidance, do not offer more than what the situation dictates. Encourage the client to expand on suggestions rather than outlining a full plan. The growth in client ability to set priorities, develop a plan with personal meaning, and establish benchmarks to measure progress stimulates self-confidence and decreases stress.

Anticipatory guidance should relate only to behaviors that can be changed. Stress-related questions about uncertainties do not qualify, for example, "If I take this chemotherapy, will I be cured, or am I going to die anyway?" The reality is that there may be no single answer. It helps to ask the client what prompted the question and to have a good idea of the client's level of knowledge before answering. Honest communication is essential, but sensitivity to the client's experience also is critical.

Social Support. *Social support* is defined as the emotional comfort, advice, and instrumental assistance that a person receives from other people in their social network (Taylor et al., 2007). The concept has three distinct functions in helping clients reduce stress levels: validation, emotional support, and correction of distorted thinking. Social support refers to both the "perceived availability of help, or support actually received" (Schwarzer and Knoll, 2007, p. 244). A person's social networks are drawn from family, friends, church, work, social groups, or school. Being able to contact family and friends when you need an emergency babysitter or an extra hand in a stressful situation immediately lessens stress. Not only does sharing with others reduce stress by "externalizing" negative emotions, but family, friends and support groups can provide a sounding board, practical assistance, and tangible encouragement. Seeking help can empower both seeker and provider of emotional support. Sharing a laugh, eating a meal with others, and being in good company helps people feel more relaxed, which, in turn, reduces stress levels.

Social support does not have the same meaning for all cultures in terms of self-disclosure. Taylor et al (2007) report that Asian American clients may be more comfortable with an implicit form of social support that does not require extensive sharing of thoughts. Examples of implicit social support include showing kindness, caring, acceptance, and positive regard for a client.

Helping Families Balance Care Activities with Self-Care. Contemporary health care environments with advanced technology, shorter stays, and multiple caregivers are complex and anxiety producing. Sources of stress for families can include "fear of death, uncertain outcome, emotional turmoil, financial concerns, role changes, disruption of routines, and unfamiliar

hospital environments" (Leske, 2002, p. 61). Families look to nurses for support and direction. Regular communication with families is a key component of stress reduction. Listen carefully to the family and put into words how you might feel in a similar situation. Statements such as "Most people would feel anxious in this situation," or "It would be hard for anyone to have all the answers in a situation like this" can normalize difficult situations.

Ongoing direct family contact can sometimes provide additional information about client preferences, health care needs, and resources. This strategy is particularly helpful when the client is unable to provide information (Davidson, 2007).

Nurses play an important role in helping families reduce their stress levels to a workable level in health care. You can explore the presence of stress by linking the immediate health situation with expected feelings: "Seeing your husband like this must be a terrible shock. I suspect you might be wondering how you are going to cope with his care at home." This type of statement normalizes feelings and introduces subjects that are difficult but necessary to talk about. Nurses can help families process complex information and address specific concerns. Topics should focus on what will happen next, how to explain the illness to others, or what the client or family is experiencing related to the stressor. Table 16-2 identifies interventions to decrease family stress.

In critical care situations, families have a strong need to remain physically close to the client; there is a strong correlation between proximity to the client and satisfaction with care (Davidson, 2007). It is important to support the presence of key family members in "every area of the hospital, including the emergency department and the intensive care unit (Leape et al., 2009, p. 426). Family members often want to provide support and comfort to critically ill clients. They want to be full "partners in care." Being able to "do something" for the client helps them feel less helpless and defuses stress. Allowing family members to provide comfort measures and participate in the client's care to whatever extent is possible for the client and comfortable for the family can be a meaningful experience for both. Even the most dedicated family members, however, need respite periods. A helpful strategy is suggesting that family members take short breaks. Family members may need "permission" to go to a movie or eat in a restaurant outside the hospital. Sometimes they

TABLE 16-2	Nursing Interventions to Decrease Family Anxiety
Recommendation	**Specific Actions**
Identify a family spokesperson and support persons involved in decision making	Choose a person the family and client trusts; establish mechanisms for contact
Identify a primary nursing contact for the family	If possible, choose the nurse most in contact with the client.
	Meet with the family within 24 hours of admission to explain roles of each health care team member.
	Provide contact number to family spokesperson.
Discuss family access to the client	Arrange for visitation based on unit protocols, client condition and needs, family preferences.
	Educate the family about visiting hours, how to reach the hospitalist, when rounds occur.
	Involve family in client care whenever possible and desired.
Call the family about any changes in client condition or treatment	Inform family of changes as they occur.
	Provide frequent status reports.
	Allow time for questions.
Provide complete data in easily understandable terms	Ask questions about what the client and family understands about the client's condition, how they are coping, what they fear.
	Check for misunderstandings, incomplete information.
	Provide information based on family needs.
	Respect cultural and personal desire for level of information disclosure.
Actively involve the client and family in all clinical decisions	Hold formal care conferences for important care decisions.
	Take into account and respect client preferences, spiritual and cultural attitudes.
	Allow time for questions.
	Strive for consensus in decisions.
Connect family with support services	Provide information about support groups, hospital-based social, spiritual, medicare, hospice, home care, and other care services as needed.
Ensure collaborative rapport and support among health care team members	Maintain clear communication among health care team members.
	Avoid conflicting messages to the family.
	Provide opportunities for staff to decompress and discuss difficult situations and feelings.

Data from Davidson J, Powers K, Hedayat K, et al.: Clinical practice guidelines for support of the family in the patient-centered intensive care unit: American College of Critical Care Medicine Task Force 2004-2005, *Crit Care Med* 35(2):605-622, 2007; Leske J: Interventions to decrease family anxiety, *Crit Care Nurs* 22(6):61-65, 2002.

will do so with an assurance that they will be called should there be any change in the client's condition.

Promoting a Healthy Lifestyle. Encouraging a healthy lifestyle is an essential but sometimes overlooked component of stress-reduction strategies. Good health habits improve stress resistance. Eating a healthy diet and avoiding emotional eating gives people a sense of control and well-being. Too much caffeine and alcohol can exacerbate stress. Laughter dissolves it, and reduces stress levels.

Adequate quality sleep is restorative. Healthy night-time habits, such as establishing a scheduled bedtime and having a small snack before bedtime, encourages sleep. Regular exercise helps the body release tension, as well as contributes to fitness. Exercise can be accomplished in a social setting, for example, hiking or biking. Certain exercise programs such as yoga or tai chi meditation, deep breathing, and muscle stretching, are well known stress reducers. Organizing time and deliberately choosing activities that energize rather than stress, balancing work with leisure activities, and eliminating unnecessary obligations reduce stress.

Therapeutic Approaches for Chronic Stress Management

Cognitive Behavioral Approaches. Cognitive-behavioral approaches have proven useful in addressing stressful negative attributions about oneself, and modifying negative core beliefs. The cognitive behavioral (CBT) model (Beck and Beck, 2011) uses a person-centered approach aimed at helping individuals troubled by faulty thinking reframe the meaning of difficult situations. According to Beck, the relationship between a person's thoughts and feelings influences behaviors. Optimistic or neutral thoughts can lead to positive emotions and tend to create cooperative constructive actions. Negative thinking does the opposite. Faulty thinking causes a person to interpret neutral situations in unrealistic, exaggerated, or negative ways. Helping people become aware of and modify negative or dysfunctional thoughts, beliefs, and perceptions (cognitive distortions) makes it possible for them to change behavior patterns. Awareness can result in a more constructive approach to a problem situation.

Stress symptoms look similar on the surface, but the cognitive beliefs supporting the stress reaction can be quite different. Cognitive restructuring is a strategy, which "involves teaching clients to question the automatic beliefs, assumptions and predictions that often lead to negative emotions and to replace negative thinking with more realistic and positive beliefs" (Schacter et al., 2010, p. 599). The focus of CBT is not on the behavior itself, but on the internal perceptions and thoughts that create and perpetuate negative self-evaluations and self-defeating behaviors.

Automatic negative thoughts are classified as **cognitive distortions**. Examples include magnifying or minimizing the impact of a single behavior as a commentary on the person. For example, failing a test is experienced as "I am stupid." Mind reading or having rigid rules about what a person "should" do is another example. Over time a person develops a set of related automatic distortions referred to as a *schema* or *schemata*. The person uses core schemas to filter incoming

information and determine its meaning related to self, others, and the world. Schemas become a template for understanding the meaning of incoming information and appraising its value to the self. They are more pervasive and hard to dislodge. Although distortions seem to be legitimate assessments, they are not valid.

Nurses help clients challenge distortions through Socratic questioning. By gathering and weighing evidence to support a different position, people are able to distinguish between a distorted perception and a realistic appraisal of its validity. Ridding oneself of unrealistic expectations and negative self-thoughts allows cognitive space for thinking about possible options and broader choices. Once a problem is appropriately categorized, solutions become more apparent. You can help clients understand that they have choices and that no matter what feeling they have, it is not permanent. Initially people have to force themselves to challenge negative thoughts and replace them with more balanced thoughts. Over time this becomes easier.

Nurses can use open-ended questions such as
- What is the worst thing that can happen?
- If_ (*worst thing*) _did happen, what could your do?

Mind-Body Therapies and Meditation. Mind-body therapies are designed to lessen the intensity of the stressor on a person once the stress response has occurred. Examples include meditation, relaxation techniques, yoga, and cognitive restructuring. Meditation is a stress-reduction strategy that people use to develop a sense of inner peace and tranquility. Meditation clears the mind of disturbing thoughts and neutralizes toxic feelings as the technique strives to center the individual on the larger picture of life. This activity helps to reduce the concentration of stress hormones attached to stressful thinking. A guide to meditation is provided in Box 16-4.

Mindfulness is a stress management tool that can be used at any point. It can be as simple as focusing on deep breathing. Focusing completely on your breathing, music, or what is happening in the current moment forces you to at least momentarily let go of stressful thoughts. It is an easy way of quieting the mind and decreasing the intensity of stressful feelings.

Biofeedback. Biofeedback is used in the management of clients with chronic stress responses affecting individual body systems (e.g., essential hypertension, migraine headaches, Raynaud disease,

BOX 16-4   Meditation Techniques

1. Choose a quiet, calm environment with as few distractions as possible.
2. Get in a comfortable position, preferably a sitting position.
3. To shift the mind from logical, externally oriented thought, use a constant stimulus: a sound, word, phrase, or object. The eyes are closed if a repetitive sound or word is used.
4. Pay attention to the rhythm of your breathing.
5. When distracting thoughts occur, they are discarded and attention is redirected to the repetition of the word or gazing at the object. Distracting thoughts will occur and do not mean you are performing the techniques incorrectly. Do not worry about how you are doing. Redirect your focus to the constant stimulus and assume a passive attitude.

Adapted from Benson H: *The relaxation response*, New York, 1975, Morrow.

and ulcerative colitis). The goal is to lower physiologic arousal and promote relaxation (Grazzi and Andrasik, 2010). Equipment used with biofeedback includes the electroencephalogram; skin temperature devices; blood pressure measures; galvanic skin resistance measurements; and the electromyogram, which measures muscle tension. Biofeedback allows clients to control a variety of physiologic activities such as their brain activity, blood pressure, heart rate, pain, migraine or tension headaches. Biofeedback provides awareness of minute-by-minute changes in biologic activity.

Progressive Relaxation. Progressive relaxation is a technique that focuses the client's attention on conscious control of voluntary skeletal muscles. Originally developed by Edmund Jacobson (1938), the technique consists of alternately tensing and relaxing muscle groups. Davis and colleagues (2008) provide an excellent step-by-step description of the basic procedure for progressive relaxation.

A variant of progressive relaxation is deep breathing. This can be accomplished anywhere and at any time a person experiences stress.

- Deeply inhale to the count of 10 and hold your breath.
- Exhale slowly, again to the count of 10.
- Concentrate as you do this exercise only on your breathing.
- Feel the tension leave your body.

Focusing the mind on the continuous rhythm of inhaling and exhaling turns the mind away from thinking about specific stressors. To experience the progressive relaxation technique, see Exercise 16-5.

Yoga and Tai Chi. Yoga is a mind-body exercise practice rooted in ancient India. The practice of yoga has proven useful as a treatment for depression and for promotion of physical and mental health (Rao et al., 2013). Yoga emphasizes correct alignment, controlled postures or poses, and regulated breathing to help people relax and reduce stress. Controlling breathing helps to quiet the mind. Some forms of yoga involve meditation and developing self-awareness. Tai chi is an exercise system consisting of stretching and rhythmic movements coordinated with controlled breathing. The postures and movements are practiced in a slow, graceful manner. The concentration required for both yoga and tai chi require a person to relax and forget distressing thoughts.

Guided Imagery. Guided imagery is a technique often used in combination with relaxation strategies for cancer pain and stress (Kwekkeboom, 2008). Imagery techniques use the client's imagination to stimulate healing mental images designed to promote stress relief. The process involves asking the client to imagine a scene, previously experienced as safe, peaceful, or beautiful. Supportive prompts to engage all of senses deepen the imagery experience. This scene can be used each time that the client begins to experience stress. Inspirational tapes and music are also used in connection with guided imagery.

Support Groups. Support groups for clients or families struggling with the same health situation or crisis can be extremely helpful in helping them defuse stress and learn coping strategies to self-manage difficult health issues. Examples include bereavement groups, cancer support groups, dementia family groups, and specialized groups for abuse or alcoholism. Psychoeducational groups with supportive interventions include the National Alliance on Mental Illness (NAMI), cardiac rehabilitation, and health promotion groups for targeted populations.

OCCUPATIONAL STRESS
Burnout

Khamisa et al (2013) notes that nurses experience a greater vulnerability to burnout because they work in high-stress service environments, helping people cope with serious life and death situations every day.

EXERCISE 16-5	Progressive Relaxation

Purpose: To help students experience the beneficial effects of progressive relaxation in reducing tension.

Procedure

This exercise consists of alternately tensing and relaxing skeletal muscles.

1. Sit in a comfortable chair with arm supports. Place the arms on the arm supports, and sit in a comfortable upright position with legs uncrossed and feet flat on the floor.
2. Close your eyes and take 10 deep breaths, concentrating on inhaling and exhaling.
3. Your instructor or a member of group should give the following instructions, and you should follow them exactly:
   - I want you to focus on your feet and to tense the muscles in your feet. Feel the tension in your feet. Hold it, and now let go. Feel the tension leaving your feet.
   - I would like you to tense the muscles in your calves. Feel the tension in your calves and hold it. Now let go and feel the tension leaving your calves. Experience how that feels.
   - Tense the muscles in your thighs. Most people do this by pressing their thighs against the chair. Feel the tension in your muscles and experience how that feels. Now release the tension and experience how that feels.
   - I would like you to feel the tension in your abdomen. Tense the muscles in your abdomen and hold it. Hold it for a few more seconds. Now release those muscles and experience how that feels.
   - Tense the muscles in your chest. The only way you can really do this is to take a very deep breath and hold it. (The guide counts to 10.) Concentrate on feeling how that feels. Now let it go and experience how that feels.

- I would like you to tense your muscles in your hands. Clench your fist and hold it as hard as you can. Harder, harder. Now release it and concentrate on how that feels.
- Tense the muscles in your arms. You can do this by pressing down as hard as you can on the arm supports. Feel the tension in your arms and continue pressing. Now let go and experience how that feels.
- I would like to you to feel the tension in your shoulders. Tense your shoulders as hard as you can and hold it. Concentrate on how that feels. Now release your shoulder muscles and experience the feeling.
- Feel the tension in your jaw. Clench your jaw and teeth as hard as you can. Feel the tension in your jaw and hold it. Now let it go and feel the tension leave your jaw.
- Now that you are in this relaxed state, keep your eyes closed and think of a time when you were really happy. Let the images and sounds surround you. Imagine yourself back in that situation. What were you thinking? What are you feeling?
- Open your eyes. Students who feel comfortable may share the images that emerged in the relaxed state.

Discussion

1. What are your impressions in doing this exercise?
2. Do you feel more relaxed after doing this exercise?
3. If applicable, after doing the exercise, in what ways do you feel differently?
4. Were you surprised at the images that emerged in your relaxed state?
5. In what ways do you think you could use this exercise in your nursing practice?

Over time, prolonged work related stress takes its toll. Freudenberger (1980) defines **burnout** as "a state of fatigue or frustration brought about by devotion to a cause, way of life, or relationship that failed to produce an expected reward" (p. 13). It develops in individuals involved with "people work" and is characterized by emotional exhaustion, depersonalization, and a sense of diminished professional accomplishment (Maslach, 2001). Although burnout shares some characteristics with depression and anxiety, it is a different syndrome, clearly linked to a work environment and personal expectations of self and others within that setting.

Burnout begins insidiously, particularly in nurses who strive for perfection. Unchecked, it is a progressive syndrome associated with emotional exhaustion and loss of meaning. Freudenberger (1980) refers to burnout as the "overachievement syndrome." High achievers and committed nurses, who are passionate about their work, are more at risk. Burnout develops from combined factors in the work environment and within the person. Six areas of organizational contributors to burnout include workload, control, reward, community, fairness, and values (Freeney and Tiernan, 2009). Sources of work-related burnout for nurses include working too

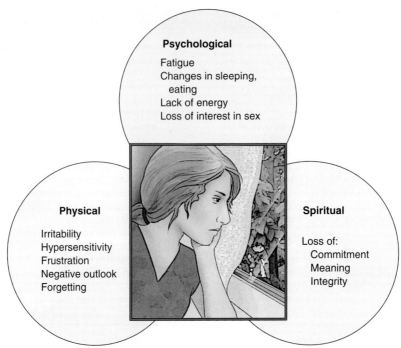

Psychological

Fatigue
Changes in sleeping,
    eating
Lack of energy
Loss of interest in sex

Physical

Irritability
Hypersensitivity
Frustration
Negative outlook
Forgetting

Spiritual

Loss of:
    Commitment
    Meaning
    Integrity

Figure 16-3   Symptoms of burnout.

many hours or at an accelerated pace with no respite, feeling unappreciated, giving too much to needy clients, trying to meet multiple demands of administrators, lack of community with coworkers, and feeling resentment, in place of the meaning that work once held.

Symptoms of Burnout. Figure 16-3 identifies common symptoms of burnout.

Khamisa et al (2013) notes typical characteristics of burnout as emotional exhaustion, depersonalization, and a reduced sense of competence. Nurses experiencing burnout usually feel disillusioned and lack zest for their work. Other signs include loss of motivation and ideals, boredom or dissatisfaction at work, irritability and cynicism, resentment of expectations, and avoidance of meaningful encounters with clients and families. Headaches, gastric disturbances, skipping meals or eating compulsively on the run, feeling irritated by the intrusion of others, and a lack of balance between a nurse's work and personal life can signal the onset of burnout. In a study of coworkers' perceptions of colleagues suffering from burnout, signs observed included a struggle to achieve unobtainable goals, wanting to manage alone, and becoming isolated from others (Ericson-Lidman and Strandberg, 2007).

Burnout Prevention Strategies. The ABCs of burnout prevention (Arnold, 2008) are presented in

Table 16-3. Reflecting on the sources of stress in your life puts boundaries on it. Think about your goals and what is important to you. Rather than simply complaining, seek role models or trusted coworkers who can offer you the support and sensitivity you need to become aware of what is going on in your life. A useful exercise is to imagine yourself a year from now and ask yourself how important the issue would be a year from now.

Identifying realistic achievable goals in line with your personal values is an excellent burnout prevention strategy. Goals should be aligned with purpose and values. Focusing on one thing at a time and finishing one project before starting another has several benefits. Achieving small related goals promotes self-efficacy and offers hope that more complex goals are achievable.

Give yourself a break! Maintaining a healthy balance between work, family, leisure, and lifelong learning activities enhances personal judgments, satisfaction, and productivity in all three spheres. Actively schedule a time for each of these activities and stick to it. You actually will be a better nurse if you choose a balanced life.

Remember---you always have choices even it is to change your attitudes to allow caring for yourself as part of providing excellent nursing care. People experiencing burnout lose sight of this fact. Life is a series of choices

TABLE 16-3	ABCs of Burnout Prevention
	Suggested Strategy
Awareness	Use self-reflection and conversations with others to sort out priorities and identify parts of life out of balance. Recognize and allow feelings.
Balance	Maintain a healthy lifestyle. Balance care of others with self-care and self-renewal needs.
Choice	Differentiate between things you can change and those you cannot. Deliberately make choices that are purpose driven and meaningful.
Detachment	Detach from excessive ego involvement and personal ambition. Share responsibility and credit for care. Use meditation to center self.
Altruistic egoism	Take scheduled time for self, learn to say no, practice meditation, and develop outside interests that enrich the spirit.
Faith	Burnout is a malaise of the spirit. Trust in a higher power or purpose to center yourself when you do not know what will happen next.
Goals	Identify and develop realistic goals in line with personal strengths. Seek feedback and support.
Hope	Hope is nurtured through conversations with others that lighten the burden and a belief in one's possibilities and personal worth in the greater scheme of things.
Integrity	Recognize that each of us is the only person who can determine the design and application of meaning in our lives.

Data from Arnold E: Spirituality in educational and work environments. In Carson V, Koenig H, editors: *Spiritual dimensions of nursing practice*, revised edition, Conshohocken, PA, 2008, Templeton Foundation Press, pp. 386-399.

and negotiations. The choices we make create the fabric of our lives. Refusing to delegate work because someone else cannot do it as well, or not going out to dinner with friends because you have too much work to do, are choices—bad options that lead to burnout.

Detachment from ego and/or taking responsibility for outcomes is a critical component of burnout prevention. It means that you do not allow emotional involvement in a task or relationship to undermine your quality of life, values, or needs. Someone once asked Mother Teresa how she was able to remain so energetic and hopeful in the midst of suffering she encountered in Calcutta. She replied that it was because she did the best she could and did not worry about the outcome because she could not control it.

It is important to pay as much attention to your own personal needs as you do to the needs of others. Although this seems obvious, nurses sometimes consider attention to their own needs as being selfish. However, one cannot give from an empty cupboard. Replenishing the self actually improves what one can give to others.

Faith is defined as an intangible connection with a larger purpose or higher power to guide and support a person during both good and bad times. Faith helps people develop an optimistic worldview and experience less distress. Nurses experiencing burnout often feel helpless and hopeless about changing their situation, other than to leave it. Hope is a powerful antidote for burnout. Exercise 16-6 provides an opportunity to think about your personal burnout potential and ways to achieve better balance in your life.

Burnout challenges personal integrity when important values are ignored or devalued. When you begin to forget who you are and try to become what everyone else expects of you, you are in trouble. Reclaim yourself! Taking responsibility for yourself and doing what is important to you helps to reverse burnout. Take the risk to be all that you are, as well as all that you can be, without worrying about what others think. Seek professional supports such as training, staff retreats, staff support networks, and job rotation to stimulate new ideas and insights. Professional support groups are effective as a means of providing encouragement to nurses in acute settings.

SUMMARY

This chapter focuses on the stress response in health care and supporting client and family coping with stress through nurse-client relationships. Stress can negatively impact client outcomes, level of satisfaction with care, and compliance with treatment. A fundamental goal in the nurse-client relationship is to empower clients and families with the knowledge, support, and resources they need to cope effectively with stress.

Stress is a part of everyone's life. Mild stress can be beneficial, but greater stress levels can be unhealthy. Concurrent and cumulative stresses increase the response level. Theoretical models address stress as a physiologic response, as a stimulus, and as a transaction

EXERCISE 16-6   Burnout Assessment

Purpose: To help students understand the symptoms of burnout.

Procedure

Consider your life over the past year. Complete the questionnaire by answering with a 5 if the situation is a constant occurrence, 4 if it occurs most of the time, 3 if it occurs occasionally, 2 if it has occurred once or twice during the last 6 months, and 1 if it is not a problem at all. Scores ranging from 60 to 75 indicate burnout. Scores ranging from 45 to 60 indicate you are stressed and in danger of developing burnout. Scores ranging from 20 to 44 indicate a normal stress level, and scores of less than 20 suggest you are not a candidate for burnout.

1. Do you find yourself taking on or being overwhelmed by other people's problems?
2. Do you feel resentful about the amount or nature of claims on your time?
3. Do you find you have less time for social activities?
4. Have you lost your sense of humor?
5. Are you having trouble sleeping?
6. Do you find you are more impatient and less tolerant of others?
7. Is it difficult for you to say no?
8. Are the things that used to be important to you slipping away from you because you do not have time?
9. Do you feel a sense of urgency and not enough time to complete tasks?
10. Are you forgetting appointments, friends' birthdays?
11. Do you feel overwhelmed and unable to pace yourself?
12. Have you lost interest in intimacy?
13. Are you overeating or have you begun to skip meals?
14. Is it difficult to feel enthusiastic about your work?
15. Do you feel it is difficult to connect on a meaningful level with others?

Tally up your scores and compare your scores with your classmates. Nursing school is a strong breeding ground for the development of burnout (demands exceed resources). To offset the possibility of developing burnout symptoms, do the following:

1. Think about the last time you took time for yourself. If you cannot think of a time, you really need to do this exercise.
2. Identify a leisure activity that you can do during the next week to break the cycle of burnout.
3. Describe the steps you will need to take to implement the activity.
4. Identify the time required for this activity and what other activities will need rearrangement to make it possible.
5. Describe any obstacles to implementing your activity and how you might resolve them.

Discussion

1. Was it difficult for you to come up with an activity? If so, why?
2. Were you able to develop a logical way to implement your activity?
3. Were the activities chosen by others surprising or helpful to you in any way?
4. How might you be able to use this exercise in your future practice?

---

between person and environment. Factors that influence the development of a stress reaction include the nature of the stressor, personal interpretation of its meaning, number of previous and concurrent stressors, previous experiences with similar stressors, and availability of support systems and personal coping abilities.

People use problem- and emotion-focused coping strategies to minimize stress. Social support is key to effectively coping with stress. Assessment should focus on stress factors the person is experiencing, the context in which they occur, and identification of coping strategies. Supportive interventions include giving information, opportunities to express their feelings, thoughts, and worries, and anticipatory guidance.

Nurses are at the forefront of health care delivery to clients and families experiencing complex health and life issues. They too can experience stress and need support to do their job effectively. Burnout prevention requires recognition and resolution of organizational and personal factors contributing to job-related stress in professional nurses.

ETHICAL DILEMMA   What Would You Do?

The mother of a client with acquired immunodeficiency syndrome (AIDS) does not know her son's diagnosis because her son does not want to worry her and fears her disapproval if she knows he is gay. The mother asks the nurse if the family should have an oncology consult because she does not understand why, if her son has leukemia, as he says he does, that an oncologist is not seeing him. What should the nurse do?

DISCUSSION QUESTIONS

1. What would you identify as tips for self-care to prevent the development of burnout?
2. Stress is characterized by physical and emotional symptoms of tension. In what ways does stress manifest itself in your client's behaviors?
3. What are some of the stress management strategies you have tried or observed that seem to work best?

REFERENCES

Aldwin CM, Levenson MR: Posttraumatic growth: a developmental perspective, *Psychol Inq* 15(1):19–22, 2004.

Aldwin CM: Culture, coping and resilience to stress. Gross National Happiness and Development - Proceedings of the First International Conference on Operationalization of Gross National Happiness, Thimphu 2004, 2010, Centre for Bhutan Studies. PP. 563–573 http://archiv.ub.uni-heidelberg.de/savifadok/volltexte/2010/1333. Accessed, March 2, 2014.

Antoni M: Psychosocial intervention effects on adaptation, disease course and biobehavioral processes in cancer, *Brain Behav Immun* 30(Suppl):S88–S98, 2013.

Arnold E: Spirituality in educational and work environments. In Carson V, Koenig H, editors: *Spiritual dimensions of nursing practice*, revised edition, Conshohocken, PA, 2008, Templeton Foundation Press, pp 368–399.

Arnold E: The stress connection: women and coronary heart disease, *Crit Care Nurs Clin North Am* 9(4):565–575, 1997.

Beck J, Beck AT: Cognitive Behavior Therapy: Basics and Beyond, New York, NY, 2011, The Guilford Press.

Benson H: *The relaxation response*, New York, 1975, Morrow.

Bippus A, Young S: Using appraisal theory to predict emotional and coping responses to hurtful messages, *Interpersona* 6(2):176–190, 2012.

Cannon WB: *The wisdom of the body*, New York, 1932, Norton Pub.

Chaboyer W,H, James H, Kendall M, et al.: Transitional care after the intensive care unit, *Crit Care Nurse* 25(3):16–27, 2005.

Davidson J, Powers K, Hedayat L, Tieszen M, Kon A, et al.: Clinical practice guidelines for support of the family in the patient-centered intensive care unit: American College of Critical Care Medicine Task Force 2004–2005, *Crit Care Med* 35(2):605–622, 2007.

Davis M, Eshelman E, McKay M, et al.: *The relaxation and stress reduction workbook*, Oakland CA, 2008, New Harbinger Publications, Inc.

Dolbier C, Smith S, Steinhardt MA, et al.: Relationships of protective factors to stress and symptoms of illness, *Am J Health Behav* 31(4):423–433, 2007.

Ericson-Lidman E, Strandberg G: Burnout: co-workers' perceptions of signs preceding workmates' burnout, *J Adv Nurs* 60(2):199–208, 2007.

Folkman S: The case for positive emotions in the stress process, *Anxiety Stress Coping* 21(1):3–14, 2008.

Freedman R: Coping, resilience, and outcome, *Am J Psychiatry* 165(12):1505–1506, 2008.

Freeney V, Tiernan J: Exploration of the facilitators of and barriers to work engagement in nursing, *Int J Nurs Stud* 46:1557–1565, 2009.

Freudenberger H: *Burn-out: the high cost of high achievement*, Garden City, NY, 1980, Doubleday.

Ganzel B, Morris P, Wethington E, et al.: Allostasis and the human brain: integrating models of stress from the social and life sciences, *Psychol Rev* 117(1):134–174, 2010.

Garcia-Dia MJ, DiNapoli JM, Garcia-Ona L, Jakuboski R, O'Flaherty D: Concept analysis: resilience, *Archives of Psychiatric Nursing* 27:264–270, 2013.

Grazzi L, Andrasik F: Non-pharmacological approaches in migraine prophylaxis: behavioral medicine, *Neurol Sci* 31(Suppl 1):S133–S135, 2010.

Grillon C: In Saddock B, Saddock V, editors: *Anxiety disorders: Psychophysiological aspects*, Philadelphia, PA, 2005, Lippincott, Williams and Wilkins, pp 1728–1739.

Haugland T, Veenstra M, Vatn M, Wahl A: Improvement in stress, general self-efficacy and health related quality of life following patient education for patients with neuroendocrine tumors: A pilot study, *Nurs Res Pract* 695820, 2013. http://dx.doi.org/10.1155/2013/695820. Epub 2013 Apr 23.

Hoff L, Hallisey B, Hoff M, et al.: *People in crisis: clinical diversity perspectives*, ed 6, New York, NY, 2009, Routledge.

Holmes, Rahe R: The social readjustment rating scale, *J Psychosom Res* 11:213–218, 1967.

Jacobson E: *Progressive relaxation*, Chicago, 1938, University of Chicago Press.

Jamieson J, Nock M, Mendes W: Mind over matter: reappraising arousal improves cardiovascular and cognitive responses to stress, *J Exp Psychol Gen* 141:417–422, 2011.

Jaser S, Faulkner M, Whittemore R, Sangchoon J, et al.: Coping, self-management, and adaptation in adolescents with type 1 diabetes, *Ann Behav Med* 43(3):311–319, 2012.

Khamisa N, Peltzer Oldenburg B: Burnout in relation to specific contributing factors and health outcomes among nurses: a systematic review, *Int J Environ Res Public Health* 10(6):2214–2240, 2013.

Keller V, Baker L: Communicate with care, *RN* 63(1):32–33, 2000.

Kwekkeboom K: Patients' perceptions of the effectiveness of guided imagery and progressive muscle relaxation, *Complement Ther Clin Pract* 14(3):185–194, 2008.

Lazarus RS, Folkman S: *Stress, appraisal and coping*, New York, 1984, Springer.

Lavoie J: Eye of the beholder: Perceived stress, coping style, and coping effectiveness of discharged psychiatric patients, *Arch Psychiatr Nurs* 27:185–190, 2013.

Lazarus R: *Psychological Stress and the Coping Process*, New York, 1991, Springer.

Leape L, Bearwick D, Clancy C, et al.: Transforming health care: A safety imperative, *Qual Saf Health Care* 18:424–428, 2009.

Lehrer P, Woolfolk R, Sime W, et al.: *Principles and practice of stress management*, New York, 2007, Guilford Press.

Leske J: Interventions to decrease family anxiety, *Crit Care Nurs* 22(6):61–65, 2002.

Lin FY, Rong JR, Lee TY: Resilience among caregivers of children with chronic conditions: a concept analysis, *J of Multidisciplinary Health Care* 6:324–333, 2013.

Marsiglia FF, Kulis S, Garcia Perez H, Bermudez-Parsai M: Hopelessness, family stress, and depression among Mexican-heritage mothers in the southwest, *Health Soc Work* 36(1):7–18, 2011.

Martin P, Lae L, Reece J, et al.: Stress as a trigger for headaches: relationship between exposure and sensitivity, *Anxiety Stress Coping* 20(4):393–407, 2007.

Maslach C: What have we learned about burnout and health? *Psychol Health* 16:607–611, 2001.

McEwen B: Allostasis, allostatic load, and the aging nervous system: role of excitatory amino acids and excitotoxicity, *Neurochem Res* 9(10):1219–1231, 2000.

McEwen B: Physiology and neurobiology of stress and adaptation: central role of the brain, *Physiol Rev* 87(3):873–904, 2007.

McEwen B: Brain on stress: How the social environment gets under the skin, *Proc Natl Acad Sci U S A* 109(suppl. 2):17180–17185, 2012.

Meyers D: *Psychology in Everyday Life*, New York, NY, 2011, Worth Publications.

Miller G, Wrosch C: You've gotta know when to fold them, *Psychol Sci* 18:773–777, 2007.

Moeini M, Taleghani F, Mehrabi T, Musarzale A: Effects of a spiritual care program on levels of anxiety in patients with leukemia, *Iran J Nurs Midwifery Res* 19(1):88–93, 2014.

Neale D, Arentz A, Jones-Ellis J, et al.: The negative event scale: measuring frequency and intensity of adult hassles, *Anxiety Stress Coping* 20(2):163–176, 2007.

Pearlin L, Schooler C: The structure of coping, *J Health Soc Behav* 19:2–21, 1978.

Pearlin L: The sociological study of stress, *J Health Soc Behav* 30(3):241–256, 1989.

Rao N, Varambally S, Gangadhar B: Yoga school of thought and psychiatry: Therapeutic potential, *Indian J Psychiatry* 55(suppl 2): S145–S149, 2013.

Reich J, Zautra A, Hall J, et al.: *Handbook of adult resilience*, New York, NY, 2010, Guilford.

Richards M, Steele R: Children's self-reported coping strategies: the role of defensiveness and repressive adaptation, *Anxiety Stress Coping* 20(2):209–222, 2007.

Samuel-Hodge C, Watkins D, Rowell K, et al.: Coping styles, well-being and self-care behaviors among African Americans with type 2 diabetes, *Diabetes Educ* 34(3):501–510, 2008.

Schacter D, Gilbert D, Wegner D: *Psychology*, 2nd Ed, New York, 2010, Worth.

Schwarzer R, Knoll N: Functional roles of social support within the stress and coping process: a theoretical and empirical overview, *Int J Psychol* 42(4):243–252, 2007.

Selye H: Stress and the general adaptation syndrome, *Br Med J* 4667:1383–1392, 1950.

Schieveld J: On grief and despair versus resilience and personal growth in critical illness, *Intensive Care Med* 35:779–780, 2009.

Sinha B, Watson D: Stress, coping and psychological illness: a cross-cultural study, *Int J Stress Manag* 14(4):386–397, 2007.

Skinner E, Edge K, Altman J, et al.: Searching for the structure of coping: a review and critique of category systems for classifying ways of coping, *Psychol Bull* 129(2):216–269, 2003.

Sterling P, Eyer J: Allostasis: a new paradigm to explain arousal pathology. In Fisher S, Reason J, editors: *Handbook of life stress, cognition and health*, New York, 1988, Wiley, pp 629–649.

Stewart J, Mishel MH: Uncertainty in childhood illness: a synthesis of the parent and child literature, *Sch Inq Nurs Pract* 14(4):299–319, 2000. discussion 321–326.

Taylor SE: Tend and befriend: biobehavioral bases of affiliation under stress, *Curr Dir Psychol Sci* 15:273–277, 2006.

Taylor SE, Welch W, Kim HS, et al.: Cultural differences in the impact of social support on psychological and biological stress responses, *Psychol Sci* 18:831–837, 2007.

Thoits P: Compensatory coping with stressors. In Avison W, Aneshensel CS, Shieman S, Weaton B, editors: *Advances in the Conceptualization of the Stress Process: Essays in Honor of Leonard I Pearlin*, Springer, 2010, pp 23–34. Chapter 2.

Yeager K, Roberts A: Differentiating among stress, acute stress disorder, crisis episodes, trauma, and PTSD: Paradigm and treatment goals, *Brief Treatment and Crisis Intervention*(3)3–25, 2003.

CHAPTER 17

Communicating with Clients Experiencing Communication Deficits

Kathleen Underman Boggs

OBJECTIVES

At the end of the chapter, the reader will be able to:

1. Identify common communication deficits.
2. Describe nursing strategies for communicating with clients experiencing communication deficits secondary to visual, auditory, cognitive, stimuli-related disabilities, or that are treatment-related.
3. Describe a specific communication deficit advocacy issue for nurses.
4. Access evidence-based databases for communication deficits and discuss application of these evidence-based practices and research findings to your clinical practice.

This chapter presents an overview of communication difficulties commonly encountered when caring for clients with communication deficits. Studies show many clients receiving care in hospitals, long-term care agencies, or in their homes have communication problems. For some, the underlying problem is related to physiological impairments making it difficult to communicate their needs. Consider the following case of Private Tim Dakota.

Case Example: Private Tim Dakota

Private Tim Dakota, age 22 years, is 3 weeks posttraumatic brain injury and has been a patient in your neurologic intensive care unit for 2 weeks.

Nurse: Good morning, Tim Dakota. I am Sue Nance, your nurse for this fine Sunday morning. I am going to give you your bath now. The water will feel a little warm to you. After your bath, your wife will be in to see you. She stayed in the waiting room last night because she wanted to be with you. (No answer is necessary if the client is unable to talk, but the sound of a human voice and attention to the client's unspoken concerns can be very healing.)

Summary of the strategies this nurse used:

- Called client by name
- Introduced self
- Established time (date, time, place would be better)
- Explained procedure before beginning
- Changed client's position frequently

Changing the client's position frequently benefits the person physiologically and offers us something to talk about. Our efforts to create a more stimulating environment, to offer reassurance and support, have later been reported to have been meaningful to the client.

As we strive to meet our QSEN competency of coordinating patient-centered care, we are also charged with using our skills to communicate client needs to the other members of the health care team. In this chapter, we describe strategies for enhancing communication for this population.

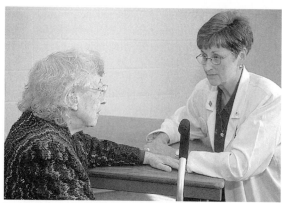

Touch, eye movements, and sounds can be used to communicate with clients experiencing aphasia.

BASIC CONCEPTS

A communication deficit is an impairment in the ability to receive, send, process, and comprehend concepts or verbal, nonverbal, and graphic symbol systems, as defined by the American Speech-Language-Hearing Association (ASLHA, 1993). These include deficits such as compromised hearing, vision, speech, language, or problems with cognitive processing (O'Halloran et al., 2012). They may be congenital or acquired; they range from mild to severe. Severe cognitive and sensory deficits interfere with communication, decrease access to health care, and lead to feelings of frustration. Overall, nearly one in six Americans has a sensory or communication deficit, which is nearly 50 million people (U.S. Department of Health and Human Services, n.d.). Improving access to care for these clients is one of the goals of *Healthy People 2020*. Many of these individuals report delays or difficulties obtaining health care.

In 2001, the World Health Organization (WHO)'s International Classification of Functioning, Disability and Health shifted away from a medical diagnosis model to a functional model (i.e., how the person with a sensory impairment functions in his or her everyday life). Under this model, a communication disability definition includes any client who has any impairment in body structure or function that interferes with communication. Specifically, the client has a communication difficulty because of impaired functioning of one or more of the five senses, or the client has impaired cognitive processing functioning. Communication deficits can also arise from the kind of sensory deprivation that occurs in some agencies and units, such as intensive care units. The degree of difficulty in communicating is an interaction between the client's type of functional impairment, personal adaptability, and the health care environment (i.e., body factors, personal factors, and environmental factors as stated in WHO's model).

Any impairment of a client's ability to send and/or receive information from health care providers may compromise his or her health, health care, and rights to make decisions. When working with these clients, you may need to modify communication strategies presented earlier in this textbook. Assess *every* client's communication abilities. Two individuals can have the same sensory impairment but not be equally communication disabled. Each person compensates for his or her impairment in different ways.

GOAL

Our primary nursing goal is to maximize our client's ability to successfully communicate and to interact with the health care system to ensure optimal health and quality of life. Evidence shows us that when nurses are unable to understand them, clients with communication disabilities become frustrated, angry, anxious, depressed, or uncertain. Some clients become so frustrated that they exhibit behavioral problems or even omit needed care. Even when care is accessed, communication deficits interfere with the therapeutic relationship and delivery of optimum care (Markov and Hazan, 2012). The client's deficit is one barrier. But other barriers may include staff's negative attitude or inability to adapt communication.

LEGAL MANDATES

In the legal system, the standard of "effective communication" is based on several statutes. The Americans with Disabilities Act (ADA) prohibits discrimination on the basis of a disability. Thus physician offices are required to provide reasonable accommodations to ensure effective communication. The Rehabilitation Act bars discrimination by those providers receiving federal monies, including Medicare. Title VI of the 1964 Civil Rights Act prohibits discrimination on the basis of national origin.

HOME-BASED HEALTH CARE

Visiting clients with communication deficits in their home allows nurses the time to engage in collaborative negotiations for which there may not have been time during acute care management. Home health nurses can build the infrastructure needed to prevent worsening of disability, as demonstrated in a study of elders by Liebel and associates (2012).

TYPES OF DEFICITS

HEARING LOSS

More than 28 million Americans have some problem hearing. Loss can be conductive, sensorineural, or functional. Causes can be genetic or acquired, such as due to infections, medication toxicity, or even due to exposure to excessive noise, such as occurs in combat. Hearing losses, especially in higher ranges, are most often found in older aged clients, as discussed in

Chapter 19. Nurses have both a legal and ethical obligation to provide appropriate care. Yet, deaf people are less likely to seek health-related information from care providers. Title III of the ADA delineates rights of the deaf and applies to communication between deaf clients and medical services.

People's sense of hearing alerts them to changes in the environment so they can respond effectively. The listener hears sounds and words, and also a speaker's vocal pitch, loudness, and intricate inflections accompanying the verbalization. Subtle variations can completely change the sense of the communication. Combined with the sound and intensity, the organization of the verbal symbols allows the client to perceive and interpret the meaning of the sender's message. The extent of your client's loss is not always appreciated because they often look and act in a normal fashion. Even mild to moderate hearing losses can lead to significant functional impairments (George et al., 2012). Deprived of a primary means of receiving signals from the environment, clients with hearing loss may try to hide deficits, may withdraw from relationships, become depressed, or be less likely to seek information from health care providers.

Children. Nearly 3 of every 1000 newborns are deaf or have hearing loss (U.S. Department of Health and Human Services, n.d.). Fortunately, many of these deficits are diagnosed at birth. Newborn hearing is tested in the nursery via auditory brainstem response tests (see the National Institute on Deafness and Other Communication Disorders web site at www.nidcd.nih.gov). **Hearing screening** is recommended for all newborn children by the U.S. Preventive Services Task Force (USPSTF) (AHRQ, 2012) and American Academy of Pediatrics.

Older Adults. As we age, we have an increased likelihood for *presbycusis*, or degeneration of ear structures, which is a sensorineural dysfunction that normally occurs with aging.

VISION LOSS

Humans rely more heavily on vision than do most species. Nearly 5 million Americans are blind or have uncorrectable visual impairments (National Eye Institute, n.d.). The majority of these are older than 50 years of age. Clients who lack vision lose a primary method to decode the meaning of messages. All of the nonverbal cues that accompany speech communication (e.g., facial expression, nodding, and leaning toward the

client) are lost to blind clients. Even with partial loss, it is important for you to assess whether your client can read directions, medication labels, and so forth.

Children. Children with visual impairments lack access to visual cues, such as the facial expressions that encourage them to develop communication skills. The USPSTF recommends testing children younger than 5 years for amblyopia, strabismus, and acuity, but traditional vision screening requires a verbal child and cannot be done reliably until age 3 years.

Older Adults. As we age, the lens of the eye becomes less flexible, making it difficult to accommodate shifts from far to near vision; this is a condition known as *presbyopia*. Macular degeneration has also become a major cause of vision loss in older adults.

IMPAIRED VERBAL COMMUNICATION SECONDARY TO SPEECH AND LANGUAGE DEFICITS

Clients who have speech and language deficits resulting from neurologic trauma present a different type of communication problem. Normal communication allows people to perceive and interact with the world in an organized and systematic manner. People use language to express self-needs and to control environmental events. Language is the system people rely on to represent what they know about the world. Early identification of children with at-risk prelinguistic skills may allow intervention to improve communication competencies. Clients unable to speak, even temporarily because of intubation or ventilator dependency, incur feelings of frustration, anxiety, fear, or even panic.

When the ability to process and express language is disrupted, many areas of functioning are assaulted simultaneously. *Aphasia* is a neurologic linguistic deficit, such as occurs after a stroke. Aphasia can present as primarily an expressive or receptive disorder. The client with *expressive aphasia* can understand what is being said but cannot express thoughts or feelings in words.

Receptive aphasia creates difficulties in receiving and processing written and oral messages. With *global aphasia*, the client has difficulty with both expressive language and reception of messages. Your client may have feelings of loss and social isolation imposed by the communication impairment. Although there may be no cognitive impairment, the client may need more "think time" for cognitive processing during a conversation.

IMPAIRED COGNITIVE PROCESSING

Impaired cognitive processing ability can interfere with the communication process and leads to anxiety and confusion. Understanding involves receiving new information and integrating it meaningfully with prior knowledge. Clients with impaired processing ability have to work harder and require more time for conceptual integration. The responsibility for assessing ability to understand, to give consent, and to overcome communication difficulties rests with both social services and health care workers. You need to continually determine the extent of your clients' understanding and even their ability to understand self-care activities. Assess their use of alternative communication aids (Gibson-Mee, 2011).

Children. Because there is a significant increase in the prevalence of children with developmental disabilities, more nurses will be caring for them both in clinical agencies and in the community (Betz, 2012). Atypical communication is often the first behavioral clue to cognitive impairment in young children, associated with conditions such as mental retardation, autism, and affective disorders. As these children grow, subtle distortions in communication may exist. For example, children with Down syndrome, have been shown to judge nonverbal facial expressions more positively than other children, which could lead to a misinterpretation of the nurses' messages.

Older Adults. Cognitively impaired older clients may have altered communication pathways. Although most older adults retain their mental acuity, we need to assess risks. Memory loss, for example, can interfere with client ability to correctly take prescribed medications.

COMMUNICATION DEFICITS ASSOCIATED WITH SOME MENTAL DISORDERS

Clients with serious mental disorders may have a different type of communication deficit resulting from a malfunctioning of the neurotransmitters that normally transmit and make sense out of messages in the brain. Thirteen million Americans have a serious, debilitating mental illness (U.S. Department of Health and Human Services, n.d.). Some of these have communication difficulties. In addition to illness-related communication problems, social isolation and impaired coping may accompany the client's inability to receive or express language signals.

Other communication problems occur with different mental disorders. As an example, some clients with mental disorders can perhaps have intact sensory channels, but they cannot process and respond appropriately to what they hear, see, smell, or touch. In some forms of *schizophrenia* there are alterations in the biochemical neurotransmitters in the brain, which normally conduct messages between nerve cells and help orchestrate the person's response to the external environment. Messages have distorted meanings. It is beyond the scope of this text to discuss the psychotic client's management. Basic communications strategies are described.

Some clients with mental disorders present with a poverty of speech and limited content. Speech appears blocked, reflecting disturbed patterns of perception, thought, emotions, and motivation. You may notice a lack of vocal inflection and an unchanging facial expression. A "flat affect" makes it difficult to truly understand your client. Illogical thinking processes may manifest in the form of illusions, hallucinations, and delusions. Common words assume new meanings known only to the person experiencing them.

ENVIRONMENTAL DEPRIVATION AS RELATED TO ILLNESS

Communication is particularly important in nursing situations characterized by sensory deprivation, physical immobility, limited environmental stimuli, or excessive, constant stimuli (Figure 17-1). Nurses need to show concern for the client in bewildering situations, such as emergency departments or intensive care units (ICUs). Clients may be frightened, in pain, and may be unable to communicate easily with others, because of intubation or other complications. Research indicates that the absence of interpersonal stimulation and the subsequent gradual decline of cognitive abilities are related. Clients with normal intellectual capacity can appear dull, uninterested, and lacking in problem-solving abilities if they do not have frequent interpersonal stimulation.

APPLICATIONS

Communication deficits may be developmental or acquired. The emphasis on patient-centered care embodies a need for clients with communication deficits to become active participants in their care. In

Developing an Evidence-Based Practice

Access some of the many databases that summarize research to compile "best practice" guidelines for adapting communication, especially pertinent for those who have communication deficits. Most sites rank the strength of the research evidence from strong to poor. Access www.guideline.gov/content. aspx?id=34160&search=best+evidence+statement +multiple+means for the "Best evidence statement (BESt). Communication of health care information to patients and caregivers using multiple means" from Cincinnati Children's Hospital Medical Center, 2011, May 15.

This group of expert clinicians created a comprehensive review to determine the most effective methods of communication about discharge with children and youth hospitalized in psychiatric facilities. Clients had referrals to occupational and speech therapy and language pathology.

Results: Based on extensive review, they found "good" evidence to recommend using standardized verbal and written discharge information, appropriate for client literacy level, limiting use of medical terminology. Results suggest it is most effective to use active verbs, short sentences, and visual aides to emphasize main points.

Application to your clinical practice: You may find it most effective to use active verbs and short sentences with all clients having communication deficits. Additionally, these findings suggest you supplement oral information with your choice of visual aids, including either pictures, PowerPoint presentations, or video.

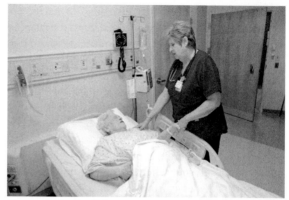

Figure 17-1   The following are situational factors that affect client responses to critical care hospital situations:
- Anxiety and fear
- Pain
- Altered stimuli—too much or too little, including unusual noises and isolation
- Sleep deprivation
- Unmet physiological needs such as thirst
- Losing track of time
- Multiple life changes
- Multiple care providers
- Immobility
- Frequent diagnostic procedures
- Lack of easily understood information

EARLY RECOGNITION OF COMMUNICATION DEFICITS

Identification of communication deficit is one aspect of your role. For example, if your 4-year-old client fails to speak at all or uses a noticeably limited vocabulary for his or her age, cannot name objects or follow your directions, would you recognize the need for further assessment? Given this history, you could urge the health team to make a referral for speech and language evaluation.

ASSESSMENT OF CURRENT COMMUNICATION ABILITIES

You need to assess each client's communication problems. Your plan of care can then be tailored to help meet identified communication needs. Provision of alternative communication methods is required by law.

COMMUNICATION STRATEGIES

Specific strategies are contained in the accompanying boxes. In general, evidence-based practice suggests you create a quiet environment, allocate more of your time

a hospital, all staff need to be aware of the client's communication disability, perhaps by posting a sign or symbol on the door. Mutual goals involve fostering effective communication with all members of the health team. Yet even when we are aware of the deficit, we sometimes lack the ability to communicate effectively with these clients. An amazing variety of communication devices have recently become available to assist in communication. Rather than reviewing all these devices, the following section primarily focuses on some basic strategies nurses can use to foster communication. Always let your client know when you cannot understand his or her communication. Aspects of your nurse role include assessment, development of strategies to facilitate communication, education, provision of psychological support, and advocacy.

to facilitate communication, take time to listen, ask yes/no questions, observe nonverbal cues, repeat back comments, effectively use communication equipment, assign same staff for care continuity, and encourage family members to be present to assist in communications (O'Halloran et al., 2012; also see the AHRQ web site).

CLIENTS WITH HEARING LOSS

Assessment of functional hearing ability is recommended for all your clients. Assessment of auditory sensory losses can provide an opportunity for referral. Your assessment should include the age of onset and the severity of the deficit. Hearing loss that occurs after the development of speech means that the client has access to word symbols and language skills. Deafness in children can cause developmental delays, which may need to be taken into account in planning the most appropriate communication strategies. Clues to hearing loss occur when clients appear unresponsive to sound or respond only when the speaker is directly facing them. Ask clients whether they use a hearing aid and whether it is working properly.

Strategies for communicating with clients who have a hearing loss depend on the severity of the deafness. Covering your face with a mask or speaking with an accent may make it impossible for a lip reader to understand you. Communication-assisting equipment should be available. We need to know how to operate auditory amplifiers such as assisted listening devices, hearing aids, and telephone attachments. Often, clients have hearing aids but fail to use them unless family or nurse assists them. Exercises 17-1 and 17-2 will help you understand what it is like to have a sensory deficit.

Refer to Box 17-1 to adapt your communication techniques. American Sign Language has been a standard communication tool for many years; however, few care providers are able to use it. Basic strategies include use of paper and pencil, use of hand signals or gestures, and use of technologic communication assistance devices, such as *speech amplifiers* (e.g., the pocket talker), communication boards, pictograph cards, and **wireless text communication** (text messaging) on cell phones. Your deaf client may also use teletypewriters (TTYs) or other devices or handheld electronics to exchange e-mail and receive instant alphanumeric

EXERCISE 17-1	Loss of Sensory Function in Geriatric Clients

Purpose: To assist students in getting in touch with the feelings often experienced by older adults as they lose sensory function. If the younger individual is able to "walk in the older person's shoes," he or she will be more sensitive to the losses and needs created by those losses in the older person.

Procedure
1. The class separates into three groups.
2. Group A: Place cotton balls in your ears. Group B: Cover your eyes with a plastic bag. Group C: Place cotton balls in your ears and cover your eyes with a plastic bag.
3. A student from Group B should be approached by a student from Group A. The student from Group B is to talk to the student from Group A using a whispered voice. The Group A student is to verify the message heard with the student who spoke. The student from Group B is then to identify the student from Group A.
4. The students in Group C are expected to identify at least one person in the group and describe to

that person what he or she is wearing. Each student who does not do the description is to make a statement to the other person and have that individual reveal what he or she was told.
5. Having identified and conversed with each other, hold hands or remain next to each other and remove the plastic bags and cotton balls (to facilitate verification of what was heard and described).

Discussion
1. How did the loss you experienced make you feel?
2. Were you comfortable performing the function expected of you with your limitation?
3. What do you think could have been done to make you feel less handicapped?
4. How did you feel when your "normal" level of functioning was restored?
5. How would you feel if you knew the loss you just simulated was to be permanent?
6. What effect do you think this experience might have on your future interactions with older individuals with such sensory losses?

Courtesy Glenn BJ, former member of the North Carolina State Health Coordinating Council Acute Care Committee, 1998.

EXERCISE 17-2   Sensory Loss: Hearing or Vision

Purpose: To help raise consciousness regarding loss of a sensory function.

Procedure
- Pair up with another student. One student should be blindfolded. The other student should guide the "blind" student on a walk around the campus.
- During a 5- to 10-minute walk, the student guide should converse with the "blind" student about the route they are taking.
  or
- Watch the first 2 minutes of a television show with the sound turned off. All students should watch the same show (e.g., the news report or a rerun of a situation comedy).

- In class, students share observations and answer the following questions.

Discussion
1. Were perceptual differences noted? What implications do you think these differences have in working with blind or deaf clients?
2. How frustrating was it for you to be sensory deprived? How did it make you feel?
3. What did you learn about yourself from this exercise that you can apply to your nursing clinical practice?

BOX 17-1   Suggestions for Helping the Client with Sensory Loss

- Assess psychological readiness to communicate.
- Introduce yourself and convey respect, an understanding of client frustrations, and your willingness to communicate.
- Be concise.
- Always maximize the use of sensory aids, such as communication boards, pictures, sign language, and electronic aids.
- Pick the means of available communication best suited to your client. Multiple pathways using both audio and visual are standard recommendations.
- Always help clients to use their assistive equipment (adjust hearing aids, glasses, smartphones for texting, etc.).

For Hearing-Impaired Clients
- Tap on the floor or table to get the client's attention via the vibration.
- Communicate in a well-lighted room and face the client to focus his or her attention, so the client can see your facial expression and can see your lips move.
- Choose a quiet, private place; close doors and turn off TVs or radios to decrease environmental noise.
- Use facial expressions, hand signals, and gestures that reinforce verbal content. Or request a sign language interpreter, perhaps a family member.
- Speak distinctly without exaggerating words. Partially deaf clients respond best to well-articulated words spoken in a moderate, even tone. Speak only as loudly as you need to; do not shout.
- Write important ideas and allow the client the same option to increase the chances of

communication. Always have a writing pad available.
- Arrange for a teletypewriter (TTY) or an amplified telephone handset for clients with partial hearing loss.
- If the client is unable to hear, rely primarily on visual materials.
- Arrange for closed-captioned television.
- Use text messaging on client's cell phone or e-mail at his or her computer.
- Encourage the client with hearing loss to verbalize speech, even if the person uses only a few words or the words are difficult to understand at first.
- Use an intermediary, such as a family member who knows sign language, to facilitate communication with deaf clients who sign.

For Vision-Impaired Clients
- Let the person know when you approach by identifying yourself, use a simple touch, and always indicate when you are leaving.
- Adapt communication to compensate for lack of nonverbal messaging.
- Adapt teaching for low vision by using large print, audiotaped information, or Braille.
- Do not lead or hold the client's arm when walking; instead, allow the person to take your arm.
- Use touch and close physical proximity while you are with the client; give the person something substantial to touch in your absence.
- Develop and use signals to indicate changes in pace or direction while walking.

messages and pages. Consider the following case example of Timmy.

Case Example: Timmy

Two student nurses were assigned to care for 9-year-old Timmy, who is deaf and mute. When they went into his room for assessment, he was alone and appeared anxious. No information was available as to his ability to read lips, the nurses were not sure what reading skills he had, and they did not know sign language. So, instead of using a pad and paper for communication, they decided to role-play taking vital signs by using some funny facial expressions and demonstrating on a doll.

CLIENTS WITH VISION LOSS

Vision assessment for impairment is recommended for all clients routinely. Nurses caring for any client with vision limitations should perform some evaluation and ensure that glasses and other equipment are available to hospitalized clients. Refer to Box 17-1 for strategies of use in caring for vision-impaired clients. Use of vocal cues (e.g., speaking as you approach) helps prevent startling the blind client. Because clients cannot see our faces or observe our nonverbal signals, we need to use words to express what the client cannot see in the message. It also is helpful to mention your name as you enter the client's presence. Even people who are partially blind appreciate hearing the name of the person to whom they are speaking. Communication-enhancing equipment for vision-impaired clients includes electronic magnifier machines, auditory teaching materials, computer screen readers with voice synthesizers, Braille keypads or cards, and video magnifying machines.

When caring for clients with macular degeneration, remember to stand to their side, an exception to the "face them directly" rule applied with clients with hearing loss. Macular degeneration clients often still have some peripheral vision. Enhanced lighting and use of light filters to reduce glare may help you communicate with clients who have reduced vision.

With blind clients, the use of touch acts as a social reinforcer and can orient the client to your presence. However, use of verbal greetings may better alert your clients. Voice tones and pauses that reinforce the verbal content are helpful. They need to be informed when you are leaving the room. Consider the following case of Ms. Shu.

Case Example: Ms. Shu

You can use words to supply additional information to counterbalance the missing visual cues. Ms. Sue Shu is a blind, elderly client who commented to the student nurse Ruth that she felt Ruth was uncomfortable talking with her and perhaps did not like her. Not being able to see Ruth, Ms. Shu interpreted the hesitant uneasiness in Ruth's voice as evidence that Ruth did not wish to be with her. Ruth agreed with Ms. Shu that she was quite uncomfortable but did not explain further. Had Ms. Shu been able to see Ruth's apprehensive body posture, she would have realized that Ruth was quite shy and ill at ease with *any* interpersonal relationship. To avoid this serious error in communication, Ruth might have clarified the reasons for her discomfort, and the relationship could have moved forward.

ORIENTATION TO ENVIRONMENTAL HAZARDS

When a blind client is being introduced to a new environmental setting, you should orient the client by describing the size of the room and the position of the furniture and equipment. When placing the client's food tray, describe the position of items, perhaps using a clock face analogy (e.g., "Carrots are at 2 o'clock, potatoes at 11 o'clock."). If other people are present, you could name each person. A good communication strategy is to ask the other people in the room to introduce themselves to the client. In this way, he or she gains an appreciation for their voice configurations. You should avoid any tendency to speak with a blind client in a louder voice than usual or to enunciate words in an exaggerated manner. This may be perceived by some clients as condescending or insensitive to the nature of the handicap. Voice tones should be kept natural.

A blind client may need guidance in moving around in unfamiliar surroundings. For example, surveyed blind clients said they needed assistance getting to and from their bathroom. One way of preserving the client's autonomy is to offer your arm to the client instead of taking the client's arm. Mention steps and changes in movement as they are about to occur to help the client navigate new places and differences in terrain. Some clients will be using wearable navigation systems.

IMPAIRED VERBAL COMMUNICATION SECONDARY TO SPEECH AND LANGUAGE DEFICITS

Assessment of speech and language is part of the initial evaluation. Difficulties arise when clients are unable to speak (**aphasia**). For these clients, an assessment of the type your client is experiencing will aid in selecting the most appropriate intervention. Expressive language problems are evidenced in an inability to find words or to associate ideas with accurate word symbols. Some clients with **expressive aphasia** can find the correct word if given enough time and support. Other clients have difficulty organizing their words into meaningful sentences or describing a sequence of events. Clients with receptive communication deficits have trouble following directions, reading information, writing, or relating data to previous knowledge. Even when your client appears not to understand, you should explain in simple terms what is happening. Using touch, gestures, eye movements, and squeezing of the hand should be attempted. Clients appreciate nurses who take the time to respond to communication attempts.

Refer to Box 17-2 for strategies to use with clients having speech deficits. Clients who lose both expressive and receptive communication abilities have *global aphasia*. Clients with these deficits can become frustrated when they are not understood. Struggling to speak causes fatigue. Short, positive sessions are used to communicate. Otherwise, the client may become nonverbal as a way of regaining energy and composure. Changes in self-image occasioned by physical changes, the

uncertain recovery course and outcome of strokes, shifts in family roles, and the disruption of free-flowing verbal interaction among family members all make the loss of functional communication particularly agonizing. Any language skills that are preserved should be exploited.

Alternative means of communication, such as pointing, gesturing, or using pictures can be used, as well as speech-generating electronic devices. Augmentive and alternative communication (AAC) methods have been found to help nurses better communicate with clients who are unable to speak (Finke et al., 2008). AAC options include communication boards, picture cards, and use of picture pain rating scales. But the preferred AAC method found by van der Meer and associates (2011) is use of **speech-generating devices**. There are several **smart phone apps** available that allow the client to touch a picture on screen causing a mechanical voice to speak, conveying the intended message.

COMMUNICATION WITH CLIENTS WHO HAVE MENTAL PROCESSING DEFICITS

Cognitive understanding involves recognition of words and integrating them into a schemata of acquired knowledge. Some clients may have difficulty ignoring irrelevant information or have difficulty organizing input meaningfully.

Clients with Learning Delays. As a nurse providing care to learning delay (LD) clients, you need to adapt your messages to an understandable level. This is crucial is all communication but especially when you are seeking to gain informed consent for treatment. To what extent should you involve your cognitively impaired client in decision making? In communicating about general health care, adaptations include simple explanations, touch, and use of familiar objects.

Communication deficits associated with some mental disorders. When working with some clients with mental disorders, you will face a formidable challenge in trying to establish a relationship. Clients with altered reality discrimination have both verbal and nonverbal communication deficits. Rarely will this client approach you directly. The client generally responds to questions, but the answers are likely to be brief, and the client does not elaborate without further probes. Although the client appears to rebuff any social interaction, it is important to keep trying to connect. People with mental disorders such as schizophrenia are easily overwhelmed by the external environment. Tremeau and colleagues (2005)

BOX 17-2	Strategies to Assist the Client with Cognitive Processing Deficits or Speech and Language Difficulties

- Speak slowly, using simple sentences; ask yes or no questions.
- Talk about one thing at a time or ask one question at a time; do not rush.
- Give clients extra time to process and formulate a response; do not interrupt.
- Avoid prolonged, continuous conversations; instead, use frequent, short talks. Present small amounts of information at a time.
- When clients falter in written or oral expression, supply needed compensatory support.
- Praise efforts to communicate.
- Provide regular mental stimulation in a nontaxing way.
- Help clients focus on the faculties still available to them for communication.
- Use visual cues; for print materials, use short, bulleted lists.
- Make referrals so clients can obtain and use augmentive and alternative communication (AAC) devices.

EXERCISE 17-3   **Schizophrenia Communication Simulation**

Purpose: To gain insight into communication deficits encountered by clients with schizophrenia.

Procedure
1. Break class into groups of three (triads) by counting off 1, 2, 3.
2. Person 1 (the nurse) reads a paragraph of rules to the client and then quizzes him or her afterward about the content.
3. Person 2 (the client with schizophrenia) listens to everything and tries to answer the nurse's questions correctly to get 100% on the test.

4. Person 3 (representing the mental illness) speaks loudly and continuously in the client's ear while the nurse is communicating, saying things like "You are so stupid," "You have done bad things," and "It is coming to get you," over and over.

Discussion
Did any client have 100% recall? Ask the client to share how difficult it is to communicate to the nurse when you are "hearing voices."

Courtesy Ann Newman, PhD, University of North Carolina, Charlotte.

demonstrated that schizophrenic clients have the same expressive deficits as do depressed clients. Keeping in mind that the client's unresponsiveness to words, failure to make eye contact, unchanging facial expression, and monotonic voice are parts of the disorder and not a commentary on your communication skills helps you to continue to engage with your client.

If your client is hallucinating or using delusions as a primary form of communication, you should neither challenge their validity directly nor enter into a prolonged discussion of illogical thinking. Often you can identify the underlying theme the client is trying to convey with the delusional statement. For example, when your client says, "Voices are telling me to do…," you might reply, "It sounds as though you feel powerless and afraid at this moment." Listening to your client carefully, using alert posture, nodding to demonstrate active listening, and trying to make sense out of the client's underlying feelings models effective communication and helps you decode nonsensical messages. Exercise 17-3 may help you gain some understanding of communication problems experienced by the client with schizophrenia.

CLIENTS EXPERIENCING TREATMENT-RELATED COMMUNICATION DISABILITIES

Communication disabilities can stem from sedative medications, mechanical ventilation, isolation in an ICU, or isolation such as occurs when older adults are in long-term care facilities. A number of recent studies of client communication in intensive care show that clients are very dependent on their nurse to institute communication. Specific recommended

skills are listed in Box 17-3. Many of the simpler items such as use of communication boards or cards are useful with ventilator-dependent clients temporarily unable to speak. Newer advances in electronic technologies are available to help clients communicate, such as **gaze-controlled communication computer programs**. A recent study confirmed that better communication leads to psychological improvements such as decreased anxiety and depression (Maringelli et al., 2013).

LACK OF COMMUNICATION DUE TO LOWERED LEVEL OF CONSCIOUSNESS

When a client is not fully alert, it is not uncommon for nurses to speak in his or her presence in ways they would not if they thought the client could fully understand what is being said, forgetting that hearing can remain acute. It is not possible to be certain about what level of awareness remains. Good practice suggests you never say anything you would not want the client to hear. Always calling your client by name; orienting to time, place, and location; explaining all procedures; and using touch are considered best practice. Consider the following case of Mr. Lopez.

Case Example: Mr. Lopez

Your client Mr. Lopez is totally paralyzed and seems unresponsive immediately after a rupture of a blood vessel in his brain. Mrs. Lopez thinks he can still blink his eyes. You say: "Mr. Lopez, you are in the emergency department of General Hospital. I am your nurse, Kathleen. I need to draw a sample of your blood. Can you feel this? Blink once for yes and twice for no."

BOX 17-3	Strategies for Communicating with Clients with Treatment-Related Communication Deficits Such as Occurs in the Intensive Care Unit

- Encourage the client to display pictures or a simple object from home.
- Orient the client to the environment, to time and place.
- Ask many questions, especially questions the client can answer with a yes or no.
- Frequently provide information about the client's condition and progress.
- Reassure the client that cognitive and psychological disturbances are common.
- Give explanations before procedures by providing information about the sounds, sights, and feelings the client is experiencing.
- Make communication assistive devices available, ranging from paper and pencil or communication cards to computerized communication.
- Always assess whether your communication to the client was successful.

For all communication-impaired clients, convey a caring, compassionate attitude, use alternative communication strategies, and give frequent orienting cues, linking events to routines (e.g., saying, "The x-ray technician will take your chest x-ray right after lunch."). When clients are unable or unwilling to engage in a dialogue, you should continue to initiate communication in a one-way mode.

REFERRALS

As the health team member having the most daily contact with a client, you may be best positioned to know when he or she is ready for a referral. For example, a client with speech loss secondary to throat cancer surgery may be ready for a referral to a speech therapist to learn alternative communication earlier than expected based on a standard clinical pathway.

CLIENT ADVOCACY

Our nurse role also includes acting as an advocate for our clients who have communication disabilities. Too often these clients are discounted. Medical treatment decisions may be made without seeking input from them. Appropriate communication aids may be withheld while the client is hospitalized. In the larger community, we need to advocate for community services designed to foster communication, including referrals to speech and language therapists.

SUMMARY

This chapter discusses the specialized communication needs of clients with communication deficits. Adapting our communication skills and projecting a caring, positive attitude are important in overcoming barriers. Basic issues and applications for communicating with clients experiencing sensory loss of hearing and sight are outlined. Sensory stimulation and compensatory channels of communication are needed for clients with sensory deprivation. All workers who come in contact with the client need to be aware of their communication impairments. We need to learn how to operate and fit equipment such as hearing aids, because hospitalized clients often need help with devices. The mentally ill client has intact senses, but information processing and language are affected by the disorder. It is important for you to develop a proactive communication approach with clients who are learning impaired or who suffer from mental disorders. For clients such as those with aphasia, you can develop alternative methods of communicating. Other clients can experience communication isolation and temporary distortion of reality. Such clients need frequent cues that orient them to time and place, as well as providing sensory stimulation. Evidence shows that we need to be careful not to associate communication disability with intellectual dysfunction. Our skill in adapting communication is important to the client.

ETHICAL DILEMMA   What Would You Do?

Working in a health department clinic, the nurse—through a Spanish-speaking translator—interviews a 46-year-old married woman about the missing results of her recent breast biopsy for suspected cancer. Because the translator is of the same culture as the client and holds the same cultural belief that suicide is shameful, he chooses to withhold from the nurse information he obtained about a recent suicide attempt. If this information remains hidden from the nurse and doctor, could this adversely affect the client? What ethical principle is being violated?

DISCUSSION QUESTIONS

As part of our QSEN patient-centered care expected competencies, what skills and attitudes would you use in the following situations?

1. Describe what you might say at your first meeting with your confused client as you begin the 3-11 shift in General Medical Centers Intensive Care Unit. (Hint: check Box 17-3.)

2. You notice your clients on the medical wing at Shangri-La Long-Term Care Facility are rarely out of their rooms and seem withdrawn. What patient-centered interventions might you use to ameliorate stimuli-related communication disabilities?

3. Reflect on opportunities for client advocacy. Identify one way in which you can advocate for a deficit issue affecting client communication.

REFERENCES

Agency for Healthcare Research and Quality (AHRQ). www.ahrq.gov/topicsobjectives2020/ Refer to Goal DH-8 and sections on hearing and other sensory or communication disorders.

American Speech-Language-Hearing Association (ASLHA). (1993). *Definitions of communication disorders and variations* [Relevant Paper]. Available from www.asha.org/policy. Accessed July 4, 2014.

Betz C: Opportunities to create nurse-directed, evidence-based services and programs for children and youth with special health care needs and developmental disabilities, *J Pediatr Nurs* 27(6):1–2, 2012.

Finke LH, Light J, Kitko L: A systematic review of the effectiveness of nurse communication with patients with complex communication needs with a focus on the use of augmentative and alternative communication, *J Clin Nurs* 17:2102–2115, 2008.

Gibson-Mee S: Communication skills to improve clients' experiences of hospital, *Learn Disabil Pract* 14(9):28–30, 2011.

George P, Farrell TW, Griswold MF: Hearing loss: Help for the young and old, *J Fam Pract* 61(5):268–270, 2012. 274-277.

U.S. Department of Health and Human Services (n.d.). Healthy People 2020: Topics and Objectives. Hearing and other sensory or communication disorders. www.healthypeople.gov/2020/topicsobjectives2020/overview.aspx?topicid=20. Accessed July 4, 2014.

Liebel DV, Powers BA, Friedman B, Watson NM: Barriers and facilitators to optimize function and prevent disability worsening: A content analysis of a nurse home visit intervention, *J Adv Nurs* 68(1):80–93, 2012.

Maringelli F, Brienza N, Scorrano F, Grasso F, Gregoretti C: Gaze-controlled, computer-assisted communication in Intensive Care Unit: "speaking through the eyes." *Minerva Anestesiol* 79(2):165–175, 2013.

Markov M, Hazan A: Advances in communication technology: Implications for new nursing skills, *J Pediatr Nurs* 27(5):1–4, 2012.

National Eye Institute. www.nei.nih.gov/. Eye Data Statistics. Accessed July 2, 2014.

O'Halloran R, Hickson L, Worrall L: Stroke patients communicating their needs in a hospital: A study within the ICF framework, *Int J Lang Commun Disord* 47(2):130–143, 2012.

Tremeau F, Malaspina D, Duval F, et al.: Facial expressiveness in patients with schizophrenia compared to depressed patients and nonpatient comparison subjects, *Am J Psychiatry* 162(1):92–101, 2005.

QSEN www.qsen.org/Assessing preferences for AAC options in communication interventions for individuals with developmental disabilities: A review of the literature. Res Dev Disabil 32(5), 1422–1431.

World Health Organization (WHO): *International classification of functioning, disability, and health Author*, Geneva, 2001, Switzerland.

Agency for Healthcare Research and Quality (AHRQ): Guide to Clinical Preventive Services: Recommendations of the U.S. *Preventive Services Task Force*, 2012. Accessed July 20, 2013. http://www.ahrq.gov/professionals/clinicians-providers/guidelines-recommendations/guide/index.html.

CHAPTER 18

Communicating with Children

Kathleen Underman Boggs

OBJECTIVES

At the end of the chapter, the reader will be able to:

1. Identify how developmental levels impact the child's ability to communicate within interpersonal relationships with caregivers.
2. Discuss evidenced-based practice applications for communicating with a child in clinical practice.
3. Describe modifications in communication strategies to meet the specialized needs of children.
4. Describe interpersonal techniques needed to interact with concerned parents of ill children.
5. Use a pediatric web site to access data for evidence-based pediatric practice.

This chapter is designed to help you recognize and apply communication concepts related to the nurse-child-family relationship in pediatric clinical situations. In mastering QSEN competency of patient-centered care, effective tools need be attitudinal, cognitive, and developmentally appropriate. For each of these domains, the child's and family's socioeconomic status and cultural background must be considered.

Communicating with children at different age levels requires modifications of the skills learned in previous chapters. By understanding the child's cognitive and functional level, you are able to select the most appropriate communication strategies. Children undergo significant age-related changes in the ability to process cognitive information and in the capacity to interact effectively with the environment. To have an effective therapeutic relationship with a child, you need to understand the feelings and thought processes from the child's perspective and convey honesty, respect, and acceptance of feelings.

Communicating with parents of seriously ill children requires a deliberate effort. Parents need explanations they can understand, need to have established trust with the nurse, and need to feel they have some control over what is happening to their child. This chapter identifies strategies to enhance communication with parents as well as children.

BASIC CONCEPTS

LOCATION

Just as there is a nationwide emphasis on outpatient procedures and home care for adults, the same is true for children. More than 70% of pediatric illness care occurs in ambulatory settings. Since 2000, inpatient care has continued to decline significantly. Hospitalization for potentially preventable acute and chronic conditions declined by 18% between 2000 and 2007 (Friedman et al., 2011).

ATTITUDE

Quality of care studies indicate that in all settings children may receive less than half of "best evidence" interventions. Could this be due to overreliance on health care providers own experience, or lack of time to access the latest data and protocols? Major changes in society are mirrored in changing health care for children. Involving children in their own health care decision making is a part of QSEN's "patient-centered care." Making the child a (limited) partner might lead to better health outcomes than treating the child as a target for our delivery of care. Do you see this as desirable?

COGNITION

Childhood is very different from adulthood. A child has fewer life experiences from which to draw and is still in the process of developing skills needed for reasoning and communicating. Every child's concept of health and illness must be considered within a developmental framework. Erikson's (1963) concepts of ego development and Piaget's (1972) description of the progressive development of the child's cognitive thought processes together form the theoretical basis for the child-centered nursing interventions described in this chapter. Both theorists say that the child's thought processes, ways of perceiving the world, judgments, and emotional responses to life situations are different from those of the adult. Cognitive and psychosocial development unfold according to an ordered hierarchical scheme, increasing in depth and complexity as the child matures.

DEVELOPMENTALLY APPROPRIATE

Piaget's descriptions of stages of cognitive development provide a valuable contribution toward understanding the dimensions of a child's perceptions and communication abilities. Cognitive development and early language development are integrally related. Although current developmental theorists expand on Piaget's theoretical model by recognizing the effects of the parent-child relationship and a stimulating environment on developing communication abilities, his work forms the foundation for the understanding of childhood cognitive development. Piaget observed cognitive development occurring in sequential stages (Table 18-1). The ages are only approximated, because Piaget himself was not specific.

Wide individual differences exist in the intellectual functioning of same-age children. Variations also occur across situations, so that the child under stress or in a different environment may process information at a lower level than he or she would under normal conditions. Because two children of the same chronologic age may have quite different skills as information processors, we need to assess level of functioning. Language alternatives familiar to one child because of certain life experiences may not be useful in providing health care and teaching with another. Integrating cognitive and psychosocial developmental approaches into communication with children at different ages enhances effectiveness.

INTERPERSONAL

GENDER DIFFERENCES IN COMMUNICATION

Some studies show school-age children are more satisfied if their health care provider is the same sex. Past studies showed that communication by female providers was more social, more encouraging, and involved speaking more often directly with the child client. Use of good age-appropriate communication strategies probably outweighs gender as a factor in successful communication with a child, but gender cannot be excluded as a factor affecting communication.

UNDERSTANDING THE ILL CHILD'S NEEDS

Difficulties arise in adult-child communication, in part, because of the child's limited experience in interpreting subtle nuances of facial expression, inflection, and word meanings. When illness and physical or developmental disabilities occur during formative years, situational stressors are added that affect the way children perceive themselves and the environment. Illness may lead to significant alterations in role relationships with family and peers. You need to assess not only the physical care needs of the child but the impact of the illness on the child's self-esteem and on his or her relationships with family and friends. Responses to hospitalization vary with the individual according to his or her age. Negative responses may include separation anxiety, night terrors, feeding disturbances, or regression to earlier developmental stage behavior. Things that affect a child's response may include the chronicity of illness, its impact on lifestyle, the child's cognitive understanding of the disease process, and the family's ability to cope with care demands.

Children with Special Health Care Needs

Some children have chronic physical, developmental, behavioral, or emotional conditions that require health services. In the United States, 1 in every 5 childrearing households has a child with a chronic health condition

TABLE 18-1	Stages of Cognitive Development		
Age	**Piaget's Stage**	**Characteristics**	**Language Development**
Birth to 2 years	Sensorimotor	Infant learns by manipulating objects. At birth, reflexive communication, then moves through six stages to reach actual thinking.	**Presymbolic** Communication largely nonverbal. Vocabulary of more than 4 words by 12 months, increases to >200 words and use of short sentences before age 2 years.
2-6 years	Preoperational	Beginning use of symbolic thinking. Imaginative play. Masters reversibility.	**Symbolic** Actual use of structured grammar and language to communicate. Uses pronouns. Average vocabulary >10,000 words by age 6 years.
7-11 years	Concrete operations	Logical thinking. Masters use of numbers and other concrete ideas such as classification and conservation.	Mastery of passive tense by age 7 years and complex grammatical skills by age 10 years
12+ years	Formal operations	Abstract thinking. Futuristic; takes a broader, more theoretical perspective.	Near adult-like skills

Adapted from Piaget J: *The child's conception of the world*, Savage, MD, 1972, Littlefield, Adams.

(DHHS, Maternal and Child Health Bureau). Many of these children previously would have died but were saved by current technology, leaving some with chronic problems.

FAMILY-CENTERED CARE

In pediatric situations, patient-centered care is really family-centered with attention to family diversity and family processes. Evidence documents relationships between such processes and child health outcomes. If the child needs to be hospitalized, this is a *situational crisis* for the child and the entire family. Hospitalization is always stressful. *Prehospitalization preparation* can be done to decrease the child's anxiety. Before elective procedures, many hospitals now offer orientation education tours to youngsters. There are many good books designed to prepare children for their hospitalization available in most public libraries.

Hospitalized children have to contend not only with physical changes but with possible separation from family and friends, as well as living in a strange, frightening, and probably painful environment. Usually a family member stays with their child. Parenting a seriously ill child has been documented to be very stressful, especially for young parents or those with illness related perceived financial hardship. Their child's suffering impairs their own coping ability (Rosenberg et al., 2013). Nurses are in a position to support parents, to identify those who are most highly stressed. The extent of responsibility the family assumes for basic care of their hospitalized child needs to be negotiated with staff. Some parents prefer to bathe or feed their child themselves. Expectations for care and information about treatment need to be clearly communicated with consistent team members. For example, in a Swedish study of neonates, parents reported miscommunication when many different nurses were involved in their child's care, or when information was incompletely transmitted during "hand-offs" shift change. Parents also expressed a desire to be present during physician rounds (Wigert et al., 2013).

With chronically ill children, the family needs to learn new interactional patterns and coping strategies that take into consideration the meaning of an illness and disability in family life. Some studies show parents taking home an infant with a life-threatening condition may have less secure attachment related possibly to insecurity about the child's survival (Rempel et al., 2013). Caring for a chronically ill child demands considerable resources.

Developing an Evidence-Based Practice

There are many evidence-based data web sites you can use to aid your pediatric practice. In addition to doing journal searches and downloading specific journal articles, the Cumulative Index to Nursing and Allied Health (CINAHL) web site, has compiled "Evidence-Based Care Sheets" you can access. For example, they have summarized the best evidence to list strategies for *pediatric pain assessment*. They describe research results showing that three-quarters of the children admitted to emergency departments are in pain, but that only half of these children receive analgesics. This may be because emergency department nurses are not all using age-appropriate visual pain scales to assess the child's pain, even though data shows self-report is the most reliable tool in children older than age 4 years.

Access CINAHL for application to your practice:
1. Which pain assessment scales are available?
2. How much time does it take to use one to assess a child's pain?
3. What reasons do nurses and physicians use to justify not giving pain relief?

APPLICATIONS

Although children historically have not been the subjects of study, research has contributed to our knowledge of child learning and development. Children are more vulnerable, and thus are entitled to extra protection as research subjects. Findings are limited because of overreliance on what parents have told us. Agencies tend to see children as similar, without consideration of differences because of age, gender, race, or culture. To give one example, many of the medicines we use to treat children have been tested only on adults by pharmaceutical companies.

Major sources of stress for parents of critically ill children include uncertainty about current condition or prognosis, lack of control, and lack of knowledge about how to best help their hospitalized child or how to deal with their child's response. Although more nursing research is being conducted on effective communication with both parents and their ill children, many of the applications we discuss are based more on experience than on research.

ASSESSMENT

Assessing a child's reaction to illness requires knowing the child's normal patterns of communication. Interactions are observed between parent and child. The child's behavioral responses to the entire interpersonal environment (including nurse and peers) are assessed. Are the child's interactions age-appropriate? Are behaviors organized, or is the child unable to complete activities? Does the child act out an entire play sequence, or is such play fragmented and disorganized? Do the child's interactions with others suggest imagination and a broad repertoire of relating behaviors, or is communication devoid of possibilities? Because children cannot communicate fully with us, we have a special responsibility to assess for problems. For example, nearly 6 million American children are reported victims of neglect, physical abuse, psychological abuse, or even sexual abuse (U.S. Department of Health and Human Services (DHHS n.d.) Health Resources and Services Administration (HRSA) Maternal and Child Bureau). Once baseline data have been collected, you can plan specific communication strategies to meet the specialized needs of the child client (Figure 18-1). An overview of nursing adaptations needed to communicate effectively with children is summarized in Box 18-1.

REGRESSION AS A FORM OF CHILDHOOD COMMUNICATION

A severe illness can cause a child to show behaviors that are reminiscent of an earlier stage of development. A certain amount of regression is normal. Common behaviors include whining, demanding undue attention, withdrawal, or having toileting "accidents." These behaviors might stem from the powerlessness the child feels in attempting to cope with an overwhelming, frightening environment. Reassuring the parent that this is a common response to the stress of illness can be helpful.

Because children have limited life experience to draw from, they exhibit a narrower range of behaviors in coping with threat. The quiet, overly compliant child who does not complain may be more frightened than the child who screams or cries. This should alert you

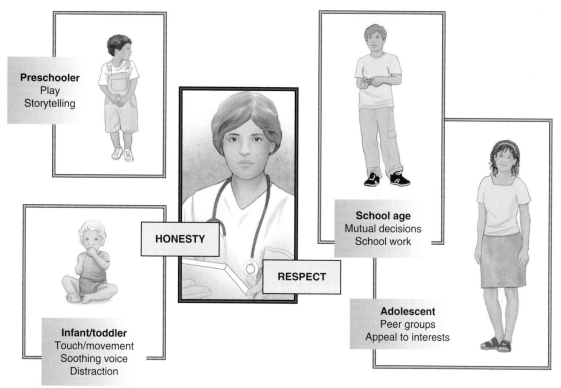

Figure 18-1 Nursing strategies must be geared toward the developmental level of the child.

to the child's emotional distress. You need to obtain detailed information regarding the usual behavioral responses of the family and child. Some behaviors that look regressive may be a typical behavioral response for the child (e.g., the 2-year-old who wants a bedtime bottle). A complete baseline history offers a good counterpoint for assessing the meaning of current behaviors.

AGE-APPROPRIATE COMMUNICATION

An assessment of vocabulary and understanding is essential in fostering communications. Whenever possible, you should communicate using words familiar to the child. Parents are valuable resources in helping interpret behavioral data. You might assist a child who is having difficulty finding the right words by reframing what he said and repeating it in a slightly different way.

The ill child's peers often have difficulty accepting individual differences created by health deviations. They lack the knowledge and sensitivity to deal with physical changes that they do not understand, as evidenced by "bald" jokes about the child receiving

chemotherapy. Children with hidden disorders such as diabetes, some forms of epilepsy, or minimal brain dysfunction are particularly susceptible to interpersonal distress. For example, it may be difficult for diabetics to regulate their intake of fast foods when all of their friends are able to eat what they want. When peer pressure is at its peak in adolescence, teenagers with newly diagnosed convulsive seizure disorders may find it difficult to tell peers they no longer can ride bicycles or drive cars. Unless the family and nurse provide appropriate interpersonal support, such children have to cope with an indistinct assault to their self-concept alone. A summary of age-appropriate strategies is provided in Box 18-2.

COMMUNICATING WITH CHILDREN WITH PSYCHOLOGICAL BEHAVIORAL PROBLEMS

One out of 10 adolescents and children in our society suffer from a mental illness. These illnesses lead to some level of interactional problems, which may be encountered by nurses in schools, hospitals, clinics, or during home visits to treat physical illnesses. Discussion

BOX 18-1	Nurse-Child Communication Strategies: Adapting Communication to Meet the Needs of the Ill Child

- Develop an understanding of age-related norms of development.
- Let the child know you are interested in him or her; convey respect and authenticity.
- Let the child know how to summon you (call bell, etc.).
- Develop trust through honesty and consistency in meeting the child's needs.
- Use "transitional objects" such as familiar pictures or toys from home.
- Assess:
  - Level of understandings
  - The child's needs in relation to the immediate situation
  - The child's capacity to cope successfully with change
- Observe for nonverbal cues.
- Use *nonverbal* communication:
  - Tactile (soothing strokes)
  - Kinesthetic (rocking)
  - Get down to the child's height; do not tower over him or her
  - Make eye contact and use reassuring facial expressions
  - Interpret the child's nonverbal cues verbally back to him
  - Instead of conversation, use some indirect age-appropriate communication techniques (e.g., storytelling, picture drawing, music, creative writing)
- Use *verbal* communication:
  - Use familiar words
  - Use age-appropriate vocabulary
  - Listen without interrupting
  - Humor and active listening to foster the relationship
  - Use open-ended questions
  - Use "I" statements
  - Help child to clarify his or her ideas and feelings ("Tell me more…"; "You got scared when…")
- Respect the child's privacy.
- Accept child's emotions.
- Help child understand the difference between thoughts and actions.
- Increase coping skills by providing play opportunities; use creative, unstructured play, medical role play, and pantomime.
- Use alternative, supplementary communication devices for children with specialized needs (e.g., sign language and computer-enhanced communication programs).

of nursing interventions with mentally ill children is beyond the scope of this textbook. An excellent source is available via Web links from the Maternal and Child Health Bureau of the U.S. Department of Health and Human Services (DHHS).

COMMUNICATING WITH PHYSICALLY ILL CHILDREN IN THE HOSPITAL AND AMBULATORY CLINIC

Overestimating a child's understanding of information about illness results in confusion, increased anxiety, anger, or sadness. Beyond physiologic care, ill children of all ages need support from every member of the health team—support that they normally would receive from parents. The nurse must provide stimulation to talk, listen, and play. Play is their language, especially because children have major difficulties verbalizing their true feelings about the treatment experience. As nurses, we adapt our communication to meet the ill child's needs. Many agencies have play therapists who serve as excellent resources for staff.

COMMUNICATION WITH INFANTS FROM BIRTH TO 12 MONTHS

Cues to assessment of the preverbal infant include tone of the cry, facial appearance, and body movements. Because the infant uses the senses to receive information, nonverbal communication (e.g., touch) is an important tool for the pediatric nurse. Tone of voice, rocking motion, use of distraction, and a soothing touch can be used in addition to or in conjunction with verbal explanations. Face-to-face position, bending or moving to the child's eye level, maintaining eye contact, and making a reassuring facial expression further help in interactions with infants.

Anticipate developmental behaviors such as "stranger anxiety" in infants between 9 and 18 months of age. Rather than reaching to pick a child up immediately, the nurse might smile and extend a hand toward the child or stroke the child's arm before attempting to hold the child. In this way, the nurse acknowledges the infant's inability to generalize to unfamiliar caregivers. If the child is able to talk, asking the child his or her name and pointing out a notable pleasant physical characteristic conveys the impression that you see the child client as a unique person. To a tiny child, this treatment can be synonymous with caring.

| BOX 18-2 | Key Points in Communicating with Children According to Age Group |

Infants
- Nonverbal communication is a primary mode.
- Infants are biologically "wired" to pay close attention to words. In first year, infants are able to distinguish all conversational sounds.
- Infants are bonded to primary caregivers only. Those older than 8 months may display separation anxiety when separated from parent or when approached by strangers.

Use Kinesthetic Communication
- Use stroking, soft touching, and holding.
- Use motion (e.g., rocking) to reassure. Allow freedom of movement and avoid restraining when possible.
- Learn specifically how the primary caregiver provides care in terms of sleeping, bathing, and feeding, and attempt to mimic these approaches.

Hold Close to Adapt to Limited Vision (20/200 to 20/300 at Birth)
- Encourage the infant's caregivers (parents) to use a lot of intimate space interaction (e.g., 8-18 inches). Mimic the same when trust is established.

Talk with Infants
- Talk with infants in normal conversational tones; soothe them with crooning voice tone.

Establish Trust
- Use parents to give care. Arrange for one or both parents to remain within the child's sight.

Shorten Your Stature
- Sit down on chair, stool, or carpet to decrease posture superiority, so as to look less imposing.

Handle Separation Anxiety When Primary Caregiver Is Absent
- Establish rapport with the caregiver (parent) and encourage the caregiver to be with child and reassure child that staff will be there if caregiver is away. At first keep at least 2 feet between nurse and infant. Talk to and touch the infant and initially smile often. Provide for kinesthetic approaches; offer self while infant is protesting (e.g., stay with the child; pick the child up and rock or walk; talk to the child about Mommy and Daddy and how much the child cares for them).

1- to 3-Year-Olds
- Child begins to talk around 1 year of age; learns nine new words a day after 18 months.

- By age 2, child begins to use phrases; should be able to respond to "what" and "where" type questions.
- By age 3, child uses and understands sentences.

Adapt to Limited Vocabulary and Verbal Skills
- Make explanations brief and clear. Use the child's own vocabulary words for basic care activities (e.g., use the child's words for defecate [poop, goodies] and urinate [pee-pee, tinkle]). Learn and use self-name of the child.
- Rephrase the child's message in a simple, complete sentence; avoid baby talk. Child should be able to follow two simple directions.

Continue to Use Kinesthetic Communication
- Allow ambulating where possible (e.g., using toddler chairs or walkers). Pull the child in a wagon often if child cannot achieve mobility.

Facilitate Child's Struggle with Issues of Autonomy and Control
- Allow the child some control (e.g., "Do you want a half a glass or a whole glass of milk?").
- Reassure the child if he or she displays some regressive behavior (e.g., if child wets pants, say, "We will get a dry pair of pants and let you find something fun to do.").
- Allow the child to express anger and to protest about his or her care (e.g., "It's okay to cry when you are angry or hurt.").
- Allow the child to sit up or walk as often as possible and as soon as possible after intrusive or hurtful procedures (e.g., "It's all over and we can do something more fun.").
- Use nondirective modes, such as reflecting an aspect of appearance or temperament (e.g., "You smile so often."), or playing with a toy and slowly coming closer to and including the child in play.

Recognize Fear of Bodily Injury
- Show hands (free of hurtful items) and say, "There is nothing to hurt you. I came to play/talk."

Accept Egocentrism and Possible Regression
- Allow child to be self-oriented. Use distraction if another child wants the same item or toy rather than expect the child to share. Some children cope with stress of hospitalization by regressing to an earlier mode of behavior, such as wanting to suck on a bottle, and so forth.

Continued

| BOX 18-2 | Key Points in Communicating with Children According to Age Group—cont'd |

Redirect Behavior to a Verbal Level
- Use a nondirective approach. Sit down and join the parallel play of the child. Reflect messages sent by toddler (nonverbally) in a verbal and nonverbal manner (e.g., "Yes, that toy does lots of interesting and fun things.").

Deal with Separation Anxiety
- Accept protesting when parent(s) leave. Hug, rock the child, and say, "You miss Mommy and Daddy! They miss you, too." Play peek-a-boo games with the child. Make a big deal about saying, "Now I am here."
- Show an interest in one of the child's favorite toys. Say, "I wonder what it does" or the like. If the child responds with actions, reflect them back.

3- to 5-Year-Olds
- Most children this age can make themselves understood to strangers.
- They speak in sentences but are unable to comprehend abstract ideas.
- Unable to recognize their own anxiety, at this age some will somaticize (i.e., complain only of stomachache, etc.)
- They begin to understand cause-and-effect relationships; should be able to understand, "If you do…, then we can…"
- Can follow a series of up to four directions unless anxious about being hurt, and so on.

Use Age-Appropriate, Simple Vocabulary
- Use simple vocabulary; avoid lengthy explanations. Focus on the present, not the distant future; use concrete, meaningful references. For example, say, "Mommy will be back after you eat your lunch" (instead of "at 1 o'clock").

Behave in a Culturally Sensitive Manner
- In some cultures, a child is unable to tolerate direct eye-to-eye contact, so use some eye contact and attending posture. Sit or stoop, and use a slow, soft tone of voice.

Attempt to Decrease Anxiety about Being Hurt
- Use brief, concrete, simple explanations. Delays and long explanations before a painful procedure increase anxiety.
- Be quick to complete the procedure; give explanations about its purpose afterward. For example, say, "Jimmy, I'm going to give you a shot," then quickly administer the injection. Then say, "There. All done. It's okay to cry when you hurt. I'd

complain too. This medicine will make your tummy feel better." Some experts suggest you create a "safe zone" in the child's bed by doing all painful procedures elsewhere, perhaps in a treatment room.

Use Play Therapy
- Explanations and education can be done using imagination (puppetry, drama with costumes), music, or drawings.
- Allow the child to play with safe equipment used in treatment. Talk about the needed procedure happening to a doll or teddy bear, and state simply how it will occur and be experienced. Use sensory data (e.g., "The teddy bear will hear a buzzing sound.").

Use Distraction and a Sense of Humor
- Tell corny jokes and laugh with the child.

Allow for Child's Continuing Need to Have Control
- Provide for many choices (e.g., "Do you want to get dressed now or after breakfast?").

5- to 10-Year-Olds
- They are developing their ability to comprehend. Can understand sequencing of events if clearly explained: "First this happens…, then…"
- They can use written materials to learn.

Facilitate Child to Assume Increased Responsibility for Own Health Care Practices
- Include the child in concrete explanations about condition, treatment, and protocols.
- Use draw-a-person to identify basic knowledge the child has and build on it.
- Use some of the same words the child uses in giving explanations.
- Use sensory information in giving explanations (e.g., "You will smell alcohol in the cast room.").
- Reinforce basic health self-care activities in teaching.

Respect Increased Need for Privacy
- Knock on the door before entering; tell the client when and for what reasons you will need to return to his or her room.

11-Year-Olds and Older
- Have an increased comprehension about possible negative threats to life or body integrity, yet some difficulty in adhering to long-term goals.

| BOX 18-2 | Key Points in Communicating with Children According to Age Group—cont'd |

- Continue to use mainly concrete rather than abstract thinking.
- They are struggling to establish identity and be independent.

Verbalize Issues in Age-Appropriate Ways
- Talk about treatment protocols that require giving up immediate gratifications for long-term gain. Explore alternative options (e.g., tell a diabetic adolescent who must give up after-school fries with friends that he or she could save two breads and four fats exchanges to have a milkshake). If you use abstract thinking, look for nonverbal cues (e.g., puzzled face) that may indicate lack of understanding; then clarify in more concrete terms. Use humor or street slang, if appropriate.

Remember That Confidentiality May Be an Issue
- Reassure the adolescent about the confidentiality of your discussion, but clearly state the limits of

this confidentiality. If, for example, the child should talk of killing himself, be clear that this information needs to be shared with parents and staff.

Foster and Allow a Sense of Independence
- Allow participation in decision making, such as wearing own clothes. Avoid an authoritarian or judgmental approach.
- Accept behaviors such as regression, but set limits on injurious behavior.
- Encourage responsibility for keeping own appointments, bedtime poutiness, administration of own medications such as insulin and so forth.

Assess Sexual Awareness and Maturation
- Demonstrate a willingness to listen. Provide value-free, accurate information.

Updated 2014, from material originally supplied by Joyce Ruth, MSN, University of North Carolina Charlotte, College of Health Sciences.

COMMUNICATION WITH CHILDREN 1 TO 3 YEARS OF AGE (TODDLERS)

Almost all small children receiving invasive treatment feel some threat to their safety and security, one of Maslow's hierarchies of human needs. This need is exaggerated in toddlers and young children, who cannot articulate their needs or understand why they are ill. To help the child's comprehension, use phrases rather than long sentences and repeat words for emphasis. Because the toddler has a limited vocabulary, you may need to put into words the feelings that the ill child is conveying nonverbally.

Evaluate the Agency Environment

Is it safe? Does it allow for some independence and autonomy? Care in the ambulatory setting is facilitated if a parent or caregiver is present. Agency policies should promote parent-child contact (e.g., unlimited visiting hours, rooming in, or use of CDs, Skype, or podcasts of a parent's voice). Familiar objects make the environment feel safer. Use transitional objects such as a teddy bear, blanket, or favorite toy to remind the alone or frightened child that the security of the parent is still available even when the parent is not physically present. Distraction is a successful strategy with toddlers in ambulatory settings.

Use of stuffed animals, windup toys, or "magic" exam lights that blow out "like a birthday candle" can turn fright into delight. The author wears a small toy bear on her stethoscope and asks the child to help listen for a heart sound from the bear, so the child focuses on the toy, making it easier to listen to the child's heart.

COMMUNICATION WITH CHILDREN 3 TO 5 YEARS (PRESCHOOLERS)

Throughout the preoperational period, young children tend to interpret language in a literal way. For example, the child who is told that he will be "put to sleep" during the operation tomorrow may think it means the same as the action recently taken for a pet dog who was too ill to live. Children do not ask for clarification, so messages can be misunderstood quite easily. Preschool children have limited auditory recall and are unable to process auditory information quickly. They have a short attention span. Verbal communication with the preschool child should be clear, succinct, and easy to understand.

Before the age of 7 years, most children cannot make a clear distinction between fantasy and reality. Everything is "real," and anything strange is perceived as potentially harmful. In the hospital, preschool children need frequent concrete reminders to reinforce reality. Assigning the same caregiver reduces insecurity. Visiting the preschooler at the same time each day and posting family pictures are simple strategies to reduce the child's fears of abandonment. You can link information to activities of daily living. For example, saying, "Your mother will come after you take your nap," rather than "at 2 o'clock" is much more understandable to the preschool client.

Children need to be assessed for misconceptions and troubling problems, preferably using free play and fantasy storytelling exercises. Egocentrism can be a normal developmental process that may prevent children from understanding why they cannot have a drink when they are fasting before a scheduled test. Explanations given a long time beforehand may not be remembered. If something is going to hurt, you should be forthright about it, while at the same time reassuring the child that he or she will have the appropriate support. Simple explanations reduce the child's anxiety. No child should ever be left to figure out what is happening without some type of simple explanation. Reinforce the child's communication by praising the willingness to tell you how he or she feels. Avoid judging or censuring the child who yells such things as, "I hate you," or "You are mean for hurting me." Not being able to recognize or communicate anxiety, the child may just complain of a physical symptom, like a headache or stomachache (Emslie, 2008). Box 18-2 can help you focus on specific communication strategies with the hospitalized preschooler.

Play as a Communication Strategy

The preschooler lacks a suitable vocabulary to express complex thoughts and feelings. Small children cannot picture what they have never experienced. Play is an effective means by which a puzzling and sometimes painful real world can be approached. Play allows the child to create a concrete experience of something unknown and potentially frightening. By constructing a situation in play, the child is able to put together the components of the situation in ways that promote recognition and make it a concrete reality. When the child can deal with things that are small or inanimate, the child masters situations that might otherwise be overwhelming. Cartoons, pictures, or puppets can be used to demonstrate actions and terminology. Dolls

with removable cloth organs help children understand scheduled operations.

Preschoolers tend to think of their illness, their separation from parents, and any painful treatments as punishment. Play can be used to help children express their feelings about an illness and to role-play coping strategies. Allowing the young child to manipulate syringes and give "shots" to a doll or put a bandage or restraint on a teddy bear's arm allows the child to act out his or her feelings. The child becomes "the aggressor." Play can be a major channel for communication in the nurse-client relationship involving a young child. Preschool children develop communication themes through their play and work through conflict situations in their own good time; the process cannot be rushed.

Play materials vary with the age and developmental status of the child. Simple, large toys are used with young children; more intricate playthings are used with older preschoolers. Clay, crayons, and paper become modes of expression for important feelings and thoughts about problems. Play can be your primary tool for assessing preschool children's perceptions about their hospital experience, their anxieties, and their fears. Play can increase their coping ability. Preschoolers love jokes, puns, and riddles; the cornier, the better. Using jokes during the physical assessment, such as "Let me hear your lunch," or, "Golly, could that be a potato in your ear?" helps form the bonds needed for a successful relationship with the preschool client.

Storytelling as a Communication Strategy

A communication strategy often used with young children is the use of story plots. As early as 1986, Gardner described a mutual storytelling technique. You ask the child whether he or she would like to help make up a story. If the child is a little reluctant, you may begin, as described in Exercise 18-1. At the end of the story, the child is asked to indicate what lesson might be learned from the story. If the child seems a little reluctant to give a moral to the story, you might suggest that all stories have something that can be learned from them. Analyze the themes presented by the child, which usually reveal important feelings. Is the story fearful? Are the characters scary or pleasing? The child should be praised for telling the story. The next step in the process is to ask yourself what would be a healthier resolution than the one used by the child. Then suggest an alternative ending. In your version of the story,

EXERCISE 18-1 | Using a Mutual Storytelling Technique

Purpose: To give practical experience with the mutual storytelling technique.

Procedure
1. Use the mutual storytelling process described in the text with a 5- to 8-year-old child in your neighborhood.
2. Write down the story the child told and suggest alternate endings.
3. Share your stories in turn during the next class period.

Discussion
1. How difficult was it for you to engage the child? If you had trouble, what alternate actions would you incorporate in using the technique again?
2. Were you surprised at the story the child produced? If so, in what ways?
3. What did you learn about the child when using this technique?
4. What conclusions might you draw from hearing the other students relate their experiences about the use of this technique? In what situations was it most effective? Least effective?

5. What did you learn about yourself as a helping person in using this technique?

Sample Answer
Nurse: Once upon a time in a land far away, there lived a...
Child: Dragon.
Nurse: A dragon who ate...
Child: Carrots.
Nurse: The dragon ate carrots and slept...
Child: In a cave.
Nurse: One day he left the cave to go out and find many sweet carrots to eat, but as he walked along he ran into a...
Child: Bike.
Nurse: He was afraid of the bike and so he...
Child: Kicked it and ran away.
Nurse: After he ran away, is there any more to the story?
Child (upset): He got hit with a stick.
Nurse: What is the message to this story? What does it tell us?
Child: About running away not to be punished.

---

the characters and other details remain the same initially, but the story contains a more positive solution or suggests alternative answers to problems. The object of mutual storytelling is to offer the child an opportunity to explore different alternatives in a neutral communication process with a helping person. Exercise 18-1 provides an opportunity to experiment with a mutual storytelling strategy.

COMMUNICATION WITH CHILDREN 6 TO 11 YEARS (SCHOOL AGE)

As children move into concrete operational thinking, they begin to internalize the reasons for illness: illness is caused by germs, or you have cavities because you ate too much candy or did not brush your teeth. In later childhood, most children become better able to work with you verbally. It still is important to prepare responses carefully and to anticipate problems, but the child is capable of expressing feelings and venting frustration more directly through words. Use Exercise 18-2 to reformulate medical technology into age-appropriate expressions.

Assessment of the child's cognitive level of understanding continues to be essential. Search for concrete examples to which the child can relate rather than giving abstract examples. If children are to learn from a model, they must see the model performing the skill to be learned. School-age children thrive on explanations of how their bodies work and enjoy understanding the scientific rationales for their treatment. Ask questions directly to the child, consulting the parent for validation.

Using Audiovisual Aids or Hobbies as a Communication Strategy

Audiovisual aids and reading material geared to the child's level of understanding may supplement verbal explanations and diagrams. Details about what the child will hear, see, smell, and feel are important. For the younger school-age child, expressive art can be a useful method to convey feelings and to open up communication. The older school-age child or adolescent might best convey feelings by writing a poem, a short story, or a letter. Written material as presented in the following case example can assist you in understanding hidden thoughts or emotions.

EXERCISE 18-2	Age-Appropriate Medical Terminology

Purpose: To help students think of terminology appropriate to use with young clients.

Procedure

This can be fun if the instructor quickly asks students, going around the room.

Reformulate the following expressions using words a child can understand:

Anesthesia	Inflammation	NPO
Cardiac catheterization	Injection	Operating room

Disease	Intake and output	Sedation
Dressings	Isolation	Urine specimen
Enema	IV needle	Vital signs
Infection	Nausea	

Discussion

Think of any experiences you might have had as a child client or may have observed. What were some of the troublesome words you remember from these experiences?

Case Example: Cary

Ashley, a first-year student nurse, becomes frustrated during the course of her conversation with her assigned client, 11-year-old Cary, admitted 5 days ago to the psychiatric unit. Despite a genuine desire to engage him in a therapeutic alliance, the client would not talk. Attempts to get to know him on a verbal level seemed to increase rather than decrease his anxiety. The nurse correctly inferred that despite his age, this adolescent needed a more tangible approach. Knowing that the client likes cars, Ashley brought in an automotive magazine. Together, they looked at the magazine; the publication soon became their special vehicle for communication, bridging the gap between the client's inner reality and his ability to express himself verbally in a meaningful way. Feelings about cars gradually generalized to verbal expressions about other situations, and Cary began describing his attitudes about himself. When Ashley left the unit, he asked to keep the magazine and frequently spoke of her with fondness. This simple recognition of his awkwardness in verbal communication and use of another tool to facilitate the relationship had a positive effect.

Mutuality in Decision Making

Children of this age need to be involved in discussions of their illness and in planning for their care. Explanations giving the rationale for care are useful. Involving the child in decision making may decrease fears about the illness, the treatment, or the effect on family life. Videos and written materials may be useful in involving the child in the management phase of care.

COMMUNICATION WITH CHILDREN OLDER THAN 11 YEARS OF AGE (ADOLESCENTS)

An understanding of adolescent developmental principles is essential in working with teens. Adolescence is the time when we clinicians encourage a shift in responsibility for health-related decisions from parent to the teen. Even teens enjoying good health are forced to deal with new health issues such as acne, menstrual problems, or sexual activity. The adolescent vacillates between childhood and adulthood, and is emotionally vulnerable. The ambivalence of the adolescent period may be normally expressed through withdrawal, rebellion, lost motivation, and rapid mood changes. A teen may look adult-like, but in illness especially may be unable to communicate easily with care providers. Identity issues become more difficult to resolve when the normal opportunities for physical independence, privacy, and social contacts are compromised by illness or handicap. All adolescents have questions about their developing body and sexuality. Ill teens have the same longings, but problems may be greater because the natural outlets for their expression with peers are curtailed by the disorder or by hospitalization. Use of peer groups, adolescent lounges (separate from the small children's playroom), and telephones, as well as provisions for wearing one's own clothes, fixing one's hair, or attending hospital school, may help teenagers adjust to hospitalization. When the developmental identity crisis becomes too uncomfortable, adolescents may project their fury and frustration onto family or staff. Identifying rage as a normal response to a difficult situation can be reassuring.

Assessment of the adolescent should occur in a private setting. Attention to the comfort and space of an adolescent will have a tremendous impact on the quality of the interaction. To the teenager, the nurse represents an authority figure. The need for compassion, concern, and respect is perhaps greater during adolescence than at any other time in the life span. Often lacking the verbal skills of adults, yet wishing to appear in control, adolescents do well with direct questions. Innocuous questions are used first to allow the teenager enough space to check the validity of his or her reactions to the nurse. In caring for a teen in an ambulatory office or clinic, conduct part of the history interview without the parent present. If the parent will not leave the examination room, this can be done while walking the teen down to the laboratory. Questions about substance use, sexual activity, and so on demand confidentiality.

To assess a teen's cognitive level, find out about the teen's ability to make long-term plans. An easy way to do this is the "three wishes question." Ask the teen to name three things he or she would expect to have in 5 years. Answers can be analyzed for factors such as concreteness, realism, and goal-directness.

Some teens lack sufficient experience to recognize that life has ups and downs and that things will eventually be better. Suicide is the second leading cause of death in teenagers and many experts think that the actual rate is greater because many deaths from the number one cause, motor vehicle accidents, may actually be attributed to this cause. Be aware of danger signs such as apathy, persistent depression, or self-destructive behavior. When faced with a tragedy, teens tend to mourn in doses with wide mood swings. Grieving teens may need periods of privacy, but also need the opportunity for relief through distracting activities, music, and games. In communicating with an ill adolescent, remember to listen. When a teen asks a direct question, he or she is ready to hear the answer. Answer directly and honestly.

Using Hobbies as a Communication Strategy

Adolescents still rely primarily on feedback from adults and from friends to judge their own competency. A teen may not yet have developed proficiency and comfort in carrying on verbal conversations with adults. The teen may respond best if the nurse uses several modalities to communicate. Using empathy, conveying acceptance, and using open-ended questions are three useful strategies. Sometimes more innovative communication strategies are needed. In the previous case example, the teen has a difficult time talking, so the use of another modality is appropriate.

DEALING WITH CARE PROBLEMS
Pain

The literature reflects major concern that pain in children is underestimated and inadequately relieved. Historically children's ability to feel pain was underrated. Lack of adequate pain relief may, in part, be due to fears of oversedating a child, but more likely is due to the child's limited capacity to communicate the nature of his or her discomfort. We need to adapt our pain assessments to be age appropriate. Infants indicate pain with physiologic changes (e.g., diaphoresis, pallor, increased heart rate, increased respirations, and decreased oxygen saturation). With other children we use one of the many child-based assessment scales, such as smiley faces or poker chips with toddlers and preschoolers. We also need to instigate protocols for preventing pain associated with treatment. Examples include use of local anesthetics for effective reduction of the pain associated with venipuncture. Effective nonpharmacologic interventions for pain include non-nutritive sucking/pacifiers, rocking, physical contact, and swaddling. Exercise 18-3 will stimulate discussion about care for children in pain.

Anxiety

Illness is often an unanticipated event. Uncertainty and even anxiety should be expected when both treatment and outcome are unknown. Young children react to unexpected stimuli, to painful procedures, and even to the presence of strangers with fear. Older children fear separation from parents, but also may fear injury,

---

EXERCISE 18-3	Pediatric Nursing Procedures

Purpose: To give practice in preparing young clients for painful procedures.

Procedure
Timmy, age 4, is going to have a bone marrow aspiration. (The insertion of a large needle into the hip is a painful procedure.) Answer the following questions:

1. What essential information does Timmy need?
2. If this is a frequently repeated procedure, how can you make him feel safe before and after the procedure?
3. How soon in advance should you prepare him?

EXERCISE 18-4	Preparing Children for Treatment Procedures

Purpose: To help students apply developmental concepts to age-appropriate nursing interventions.

Procedure
Students divide into four small groups and design an age-appropriate intervention for the following situation. As a large group, each small group spokesperson writes the intervention on the board under the label for the age group.

Situation
Jamie is scheduled to go to the surgical suite later today to have a central infusion catheter inserted for hyperalimentation. This is Jamie's first procedure on the first day of this first hospitalization experience.

Discussion
Group focuses on comparing interventions across the age spans.
1. How does each intervention differ according to the age of the child? (Describe age-appropriate interventions for preschooler, school-age child, and adolescent.)
2. What concept themes are common across the age spans? (education components; assessing initial level of knowledge; assessing ability to comprehend information, readiness to receive information; adapting information to cognitive level of child)
3. What formats might be best used for each age group? (Role-play with tools such as dolls, pictures, comic books, educational pamphlets, and peer group sessions.)

loss of body function, or even just being perceived by friends as different because of their illness. Exercise 18-4 helps develop age-appropriate explanations that may reduce anxiety.

Acting-Out Behaviors

Behavior problems present a special challenge to the nurse. Clear communication of expectations, treatment protocols, and hospital rules is of value. As much as possible, adolescents should be allowed to act on their own behalf in making choices and judgments about their functioning. At the same time, limits need to be set on acting-out behavior. Limits define the boundaries of acceptable behaviors in a relationship. Initially determined by the parents or the nurse, limits can be developed mutually as an important part of the relationship as the child matures. Determining consequences has a positive value in that it provides the child with a model for handling frustrating situations in a more adult manner.

Once the conflict is resolved and the child has accepted the consequences of his or her behavior, the child should be given an opportunity to discuss attitudes and feelings that led up to the need for limits, as well as reaction to the limits set. Serious symptoms such as substance abuse require specialist interventions. Estimates are that 75% of abusers have serious mental adjustment problems, especially depression (Griswold et al., 2008).

Although communication about limits is necessary for the survival of the relationship, it needs to be balanced with time for interaction that is pleasant and positive. Sometimes with children who need limits set on a regular basis, discussion of the restrictions is the only conversation that takes place between nurse and client. When this is noted, nurses might ask themselves what feelings the child might be expressing through his or her actions. Putting into words the feelings that are being acted out helps children trust the nurse's competence and concern. Usually it is necessary for the entire staff to share this responsibility. Box 18-3 presents ideas for setting limits within the context of the nurse-client relationship.

MORE HELPFUL STRATEGIES FOR COMMUNICATING WITH CHILDREN

Adapting the general communications strategies presented earlier in this book to interactions with children requires some imagination and creativity. Working with children is rewarding, hard work that sometimes must be evaluated indirectly. For example, George was the primary care nurse who had worked very hard with a 13-year-old girl over a 6-month period while the girl was on a bone marrow transplant unit. He felt bad when, at discharge, the girl stated, "I never want to see any of you people again." However, just before leaving, the nurse found her sobbing on her bed. No words were spoken, but the child threw her arms around George and clung to him for comfort. For this nurse, the child's expression of grief was an acknowledgment of the meaning of the relationship. Children, even

| BOX 18-3 | Guidelines for Developing Workable Limit-Setting Plan |

1. Have the child describe his or her behavior.
   Key: Evaluate realistically.
2. Encourage the child to assess behavior. Is it helpful for others and him- or herself?
   Key: Evaluate realistically.
3. Encourage the child to develop an alternative plan for governing behavior.
   Key: Set reasonable goals.
4. Have the child sign a statement about his or her plan.
   Key: Commit to goals.
5. Consequences for unacceptable behavior are logical and fit the situation.
   Key: Consequences are known.
6. At the end of the appropriate time period, have the child assess his or her performance.
   Key: Evaluate realistically.
7. Consequences are applied in a matter-of-fact manner, without lengthy discussion.
   Key: Consequences immediately follow the transgression.
8. Provide positive reinforcement for those aspects of performance that were successful.*
   Key: Evaluate realistically.
9. Encourage the child to make a positive statement about his or her performance.
   Key: Teach self-praise.

*If the child's performance does not meet the criteria set in the plan, return to Step 3 and assist the child in modifying the plan so that success is more possible. If, conversely, the child's performance is successful, help him or her to develop a more ambitious plan (e.g., for a longer period or for a larger set of behaviors).

those who can use words, often communicate through behavior rather than verbally when under stress.

Active Listening

The process of active listening takes form initially from watching the behaviors of children as they play and interact with their environments. As a child's vocabulary increases and the capacity to engage with others develops, listening begins to approximate the communication process that occurs between adults, with one important difference: Because the perceptual world of the child is concrete, the nurse's feedback and informational messages should coincide with the child's developmental level.

Authenticity and Veracity

Sometimes adults ignore children's feelings or else deceive them about procedures, illness, or hospitalization in the mistaken belief that they will be overwhelmed by the truth. Just the opposite is true. Children, like adults, can cope with most stressors as long as they are presented in a manner they can understand and given enough time and support from the environment to cope. Teens rate honesty, attention to pain, and respect as the three most important factors in their quality of care. Completing Exercise 18-5 may stimulate some discussion.

You should never allow any individual, even a parent, to threaten a child. For example, a few parents have been heard to say, "You be good or I'll have the nurse

| EXERCISE 18-5 | **Working with the Newly Diagnosed HIV-Positive Teenager** |

Purpose: To stimulate class discussion about how to deal with the adolescent with whom it is difficult to communicate.

Procedure
Read the case situation and answer the questions. Use class time to summarize discussion.

Situation
Bill, age 17, seeks treatment for gonorrhea. He is hospitalized for further testing after his initial workup reveals he is seropositive for human immunodeficiency virus (HIV) type 1. For 2 days on the unit he has cried, cursed, and been uncooperative. Staff tends to avoid him when possible. A team of residents begins a bone marrow aspiration procedure in the treatment room after obtaining his absent mother's permission. (She has expressed condemnation and has not yet been

to visit.) A technician walks in and out of the room to obtain supplies while the doctors concentrate on completing the procedure. A student nurse is asked to come in to help restrain Bill, who is alternately screaming, crying, and being very quiet.

1. What communication strategies could this student use while squeezing into this small room? (Clue: Verbal and nonverbal directed to the client and to the doctors)
2. What assessment might the nurse want to make? (Clue: What are Bill's feelings about his diagnosis?)
3. What can be inferred about Bill's current behavior?
4. What additional data are needed before attempting any teaching about acquired immuno deficiency syndrome (AIDS)?

give you a shot." It is appropriate to interrupt this parent. Children respect honest expression of emotions in adults. Being truthful and trustworthy with children is a crucial factor in the development of a therapeutic relationship.

Conveying Respect

It is easy for adults to impose their own wishes on a child. Respecting a child's right to feel and to express his or her feelings appropriately is important. Providing truthful answers is a hallmark of respect. When interacting with the older child, using the concept of mutuality will promote respect and should foster more positive and lasting health care outcomes. Confidentiality needs to be maintained unless the nurse judges that revealing information is necessary to prevent harm to the child or adolescent. In such cases, the child needs to be advised of the disclosure.

Providing Anticipatory Guidance to the Child

The nursing profession advocates client education for children, as do pediatricians. The American Academy of Pediatrics has published suggestions for giving caretakers health promotion information at appropriate ages. Managed care has brought an increased focus on the role a child can assume in being responsible for his or her own health care. It is never too early to begin. For example, written handouts for incorporating violence prevention can be incorporated into well-child visits. A shift in placing responsibility for good health practices onto the individual is in line with recommendations in *Healthy People 2020*. In fact one of the stated objectives is to increase the proportion of time that the health care worker provides needed information.

FORMING HEALTH CARE PARTNERSHIPS WITH PARENTS

Having an ill child is stressful for parents. Evidence shows that loss of the ability to act as the child's parent, to alleviate their child's pain, and to offer comfort, is more stressful than factors connected with the illness, including coping with uncertainty over the outcome. Studies point to a lack of needed information and support from professionals as being a top stressor. It is essential that we work in partnership with families, especially if we assess risk factors that endanger the child (Banner, 2012). Most parents want to participate in their child's care during acute hospitalizations but need information, advice, and clarification as to their role—that is, what is okay to do. They need to feel valued but not pressured into doing tasks they are uncomfortable with or do not want to do.

Parents often have questions about discussing their child's illness or disability with others. Telling siblings and friends the truth is important. For one thing, it provides a role model for the siblings to follow in answering the curious questions of their friends. Remember, however, that older children have a need for confidentiality and respond better if the nurse interviews and treats them away from parents' presence. Consider the ethical dilemma provided in this chapter.

More frustrating to nurses are parents who are critical of the nurse's interventions, displacing the anger they feel about their own powerlessness onto the nurse (Box 18-4). The nurse may be tempted to become defensive or sarcastic or simply to dismiss the comments of the parent as irrational. However, a more helpful response would be to place oneself in the parents' shoes and to consider the possible issues. Asking the parents what information they have or might need, simply listening in a nondefensive way, and allowing the parents to vent some of their frustrations facilitate the possibility of dialogue about the underlying feelings. Use of listening strategies is helpful. Sometimes a listening response that acknowledges the legitimacy of the parent's feeling is helpful: "I'm sorry that you feel so bad," or "It must be difficult for you to see your child in such pain." These simple comments acknowledge the very real anguish parents experience in health care situations having few palatable options. If possible, parental venting of feeling should occur in a private setting out of hearing range from the child. It is very upsetting to children to experience splitting in the parent-nurse relationship. Guidelines for communicating with parents are presented in Box 18-5.

COMMUNICATING WITH PARENTS OF SPECIAL HEALTH CARE NEEDS CHILDREN

Many American children have a chronic health condition requiring additional services. Caring for these children requires parental time and alters family communication patterns. Studies show these families have less time for communication (Bransletter et al., 2008). Nurses need to provide care and information about the child's condition, time for discussions about balancing family needs with care for this child, suggest strategies for moving the child toward

| **BOX 18-4** | Representative Nursing Problem: Dealing with a Frightened Parent |

During report, the night nurse relates an incident that occurred between Mrs. Smith, the mother of an 8-year-old admitted for possible acute lymphocytic leukemia and the night supervisor. Mrs. Smith told the supervisor that her son was receiving poor care from the nurses and that they frequently ignored her and refused to answer her questions. While you are making rounds after the report, Mrs. Smith corners you outside her son's room and begins to tell you about all the things that went wrong during the night. She goes on to say, "If you people think I'm going to stand around and allow my son to be treated this way, you are sadly mistaken."

Problem

Frustration and anger caused by a sense of powerlessness and fear related to the son's possible diagnosis

Nursing Diagnosis

Ineffective Coping related to hospitalization of son and possible diagnosis of leukemia

Nursing Goals

Increase the mother's sense of control and problem-solving capabilities; help the mother develop adaptive coping behaviors.

Method of Assistance

Guiding; supporting; providing developmental environment

Interventions

1. Actively listen to the client's concerns with as much objectivity as possible; maintain eye contact with the client; use minimal verbal activity, allowing the client the opportunity to express her concerns and fears freely.
2. Use reflective questioning to determine the client's level of understanding and the extent of information obtained from health team members.
3. Listen for repetitive words or phrases that may serve to identify problem areas or provide insight into fears and concerns.
4. Reassure the mother when appropriate that her child's hospitalization is indeed frightening and it is all right to be scared; remember to demonstrate interest in the client as a person; use listening responses (e.g., "It must be hard not knowing the results of all these tests.") to create an atmosphere of concern.
5. Avoid communication blocks, such as giving false reassurance, telling the client what to do, or ignoring the concerns; such behavior effectively cuts off therapeutic communication.
6. Keep the client continually informed regarding her child's progress.
7. Involve the client in her son's care; do not overwhelm her or make her feel she has to do this; watch for cues that tell you she is ready "to do more."
8. Acknowledge the effect this illness may have on the family; involve the health team in identifying ways to reduce the client's fears and provide for continuity in the type of information presented to her and to other family members.
9. Assign a primary nurse to care for the client's son and serve as a resource to the client. Identify support systems in the community that might provide help and support to the client.

From M. Michaels, University of Maryland School of Nursing, Baltimore.

future independence, and refer parents to community resources. We need to recognize that as the child reaches developmental milestones, this can be a time of increased family stress, requiring additional support from us.

Community

Partnering with the family can be the best method you have to address the complex health care needs of children. Parents are the central figures in care planning, especially for chronically ill children. We need to help provide information about which community agencies, networks, and professionals will be mobilized to provide care to their child. For example, school nurses often act as case managers by communicating about the child's needs among parent, care providers, teachers, and other resource personnel. By law in the United States, children with special needs in the educational system are required to have an Individualized Education Program. A part of this may be the health plan for children who need medical intervention or treatment during school.

Anticipatory Guidance in the Community. Because the parents usually assume responsibility for the child's care after they leave the hospital, it is essential to encourage active involvement from the very beginning of treatment. Parents may also need facts about normal development and milestones to expect, as well as information about prevention of illness.

BOX 18-5	Guidelines for Communicating with Parents

- Present complex information in informational chunks.
- Repeat information and allow plenty of time for questions.
- Keep parents continually informed of progress and changes in condition.
- Involve parents in determining goals; anticipate possible reactions and difficulties.
- Discuss problems with parents directly and honestly.
- Explore all alternative options with parents.
- Share knowledge of community supports; help parents role-play responses to others.
- Acknowledge the impact of the illness on finances; on emotions; and especially on the family, including siblings.
- Use other staff for support in personally coping with the emotional drain created by working with very ill children and their parents.

Community Support Groups

Community groups have organized to assist families. Often information about the groups' meeting times can be obtained from health care providers, from the national or local organization, or even from the phone book. For parents who cannot travel to meetings, a new form of support may be available via the Internet as described in Chapter 26.

NURSE AS ADVOCATE FOR CHILDREN IN THE COMMUNITY

Because children cannot communicate their needs to policy makers, we need to broaden our advocacy to fight for better child health at local and national levels. Children's access to health care is affected by their neighborhood, the level of their parent's education, their insurance status and problems with referrals (Larson and Halfon, 2010; Tesher and Onel, 2012). Poverty is associated with poorer child health status, lack of a regular care provider, lack of dental care, and a myriad of other health problems. Part of our advocacy role is to become actively involved in improving access to care and to focus public attention on pediatric health problems. For example, *Healthy People 2020* has designated obesity and physical activity as priorities for action, stating that only 1 in 10 American youth meet national guidelines for exercise (1 hour per day). Child obesity is causing a huge increase in related health problems such as diabetes. Related nursing advocacy

interventions include organizing campaigns to eliminate sale of junk food in schools, reinstituting recess and physical education opportunities, and joining community activist groups advocating restructuring of community neighborhoods to allow for increased exercise with sidewalks to school and safe bike paths.

SUMMARY

Communicating with ill children requires patience, imagination, and creative applications of therapeutic communication strategies. Children's ability to understand and communicate with you is largely influenced by their cognitive developmental level and their limited life experiences. We need to develop an understanding of feelings and thought processes from the child's perspective, and our communication strategies with children should reflect these understandings. Various strategies for communicating with children of different ages are suggested, as are strategies for communicating with their parents. A marvelous characteristic of children is how well they respond to caregivers who make an effort to understand their needs and take the time to relate to them.

ETHICAL DILEMMA	What Would You Do?

You are caring for Mika Soon, a 15-year-old adolescent. She has confided to you that she is being treated for chlamydia. Her mother approaches you privately and demands to know if Mika has told you if she is sexually active with her boyfriend. Because Mika is a minor and Mrs. Soon is paying for this clinic visit, are you obligated to tell her the truth?

DISCUSSION QUESTIONS

1. How would your assessment of pain in an infant differ from assessing pain in a 5-year-old hospitalized child?
2. In Exercise 18-5, describe interventions that you would use to initiate interaction with Bill's single mother in an initial post-discharge visit to their home.

REFERENCES

Banner J: Addressing safeguarding concerns through better communication, *Nurs Manage* 19(2):28–31, 2012.

Bransletter JE, Domain EW, Williams PD, et al.: Communication themes in families of children with chronic conditions, *Issues Compr Pediatr Nurs* 31(4):171–184, 2008.

Cumulative Index to Nursing and Allied Health (CINAHL) Database. www.ebscohost.com. [Subscription only, at Nursing Libraries].

Emslie GJ: Pediatric anxiety-under recognized and under treated, *N Engl J Med* 359(26):2835–2836, 2008.

Erikson EH: *Childhood and society*, Norton, 1963, New York.

Fisher MJ, Broome ME: Parent-provider communication during hospitalization, *J Pediatr Nurs* 26(1):1–12, 2011.

Friedman B, Berdahl T, Simpson LA, McCormick MC, Owens PL, Andrews R, Romano PS: Annual report on health care for children and youth in the United States: Focus on trends in hospital use and quality, *Acad Pediatr* 11(4):263–279, 2011.

Gardner R: *Therapeutic communication with children*, Ed 2, New York, 1986, Science Books.

Griswold KS, Aronoff H, Kernan JB, Kahn LS: Adolescent substance use and abuse: recognition and management, *Am Fam Physician* 77(3):331–336, 2008.

U.S: *Department of Health and Human Services (DHHS). 2011*, Health Resources and Services Administration (HRSA), August 2, 2013. Accessed www.HRSA.gov.

Data Resource Center for Child and Adolescent Health. 2012: Child and Adolescent Health Measurement Initiative. Cooperative Agreement 1-U59-MC06980-01 U.S. Department of Health and Human Services, *Health Resources and Services Administration and Maternal and Child Health Bureau*, August 2, 2013. Accessed www.childhealthdata.org.

U.S: Department of Health and Human Services (DHHS). In *Healthy People 2020*, Adolescent Health, 2014. http://healthypeople.gov/2020/topicsobjectives2020/overview.aspx?topicid=2.

Larson K, Halfon N: Family income gradients in the health and health care access of US children, *Matern Child Health J* 14(3):332–342, 2010.

U.S. Department of Health and Human Services (DHHS). (n.d.). Health Resources and Services Administration (HRSA). Maternal and Child Health Bureau. www.HRSA.gov.

Piaget J: *The child's conception of the world, Littlefield*, Savage, MD, 1972, Adams.

Rempel GR, Ravindran V, Rogers LG, Magill-Evans J: Parenting under pressure: A grounded theory of parenting young children with life-threatening congenital heart disease, *J Adv Nurs* 69(3):619–630, 2013.

Rosenberg AR, Dussel V, Kang T, Geyer JR, Gerhardt CA, Feudtner C, Wolfe J: Psychological distress in parents of children with advanced cancer, *JAMA Pediatr* 167(6):537–543, 2013.

Tesher MS, Onel KB: The clinical spectrum of juvenile idiopathic arthritis in a large urban population, *Curr Rheumatol Rep* 14(2):116–120, 2012.

Wigert H, Dellenmark MB, Bry K: Strengths and weaknesses of parent-staff communication in the NICU: A survey instrument, *BMC Pediatr* 13(71), 2013. www.ncbi.nlm.nih.gov/pubmed/23651578/.

CHAPTER 19

Communicating with Older Adults

Elizabeth C. Arnold

OBJECTIVES

At the end of the chapter, the reader will be able to:

1. Discuss concepts of normal aging.
2. Identify theoretical frameworks used in the care of older adult clients.
3. Describe client-centered assessment strategies for older adults.
4. Discuss empowerment and supportive self-management care strategies with older adults.
5. Describe client-centered care and communication strategies for cognitively impaired adults.

The purpose of Chapter 19 is to describe the nature of therapeutic interpersonal relationships with older adults. This charge takes on additional dimensions when considering that older adults are the fastest growing segment of the U.S. population. More people older than 65 years of age appear in the 2010 census than in any preceding census and it is estimated that by 2030, 1 in 8 people will be in this age group (Werner, 2010; Leuven, 2012).

Chapter 19 focuses on issues of aging and ways to support this important segment of the population using communication. It addresses features of the aging processes, identifies selected theory frameworks, and discusses how nurses can effectively communicate with older adults to promote health and well-being. Supports that older adults need to successfully live safely and independently are represented. The chapter concludes with current understandings of dementia and related communication strategies with cognitively impaired clients.

BASIC CONCEPTS

In part because people are living much longer, the term *older adult* or *senior* citizen is broken down into three age cohorts: young old (65 to 74 years), old-old (75 to 84 years), and oldest-old (85 years and older) (Moody, 2010). Of those older than the age of 65 years, 85% will have at least one chronic disease and 50% will have more than one chronic condition. Older adults become frailer as they enter their mid-80s, but frailty is not a disease (Mitty, 2010). Many retain a high level of physical, social, and intellectual function until close to their death. With supplementary supports and accommodations, healthy adults can "age in place" with a good quality of life.

CONCEPTS OF AGING

Aging is described as a universal life process of "advancing through the life cycle, beginning at birth and ending at death" (Pankow and Solotoroff, 2007, p. 19). As a dynamic physiologic process, aging affects physical strength, stamina, and flexibility, and ultimately, an individual's ability to independently negotiate the physical environment. Aging is accompanied to a greater or lesser degree by changes in appearance and energy levels, diminishing organ functioning, a weaker immune system, sensory losses, and decreased functional capacity related to mobility.

It also is a time for new possibilities for personal growth and well-being. The purpose of the chapter is to suggest ways that you as a nurse can help make this happen. Learning adaptive self-management strategies can make a major difference in the older adult's overall health and quality of life.

Each person's experience of the aging process reflects his or her genetic makeup, personality, motivation, life experiences, environmental and cultural factors, and engagement with health promotion activities. How fast a person ages is influenced by many factors, some of which are preventable or reversible. Resilience to accept aging changes that cannot be altered and to effectively manage conditions that can be improved such that it is possible to live a meaningful life despite adversity is key (Ebrahim et al., 2013).

ACTIVE AGING

The World Health Organization (WHO) (2002) defines *active aging* as ""the process of optimizing opportunities for health, participation, and security in order to enhance quality of life as people age." (p.12) Fundamental aspects of active aging include the *autonomy* to make decisions and to cope with daily life in line with personal preference and the capacity to *live independently* in the community with little or no assistance from others and a personally satisfying *quality of life* and (Constanca et al., 2012).

Quality of life remains important to people in their later years. It is a transitional time in terms of uncertainty about the personal meaning of age-related changes in appearance and functional capabilities. There are alterations in role responsibilities and expectations; Some are desired and are enthusiastically embraced. Others are not chosen and represent unwanted changes. People's interests change, as they grow older.

Cotter and Gonzalez (2009) describe "*successful aging* as the ability to adapt flexibly to age-related changes without relinquishing the central components of self-definition" (p. 335). This definition invites older adults to take charge of their aging process. Empowering older adults to restructure everyday life routines to accommodate and minimize deficits helps them to lead a purposeful life, with optimal functioning. Staying actively engaged with life to whatever extent is possible is an important component of successful aging because social interaction validates a connection between self and others and the larger universe (Ebrahimi et al., 2013). Nurses play a critical role in helping clients embrace new roles that allow them to make creative life choices.

Becoming a senior citizen calls for new coping skills, fresh expectations for self, and often, different relationships. Bortz (1990) suggests that our attitude toward aging influences how we respond to growing old.

> If we dread growing old, thinking of it as a time of forgetfulness and physical deterioration, then it is likely to be just that. On the other hand, if we expect it to be full of energy and anticipate that our lives will be rich with new adventures and insight; then that is the likely reality. We prescribe who we are. We prescribe what we are to become. (p. 55).

Older adults will experience functional limitations as they age, but much more is possible than one might think. Some articles detail the degenerative changes of aging, without paying attention to what works, and what older adults do to enhance quality of health and well-being. Biggs (2001) notes that positive stories of aging need to be told and incorporated into contemporary social policy. Staying as active as possible and as engaged in life with supportive relationships is key to thriving as an older adult. Exercise 19-1, What Will It Be Like to Be Old?, provides you with an opportunity to explore your personal ideas about aging.

AGING AND HEALTH

Chronic diseases largely associated with aging have replaced acute infectious conditions as a source of health care burden (Avolio et al., 2013). Older adults disproportionately experience a larger number of chronic conditions and diseases. They are vulnerable to a variety of age-related diseases, such as cancer, macular degeneration, and glaucoma, cardiac and circulatory problems, stroke, and degenerative bone loss. Franklin and colleagues (2006) notes that older adults are likely to gradually lose control over body functions and movements, which can interfere with their sense of dignity and self-image. Older adults are the largest users of health services (Scholder et al., 2004; Institute of Medicine (2008)).

Barriers to Treatment

Initially described by Dr. Robert Butler in 1969, ageism is still an issue in health care. Older adults can experience discrimination in accessing health care,

EXERCISE 19-1	What Will It Like to Be Old?

Purpose: To stimulate personal awareness and feelings about the aging process.

Procedure

Think about and write down the answers to the following questions about your own aging process:

1. What do you think will be important to you when you are 65 years of age?
2. Prepare a list of the traits, qualities, and attributes you hope you will have when you are this age.
3. What do you think will be different for you in terms of physical, emotional, spiritual, and social perceptions and activities?
4. How would you like people to treat you when you are an older adult?

Discussion

In groups of three to four students, share your thoughts. Have one-person act as a scribe and write down common themes. Students should ask questions about anything they do not understand.

1. In what ways did doing this exercise give you some insight into what the issues of aging might be for your age group?
2. In what ways might the issues be different for people in your age group and for people currently classified as older adults?
3. How could you use this exercise to better understand the needs of older adults in the hospital, long-term setting, or home?

level of screening, and choice of treatment options. Health care providers are less likely to use extensive diagnostic testing or aggressive treatment with older adults for reasons of age rather than health or function. Kagan (2012) writes, "Discrimination on the basis of chronological age is perhaps the most pervasive unacknowledged prejudice in our society (p. 60).

Other barriers include navigating the complexity of the medical system and limitations and gaps in services for chronic health care conditions. This obstacle is particularly challenging for dementia clients and their families (Murray and Boyd, 2009). The decreasing number of physicians and other health care providers accepting Medicare clients is another factor. On a positive note, Medicare recently introduced initial preventative physical exams (IPPEs) and subsequent annual wellness visits (AWVs). These services, plus annual screening mammograms and pelvic exams are exempt from deductibles or co-pays (Resnick, 2013).

CONTEMPORARY OLDER ADULTS

Contemporary older adults are living longer and experiencing less disability for shorter periods of time before death. They represent a health conscious and better informed cohort than even a decade ago. Many are living into their 90s because of advances in medicine and technology. They eat better, exercise more, actively engage with life, and take personal responsibility for their health and well-being. Many are retiring later. Health care reform, long-term care, the future of Medicare, and new images of health and well-being in

this population are important issues health care professionals to consider. Exercise 19-2.

THEORETICAL FRAMEWORKS

ERIK ERIKSON'S EGO DEVELOPMENT MODEL

Erikson's (1982) model specifically addresses stage development in later adulthood (older than 60 years). He identifies ego integrity versus ego despair as the ego strength associated with the final stage of life. **Ego integrity** relates to the capacity of older adults to look back on their lives with satisfaction and few regrets. Integrity involves acceptance of "one's one and only life cycle as something that had to be and that by necessity permitted of no substitutions" (Erikson, 1980, p. 104). Acceptance develops through self-reflection and dialogue with others about the meaning of one's life. Nurses can frame the older adult's illness story, recognition of social supports, and patterns of psychosocial responses in ways that help them reflect on the personal meaning of life. Nursing strategies encouraging life review and reminiscence groups facilitate the process. **Ego despair** describes the failure of a person to accept one's life as appropriate and meaningful. Left unresolved, despair leads to feelings of emotional desolation and bitterness.

Wisdom, the virtue associated with this stage of ego development is a form of "knowing" about the meaning and conduct of life, and being willing to share one's wisdom with others. Le (2008) discusses two forms of wisdom: practical wisdom and transcendent wisdom.

Purpose: To provide an understanding of changes needed to provide quality health care for baby boomers.

Procedure

Break class into groups of four to six students. Allow yourself to go beyond the facts and think about your personal response.

Answer the following questions:

1. How do you think the influx of baby boomers will affect health care?
2. What types of challenges do you see the health care system facing with the anticipated dramatic increase in numbers of older adults?
3. What are your ideas as a health professional to resolve the health care issues of the future related to care of older adults?

EXERCISE 19-3 | **The Wisdom of Aging**

Purpose: To promote an understanding of the sources of wisdom in the older adult.

Procedure

1. Interview an older adult (65 years or older) who, in your opinion, has had a fulfilling life. Ask the person to describe his or her most satisfying life events, and what he or she did to accomplish them. Ask the person to identify his or her most meaningful life experience or accomplishment. Immediately after the interview, write down your impressions, with direct quotes if possible to support your impressions.
2. Reflect on the person's comments and your ideas of what strengths this person had that allowed

him or her to achieve a sense of well-being, and to value his or her accomplishments.

Discussion

1. Were you surprised at any of older adults' responses to the question about most satisfying experiences? Most meaningful experiences?
2. On a blackboard or flip chart, identify the accomplishments that people have identified. Classify them as work-related or people-related.
3. What common themes emerged in the overall class responses that speak to the strengths in the life experience of older adults?
4. How can you apply what you learned from doing this exercise in your future nursing practice?

Practical wisdom emphasizes good judgment and the capacity to resolve complex human problems in the real world. Transcendent wisdom focuses on existential concerns and self-knowledge that allows a person to transcend subjectivity, bias, and self-centeredness. Wisdom allows older adults to share their understanding of life with those who will follow. Exercise 19-3, The Wisdom of Aging, explores the relationship of life experiences to development of wisdom.

FUNCTIONAL CONSEQUENCES THEORY

Functional consequences theory is conceptually linked to establishing and maintaining therapeutic relationships with older adults in that quality of life correlates with functional capacity and an elder's ability to meet dependency needs (Miller, 2011). The framework helps nurses to assess clients across a continuum of functioning, from high functioning to frail older adults. The framework emphasizes interventions that build functional self-management. Activities considered essential to self-regulating functional capacity include self-care,

mobility, interaction and relationships with others, cognitive reasoning ability, and engagement with life tasks.

ABRAHAM MASLOW'S BASIC NEEDS MODEL

Maslow's (1954) hierarchy of needs (see Chapters 1 and 2) helps nurses prioritize nursing actions, beginning with basic survival needs. Physiologic integrity, followed by safety and security, emerge as the most basic critical issues for clients, and need to be addressed first. For example, Touhy and Jett (2012) note that an agitated client with dementia looking for a toilet, and not being able to find it will not respond to a nurse's comfort or redirection strategies until the toileting need is met. Love and belonging needs in older adults are challenged by increased losses associated with death of important people. Esteem needs, especially those associated with meaningful purpose, and independence remain important issues in later life. Abraham Maslow believed that self-actualization occurs more often in middle-aged and older adults (Moody, 2010).

Developing an Evidence-Based Practice

Reichstadt M, Sengupta G, Depp C, Palinkas L, Jeste D: Older adults' perspectives on successful aging: qualitative interviews, *Am J Geriatr Psychiatry* 18(7):567-575, 2010.

Objectives: This aim of this qualitative study was to obtain the perspectives of older adults about their experiences of successful aging and their views about the interventions needed to support successful aging.

Methods: A purposive sample of 22 older adults (mean age 80 years; range 64-96) were recruited, and interviewed. Transcripts of the interviews were analyzed using a "coding consensus, co-occurrence, and comparison" grounded theory framework.

Results: Primary themes of self-acceptance and self-contentment were identified, with subthemes of realistic self-appraisal, "making the best of what you have," a focus on living in the present, and engagement with life exemplified in social interactions, trying new things, giving to others, and a positive attitude.

Application to your clinical practice: The authors note that the elicited perspectives support the validity of Erikson's concept of wisdom as a major contributor to the experience of successful aging. Nurses can use strategies to foster productive social engagement with life and promote self-acceptance through life review and empowering clients through realistic self-appraisal.

BOX 19-1   *Healthy People 2020* Objectives Related to Care of Older Adults

- Increase the proportion of older adults who use the Welcome to Medicare Benefit.
- Increase the proportion of older adults who are up to date on a core set of clinical preventive services.
- Increase the proportion of older adults with one or more chronic health conditions who report confidence in managing their conditions.
- Reduce the proportion of older adults who have moderate to severe functional limitations.
- Increase the proportion of older adults with reduced physical or cognitive function who engage in light, moderate, or vigorous leisure-time physical activities.

U.S. Department of Health and Human Services: 2010. *Healthy People 2020.* Available online: http://www.Healthypeople2020. Accessed July 19, 2013.

APPLICATIONS

Selected objectives from *Healthy People 2020* specifically address the health and well-being of older adults as identified in Box 19-1.

ASSESSMENT STRATEGIES WITH OLDER ADULT CLIENTS

New situations can cause transitory confusion for older adults, apart from cognitive impairment. Many clients are aware of the stereotypes associated with aging and are reluctant to expose themselves as inadequate in any way. They may stumble over questions when unusually stressed. When this occurs, the presence of family members can be helpful in giving the health care team a verbal picture of the client's pre-illness state. Family members can also be helpful in calming and normalizing care situations (Happ, 2010).

Older adults tend to be more responsive when time is taken to establish a supportive environment before conducting a formal assessment. Sensitive issues such as loneliness, abuse and neglect, caregiver burden, fears about death or frailty, memory loss, incontinence, alcohol abuse, and sexual dysfunction will only be discussed within a trustworthy relationship (Adelman et al., 2000). Continuity of care with one primary caregiver, when possible, helps foster the development of a comfortable nurse-client relationship. Older adults appreciate having the nurse provide structure to the history-taking interview by explaining the reasons for it and what it will involve (Cochran, 2005). Nurses can proactively provide this information.

Moody (2010) maintains that old age "is shaped by a life time of experience" (p. 2). Asking clients to share something about themselves and their life history, apart from the reasons for the health visit or admission, helps to establish rapport and increases the client's comfort level. Nurses get to know the client as a person, rather than categorically as an "older adult." Box 19-2 identifies communication guidelines for assessment interviews.

Assessment of older adult clients begins with their story of what brought them to the hospital or health care center. Allowing them to tell the story in their own way provides information you might otherwise not get. As clients relate their story, look for value-laden psychosocial issues (e.g., independence, fears about being a burden, role changes, and vulnerability)

BOX 19-2	Communication Guidelines for Assessment Interviews

- Establish rapport.
- Use open-ended questions first, followed by focused questions.
- Ask one question at a time.
- Elicit client perspectives first.
- Elicit family perspectives, if indicated.
- Invite ideas and feelings about diagnosis and treatment.
- Acknowledge feelings and emotions.
- Communicate a willingness to help.
- Provide information in small segments.
- Summarize the problem or condition discussed in the interview.
- Validate with the client and/or family for accuracy.
- Provide contact information for further questions or concerns.

and client preferences. These are significant issues for many older adults; without prompting, they may not be expressed. Look for client strengths, and affirm them. Help clients identify sources of social support, personal and financial resources, and coping strategies.

Case Example

Nurse: You seem concerned that your stroke will have a major impact on your life.

Client: Yes, I am. I'm an old woman now, and I don't want to be a burden to my family.

Nurse: In what ways do you think you might be a burden?

Client: Well, I obviously can't move around as I did. I can't go back to doing what I used to do, but that doesn't mean I'm ready for a nursing home.

Nurse: What were some of the things you used to do?

Client: Well, I raised three children, and they're all married now with good jobs. That's hard to do in this day and age. I did a lot for the church. I held a job as a secretary for 32 years and I got several awards for my work.

Nurse: It sounds as though you were very productive and were able to cope with a lot of things. Those coping skills are still a part of you and can be used in a different way now."

Exercise 19-4, The Story of Aging, provides a glimpse into personal life stories of older adults.

ASSESSING AGE-RELATED SENSORY CHANGES

Sensory changes occur with normal aging. Hearing and vision changes have a direct and significant impact on communication. Compensatory enhancements are essential to ensuring client safety and staying connected with others (Bonder and Dal Bello-Haas, 2009; Gonsalves and Pichora-Fuller, 2008). Because vision and hearing decline are accepted as a normal fact of aging, its significance is not always addressed as vigorously as it should be. Anderson (2005) notes that addressing common causes of sensory impairment and providing sensory cues can help reduce confusion.

Hearing

According to the National Institute on Deafness and Other Communication Disorders (NIDCD, 2013), one in three people older than 60 years of age, and half of those older than 85 years of age will experience hearing loss. Hearing loss associated with normal aging begins after age 50 years, due to loss of hair cells (which are not replaced) in the organ of Corti in the inner ear. This change leads initially to a loss in the ability to hear high-frequency sounds (e.g., *f, s, th, sh, ch*), with later losses related to frequency vowel sounds (Gallo, 2000). Older adults have special difficulty in distinguishing sounds from background noises, fully hearing people talking with an accent, and following fast-paced speech. Hearing problems diminish an older person's ability to interact with others, attend concerts and other social functions, and understand medical directions.

Kochkin (2009) notes that less than 25% of older adults with significant hearing loss use hearing aids. Many older adults with hearing aids do not use them consistently or get easily frustrated with their limitations. Others simply cannot afford them and do not use them at all.

Communication breakdowns with hearing loss are frustrating for both speaker and listener. Difficulties can occur because of environmental factors such as background noise, half hearing or misinterpreting conversations, or by incorrectly manipulating an ear piece (Pryce and Gooberman, 2012). This does not have to happen. There are hearing aid programs for people with limited income that can help with financial costs. The Department of Rehabilitation Services and nonprofit hearing aid programs have hearing aids available for free or at a discount (see http://savvysenior.org).

Adaptive Strategies for Hearing Loss. Communication with the hearing-impaired older adult need not be significantly different from one with a client without age-related hearing loss. Ideally, you should position yourself at the same level as the client. It is

EXERCISE 19-4	The Story of Aging

Purpose: To promote an understanding of older adults.

Procedure
1. Interview an older adult in your family (minimum age, 65 years). If there are no older adults in your family, interview a family friend whose lifestyle is similar to your family's.
2. Ask this person to describe what growing up was like, what is different today from the way it was when he or she was your age, what are the important values held, and if there have been any changes in them over the years. Ask this person what advice he or she would give you about how

to achieve satisfaction in life. If this person could change one thing about our society today, what would it be?

Discussion
1. Were you surprised at any of the answers older adults gave you?
2. What are some common themes you and your classmates found that related to values and the type of advice older adults gave each of you?
3. What implications do the findings from this exercise have for your future nursing practice?

important to speak with a normal or only slightly louder than normal voice tone. You do not need to shout. Other strategies include the following:

- Address the client by name before beginning to speak; it focuses attention.
- If the client has a "better" ear, sit or stand on the side with the more functional ear.
- Speak slowly, distinctly, and use a slightly louder voice. Annunciate your words; use active lip formation of words.
- If your voice is high-pitched, lower it.
- Make sure the client can see your facial expression and/or read your lips to enhance comprehension. *Keep the client's view of your mouth unobstructed.*
- Help clients adjust hearing aids; some may not be able to insert aids correctly to amplify hearing. Make sure hearing aids are turned on. If difficulties persist, check the batteries. Clients with hearing aids should always have extra batteries readily accessible.
- Keep background noise to a minimum (e.g., radio or television, competing conversations, high-activity locations, children running around, sudden noises).
- Check in with the client frequently. Solicit feedback to monitor how much and what the person has heard. Sometimes you can tell from a vague facial expression or inappropriate response that a message was misheard.

Age-Related Vision Loss

Vision normally declines as a person ages (Whiteside et al., 2006). Colors become dimmer and images less

clear. Brighter lighting and larger print help. More serious age-related vision problems such as cataracts, glaucoma, and age-related macular degeneration can cause blindness in the elderly, if left untreated. Loss of visual acuity is gradual, but progressive, associated with age-related changes in the support structures of the eye and the visual pathway (Mauk, 2010). The level and type of impairment differ from vision loss identified in Chapter 17.

Poor vision has implications for effective communication, safety, and functional ability. Older adults with progressive vision loss may not see you shaking your head or nodding. They may see changes in emotional facial expressions. Impaired vision can affect a person's ability to perform everyday activities (e.g., dressing, preparing meals, taking medication, driving, handling the checkbook, and seeing phone numbers). It disturbs functional ability to engage in hobbies or leisure activities requiring vision (e.g., reading, doing handwork, and watching television).

Reduced visual acuity, loss of contrast sensitivity, and loss of depth perception create a major safety issue related to falls. Lord (2006) notes that vision plays a significant role in postural stability because it provides the nervous system with information regarding the individual's position and movement in relation to the environment. Mobility slows as a person ages and this combined with decreased vision can lead to increased risk for falling.

Adaptive Strategies for Vision Loss. Common adaptive devices that older adults use are prescription glasses and handheld magnifiers. Nurses can support the independence of the visually impaired client with the following strategies:

- If eyeglasses are worn, make sure they are clean, and in place. Glasses can be cleaned with a soft cloth and water.
- Check that the older adult's glasses prescription gets updated as vision decreases. Regularly scheduled eye exams are vital. "Mature" eyes undergo age-related structural changes that affect vision.
- Assist the older adult on stairs, particularly descent, on curbs and on uneven terrain.
- Verbally note changes in the physical environment that could cause mobility problems *before* clients approach them.
- Face the client directly. They may see your form even when features are indistinct.
- Verbally explain all written information, allowing time for the client to ask questions.
- Provide bright lighting with no glare.
- When using written materials, consider font and letter size (14 point) for readability. Use upper and lowercase letters rather than all capitals. Use solid paper, with sharp contrasting writing, and a lot of white space.
- Encourage older adults to use audio books or electronic readers that enlarge print.

ASSESSMENT OF COGNITIVE CHANGES

Healthy older clients should not require modifications in communication related to cognition (Moody, 2010). Without the ravages of neurological disease, older adults may only require more time to complete verbal tasks or process information. Older adults are more cautious. They may hesitate or not respond as well if they are under time pressure to perform. Otherwise, there should be no difference in functioning.

Approximately 6% to 8% of the population older than 65 years and more than 30% of those who reach the age of 85 years will experience profound progressive cognitive changes associated with dementia (Yuhas et al., 2006). Dementia is characterized by memory loss, personality changes, and a deterioration in intellectual functioning that affects every aspect of the person's life. A small percentage of abnormal cognitive changes are caused by other organic problems (e.g., drug toxicity, metabolic disorders, and depression); these may be reversed with treatment.

Appraisal of serious cognitive changes is a critical assessment with older adults, because it has the most effect on a person's ability to perform activities of daily

BOX 19-3	Guide for Mental Status Testing with Older Adults

1. Select a standardized test such as the Mini-Mental State Examination
2. Administer the test in a quiet, nondistracting environment at a time when the client is not anxious, agitated, or tired.
3. Make sure the client has eyeglasses and/or hearing aids, if needed, before testing.
4. Ask easier questions first and provide frequent reassurance that the client is doing well with the testing.
5. Determine the client's level of formal education. If the client never learned to spell, it will be impossible to spell "world" backward. Saying the days of the week backward is a good alternative.
6. Document your findings clearly in the client's record, including the client's response to the testing process, so that future comparisons can be made.

living (Moody, 2010). Performing a mental status assessment early in the interview helps with an accurate diagnosis. The Mini-Mental State Examination (Folstein et al., 1975) measures several dimensions of cognition (e.g., orientation, memory, abstraction, and language). An abnormal score (less than 26) suggests dementia and the need for further evaluation of cognition. Guides for mental status testing are presented in Box 19-3.

ASSESSMENT OF FUNCTIONAL STATUS

Functional status refers to a broad range of purposeful abilities related to physical health maintenance, role performance, cognitive or intellectual abilities, social activities, and level of emotional functioning. Functional abilities range from vigorous, active, and independent, to frail and dependent with serious physical, cognitive, psychological, and sensory deficits (Bonder and Dal Bello-Haas, 2009). More than any other factor, impaired functional status is a determinant of an older adult's inability to live independently. Stress, acute and chronic illness, and age-related physiologic changes will influence a person's functional status (Zysberg et al., 2009).

Functional status rather than chronologic age should be the stronger indicator of disability-related needs in older adults, as functional impairment is not associated solely with age. Burke and Laramie (2004) note that a chronically ill 50-year-old with no support system may have more disabling symptoms of aging than a healthy, active 75-year-old with a strong social support system in place.

Evaluation of functional abilities helps determine the type and level of care an older adult requires. Essential activities of daily living (ADLs) refer to six areas of essential function: toileting, feeding, dressing, grooming, bathing, and ambulation (Miller, 2011). Instrumental activities of daily living (IADLs) are more complex than basic ADLS and refer to tasks older adults have to cope with on a daily basis. These tasks include cooking, cleaning, shopping, managing medications, getting to places beyond walking, using a telephone, and paying bills (Kleinpell, 2007). Although age robs older adults of some of life's vigor, healthy cognitively intact older adults are able to perform ADLs independently or with minimum assistance. Usually there is decline in IADLs prior to ADL performance failures.

ASSESSMENT OF PAIN

It is a common concern of older adults, related to chronic conditions such as osteoarthritis, diabetic peripheral neuropathy, constipation, among others (Jansen, 2008). Both client and health care professionals can assume that moderate or episodic pain associated with chronic disorders of aging occurs more frequently than not and needs to be addressed.

Persistent pain is reported in over 50% of the elderly (Herr, 2013). Pain limits an older adult's functional ability and compromises well-being. Although pain is a component of many chronic conditions associated with aging, it should not be considered a normal consequence of aging (Cavalieri 2005). He reports that pain in the older adult is often under reported because people equate pain with being a natural part of the aging process. Once identified, reducing pain to improve function should be the goal of treatment (Herr, 2010). There is no more reason for an older adult client to suffer with chronic pain than there is for younger clients

Chronic coexisting disorders such as depression or dementia can also limit an older adult's ability to report and correctly interpret underlying causes of pain. For example, undiagnosed depression may present as neck or shoulder pain, severe enough to interfere with sleep or activity. Liberal dispensing of analgesics to older adults for pain relief without full assessment of the nature of the pain can lead to undesired outcomes. Rowan and Faul (2007) label prescription drug abuse as one of the fastest growing public health problems among older adults in the United States.

Whereas clients can report whether their pain interferes with daily functioning, identifying pain levels on a linear scale is more of a challenge (Gloth, 2004). A comprehensive pain assessment for older adults should ask the client to

- Specify the quality and nature of the pain, for example, aching, burning, pressure, acute, or stabbing. (Some older adults will use the word *discomfort* instead of *pain*.)
- Identify when the pain occurs and under what circumstances.
- Identify specific pain patterns and/or changes in pain intensity.
- Describe how the pain affects the client's physical, psychological, and social functioning.
- Define the area of the body where the pain occurs, whether it is deep or superficial, localized or radiating (Feldt, 2008).

Assessment of pain in cognitively impaired clients and in those who cannot communicate verbally is accomplished through behavioral observation. Behaviors suggestive of pain include grimacing, tightened muscles, groaning, crying, agitation, lethargy, and unwillingness to move.

Depression can make pain more intense. Older adults who are socially isolated or depressed can experience greater pain than those who remain connected with a social support system.

It is important to ask about recent losses and changes. Loss is a reoccurring issue for older adults. Most will suffer losses of people, activities, and functions of importance to them. Depression can be untreated problem in older adults. Unlike symptoms of depression in younger people, somatization with vague physical complaints is often a presenting sign (Arnold, 2005). Older adults, particularly white males, are at higher risk for suicide. Comments reflecting hopelessness such as "life doesn't hold much for me" or "sometimes I just wish God would take me" should never be taken lightly.

EMPOWERMENT: BUILDING ON CLIENT STRENGTHS

Older adults face many negative situational stressors; they also possess a lifetime of strengths Reminiscence is an empowerment strategy that reminds them of personal strengths that so many of them still possess. Asking simple concrete questions about the older adult's life, where the person grew up, and what was most important to him or her is a prompt you can use to initiate conversation, or when communication stalls. Notice as clients talk if his or her face brightens at any point in the conversation. These topics usually have special meaning that you can help the client explore.

General nursing care for cognitively intact older adult clients in the community centers around providing supports related to self-management of chronic illness and promoting healthy lifestyles. Sometimes it is simply a lack of information. They may not be aware of elder care services: transportation, meals on wheels, church-sponsored friendly visitors, aging in place initiatives, and so forth. Others know of elder support services, but do not know how to access available resources.

Several studies indicate that many older adults experience higher psychosocial well-being compared with younger counterparts (Windsor and Anstey, 2008). This sounds counterintuitive, but older adults are more likely to seek and enjoy emotionally meaningful activities in the present moment. They are less concerned with high achievement. Older adults appreciate short, frequent conversations. Like everyone else, the need to be acknowledged is paramount to older adults' sense of self-esteem.

The *level* of social support people use depends on personal preference, individual, financial, and social resources, what older adults have at their disposal and are willing and able to use. Asking questions such as "Can you tell me who visits you" or "Who have you visited in the last couple of weeks?" or "If you needed immediate help, whom would you call?" are useful ways to gain the client's perception of social supports. In the process of asking questions, clients sometimes come up with relationships that they had not thought about.

Heliker (2009) describes story sharing as "a reciprocal give-and-take process of respectful telling and listening that focuses on what matters to the individual and minimizes the power of one over another" (p. 44). Stories become a shared experience reminding clients of a valued social identity that goes beyond descriptions of their health. Each time older adults tell their story, they remember how they saw themselves as valued, productive members of society. They know someone cares to listen. Nurses can teach and model this communication strategy with nursing assistants.

The conversational world for older adults may narrow for many reasons; mobility, death of friends, distance, or transportation. Current events to draw from as a means of starting a conversation are not as available so even cognitively intact older adults repeat stories. Repetitive stories can be frustrating for nurses. Rather than thinking, "Oh my, here he goes again with that old 'Model T' car story," it is better to respond to the story and enter the conversation as fully as possible. Each conversation becomes an opportunity to gain insight into the person, such as what the person values, what aspirations and dreams were fulfilled or unfulfilled, what contributions are valued, and what goals are yet to be attained. Focusing on what a person considers important enhances well-being among older adults, particularly the homebound.

LIFE REVIEW

Life review is a useful intervention with older adult clients. Gentle prompts and relevant questions for clarification are required. Sharing recollections from youth or early adulthood days with a compassionate listener helps older adults review their life, establish its meaning, Sometimes, it provides opportunities for older adults to reconcile long-standing conflicts (Bohlmeijer et al., 2009).

REMINISCENCE GROUPS

Interpersonal contact in groups can be therapeutic for lonely, isolated older adults (Henderson and Gladding, 2004). A specialized group for older adults in long-term settings is the reminiscence group. Minardi and Hayes (2003) differentiate between life review, which explores life events in depth, and **reminiscence groups**, which focus on sharing life experiences as simple stories. Reminiscence groups follow a structured format, with themes decided beforehand. Examples include special times in childhood or adolescence, child-rearing or work experience, and handling of a crisis. The leader guides the group in telling their stories, asking questions, and points out common themes to stimulate further reflections. Members create for themselves a shared reality by revealing to one another what life has meant and can be for them. In the process of remembering critical incidents, they reconnect with forgotten moments that held meaning for them, thus giving them a sense of continuity with their current circumstances (Jonsdottir et al., 2001). Guidelines for working with older adult groups are presented in Box 19-4.

SOCIAL AND SPIRITUAL SUPPORTS

Older adults have the same need for meaningful activity and personal relationships as younger cohorts

BOX 19-4 | Working with Older Adult Groups

- Affirm the dignity, intelligence, and pride of elderly group members.
- Ask group members to introduce themselves and ask how they would like to be called.
- Make use of humor, but never at the expense of an individual group member.
- Keep the communication simple, but at an adult level.
- Ask relevant questions at important points in a client's story.
- Call attention to the range of life experiences and personal strengths when they occur.
- Allow group members to voice their complaints, even when nothing can be done about them, and then refocus on the group task.
- Avoid probing for the release of strong emotions that neither you nor they can handle effectively in the group sessions.
- Thank each person for contributing to the group and summarize the group activity for that session.

Adapted from Corey M, Corey G: Groups for the elderly (p. 394-396), ed 9, Belmont, CA, 2013, Thompson/Brooks Cole.

(Potempa et al., 2010). But as age-related changes in eyesight, hearing, and mobility make it more difficult to do the things the older adult could do at an earlier age, some lose confidence and begin to disengage socially.

Staying engaged with life and stimulating the mind is essential to the health and well-being of older adults (Reichstadt et al., 2010). It is amazing how much an older adult perks up when someone takes the time to visit, suggests lunch, or frequently calls. Encouraging family members to proactively give this gift of self is helpful to all concerned.

The amount of socialization depends to some extent on inclination and personality factors, but social isolation compromises the health and well-being of older adults (Strine et al., 2008). In many cases, social support needs to be proactive due to mobility issues. For people who have lost a "people" support system, for age-related reasons, a connection with a personal God or church community can become an important source of social and spiritual support. Bishop (2008) notes, "Social and spiritual ties share an interdependent link to positive psychological well-being in late adulthood (p. 2). In the following case example, note the interaction between social and spiritual connections.

Case Example

Lois visits a client with dementia weekly. The woman is mostly mute with little natural speech. One day Lois read her the 23rd Psalm. The woman spontaneously repeated the psalm from a different version, smiling broadly when finished. She could not respond in the present; she could in the past about something familiar to her.

Existential awareness of a shortened life span promotes thinking about death and the meaning of life. Spiritual interventions relevant to the care of older adults include instilling hope, prayer, use of spiritual hymns or readings, and talking about the client's spiritual concerns. Helping clients cope with unfinished business is an important nursing intervention (Delgado, 2007).

ENVIRONMENTAL SUPPORTS

Independence is something most people take for granted as a younger adult; it becomes a significant issue for older adults and their caregivers. Corey and Corey (2006) note, "As we age, we have to adjust to an increasingly external locus of control when confronted with losses over which we have little control" (p. 403). Nurses need to be sensitive to often unexpressed fears of older adults around surrendering their independence. For example, an older adult awaiting discharge from the hospital told his nurse that he had a bedside commode and no stairs in his home. When the nurse visited the home, there was no commode, and the client's home had a significant number of stairs. The client told her that he was afraid she would insist he move to a nursing home if these facts were known. Formal support services in the community, home health aides, and informal family supports can be critical factors in enabling frail older adults to remain independent. Nurses can help clients access these services.

SAFETY SUPPORTS

There may be a delicate balance between the client's perceived and actual need for safety in health care. Restrictions and supports needed for safety can and should be negotiated, not simply imposed. Interventions to promote independence include the following:

- Allowing elders personal choices about their bedtime, within reason.
- Respecting choices in food selection.
- Providing chair risers, walkers, and canes as needed.

- Safety modifications in the home (e.g., bath-tub/shower grip bars, scatter rug removal, night lights). Increased frailty may make independent showering a safer option than a bath.
- Including elder clients in decision making about health care and giving them the information they need to make responsible choices.
- Installing home security, health alarm monitors, giving trusted neighbors or relatives keys and emergency phone numbers.

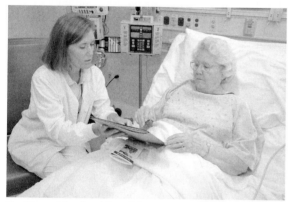

Health teaching for older adults is critical to a healthy life style.

MEDICATION SUPPORTS

Polypharmacy is a fact of life for older adults with multiple chronic conditions. Older adults are at risk for side effects and drug interactions because of the variety they take and age-related changes in metabolism (Cochran, 2005). Medications in general have a stronger effect on the older population and take longer to eliminate from the body.

Unmonitored polypharmacy is a major contributor to falls and hip fractures, and medication mismanagement is often a formal reason for hospital or nursing home admissions. Providing a weekly pillbox for multiple medications decreases errors. Other obstacles include having more than one prescribing provider. With limited knowledge of a client's full profile, including over-the-counter medications, dangerous interactions can occur. Important questions you can ask include:

- "What do you take each medication for?
- How and when do you take it?
- What kind of problems are you having?" (Gould and Mitty, 2010, p. 294).

Encourage clients and family to keep a written list of all medications to be shared with each provider. Poor self-management of medications include complexity of taking multiple medications, difficulty removing safety tops, using incorrect techniques, improper medication storage, level of health literacy, cost of medications factors, and poor eyesight.

Asking about medications including over-the-counter and herbal medications is a safety question you should ask during initial assessment and each health-related home visit. Ownby (2006) recommends using an open-ended question, such as "Tell me how you take your medications," rather than asking, "Are you taking your medication as prescribed?" (p. 33). Box 19-5 covers key areas for medication assessment. Visually checking medications with the client and talking about how the medication is working with the client and/or primary caretaker is essential in home care.

Health teaching helps clients establish and maintain appropriate self-management of medications (Curry et al., 2005). Simplifying the medication regimen and regular checking of expiration dates enhance medication management and lessen the possibility of adverse reactions. The adage "start low, and go slow" (Miller, 2011), plus regular communication with prescribers, is essential. Careful instruction as to the purpose, dosage, anticipated outcomes, and side effects can increase medication compliance. Establish a system with the client or family for medication administration, for example, prefilled medication dispensers or a medication calendar. Use a teach-back strategy to ensure that instructions are understood and the client or family feels comfortable with their knowledge and capacity to implement administration.

ELDER ABUSE

Elder abuse represents a major threat to the safety and well-being of older adults. The term refers to the mistreatment of vulnerable older adults, usually at the hands of caregivers, including professional personnel. Box 19-6 identifies fundamental rights of older adult.

The most common form of elder abuse is neglect, both passive and active. Active neglect is deliberate. Passive neglect occurs when clients, most notably those with dementia, lack properly supervised care or essential supports related to implementing instrumental or basic activities of daily living.

Elder abuse is a difficult problem to identify and treat. Diminished mental capacity compromises an older adult's ability to even understand what is happening, let alone take constructive actions to stop the abuse or to use any community services available to them (Nerenberg, 2008). Alternative options for older adults are not readily available and older adults are reluctant to consider a nursing home as an option. Pride, embarrassment, and a desire to protect family members prevent vulnerable older adults from wanting to prosecute a family member for abuse or neglect. If the nurse identifies abuse or neglect, it must be reported to appropriate social and legal protective services.

ADVOCACY SUPPORT

Fundamental rights of older adults in health care settings are identified in Box 19-5. Nurses play an important service in explaining treatment to clients and families, helping them frame questions for physicians and hospitalists, and arranging for continuity of care with community agencies. Role modeling is an indirect form of advocacy, which nurses provide in institutional settings. Treating older clients with respect, not becoming impatient with primitive behaviors, and providing excellent care is noted by family and non-professionals. Holding nursing assistants accountable for maintaining quality care is a nursing responsibility.

Health Promotion for Older Adults

Health-damaging behaviors such as poor nutrition, inactivity, and alcohol and tobacco abuse contribute heavily to the onset of disability in the elderly. The Centers for Disease Control and Prevention (CDC) recommends an integrated health promotion approach to address common risk factors and comorbidities in older adults (Lang et al., 2005). Older adults benefit from health promotion activities tailored to their stage of life. It is never too late to practice good nutrition; engage in healthful exercise such as strength training, walking, and yoga; connect with social relationships on a regular basis; and improve safety factors. Most urban communities have groups specifically for older adults.

At the same time, healthy older adults are not young people. Health requirements change as a person ages such that their nutrition, exercise, sleep and other health needs are different. Health promotion strategies need to be modified to meet the unique requirements of aging adults (Nakasato and Carnes, 2006). Box 19-7 identifies areas of relevant health promotion activities for older adults.

Nurses can engage older adults in health promotion activities by appealing to their interests and by incorporating cultural values in the presentation. Examples of relevant activities can include:

- Preparing examples of healthy ethnic food (e.g., "soul cooking the healthy way")
- Assigning blocks of time for preventive screening, specifically for older adults

---

BOX 19-5	Teaching Medication Self-Management

Areas of Assessment:

- List of current and previously taken medications, herbal and over-the-counter medications
- Medications taken episodically for insomnia, pain, intestinal upsets, colds, and coughs
- Allergies (include exact symptoms)
- Determine if the client know what each medication is for, storage, what to do for missed doses, drug interactions, side effects
- Ability to read medication labels or printed instructions
- Motor difficulties with appropriate medication administration
- Expiration dates, brown bag syndrome (having older adult bring all medications in a brown bag for clinic visit observation)
- Determination of family responsibility, and availability if medication administration support is needed

---

BOX 19-6	Fundamental Older Adult Rights

Older adults need to be able to:

- Live in safe and appropriate living environments.
- Establish and maintain meaningful relationships and social networks.
- Have equal access to health care, legal, and social services consistent with their needs.
- Have the right to make decisions about their care and quality of life.
- Have their rights, autonomy, and assets protected.
- Have appropriate information to make reasoned decisions.
- Have their personal, cultural, and spiritual values, beliefs, and preferences respected.
- Participate in all aspects of their care plan, including care decisions to the fullest extent possible.
- Expect confidentiality of all communication and clinical records related to their care.
- Be involved in advocacy and the formulation of policies that directly impact their health and well-being.

- Combining multiple prevention services into one clinical visit
- Providing free flu and pneumonia immunizations at convenient times in traditional and non-traditional settings (Lang et al., 2005; Penprase, 2006)

Health Teaching

Moody (2010) notes that health teaching for the elderly is critical if they are to master the tasks of old age and maintain their health. Healthy older adult learning capabilities remain intact for needing more time to think about how they want to handle a situation. The sensitive nurse observes the client before implementing teaching and gears teaching strategies to meet the individual learning needs of each client. Four aspects of successful aging: fall prevention, adequate nutrition, socialization, and medication management lend themselves to health teaching formats.

Exercise 19-5 provides an opportunity to think about health teaching for older adults.

Assuming that cognitively intact older adults lack the capacity to understand instructions is a common error. Health care providers often direct instruction to the older adult client's younger companion, even when the client has no cognitive impairment. This action invalidates the client and diminishes self-worth. Mauk (2006) identifies simple modifications to reduce age-related barriers to learning when teaching older adults. Suggestions include:

- Explain why the information is important to the client.
- Use familiar words and examples in providing information.
- Draw on the client's experiences and interests in planning your teaching.
- Make teaching sessions short enough to avoid tiring the client and frequent enough for continuous learning support.
- Speak slowly, naturally, and clearly.

BOX 19-7	Areas of Relevant Health Promotion Activities

- Health protection: public health approaches promoting flu vaccines
- Health prevention: environmental or home assessments to prevent falls
- Health education: information about healthy eating and exercise
- Health preservation: promoting optimal levels of functioning by increasing the control older adults have over their lives and health

Adapted from Bernard M: Promoting health in old age, Buckingham, England, 2000, Open University Press; Sanders K: Developing practice for healthy aging, *Nurs Older People* 18(3):18-21, 2006.

RELATIONSHIPS WITH COGNITIVELY IMPAIRED OLDER ADULTS

Mild cognitive impairment (MCI) and dementia are neurological disorders characterized by a progressive

EXERCISE 19-5	Health Promotion Teaching for Older Adults

Purpose: To provide a health teaching segment for an older adult.

Procedure

1. Develop a step-by-step mini teaching plan related to fall prevention for a cognitively intact older adult.
   a. Consider what person-centered information you will need from the client to effectively provide tailored content.
   b. Identify specific content you will need to include in your presentation.
   c. Describe teaching strategies you will use.
   d. What accommodations will you need to make?
   e. How will you evaluate the client's understanding of the material?

2. Implement the teaching plan
3. Share your experience with other students in small groups of three to six students.

Discussion

1. Were there any similarities/differences in themes, or client responses to the teaching session?
2. Were you surprised at anything you found in preparing for the teaching session versus what occurred during the session?
3. If you had to provide client education on another topic relevant to the older adult, what would you do differently, if anything?
4. What did you learn from doing this exercise that you could use in future practice with older adults?

TABLE 19-1	Sorting Out the Three D's: Delirium, Dementia, Depression		
Disorder	**Delirium**	**Dementia**	**Depression**
Onset	Acute, over hours, days	Insidious, over months, years	Relatively rapid, over weeks to months
Acuity	Acute symptoms, medical emergency	Chronic symptoms, progresses slowly	Episodic symptoms, coincides with losses
Course	Short term; resolves with identification of cause, treatment	Gradual, progressive deterioration, memory loss	Self-limiting; recurrent symptoms; resolves with treatment
Duration	Lasts hours to weeks, resolves with treatment	Progressive and irreversible, ends in death	At least 2 weeks, may last months to years, responds to treatment
Alertness or consciousness	Fluctuates, intervals of lucidity and confusion, worse at night	Clear, stable during day, sundown syndrome	Clear, thinking may appear slowed; decreased alertness because of lack of motivation
Attention	Trouble focusing, short attention span, fluctuates	Usually unaffected	Minimal deficit, difficulty concentrating
Orientation	Disoriented to time and place, but not to person	Impaired as disease progresses; inability to recognize familiar people or objects, including self	Selective disorientation
Memory	Recent and immediate impaired	Impaired memory for immediate/recent events; unconcerned about memory deficits	Selective impairment, concerned about memory deficits
Thinking	Incoherent, global disorganization	Impoverished, inability to learn, trouble word finding	Intact, negative themes
Perception	Gross distortions; illusions, visual, tactile hallucinations	Prone to hallucinations as disease progresses	Intact, but colored by negative themes
Speech	Incoherent, disorganized, loud, belligerent	Impoverished, tangential, repetitive, superficial, confabulations	Quiet, decreased, can be irritable, language skills intact
Sleep/Wake cycle	Disturbed; changes hourly	Disturbed; day/night reversal	Disturbed; early morning wakening, hypersomnia during day
Contributing factors	Underlying medical cause; toxicity, fever, tumor, infection, drugs	Degenerative disorder associated with age, cardiovascular deficits, substance dependence	Significant or cumulative loss; drug toxicity, diabetes, myocardial infarction

Adapted from Arnold E: Sorting out the three D's: delirium, depression, dementia, *Holist Nurs Pract* 19(3):99-104, 2005.

decline in intellectual and behavioral functioning. When a person suffers with dementia, others tend to focus on the cognitive and behavioral deficits and overlook the psychosocial, emotional, and spiritual personality components that make up the whole person (MacKinlay, 2012).

Symptoms of cognitive impairment and communication difficulties in older adults can be similar in clients suffering from depression, delirium, and dementia, so accurate diagnosis is important. Communicating with a client suffering from dementia requires a different set of strategies than for the client with depression. Table 19-1 identifies important differences between the three disorders in older adults. Secondary clinical depression and/or delirium can be superimposed on dementia, making a difficult situation even more challenging. Exercise 19-6 provides an opportunity to distinguish between dementia, delirium, and depression, using a case study.

SUPPORTING ADAPTATION TO DAILY LIFE

Box 19-8 outlines early cognitive changes seen with dementia. Memory loss is a consistent finding. Structure and consistency in the environment are important themes to consider. In the early stages, nurses can help

EXERCISE 19-6	Distinguishing Between Dementia, Delirium, and Depression in the Older Adult

Purpose: To differentiate between the 3 D's.

Mrs. S. is a recently widowed 78-year-old woman living alone in a senior apartment complex in a suburban community. Her son and his wife live nearby and visit weekly. Over the last month, the family has noticed that Mrs. S. "has not been herself." Once a meticulous dresser, she shows no current interest in dressing and grooming. She has had difficulty keeping doctor appointments and getting medications refilled. When approached by the family regarding her change in behavior, Mrs. S. says that she "doesn't know—if I could just get a good night's sleep, I would feel better."

Discussion

What distinguishing alterations in cognition does Mrs. S exhibit to suggest a depression or a dementia?

What additional questions would you like to ask to support your observations?

What screening tools are appropriate?

What approaches would you suggest for communicating with Mrs. S?

Identify ways to improve Mrs. S.'s ability to function safely and independently

What sources of support can you identify to help Mrs. S and her family cope?

Developed by AM Spellbring, PhD, RN, FAAN, February 9, 2010.

BOX 19-8	Signs of Early Cognitive Changes with Dementia

- Difficulty remembering appointments
- Difficulty recalling the names of friends, neighbors, and family members
- Using the wrong word when talking
- Jumbling words: mixing up or missing letters in words when talking
- Not following the conversation of friends or coworkers
- Not understanding an explanation or story
- Difficulty recalling whether a task was just completed the day or week before
- Difficulty keeping up with all the steps to a task
- Difficulty planning and doing an activity such as a board meeting or family reunion
- New difficulty filling out complicated forms such as income tax forms
- Different behavior: restless, quick to get angry, constant hunger (especially for sweets), quiet or withdrawn, and so forth
- Buying items and forgetting there is plenty at home
- Struggling with work or home tasks that used to be routine and easy
- Loss of interest in meeting with friends or doing activities

vocabulary seem intact is a common feature of dementia. The person appears to register on a command but acts in ways that suggest he or she has little understanding of what transpired verbally. In the following case example, the caregiver observes the client's difficulty. Notice how her response supports his ability to function.

Case Example

The care staff member noticed I.A.'s restlessness as he struggled to figure out which shoes to put on. I.A. began looking around with darting eyes, quickly shifting his gaze from here to there. The care staff member said, "I am sorry. I have put two pairs of shoes here and it is confusing. Please put these on." I.A. looked relieved, put on the shoes, and moved to a table where the care staff member placed a box that had many small articles brought from I.A.'s company. The care staff member said, "Would you help us, president?" I.A. smiled and said, "Okay... I can see you need help here," as he began to organize the articles into piles. He did not wander on that day (Ito et al., 2007, p. 14).

SUPPORTING COMMUNICATION

Difficulty with purposeful communication is a hallmark of dementia. The client's loss is a gradual process initially so many clients can maintain superficial conversation, with empathetic support. Miller (2008) notes that dementia affects basic receptive (decoding and understanding) and expressive (conveying information) forms of communication. These deficits impact the person's capacity to think

clients develop reminder strategies such as making notes to themselves and using colored labels, alarms, or calendars. Focusing on what the client can do, rather than on deficits, taps into the functions still available to the client and decreases feelings of hopelessness (Cotter, 2009).

Apraxia, defined as the loss of the ability to take purposeful action even when the muscles, senses, and abstractly and solve problems. Although clients may speak in fragments, they are still capable of interacting with prompts, and especially when given your full attention.

Providing verbal cues helps older adults with short-term memory impairment. Word retrieval occurs frequently. Clients may stop in mid-sentence, ask for help with a word, or continue with phrases that have little to do with the intended meaning (Mace and Rabins, 2011). Nurses can support clients by suggesting obvious missing words or a simple meaning. Check with the client that your interpretation is accurate. Sometimes you can grasp what the word might be from the context. For example, one client could not retrieve the word "Halloween." Instead she said, "When people dress in costumes." The nurse said, "You mean Halloween?" the client said yes, and the conversation continued. You also can ask the client to point to an object or describe something similar if you do not understand what the client is referencing (Miller, 2008).

Short-term memory allows people to follow a conversation when the topic changes. Cognitively impaired clients lack short-term memory, so topic transitions can be difficult (McCarthy, 2011). Restate ideas using simple words and sequence and validate the meaning of a client's response. Instead of using abstract prompts (such as a specific time), use words directly applicable to daily routines, such as "before lunch" to anchor the client's recognition of time frames. If a client rambles, you can refocus attention by selecting a relevant thought from the stream of ideas. Use questions that can be answered with a yes or no for clients with less verbal skill. Note whether the client's behavior is consistent with the answer and follow up if the behavior is incongruent with the words. Be aware that the client is acutely aware of your body language and looks at it as a measure of your acceptance. Your goal is to try and make each conversation a "person-centered" verbal connection. Box 19-9 summarizes communication guidelines for communicating with cognitively impaired clients.

Cognitively impaired clients often have trouble following instructions consisting of multiple steps. Breaking instructions into single steps helps these clients master tasks that otherwise are beyond their comprehension. Keep the conversation simple, and focused only on one step at a time.

Case Example

A young woman in a dementia support group for family members spoke of a meaningful experience with her grandmother. As she went to make a tuna fish sandwich for her grandmother, she decided to involve her in the process. She gave her grandmother step-by-step verbal instructions (e.g., "Get the tuna fish out of the cabinet," "Get the knife from the drawer"), all of which her grandmother was able to do with structured guidance. As the granddaughter was spreading the mayonnaise, her grandmother said, "Now don't forget the onions." It was a priceless moment of connection for the granddaughter.

Do not explain why or what will happen if the directions are not followed. This makes it harder for the client to follow. If the client does not do a task or follow directions incorrectly, keep the words simple, "please stop," in pleasant calm tones. Scolding can exacerbate confusions. Unlike children who can learn from a mistake, the dementia client cannot.

Asking mild to early moderate cognitively impaired older adults about their past life experiences is a way to connect verbally with those who might have difficulty telling you what they had for breakfast 2 hours ago. Remote memory (recall of past events) is retained longer than memory for recent events. When cognitively impaired adults share memories, they are giving a gift to the nurse by sharing part of themselves when they may have very little else to give.

Family members can be encouraged to reminisce with dementia clients. Even if the client cannot respond verbally, sometimes behaviors will show through facial expression or garbled words an appreciation for the connection. Sometimes this occurs when least expected.

Case Example

Mary was visiting her sister with dementia. She had traveled from Ohio to Maryland to visit her. Her sister was unresponsive to her and Mary was upset that she didn't seem to realize that she was her sister. A few days after Mary returned home, her sister told the nurse, "You know, my sister Mary was here last week." Things register with dementia clients that are not always visible. This is important information to share with family members.

Touch

Touch is something clients with dementia can no longer ask for, create for themselves, or tell another of its

BOX 19-9	Communication Do's and Don'ts with Dementia Clients

Communication Do's

1. Simplify environmental stimuli before beginning to converse.
2. Look directly at the client when talking.
3. Ask the client what he or she would like to be called.
4. Try to identify the emotions behind the client's words or behavior.
5. Identify and minimize anything in the environment that creates anxiety for the client
6. Watch your body language; convey interest and acceptance.
7. Repeat simple messages slowly, calmly, and patiently.
8. Give clear, simple directions one at a time in a step-by-step manner.
9. Direct conversation toward concrete, familiar objects.
10. Communicate with touch, smiles, calmness, and gentle redirection.
11. Structure the environment and routines, to allow freedom within limits
12. Use soft music or hymns when the client seems agitated.

Communication Don'ts

1. Don't argue or reason with the client; instead, use distraction.
2. Avoid confrontation.
3. Don't use slang, jargon, or abstract terms.
4. If attention lapses, don't persist. Let the client rest a few minutes before trying to regain his or her attention.
5. Don't focus on difficult behavior; look for the underlying anxiety and redirect.
6. Avoid hand restraints if at all possible.
7. Avoid small objects that could be a choking hazard.

meaning. Touch is a form of communication, used to reinforce simple verbal instructions with cognitively impaired adults and as a primary form of communication. It is experienced "not only physically as sensation, but also affectively as emotion and behavior" (Kim and Buschmann, 2004, p. 35). As dementia progresses, gentle touch can anchor an anxious or disoriented person in present time, space, and humanity. When used to gain a client's attention or to guide a person toward an activity, touch can acknowledge a client's stress, calm an agitated client or provide a sense of security. In general, clients with dementia appreciate the use of touch. But to some, it can be frightening if the client perceives the caregiver as threatening. You can usually tell when a client thinks you are entering his or her personal space by looking at facial expression. Before using touch, make sure that the client is open to it.

Putting lotion on dry skin, giving back rubs, and warming cold hands or feet can be meaningful to the dementia client, as is something as simple as holding the client's hand.

When a person is no longer able to recognize familiar caregivers by name, nurturing touch provides a touchstone with the physical reality of someone who cares about the client. It may be his or her only remaining opportunity for human interaction.

REALITY ORIENTATION GROUPS

Reality orientation groups are used with older adults experiencing moderate-to-severe cognitive impairment. Focusing on their personal environment, these groups keep people in touch with time, place, and person. Topics can include landmarks in the dining room, routes to the dining room or bathroom, the date, time and weather, what people would like to wear, and so on. Reality orientation groups may be conducted daily or weekly with three to four clients (Minardi and Hayes, 2003).

VALIDATION THERAPY

Validation describes a therapeutic communication process used in later stages of dementia. Developed by Naomi Feil, validation recognizes that a client is responding to a different reality related to time, place, or person (Minardi and Hayes, 2003). Rather than confronting dementia clients with "facts"—that people they knew or places they have lived are no longer available to them—focus on the personal meaning events, and people hold for the client. For example, you might say, "Tell me about Chris," or "What was it like living on M street?"

DEFUSING CATASTROPHIC REACTIONS

Older adults with memory loss lack the cognitive ability to develop alternatives. They emotionally overreact to situations, and can have what look like temper tantrums in response to real or perceived frustration. These behavioral outbursts are called **catastrophic reactions**. Usually there is something in the immediate environment that precipitates the reaction. Fatigue, multiple demands, overstimulation, misinterpretations, or an inability to meet expectations are contributing factors (Mace and Rabins, 2011). The emotion may be appropriate, even if the way it is expressed is not. Warning signs of an impending catastrophic reaction include restlessness, body stiffening, verbal or nonverbal refusals, and general uncooperativeness.

Instead of focusing on the behavior, try to identify and eliminate the cause(s) (Hilgers, 2003). Use distraction to move the client away from the offending stimuli in the environment; use postponement. For example, you could say, "We will do that later; right now, it's time to go out on the porch," while gently leading the person away. Direct confrontation and an appeal for more civilized behavior usually serve to escalate rather than diminish the episode.

Sundowning describes behavioral symptoms occurring later in the day with dementia clients. Common behaviors include fretfulness, anxiety, and demanding behaviors. Days and nights are reversed. Keeping the client active during the day helps. Small doses of medication are used to alleviate symptoms. Caution is needed to avoid over sedating the client and preventing medication build up, which can occur when medications are metabolized more slowly.

ADVOCATING FOR THE CLIENT WITH DEMENTIA

Frail older adults, and particularly clients with dementia, usually need legal protection to safeguard their personal and financial affairs and to allow others by proxy to make health care decisions when they are unable to do so. Nurses can be advocates for clients and families in discussing health-related personal legal matters.

Advance directives and a durable power of attorney for health care (proxy) provide direction for the client's health care wishes. For financial and property manners, the client needs a durable power of attorney, a living trust, and/or a will. Power of attorney documents are subject to state laws and are only in effect when people are unable to manage their own affairs. Under federal guidelines, state laws determine qualifications for Medicaid and property distribution if a person dies with no will or trust. Medicaid qualifications may be important for families needing long-term care for a family member.

The time to execute legal documents to client rights is *before* clients become unable to cognitively assign decision-making authority to someone they trust. Clients in the early stages of dementia usually have sufficient mental competence to participate in legal decisions regarding their health care and finances. Later, they may not be able to execute the documents.

Consultation with a lawyer regarding wills, durable and health powers of attorney, and living wills should be initiated at this time (Arnold, 2005).

Once cognitive capacity is lost, a court procedure is necessary to establish a conservatorship or guardianship. This action is costly and emotionally painful for most families, as it requires legally certifying the person as incompetent. Mental incompetence is a medicolegal determination that identifies a person's inability to manage his or her personal affairs because of injury, disease, or disability. Health incompetence refers to a person's inability to make appropriate health care decisions or to carry them out, as determined by a physician or qualified health care practitioner.

Nurses should refer client family members to local Alzheimer disease and related dementia support groups. Support groups provide a place to talk about the challenges of caring for their family member. The *36-Hour Day* (Mace and Rabins, 2011), developed from the insights of family members coping with dementia in a loved one, is an excellent resource.

Caring for Clients with Advanced Dementia

Dementia is a progressive disease; clients gradually lose control over body functions and the capacity to handle even simple tasks. Meaningful verbal communication terminates. Attempts to communicate through behavior are primitive and not easily understood.

Is the self still there? It is, but in a compromised form. Dementia clients have increasingly limited ways to connect with their environment and people in a meaningful way. Touch, smiling, gentle kind approaches are meaningful. Just think what that would be like if you could no longer communicate. Family members often speak of two deaths they experience with their dementia afflicted family members—"the death of self and the actual death." Since long term memory is retained longer than short term, it is helpful to remind family members that talking or asking questions about past memories may stimulate conversations that otherwise would not be available to the dementia client. Treatment goals for clients with advanced dementia should emphasize dignity, quality of life, and supportive comfort strategies (Rabins et al., 2006). Table 19-2 identifies common neuropsychiatric symptoms associated with advanced dementia, with suggested behavioral communication interventions.

TABLE 19-2	Symptoms of Dementia with Suggested Behavioral Communication Interventions
Dementia Symptom Pattern	**Suggested Intervention**
Agitation	Identify and remove cause Assess for physical problems Reduce stimuli, suggest a walk Use simple repetitive activities: folding towels, rolling socks Use soothing music, Bible verses Look for patterns that trigger agitation
Aggression: grabbing, hitting	Recognize that the client is frightened Decrease stimuli, move client to a quiet place Do not take the client's behavior personally Respect and enlarge the client's personal space Identify and minimize cause Make eye contact; speak in a calm voice Acknowledge frustration; do not reprimand Check medications
Withdrawal: decreased socialization, apathy, social isolation	Use simple activities Find simple socialization opportunities and support client involvement
Refusal or resistance to suggestions	Drop the topic or activity and reintroduce it later
Disturbed motor activity: wandering, pacing, raiding waste cans, shadowing caregiver	Keep the environment safe Remove trash Use medical alert bracelets Label drawers, room (photos help) Use locks on doors at home
Sleep disturbances: day/night sleep reversal, calling out/moaning in sleep	Keep active during the day Toilet client as needed during night without conversation Control wandering at night; lead back to bed; avoid use of restraints
Hallucinations, delusions, illusions	Respond to the emotion, not content Reduce stimuli Use good nonglare lighting Use distraction, e.g., walk, simple activity Use touch, reassurance, postponement
Disinhibition: inappropriate speech, touching, improper body exposure, entering other people's space	Do not reprimand Respond to the emotion Redirect client to other activities
Incontinence: urine, feces, eliminating in wrong places	Check for bladder infection, fecal impaction Note elimination pattern; establish corresponding toileting timetable Schedule toileting at frequent intervals Toilet before bedtime Take client to bathroom, verbally cue Use washable clothing, Velcro closings
Swallowing difficulty: choking, stuffing mouth, not swallowing	Cut food into small pieces, offer small quantities of liquid at one time Check medications for size, modify as needed Sit with client while eating Verbally cue to chew and swallow
Agnosia: difficulty recognizing faces, including one's own	Remove or cover mirrors if client is frightened by self-image Verbally identify familiar people and their relationship to the client

SUMMARY

Communicating with older adults should be a central concern of all health care providers. Statistics reveal that older adults constitute the fastest growing population group in the United States. Aging is a universal life process with distinctive features. Although aging is associated with a progressive decline in sensory and motor functions, with appropriate supports, older adults can expect to live longer and enjoy a better quality of life than in previous generations.

Erikson's theory of psychosocial development identifies integrity versus despair as the central crisis of old age. People who believe that their lives have purpose and meaning and that they have few or no regrets about a well-lived life demonstrate the ego strength of integrity. Supportive communication and empowerment strategies assist clients in maximizing their health and well-being.

Chapter 19 presents current understandings about the course of dementia and discusses related communication strategies with clients and families. Differential assessment of depression, delirium, and dementia is important, as symptoms can appear similar. Communication strategies with clients with dementia emphasize verbal supports. Helping clients tell their story, promoting client autonomy, using a proactive approach in conversations, acting as a client advocate, and treating older adults with dignity are proposed. Health promotion activities that take into account the unique needs and cultural values of older adults are more likely to be successful. As a primary provider in long-term care and in the community, the nurse is in a unique role to support and meet the communication needs of older adult clients.

ETHICAL DILEMMA | What Would You Do?

Mrs. Allan is an accomplished 82 year old woman, living alone. She treasures her independence. While she realizes she is more frail, she does not want to leave her home or lose her independence. Her daughter is worried about her and wants her to move to assisted living. During your initial assessment for a recent fall, Mrs. Allen confides that she too is worried about memory lapses, but she can't bear the idea of what assisted living will mean for her independence and quality of life. She asks you to keep her confidence. You can understand Mrs. Allen's concerns but you also know that keeping silent may not be in her best interest. How could you balance the ethical concept of beneficence with your client's concerns. What would you do?

DISCUSSION QUESTIONS

1. What are some examples of ageism affecting older adults?
2. How is ageism perpetuated?
3. From an advocacy perspective, how could you as a nurse help create a more positive image of older adults?

REFERENCES

Adelman M, Greene M, Ory M, et al.: Communication between older patients and their physicians, *Clin Geriatr Med* 16(1):1–24, 2000.

Anderson D: Preventing delirium in older people, 73-74 *Br Med Bull* 25–34, 2005.

Arnold E: Sorting out the 3 D's: delirium, dementia, depression, *Holist Nurs Pract* 19(3):99–104, 2005.

Avolio M, Montagnoli S, Marino D, et al.: Factors influencing quality of life for disabled and nondisabled elderly population: The results of a multiple correspondence analysis, *Curr Gerontol Geriatr Res* 2013:258–274, 2013. http://dx.doi.org/10.1155/2013/258274. Epub 2013 Jun 27.

Biggs S: Toward critical narrativity: stories of aging in contemporary social policy, *J Aging Stud* 15(4):301–316, 2001.

Bishop A: Stress and depression among older residents in religious monasteries: do friends and God matter? *Int J Aging Hum Dev* 67(1):1–23, 2008.

Bohlmeijer E, Kramer J, Smit F, et al.: The effects of integrative reminiscence on depressive symptomatology and mastery of older adults, *Community Ment Health J* 45:476–484, 2009.

Bonder BR, Dal Bello-Haas V: *Functional performance in older adults*, ed 3, Philadelphia, 2009, FA Davis.

Bortz W: Use it or lose it, *Runner's World* 25:55–58, 1990.

Burke M, Laramie J: *Primary care of the older adult: a multidisciplinary approach*, ed 2, St. Louis, 2004, Mosby.

Cavalieri T: Management of pain in older adults, suppl *J AM Osteopath Assoc* 105(3):12S–17S, 2005.

Constanca P, Ribeiro O, Teixeira L: Active ageing: An empirical approach to the WHO model, *Curr Gerontol Geriatr Res*. 2012: 382–972. http://dx.doi.org/10.1155/2012/382972. Epub 2012 Oct 31.

Cochran P: Acute care for elders prevents functional decline, *Nursing* 35(10):70–71, 2005.

Corey M, Corey G: Groups for the elderly. *Groups: process and practice*, ed 7, Belmont, CA, 2006, Thompson Brooks/Cole.

Cotter V: Hope in early-stage dementia: a concept analysis, *Holist Nurs Pract* 23(5):297–301, 2009.

Cotter V, Gonzalez E: Self-concept in older adults: an integrative review of empirical literature, *Holist Nurs Pract* 23(6):335–348, 2009.

Curry L, Walker C, Hogstel M, et al.: Teaching older adults to self-manage medications: preventing adverse drug reactions, *J Gerontol Nurs* 31(4):32–42, 2005.

Delgado C: Meeting clients' spiritual needs, *Nurs Clin North Am* 42(2):279–293, 2007.

Ebrahimi Z, Wilhelmson K, Moore C, Jakobsson A: Health despite frailty: Exploring influences on frail older adults experiences of health, *Geriatr Nurs* 34:289–294, 2013.

Erikson E: *Identity and the Life Cycle*, New York, 1980, Norton.

Erikson E: *The life cycle completed: A Review*, New York, 1982, Norton.

Feldt K: Pain assessment in older adults. In Jansen M, editor: *Managing pain in older adults*, New York, 2008, Springer, pp 35–54.

Folstein M, Folstein S, McHugh PR, et al.: Mini-mental state: a practical method for grading cognition state of clients for the clinician, *J Psychiatr Res* 12:189–198, 1975.

Franklin LL, Ternestedt BM, Nordenfelt L: Views on dignity of elderly nursing home residents, *Nurs Ethics* 13(2):130–146, 2006.

Gallo J: *Handbook of geriatric assessment*, ed 3, Gaithersburg, MD, 2000, Aspen.

Gloth F: *Handbook of pain relief in older adults*, Totowa, NJ, 2004, Humana Press.

Gonsalves C, Pichora-Fuller MK: The effect of hearing loss and hearing aids on the use of information and communication technologies by community-living older adults, *Can J Aging* 27(2):145–157, 2008.

Gould E, Mitty E: Medication adherence is a partnership, medication compliance is not, *Geriatr Nurs* 31:290–298, 2010.

Happ MB: Individualized care for frail older adults: Challenges for health care reform in acute and critical care, *Gerontol Nurs* 31(1):63–65, 2010.

Heliker D: Enhancing relationships in long-term care: through story sharing, *J Gerontol Nurs* 35(6):43–49, 2009.

Henderson DA, Gladding ST: Group counseling with older adults. In DeLucia-Waack JL, Gerrity DA, Kalodner CR, editors: *Handbook of group counseling and psychotherapy*, Thousand Oaks, CA, 2004, Sage.

Herr K: Pain in the older adult: An imperative across all health care settings, *Pain Manag Nurs* 11(2 suppl):S1–10, 2010.

Herr K: *Retooling pain assessment for older adults. Presentation at the American pain Society, 32nd Annual Scientific Meeting*, New Orleans, 2013, Louisiana. May 14, 2013.

Hilgers J: Comforting a confused client, *Nursing* 33(1):48–50, 2003.

Institute of Medicine: *Retooling for an Aging America: Building the Health Care Workforce*, Washington, DC, 2008, National Academies Press.

Ito M, Takahashi R, Liehr P, et al.: Heeding the behavioral message of elders with dementia in day care, *Holist Nurs Pract* 21(1):12–18, 2007.

Jansen M: Common pain syndromes in older adults. In Jansen M, editor: *Managing pain in older adults*, New York, 2008, Springer, pp 17–34.

Jonsdottir H, Jonsdottir G, Steingrimsdottir E, et al.: Group reminiscence among people with end-stage chronic lung diseases, *J Adv Nurs* 35(1):79–87, 2001.

Kagan S: Gotcha! Don't let ageism sneak into your practice, *Geriatr Nurs* 33(1):60–62, 2012.

Kim E, Buschmann M: Touch—stress model and Alzheimer's disease, *J Gerontol Nurs* 30(12):33–39, 2004.

Kleinpell R: Supporting independence in hospitalized elders in acute care, *Crit Care Nurs Clin North Am* 19(3):247–252, 2007.

Kochkin S: MarkeTrak VIII: 25-year trends in the hearing health market, *Hearing Rev* 16(11):12–31, 2009.

Lang J, Moore M, Harris A, et al.: Healthy aging: priorities and programs of the Centers for Disease Control and Prevention, *Generations* 29(2):24–29, 2005.

Le T: Cultural values, life experiences, and wisdom, *Int J Aging Hum Dev* 66(4):259–281, 2008.

Leuven K: Population aging: implications for nurse practitioners, *JNP* 8(7):554–559, 2012.

Lord S: Visual risk factors for falls in older people, *Age Ageing* 35(Suppl 2): ii42–ii45, 2006.

Mace N, Rabins P: *The 36-hour day: a family guide to caring for people with Alzheimer's disease, other dementias, and memory loss*, ed 5, Baltimore, MD, 2011, Johns Hopkins University.

MacKinlay E: Resistance, resilience, and change: The person and dementia, *J Religion Spirituality Aging* 24:80–92, 2012.

Maslow A: *Motivation and personality*, New York, 1954, Harper & Row.

Mauk KL: Healthier aging: reaching and teaching older adults, *Holist Nurs Pract* 20(3):158, 2006.

Mauk KL: *Gerontological Nursing: Competencies for Care*, Boston, 2010, Jones & Bartlett.

McCarthy B: *Hearing the person with dementia: person centered approaches*, Philadelphia PA, 2011, Jessica Kingsley.

Miller C: Communication difficulties in hospitalized older adults with dementia, *Am J Nurs* 108(3):58–66, 2008.

Miller C: *Nursing for wellness in older adults*, ed 6, Philadelphia, 2011, Lippincott Williams & Wilkins.

Minardi H, Hayes N: Nursing older adults with mental health problems: therapeutic interventions—part 2, *Nurs Older People* 15(7):20–24, 2003.

Mitty E: Iatrogenesis, frailty, and geriatric syndromes, *Geriatr Nurs* 31:368–374, 2010.

Moody H: *Aging: concepts and controversies*, Thousand Oaks, CA, 2010, Pine Forge Press.

Murray LM, Boyd S: Protecting personhood and achieving quality of life for older adults with dementia in the U.S. health care system, *J Aging Health* 21:350–373, 2009.

Nakasato Y, Carnes B: Health promotion in older adults: promoting successful aging in primary care settings, *Geriatrics* 61(4):27–31, 2006.

Nerenberg L: *Elder abuse prevention: emerging trends and promising strategies*, New York, 2008, Springer.

National Institute on Deafness and Other Communication Disorders (NIDCD): *Hearing loss and older adults*, . Available at www.nidcd.nih .gov/health/hearing/older.asp, 2013. Accessed August 23, 2014.

Ownby R: Medication adherence and cognition: medical, personal and economic factors influence level of adherence in older adults, *Geriatrics* 61(2):30–35, 2006.

Pankow L, Solotoroff J: *Biological aspects and theories of aging. Handbook of gerontology: evidence-based approaches to theory, practice, and policy*, Hoboken, NJ, 2007, Wiley. 19–56.

Penprase B: Developing comprehensive health care for an underserved population, *Geriatr Nurs* 27(1):45–50, 2006.

Potempa K, Butterworth S, Flaherty-Robb, Gaynor W: The healthy ageing model: health behaviors for older adults, *Collegian* 04(008):51–55, 2010.

Pryce H, Gooberman R: There's a heal of a noise: Living with a hearing loss in residential care, *Age Ageing* 41:40–46, 2012.

Rabins P, Lyketsos C, Steele C, et al.: *Practical dementia care*, ed 2, New York, 2006, Oxford University Press.

Rowan N, Faul A A: Substance abuse. In Blackburn J, Dulmus C, editors: *Handbook of gerontology: evidence-based approaches to theory, practice, and policy*, Hoboken, NJ, 2007, Wiley, pp 309–332.

Reichstadt M, Sengupta G, Depp C, Palinkas L, Jeste D: Older adults' perspectives on successful aging. Qualitative Interviews, *Am J Geriatr Psychiatry* 18(7):567–575, 2010.

Resnick B: New and exciting opportunities to promote health among older adults, *Geriatr Nurs* 34:9–11, 2013.

Schearer NB: Health empowerment theory as a guide for practice, *Geriatr Nurs* suppl 2:4–10, 2009.

Scholder J, Kagan S, Schumann MJ, et al.: Nursing competence in aging overview, *Nurs Clin North Am* 39:429–442, 2004.

Strine T, Chapman D DP, Balluz L, et al.: Health-related quality of life and health behaviors by social and emotional support: their relevance to psychiatry and medicine, *Soc Psychiatry Psychiatr Epidemiol* 43:151–159, 2008.

Touhy T, Jett K: *Ebersole and Hess' Toward healthy aging: Human needs and nursing response*, St. Louis, MO, 2012, Elsevier.

U.S. Department of Health and Human Services (DHHS). (2010) *Healthy People 2020*. Available at http//www.Healthypeople2020. Accessed July 19, 2013.

Werner C. (2010) *The older population: 2010. 2010 census briefs*. U.S. Department of Commerce Economics and Statistics Administration http://www.census.gov/prod/cen2010/briefs/c2010br-09.pdf

Whiteside M, Wallhagen M, Pettengill E, et al.: Sensory impairment in older adults: part 2: vision loss, *Am J Nurs* 106(11):52–61, 2006.

Windsor T, Anstey K: Volunteering and psychological well-being among young-old adults: how much is too much, *Gerontologist* 48(1):59–70, 2008.

World Health organization (WHO): *Active Ageing: A Policy Framework*, . http://whqlibdoc.who.int/hq/2002/WHO_NMH_NPH_02.8.pdf, 2002.

Yuhas N, McGowan B, Fontaine T, et al.: Interventions for disruptive symptoms of dementia, *J Psychosoc Nurs* 44(11):34–42, 2006.

Zysberg L, Young H, Schepp: Trait routinization, functional and cognitive status in older adults, *Int J Aging Hum Dev* 69(1):17–29, 2009.

Communicating with Clients in Crisis

Elizabeth C. Arnold

OBJECTIVES

At the end of the chapter, the reader will be able to:
1. Define crisis and related concepts.
2. Discuss theoretical frameworks related to crisis and crisis intervention.
3. Identify and apply structured crisis intervention strategies in the care of clients experiencing a crisis state.
4. Apply crisis intervention strategies to mental health emergencies.
5. Discuss crisis management strategies in disaster and mass trauma situations.

The purpose of Chapter 20 is to describe communication strategies nurses can use with clients and families experiencing a crisis situation. The chapter describes the nature of crisis and identifies its theoretical foundations. The application section provides practical guidelines nurses can use with clients in crisis, mental health emergencies, and disaster management.

BASIC CONCEPTS

DEFINITIONS

CRISIS

Flannery and Everly (2000) state, "A *crisis* occurs when a stressful life event overwhelms an individual's ability to cope effectively in the face of a perceived challenge or threat" (p. 119). People in a crisis state experience an actual or perceived overwhelming threat to self-concept, an insurmountable obstacle or a loss that conventional coping measures cannot handle. Unabated, the resulting tension continues to increase, creating major personality disorganization and a crisis state.

The word *crisis* comes from the Greek root word *krinen,* meaning "to decide, and in Latin, crisis means the turning point of a disease" (MacNeil Vroomen et al., 2013, p. 10). Personal responses to crisis can be adaptive or maladaptive. Nurses can help clients with restorative coping strategies to lessen the damaging impact of crisis. Successfully working through a crisis has the potential to strengthen people's coping responses and encourage a sense of self-efficacy. Maladaptive responses can result in the development of acute or chronic psychiatric symptoms.

Crisis State

Everly (2000) defines a ***crisis state*** as an acute *normal* human response to severely abnormal circumstances. A crisis state is *not* a mental illness, although individuals with mental illness can experience a crisis state associated with their disorder. Crisis is a complex concept, which can defy easy cause/effect explanations (James, 2008). Because a crisis state represents a personal response, two people experiencing the same crisis event will respond differently to it. Understanding the client's personal response to a crisis rather than an objective crisis stressor is critical to successful crisis intervention.

A crisis state creates a temporary disconnect from attachment to others, loss of meaning, and disruption of previous mastery skills (Flannery and Everly, 2000).

Individuals feel vulnerable. Crisis intervention strategies are designed to help support people experiencing crisis achieve psychological homeostasis. A favorable outcome depends on the person's combined interpretation of the crisis, perception of coping ability, resources, and level of social support.

TYPES OF CRISIS

Developmental Crises

A crisis is classified as developmental or situational. Erik Erikson's (1982) stage model of psychosocial development forms the basis for exploring the nature of developmental crisis. Developmental crisis can occur as individuals negotiate developmental age-related milestones in their life, for example becoming a parent or retiring from long-term employment. Normative psychosocial crisis are used as benchmarks for assessing signs and symptoms of developmental crisis. When a situational crisis is superimposed on a normative developmental crisis, the crisis experience can be more intense. For example, a woman losing a spouse at the same time she is going through menopause can experience a more intense impact.

Situational Crises

A situational crisis refers to an unusually stressful life event, which exceeds a person's resources and coping skills. Examples include unexpected illness or injury, rape, car accident, loss of home, spouse, or being laid off from a job. When the crisis impacts a large number of people simultaneously, for example, a disaster, it is referred to as an *adventitious crisis* (Michalopoulos and Michalopoulos, 2009). A situational crisis is *not* defined by the life event itself, but by the individual's personal response to it (Hoff, 2009). How successfully a person responds to a crisis can depend on

- Previous experience with crises, coping, and problem solving
- Perception of the crisis event
- Level of help or obstruction from significant others
- Developmental level and ego maturity
- Concurrent stressors

Behavioral Emergencies

James and Gilliland (2013) state that a ***behavioral emergency*** occurs "when a crisis escalates to the point that the situation requires immediate intervention to avoid injury or death" (p. 8). Examples include any type of violent interpersonal behavior, psychotic crisis, intentional or passive suicide, or homicide, in short, any type of thinking or behavior that places an individual in an immediate potentially injurious or lethal situation. A behavioral emergency is always an emotionally charged, unpredictable situation (Kleespies, 2009).

CRISIS INTERVENTION

Crisis intervention represents a systematic application of theory-based problem-solving strategies designed to help individuals and families resolve a crisis situation quickly and successfully. The desired clinical outcome is a return to an individual's pre-crisis functional level (Roberts and Yeager 2009). Crisis intervention strategies should be adapted to fit each client's preferences, beliefs, values, and individual circumstances. As a nurse, you cannot always change the nature of a crisis situation, but you can help defuse a client's emotional reaction to it with compassionate professional support and guidance.

Crisis intervention is a *time-limited* treatment. Four to six weeks is considered the standard time frame for crisis resolution. Interventions should be present-focused and action-oriented. The emphasis is on *immediate problem solving* and *strengthening personal resources* of clients and their families. Full recovery can take a much longer period of time, particularly from a disaster crisis (Callahan, 1998). Nurses function as advocates, resources, partners, and guides in helping clients resolve crisis situations, usually as part of a larger crisis intervention team.

THEORETICAL FRAMEWORKS

Erich Lindemann (1944) and Gerald Caplan (1964) developed the most widely used models of crisis and crisis intervention. Lindemann's (1944) study of bereavement provides a frame of reference for understanding the stages involved in resolving emotional crisis and bereavement. His findings suggest, "Proper psychiatric management of grief reactions may prevent prolonged and serious alterations in the patient's social adjustment, as well as potential medical disease" (p. 147).

Caplan broadened Lindemann's model to include developmental crisis and personal crisis (Roberts, 2005). Although the focus of crisis intervention is on secondary prevention because the crisis state is already in motion, Caplan's model of preventive psychiatry starts in the community. He introduced practical crisis intervention strategies, for example, crisis telephone lines, training for community workers, and early response strategies. He viewed nurses as key service providers in crisis intervention.

Caplan discusses a crisis response pattern. He identifies a person's initial response to a crisis state as *shock*, with varied emotions, ranging from anger, laughing, hysterics, crying, and acute anxiety to social withdrawal. Then follows an extended period of adjustment, a period of *recoil*, which can last from 2 to 3 weeks. Behavior appears normal to outsiders, but clients describe nightmares, phobic reactions, and flashbacks of the crisis event.

Restoration or reconstruction describes the final phase of crisis intervention. This phase involves developing a plan and taking constructive actions to resolve the crisis situation. If successfully negotiated, the person returns to a pre-crisis functional level, which is the desired clinical outcome. Maladaptive coping strategies such as drug or alcohol use, violence, or avoidance, prevents restoration and places the client person is at risk for further problems.

The nursing model developed by Donna Aguilera (1998) approaches crisis intervention from a balancing perspective between a crisis situation and a client's capacity to resolve it. The model proposes that a crisis state develops because of a distorted perception of a situation or because the client lacks the resources to cope successfully with it. Balancing factors include a realistic perception of the event, the client's internal resources (beliefs or attitudes), and the client's external (environmental) supports. These factors can minimize or reduce the impact of the stressor, leading to the resolution of the crisis.

Absence of adequate situational support, lack of coping skills, and a distorted perception of the crisis event can result in a crisis state, leaving individuals and families feeling overwhelmed and unable to cope. Interventions are designed to increase the balancing factors needed to restore a client to pre-crisis functioning. Exercise 20-1 provides insight into the nature of crisis.

Developing an Evidence-Based Practice

Patel A, Roston A, Tilmon S, et al: Assessing the extent of provision of comprehensive medical care management for female sexual assault patients in US hospital emergency departments, *Int J Gynaecol Obstet* 123(1):24-28, 2013.

Purpose: This cross-sectional study was conducted to identify the level and quality of emergency medical services provided to sexual assault patients in U.S. emergency departments. Using a telephone survey, the researchers assessed provision of emergency department services to sexual assault survivors across 582 U.S. hospital emergency departments.

Results: All emergency departments provided acute medical care, but only 17.4% provided all 10 elements of comprehensive medical care management (CMCM), and only 40% provided rape crisis counseling.

Application to your clinical practice: Because the emergency department is the primary point of care for most sexual assault victims, this study strongly suggests the need for quality comprehensive rape crisis care. What implications do you see in your nursing practice for promoting safe, effective client-centered care in the emergency department?

EXERCISE 20-1 Understanding the Nature of Crisis

Purpose: To help students understand crisis in preparation for assessing and planning communication strategies in crisis situations.

Procedure

1. Describe a crisis you experienced in your life. There are no right or wrong definitions of a crisis, and it does not matter whether the crisis would be considered a crisis in someone else's life.
2. Identify how the crisis changed your roles, routines, relationships, and assumptions about yourself.
3. Apply a crisis model to the situation you are describing.
4. Identify the strategies you used to cope with the crisis.
5. Describe the ways in which your personal crisis strengthened or weakened your self-concept and increased your options and your understanding of life.

Discussion

What did you learn from doing this exercise that you can use in your clinical practice?

APPLICATIONS

The goal of crisis intervention is to return the client to his or her previous level of functioning. This goal is evidenced by

- Stabilization of distress symptoms
- Reduction of distress symptoms
- Restoration of functional capabilities
- Referrals for follow-up support care, if indicated (Everly, 2000, pp. 1-2)

STRUCTURING CRISIS INTERVENTION STRATEGIES

Roberts (2005) provides a seven-stage sequential blueprint for clinical intervention, which can be used to structure the crisis intervention process in nurse-client relationships. This model is compatible with the nursing process sequence of assessment, planning, implementation, and evaluation.

STEP 1 (ASSESSMENT): ASSESSING LETHALITY AND MENTAL STATUS

Initially, assessment should focus on determining the severity a client's current danger potential—both to self and to others. Box 20-1 presents a field expedient

BOX 20-1	Field Expedient Tool to Assess Dangerousness to Self or Others

Depression/suicidal
Anger/agitation, aggressive
Noncompliance with requests/taking medication
General appearance/inappropriate dress/poor hygiene
Evidence of self-inflicted injury
Responding/reacting to delusions or hallucinations
Owns/displays weapon(s)
Unorganized thoughts/appearance/behavior
Speech pattern/substance/rate (too fast, too slow, jumps all over)
Paranoid
Erratic or fearful behavior
Recent loss of job/loved one/home
Substance abuse
Orientation to date/time/location/situation/insight into illness
Number and type of previous contacts with police, mental health, or crisis workers

From Officer Scott A Davis, Crisis Intervention Team (CIT) Coordinator: *Field expedient tool to assess dangerousness to self or others*, Rockville, MD, February 2010a, Montgomery County Police Department.

tool for initial assessment of a potential behavioral emergency. Crisis intervention teams (CIT) developed and use this tool to assess potential dangerous client behaviors. Psychotic individuals and those under the influence of drugs, who are severely agitated or temporarily out of control for medical reasons, require immediate triage to stabilize their physical and mental condition. Crisis states complicated by delirium or nonlethal self-harm necessitate high-priority medical attention before addressing crisis intervention issues. With the downturn in the economy, more clients are presenting in the community as mental health emergencies.

STEP 2: ESTABLISHING RAPPORT AND ENGAGING THE CLIENT

Once the initial triage assessment of a client in crisis is completed, the nurse performs a more comprehensive crisis appraisal. This assessment should be specific to the client's current state and circumstances. Clients in crisis look to health professionals to structure interactions. Introduce yourself briefly, and quickly orient the client to the purpose of the crisis questions and how the information will be used. Health Insurance Portability and Accountability Act (HIPAA) of 1996 regulations require confidentiality. If clients expect family members to give or receive information to health providers when the client is not present, the client needs to sign a consent form.

Clients experiencing a crisis state require a compassionate, flexible, but clearly directive calm approach from nurses. Place the client in a quiet, lighted room with no shadows, away from the mainstream of activity. Avoid the use of touch, as the client may be supersensitive to any form of unexpected response from a health professional. If there is a need to restrain a client temporarily, explain what is happening simply and directly. Use fewer rather than more words to explain.

Only a minimum number of people should be involved with the client, until the client has calmed down. If the client is unable to cooperate, for safety reasons, more than one professional may be needed to stabilize the situation. Depending on the nature of the crisis and client's personal responses, a trusted family member may be included.

Speak calmly and use short, clear, direct phrases and questions. James and Gilliland (2013) advocate the use of closed-ended questions in the *early* stages of crisis intervention related to safety issues, requesting specific information, and eliciting a client commitment to immediate action needed to stabilize the crisis situation.

Careful, accurate listening skills are essential. It is important to find out the client's perception of the crisis—how it developed, how it impacts the client's life, is this a first encounter with a serious crisis, or one of many that the client has experienced? Questions to assess the client's perception of his or her emotional coping strength are important. James (2008) suggests asking question such as "How were you feeling about this before the crisis got so bad?" "Where do you see yourself headed with this problem?" (p. 51).

Use reflective listening responses to identify feelings (e.g., "It sounds as if you are feeling very sad [angry, lonely] right now."). You can help clients focus on relevant points by repeating a phrase, asking for validation or clarification to focus the discussion. Family and significant others can provide essential data related to the client's current crisis state (e.g., documenting changes in behavior, ingestion of drugs, or medical history) if the client is unable to do so.

Exercise 20-2 offers an opportunity to understand reflection as a listening response in crisis situations.

STEP 3 (ASSESSMENT): IDENTIFYING MAJOR PROBLEMS

Keep the focus on the here and now. Questions should be short and relevant to the crisis.

Request more specific details (e.g., ask who was involved, what happened, and when it happened) if this information is needed.

Ask about the feelings associated with the immediate crisis.

Responses to clients should be brief, empathetic, and clearly related to the client's story.

Note changes in expression, body posture, and vocal inflections as clients tell their story and at what points they occur. Be alert for escalation of agitation or verbal outbursts.

Identify central emotional themes in the client's story (e.g., powerlessness, shame, hopelessness) to provide a focus for intervention.

Proceed slowly with a calm tone and direct communication.

Affirm client efforts and offer encouragement.

Summarize content often and ask for validation so that you and your client are on the same page, with a comprehensive understanding of major issues. Periodically ask the client to summarize thoughts. Check for personal reservations about part or the entire plan.

Identifying Feelings

Clients can have difficulty putting crisis emotions into words because of high anxiety. Nurses can help clients clarify important feelings with observations about client response (e.g., "I wonder if because you think your son is using drugs [*precipitating event*], you feel helpless and confused [*client emotional response*], and don't know what to do next [*client behavioral reaction*].")."Does that capture what is going on with you?" Checking in with clients helps ensure that your interpretations represent the client's truth.

Clients in crisis tend to develop tunnel vision (Dass-Brailsford, 2010). Often, they feel there is no solution. Losing sight of personal assets and potential reserves, which could be used to defuse the crisis, some clients are frightened by the intensity of their emotional

---

| EXERCISE 20-2 | Using Reflective Responses in a Crisis Situation |

Purpose: To provide students with a means of appreciating the multipurpose uses of reflection as a listening response in crisis situations.

Procedure
Have one student role-play a client in an emergency department situation involving a common crisis situation (e.g., fire, heart attack, auto accident). After this person talks about the crisis situation for 3 to 4 minutes, have each student write down a reflective listening response that they would use with the client in crisis. Have each student read their reflective response to the class. (This can also be done in small groups of students if the class is large.)

Discussion
1. Were you surprised at the variety of reflective themes found in the students' responses?
2. In what ways could differences in the wording or emphasis of a reflective response influence the flow of information?
3. In what ways do reflective responses validate the client's experience?
4. How could you use what you learned from doing this exercise in your clinical practice?

reactions Clients appreciate hearing that most people experience powerful and conflicting feelings in crisis situations. The message you want to get across is "you are not alone, and together we can come up with a plan to deal with this difficult situation." Global reassurance is not helpful, but specific supportive comments that recognize client efforts can help clients to de-escalate a crisis event to workable proportions.

Affirming Personal Strengths

Compassionate witnessing defined as "noticing and feeling empathy for others" (Powley, 2009, p. 1303) helps to broaden a client's perspective. When combined with social supports and community resources, professional compassionate witnessing of the situation and calling attention to personal strengths can significantly enhance coping skills. For example, financial resources and knowledge about accessing health care services are critical assets people lose sight of in crisis situations. Reinforce personal strengths as you observe them or as the client identifies them. Exercise 20-3 provides an opportunity to experience the value of personal support systems in crisis situations.

Providing Explicit Information

Being truthful about what is known and unknown and updating information as you learn about it helps build trust with clients in crisis. Even with unknowns, people cope better when uncertainty is briefly acknowledged, rather than not mentioned. Explain what is going to happen, step by step. Letting clients know

as much as possible about progress, treatment, and the consequences of choosing different alternatives allows clients to make informed decisions and reduces the heightened anxiety associated with a crisis situation.

STEP 4 (PLANNING): EXPLORING ALTERNATIVE OPTIONS AND PARTIAL SOLUTIONS

Step 4 strategies focus on broadening client perspective by looking at partial solutions. Breaking tasks down into small, achievable parts empowers clients. Proposed strategies should accommodate both the immediate problems and client resources. You can assist clients in discussing the consequences, costs, and benefits of choosing of one action versus another (e.g., "What would happen if you choose this course of action as compared with…?" or "What is the worst that could happen if you decided to…?"). Making autonomous choices helps clients reestablish control. Even a small decision encourages clients to become invested in the solution-finding process and hopeful about finding a resolution to a crisis situation.

Involving Immediate Support Systems and Community Resources

Accessing immediate social supports, and available community resources provide a buffer and can act a source of information and sounding board for individuals in a crisis state. *Support networks* provide practical advice and a sense of security. They are a source of encouragement that can reaffirm a client's worth and help defuse anxiety associated with the uncertainty of

---

| EXERCISE 20-3 | **Personal Support Systems** |

Purpose: To help students appreciate the breadth and importance of personal support systems in stressful situations.

Procedure
All of us have support systems we can use in times of stress (e.g., church, friends, family, coworkers, clubs, recreational groups).
1. Identify a support person or system you could or do use in a time of crisis.
2. Reflect on why you would choose this person or support system.
3. What does this personal support system or person do for you (e.g., listen without judgment; provide honest, objective feedback; challenge you to think; broaden your perspective; give

unconditional support; share your perceptions)? List everything you can think of.
4. What factors go into choosing your personal support system (e.g., availability, expertise, perception of support)? Which is the most important factor?

Discussion
1. What types of support systems were most commonly used by class or group members?
2. What were the most common reasons for selecting a support person or system?
3. After doing this exercise, what strategies would you advise for enlarging a personal support system?
4. What applications do you see in this exercise for your nursing practice?

a crisis situation. In addition to inquiring about the number and variety of people in the client's support network, find out, "who does the client and/or family trust" and "who would the client be most comfortable telling about their situation." It is helpful to learn when the client and/or family last had contact with the identified person. In crisis situations, many clients and families temporarily withdraw from natural support systems and may need encouragement to reconnect.

STEP 5 (PLANNING): DEVELOP A REALISTIC ACTION PLAN

Crisis intervention "is action-oriented and situation focused" (Dass-Brailsford, 2010, p. 56). Formulating a realistic action plan starts with prioritizing identified problems and related essential action steps. An effective crisis plan should have a practical, here-and-now, therapeutic, short-term focus and should reflect the client's choices about best options. Stabilization of the client through guidance, careful listening, and developing small viable plans helps defuse the sense of helplessness in a crisis situation.

Focus on the Present

Help your clients to think in terms of short time intervals and immediate next steps (e.g., "What can you do with the rest of today just to get through it better"?) Examples include getting more information, gathering essential data, taking a walk, calling a family member, taking time for self. When people begin to take even the smallest step, they gain a sense of control, and this stimulates hope for future mastery of the crisis situation. Thinking about crisis resolution as a whole is counterproductive.

Incorporate Previously Successful Coping Strategies

Looking at past coping strategies can sometimes reveal skills that could be used in resolving the current crisis situation. Ask, "What do you usually do when you have a problem?" or "To whom do you turn when you are in trouble?" Explore the nature of tension-reducing strategies the client has used in the past (e.g., aerobics, Bible study, calling a friend). If the client seems immobilized and unable to give an answer about usual coping strategies, you can offer prompts such as "Some people talk to their friends, bang walls, pray, go to church..." Usually, with verbal encouragement, clients begin to identify successful coping mechanisms, which can be built on, for use in resolving the current crisis.

STEP 6 (IMPLEMENTATION): DEVELOPING AN ACTION PLAN
Developing Reasonable Goals

Crisis offers clients an opportunity to discover and develop new self-awareness about things that are important to them. Developing realistic goals is a critical component of crisis intervention. This process includes becoming aware of choices, letting go of ideas that are toxic or self-defeating, and making the best choice among the viable options. Goal-directed activities should reflect the client's strengths, values, capabilities, beliefs, and preferences. Tangible, achievable goals give clients and families hope that they can get to a different place with resolving their crisis. Goals with meaning to the client are more likely to be accomplished.

Designing Achievable Tasks

Help clients choose tasks that are within their capabilities, circumstances, and energy level. Achievable tasks can be as simple as getting more information or making time for self. You can suggest, "What do you think needs to happen first?" or "Let's look at what you might be able to do quickly." Engaging clients in simple problem solving reduces crisis-related feelings of helplessness and hopelessness. Problem-solving tasks that strengthen the client's realistic perception of the crisis event, incorporate a client's beliefs and values, and integrate social and environmental supports offer the best chance for success. Greene and colleagues (2005) suggest that helping clients tap into and use their personal resources to achieve goals facilitates crisis resolution and provides individuals with tools for further personal development.

Providing Structure and Encouragement

Clients need structure and encouragement as they perform the tasks that will move them forward. Setting time limits and monitoring task achievement is important.

Resolving a crisis state is not a straightforward movement. There will be setbacks. Clients need ongoing affirmation of their efforts. Supportive reinforcement includes validation of the struggles clients are coping with, anticipatory guidance regarding what to expect, and discussion of ambivalent feelings, uncertainty, and fears surrounding the process. Comparing progressive functioning with baseline admission presentations helps nurses and their clients mutually evaluate progress, foresee areas of necessary focus, and monitor progress toward treatment goals.

Providing Support for Families

Crisis intervention strategies should include support for family members. A crisis affects family dynamics, such that each family member is coping with some sort of emotional fallout brought about by the client's crisis. Additionally, there may be issues requiring family response to an unstable home environment created by the client's absence or an inability to function in their previous roles. There may be legal or safety issues that family members also have to address.

Individual family members experience a crisis in diverse ways, so different levels of information and support will be required. Bluhm (1987) suggests picturing the family as "a group of people standing together, with arms interlocked. What happens if one family member becomes seriously ill and can no longer stand? The other family members will attempt to carry their loved one, each person shifting his weight to accommodate the additional burden" (p. 44). Giving families an opportunity to talk about the meaning of the crisis for each family member and offering practical guidance about resources they can use to support the client and take care of themselves are important strategies nurses can use with families. Communication strategies the nurse can use to help families in crisis are presented in Box 20-2.

STEP 7 (EVALUATION): DEVELOPING A TERMINATION AND FOLLOW-UP PROTOCOL

Kavan and colleagues (2006) note, "Follow-up provides patients with a lifeline and improves the likelihood that they still follow through with the action plan" (p. 1164). Clients should receive verbal instructions, with *written* discharge or follow-up directives, and phone numbers to call for added help or clarification. Although acute symptoms subside with standard crisis intervention strategies, many clients will need follow-up for residual clinical issues.

Mobilize community resources to provide essential supports. Some clients are reluctant to use social services, medications, or mental health services, even short term, because of the stigma they feel about their use. Others are cautious about the need for follow up. Nurses can help clients and families sort out their concerns, assess their practicality, and develop viable contacts. If indicated, nurses can facilitate the referral process by sharing information with community agencies and by giving clients enough information to follow through on getting additional assistance. Having written referral information available regarding eligibility requirements, location, cost, and accessibility can make a difference in client interest and compliance. Exercise 20-4 provides an opportunity to practice crisis intervention skills.

MENTAL HEALTH EMERGENCIES

Mental health emergencies present significant challenges for nurses. Whether encountered in the community, or with clients admitted to an emergency department, these clients often present as a danger to themselves or others. They present with chaotic distress behaviors, which are not under the client's control.

In addition to mental health emergencies, nurses should be aware of the presentation of co-occurring disorders. A person with a co-occurring disorder presents with both a mental illness and a substance use disorder (SUD). Often these clients will stop taking their prescribed psychotropic medications and instead self-medicate with other, non-prescribed medications (sometimes from other family or friends) or illicit drugs or alcohol. Clients may feel their psychiatric symptoms subside or even go away for a while when they self-medicate. The problems arise with the propensity of overdose and the possibility of going into drug-induced delirium (also known in the law enforcement field as "excited delirium") or other somatic (heart issues) or drug-induced effects (difficulty driving, impulsive behavior, etc.). Nurses should be aware that these patients may present at the emergency department sometimes seeking legitimate care for their symptoms or may present to "Doc Shop" and obtain medications (narcotics, benzodiazepines) that they are either out of, or abuse regularly which in turn, can counter or repress their psychiatric symptoms (Davis, 2014).

Mental health emergencies require an *immediate* coordinated response designed to alleviate the potential for harm and restore basic stability. Examples of a mental health emergency include suicidal, homicidal, or threatening behavior, self-injury, severe drug or alcohol impairment, and highly erratic or unusual behavior associated with serious mental disorders. Unpredictability, acute emotions, and acting

| BOX 20-2 | Interventions for Initial Family Responses to Crisis |

Anxiety, Shock, Fear

- Give information that is brief, concise, explicit, and concrete.
- Repeat information and frequently reinforce; encourage families to record important facts in writing.
- Determine comprehension by asking family to repeat back to you what information they have been given.
- Provide for and encourage or allow expression of feelings, even if they are extreme.
- Maintain constant, nonanxious presence in the face of a highly anxious family.
- Inform family as to the potential range of behaviors and feelings that are within the "norm" for crisis.
- Maximize control within hospital environment, as possible.

Denial

- Identify what purpose denial is serving for family (e.g., Is it buying them "psychological time" for future coping and mobilization of resources?).
- Evaluate appropriateness of use of denial in terms of time; denial becomes inappropriate when it inhibits the family from taking necessary actions or when it is impinging on the course of treatment.
- Do not actively support denial, but do not dash hopes for the future (You might say, "It must be very difficult for you to believe your son is nonresponsive and in a trauma unit.").
- If denial is prolonged and dysfunctional, more direct and specific factual representation may be essential.

Anger, Hostility, Distrust

- Allow for venting of angry feelings, clarifying what thoughts, fears, and beliefs are behind the anger; let the family know it is okay to be angry.
- Do not personalize family's expressions of these strong emotions.
- Institute family control within the hospital environment when possible (e.g., arrange for set times and set person to give them information in reference to the patient and answer their questions).
- Remain available to families during their venting of these emotions.

- Ask families how they can take the energy in their anger and put it to positive use for themselves, for the patient, and for the situation.

Remorse and Guilt

- Do not try to "rationalize away" guilt for families.
- Listen and support their expression of feeling and verbalizations (e.g., "I can understand how or why you might feel that way; however...").
- Follow the "however's" with careful, reality-oriented statements or questions (e.g., "None of us can truly control another's behavior"; "Kids make their own choices despite what parents think and want"; "How successful were you when you tried to control _____'s behavior with that before?"; "So many things happen for which there are no absolute answers").

Grief and Depression

- Acknowledge family's grief and depression.
- Encourage them to be precise about what it is they are grieving and depressed about; give grief and depression a context.
- Allow the family appropriate time for grief.
- Recognize that this is an essential step for future adaptation; do not try to rush the grief process.
- Remain sensitive to your own unfinished business, and hence comfort or discomfort with family's grieving and depression.

Hope

- Clarify with families their hopes, individually and with one another.
- Clarify with families their worst fears in reference to the situation. Are the hopes/fears congruent? Realistic? Unrealistic?
- Support realistic hope.
- Offer gentle factual information to reframe unrealistic hope (e.g., "With the information you have or the observations you have made, do you think that is still possible?").
- Assist families in reframing unrealistic hope in some other fashion (e.g., "What do you think others will have learned from _____ if he doesn't make it?" "How do you think _____ would like for you to remember him/her?").

Adapted from Kleeman K: Families in crisis due to multiple trauma, *Crit Care Nurs Clin North Am* 1(1):25, 1989.

Purpose: To give students experience in using the three-stage model of crisis intervention.

Procedure
1. Break class up into groups of three. One student should take the role of the client and one the role of the nurse; the third functions as observer.
2. Using one of the following role plays or one from your current clinical setting, engage the client and use the crisis intervention strategies presented in this chapter to frame your interventions.
3. The observer should provide feedback.
   (This exercise can also be handled as discussion points rather than a role play with small group or class feedback as to how students would have handled the situations.)

Role Play
Julie is a 23-year-old graduate student who has been dating Dan for the past 3 years. They plan to marry within the next 6 months. Last summer she had a brief affair with another graduate student while Dan was away but never told him. She is seeing you in the clinic having just found out that she has herpes from that encounter.

Sally is a 59-year-old postmenopausal woman admitted for diagnostic testing and possible surgery. She has just found out that her tests reveal a malignancy in her colon with possible metastasis to her liver. You are the nurse responsible for caring for her.

Bill's mother was admitted last night to the intensive care unit (ICU) with sepsis. She is on life support and intravenous antibiotics. Bill had a close relationship with his mother earlier in his life, but he has not seen her in the past year. You are the nurse for the shift but do not yet know her well.

Discussion
1. What would you want to do differently as a result of this exercise when communicating with the client in crisis?
2. What was the effect of using the three-stage model of crisis intervention as a way of organizing your approach to the crisis situation?

out behaviors increase the intensity of mental health emergencies. Myer and Conte (2006) describes a triage assessment system (TAS) for mental health crises that can help nurses understand a client's responses across three domains: affective, behavioral, and cognitive. All three response domains are interrelated, but Meyer suggests that clinicians first focus on the client's affective reaction, for example, client anger, fear, or sadness. Box 20-3 provides de-escalation tips for use with clients presenting in the community with mental health emergencies.

Model respect in communicating with mentally ill clients experiencing a meltdown or acute anxiety to avoid traumatizing individuals already experiencing a chaotic, distressed state. Mentally ill clients respond best to respectful, calmly presented suggestions rather than commands. They usually need additional space. Keep communication calm, short, compassionate, and well defined. Do not indicate you feel threatened or argue the logic of a situation. Avoid intimidating the client, but set reasonable limits. Proceed slowly with purpose and avoid sudden movements. Whenever possible, offer simple choices with structured coaching. Psychiatric emergency clients usually require medication for stabilization of symptoms and close supervision.

TYPES OF MENTAL HEALTH EMERGENCIES
Callahan (2009) identifies three types of mental health emergencies in health care: violence, suicidal behavior and interpersonal victimization, each of which requires emergency intervention.

Violence
Violence is a mental health emergency, which creates a critical challenge to the safety, well-being, and health of the clients and others in their environment. Nurses should always assume an organic component (drugs, alcohol, psychosis, or delirium) underlying the aggression in clients presenting with disorganized impulsive or violent behaviors, until proven otherwise.

Client body language offer clues to escalating anxiety, particularly agitation, threatening gestures, or darting eye movements. Table 20-1 presents indicators of increasing tension as precursors to violence. A history of violence, childhood abuse, substance abuse, mental retardation, problems with impulse control, and psychosis, particularly when accompanied by command hallucinations, are common contributing factors.

Treatment of violent clients consists of immediately providing a safe, nonstimulating environment for the client. Often clients calm down if taken to an area with less sensory input. The client should be checked

BOX 20-3	De-escalation Tips for Mental Health Emergencies

- Use a nonthreatening stance—open, but not vulnerable. Have them "take a seat."
- Eye contact—not constant, brief to show concern.
- Commands—brief, slow, with simple vocabulary, only as loud as needed, repeat as needed.
- Movement—not sudden, announce actions when possible, keep hands where they can be seen.
- Attitude—calm, interested, firm, patient, reassuring, respectful, truthful.
- Acknowledge legitimacy of feelings, delusions, hallucinations as being real to the client "I understand you are seeing or feeling this, but I am not."
- Remove distractions, upsetting influences.
- Keep the client talking/focused on the here and now.
- Ignore rather than argue with provocative statements.
- Allow verbal venting within reason.
- Be sensitive to personal space/comfort zone.
- Remove client to a quiet space; remove others from immediate area (avoid the "group spectators").
- Give some choices or options, if possible.
- Set limits if necessary.
- Limit interaction to just one professional and let that person do the talking.
- Avoid rushing—slow things down.
- Give yourself an out; do not put the client between yourself and the door.

Adapted from Officer Scott A Davis, Crisis Intervention Team (CIT) Coordinator: *De-escalation tips*, Rockville, MD, February 10, 2010b, Montgomery County Police Department.

TABLE 20-1	Behavioral Indicators of Potential Violence
Behavioral Categories	**Potential Indicators**
Mental status	Confused
	Paranoid ideation
	Disorganized
	Organic impairment
	Poor impulse control
Motor behavior	Agitated, pacing
	Exaggerated gestures
	Rapid breathing
Body language	Eyes darting
	Prolonged (staring) eye contact or lack of eye contact
	Spitting
	Pale, or red (flushed) face
	Menacing posture, throwing things
Speech patterns	Rapid, pressured
	Incoherent, mumbling, repeatedly making the same statements
	Menacing tones, raised voice, use of profanity
	Verbal threats
Affect	Belligerent
	Labile
	Angry

Data adapted from Keely B: Recognition and prevention of hospital violence, *Dimens Crit Care Nurs* 21(6):236-241, 2002; Luck L, Jackson D, Usher K: STAMP: components of observable behaviour that indicate potential for patient violence in emergency departments, *J Adv Nurs* 59(1):11-19, 2007.

thoroughly for potential weapons and physically disarmed, if necessary. Short-term medication usually is indicated to help defuse potentially harmful behaviors. The nurse should briefly identify why the med is being given, and the client should be carefully monitored for physical and behavioral responses.

Sexual Assault

Sexual assault and rape is a serious form of interpersonal victimization, which violates the core of self, in ways that are probably only second to murder. The client's subjective stress is intense and long lasting. In the immediate aftermath of a sexual assault, everything should be done to help the client feel safe and supported. The client should be taken to a private room and should not be left alone. Evidence, if it is to be collected, requires that the client not shower or douche

prior to being examined. Larger emergency departments have a Sexual Assault Nurse Examiner (SANE) program, staffed by a specially trained nurse who provides first response medical care and crisis intervention (James and Gilliland, 2013).

Adapting psychological first aid (PFA) to rape and sexual assault victims is a helpful comprehensive action-oriented intervention. PFA consists of eight core actions:

1. Contact and engagement
2. Safety and comfort
3. Stabilization
4. Information gathering

5. Practical assistance
6. Connection with social supports
7. Information on coping support
8. Linkage with collaborative services (Ruzek et al., 2007).

In a sexual assault situation, there should be no blame or conjecture about the victim's role in attracting a perpetrator. Sexual assault is always an act of violence and control. It is not a voluntary sexual act, even if the perpetrator and victim are known to each other. Follow-up referral to a mental health professional can help clients cope with stress symptoms, shame, and the intrusive thoughts that frequently develop in the days and weeks following the assault.

Psychosis

An acute psychotic break represents a serious mental health behavioral emergency. Psychotic and delirious clients have disorganized thinking, reduced insight, and limited personal judgment. Clients experiencing "command" hallucinations are at higher risk for suicide. Medication is almost always indicated to manage acute psychotic symptoms, and one-to-one supervision is required. Allow the client sufficient space to feel safe, and never try to subdue a client by yourself. Remain calm and positive. Use less, rather than more words. An open expression, eye contact, a calm voice, and simple concrete words invite trust. Do not use touch, as it can be misinterpreted.

Suicide

Suicide is the 10th leading cause of death in the United States, and for every person who commits suicide, there are 30 other suicide attempts (Office of the Surgeon General, 2012). Defined as any self injurious behavior that results in the death of an individual, and classified as a behavioral emergency, completed suicide is the ultimate personal crisis because there is no second chance. The Joint Commission (2010) identifies suicide as a "sentinel event," and calls for appropriate screening in medical surgical units and the emergency department to avert suicide completion. People turn to suicide as an option in times of acute distress, or when under the influence of drugs, or when they believe there are no other alternatives. Impulsiveness and hopelessness often go together with suicidal behaviors. Behavioral indicators of escalating suicidal ideation include a noteworthy change in behavior, often characterized by a burst of energy.

Examples of changes in behavior of successful suicide completers include

- A father gave away all of his deceased wife's jewelry 2 weeks before his death.
- An 18-year-old young man went door to door in his neighborhood apologizing for his "past" erratic behavior 3 days before he shot himself.
- A chronically ill mentally ill outpatient shared personal information and talked extensively in group therapy for the first time the week before he jumped off a bridge.

Completed suicide has long-lasting effects, for families, friends, co-workers and the larger community. Vannoy (2010) refers to suicide as a "stigmatized behavior" (p. 34). People do not know how to respond, so they are hesitant to talk about their feelings. People who talk about harming themselves are not necessarily at less risk, but there is more opportunity to prevent suicide. Every suicidal statement, however indirect, should be taken seriously. Even with clients who indicate that they are "just kidding," the fact that they have verbalized the threat places them at greater risk.

Passive suicidal wishes and actions such as not taking medications, not practicing safe sex, drinking too much, driving too fast, and not caring if you are in an accident warrant exploration. Pay attention to statements such as "I don't think I can go on without...," "I sometimes wish I could just disappear," or "People would be better off without me" are examples of suicidal ideation. Such statements require further clarification (e.g., "You say you can't go on without... Can you tell me more about what you mean?"). Nurses should ask directly: "Do you have any thoughts of hurting yourself?" (include frequency and intensity of thoughts). If the answer is yes, you need to follow up with the following line of questioning:

- Do you have a plan? Individuals with a detailed plan and the means to carry it out are at greatest risk for suicide. Assess the lethality of the plan, inquire about the method, and the client's knowledge and skills about its use (Roberts et al., 2008).
- What do you hope to accomplish with the suicide attempt? (look for *hopelessness*, including severity and duration)
- Have you thought about when you might do this? (immediate vs. chronic thinking)
- Who are you able to turn to when you are in trouble? (social support)

Risk Factors

Clients with mental illnesses, particularly bipolar disorder, schizophrenia with command hallucinations, and comorbidity with substance abuse are more at risk for *completed* suicide. Clients with antisocial or borderline personality disorders demonstrate more increased suicide *attempts*. Although psychiatric diagnosis is a risk factor for suicide, many successful suicide completers on general hospital units have no previous psychiatric history and no evidence of prior suicide attempts (Rittenmeyer, 2012).

Suicide rates are greater for older adults than among any other age group, and particularly for white men (Struble, 2014). Men are more likely to complete suicide, whereas more women attempt suicide (American Psychiatric Association, 2003).

Other high-risk factors include
- Previous attempts or family history of suicide
- Major physical illness
- Social isolation, lack of social support
- Recent major loss
- History of trauma
- A sense of hopelessness

Stabilization of symptoms and client safety are the most immediate concerns with clients experiencing suicidal crisis. Possible weapons (e.g., mirrors, belts, knitting needles, scissors, razors, medications, clothes hangers) should be confiscated. Explain in a calm, compassionate manner the reason why the items should not be in the client's possession and where they will be kept. Clients need to be assured that the items will be returned when the danger of self-harm resolves. Connectedness with others is considered a key protective factor in suicide prevention (Rodgers, 2011).

In the general hospital, completed suicides occur more frequently than one would suppose. Bostwick and Rackley (2007) emphasize notable differences between suicidal behavior in psychiatric settings and on general hospital units. On general units, suicides are almost always impulsive acts. Clients experiencing intense pain, terminal prognosis, substance abuse and recent bereavement are at higher risk. Clients have greater access to potentially lethal means to commit suicide, and health personnel do not immediately think of suicide in medical health situations. Characteristic of suicide completers on general units is the presence of acute agitation, often both physical and psychological in a disturbed client.

Documentation of the suicidal risk assessment, interventions, and client responses is essential. Included in the documentation should be quotes made by the client, details of observed behavior, review of identified risk factors, and client responses to initial crisis intervention strategies. The names and times of anyone you notified and contacts with family should be documented. The Joint Commission requires that any death, which is not consistent with a client's disease process, or any permanent loss of function occurring as a consequence of an attempted suicide in a hospital be reported as a sentinel event (Captain, 2006).

Most psychiatric inpatient settings and emergency departments have written suicide precaution protocols that must be followed with clients presenting with suicidal ideation. Clients exhibiting high-risk behaviors require one-to-one constant staff observation; a potentially suicidal client should never be left alone. Monitoring of suicidal clients ranges from constant 1:1 observation, to 15- or 30-minute observational checks. Less restrictive checks can include supervised bathroom, unit restriction or restriction to public areas, and supervised sharps (Jacobs, 2007). The frequency and type of observation is dependent on the suicidal assessment of the client.

Consistent with high risk for suicidal behavior is a sense of hopelessness, lack of meaningful connection with others, and the feeling of being a burden to others (Stellrecht et al., 2006). Acceptance of the client is a critical element of rapport. Nurses need to explore their own feelings about suicide behaviors as the basis for understanding the client in danger of self-injury.

Suicidal ideation waxes and wanes, so careful observation is critical even after the acute crisis has subsided. Captain (2006) suggests reassessing a client's suicidal intent every shift, using a 10-point scale and asking the client to "rate your level of suicidal intent on a 0-to-10 scale, with 0 meaning no thoughts of suicide and 10 meaning constant thoughts of suicide" (p. 47). Assessments should be repeated any time changes in behavior are noted and again before discharge.

CRISIS INTERVENTION TEAMS (CIT)

In the community, police with special training are important first responders in behavioral health emergencies (Miller, 2010). Community based crisis intervention teams (CIT) offers a successful model of collaborative pre-booking interventions between specially trained law enforcement officers and mental health care providers designed to treat rather than punish mentally ill clients with comorbid behavioral emergency symptoms (Watson and Fulambarker, 2012). Emergency nurses are important stakeholders and collaborators with CIT-trained law enforcement (Ralph, 2010). Officer Scott Davis (2014), crisis intervention team (CIT) coordinator with the Montgomery County Police Department shares a field expedient tool, using the acronym "DANGEROUS PERSON" (see Box 20-1), to assess dangerousness to self or others in clients presenting as a mental health emergency.

Clients experiencing mental health emergencies may perceive necessary medical procedures as being intrusive and threatening. Perry and Jagger (2003) advise that before starting any procedure, you should tell the client exactly what you are going to do and why the procedure is necessary, with a request to cooperate. If the client refuses, do not insist, but explain the reason for doing the procedure in a calm, quiet voice. If you can help clients regain a sense of control, they are more likely to cooperate with you. Your movements should be calm, firm, and respectful.

DISASTER MANAGEMENT

DISASTER AND MASS TRAUMA SITUATIONS

A **disaster** is defined as "a calamitous event of slow or rapid onset that results in large-scale physical destruction of property, social infrastructure, and human life" (Deeny and McFetridge, 2005, p. 432). Recent years have borne witness to more unprecedented natural disasters, terrorism, and barbaric war than the world has seen in many decades. The September 11th terrorist attack on the World Trade Center in 2001, the Oklahoma City bombing, and the devastation of Hurricane Katrina, which demolished a thriving city in a matter of days, stimulated a fresh awareness of the need for community and national planned responses to mass trauma events that can happen anywhere and at any time to innocent masses of people. Webb (2004) identifies the components of mass trauma events in Table 20-2.

Myer and Moore (2006) note, "Crises do not happen in a vacuum, but are shaped by the cultural and social contexts in which they occur" (p. 139). From the perspective of its victims, terrorism is a random event, which reinforces insecurity, creates lingering anxiety,

TABLE 20-2	Assessing Elements of Mass Trauma Events
Element	**Example**
Single vs. recurring traumatic event	Type I (acute) trauma
	Type II (chronic or ongoing) trauma
Proximity to the traumatic event	On site
	On the periphery
	Through the media
Exposure to violence/ injury/pain	Witnessed and/or experienced
Nature of losses/ death/destruction	Personal, community, and/or symbolic loss
	Danger, loss, and/or responsibility traumas
	Loved one, missing or no physical evidence
	Death determined by retrieval of body or fragment
	Loss of status/employment/ family income
	Loss of a predictable future
Attribution of causality	Random
	Act of God or deliberate
	Human-made

From Webb N: The impact of traumatic stress and loss on children and families. In Webb N, editor: *Mass trauma and violence: helping families and children cope*, New York, 2004, Guilford, p. 6. Reprinted by permission.

and increases avoidant behaviors around potential risks. The idea of a reciprocal relation between social forces and disaster crisis is supported by the Butler and colleagues (2003).

PLANNING FOR DISASTER MANAGEMENT

In the United States, the Federal Emergency Management Agency (FEMA) is responsible for setting forth recommendations related to creating an effective disaster plan (Hendriks and Bassi, (2009). FEMA recommendations provide guidelines for the creation of local disaster planning teams. Community-based governments and businesses, first responders, hospitals, and health providers are expected to be actively involved in community disaster planning. Around the globe, tsunamis in Indonesia, earthquakes occurring in rapid succession in China, Iceland, and South America, the threat of nations developing nuclear weapons, pandemic flu, and severe acute respiratory syndrome (SARS) remind us of a global approach to emergency preparedness.

Strategies for creating and sustaining community-wide emergency preparedness are published by The Joint Commission (2003), which states, "It is no longer sufficient to develop disaster plans and dust them off if a threat appears imminent. Rather, a system of preparedness across communities must be in place every day" (p. 5). Disaster planning can act as a deterrent to terrorist activity, as well as immediate resource in a disaster situation.

DISASTER INTERVENTION PROTOCOLS

Disaster intervention protocols focus on treating injury and acute illness, rather than chronic health conditions (Spurlock et al., 2009). Crisis intervention responses must be embedded in community systems and should be consistent with societal norms and available community resources. Not everyone can be saved. *Triage* is a tem used to describe how health workers sort out the severity of client needs and determine the priority of client treatments in a mass emergency or disaster situation. In the recent Haitian earthquake disaster, Merin and colleagues (2010) report that a three-question algorithm was used to provide an equitable triage process:

1. "How urgent is this patient's condition?
2. Do we have adequate resources to meet this patient's needs?
3. Assuming we admit this patient and provide the level of care required, can the patient's life be saved ?" (Jose, 2010, p. 459).

Disaster management requires providing immediate physical and emotional first aid. Instead of initially eliciting details of the experience, Everly and Flynn (2006) stress promotion of adaptive functioning and stabilization as a first response. They use the acronym BICEPS, which stands for brevity, immediacy, contact, expectancy, proximity, and simplicity to describe the type of psychological first aid needed in mass disaster situations.

CRITICAL INCIDENT DEBRIEFING

Disasters, deliberate violence, and terrorist attacks are random events producing permanent changes in people's lives and shaking their perception of being in charge of their lives. **Critical incident debriefing** is used to help a group of people who have witnessed or experienced a mass trauma crisis event externalize and process its meaning. Guided group sharing of the crisis experience by those most impacted by it can be healing. The debriefing allows the people involved in a traumatic situation to achieve a sense of psychological closure. The debriefing team also teaches participants about the nature of distress reactions and offers helpful hints to reduce their effects (Dietz, 2009).

Critical Incident Stress Debriefing Process

A specially trained professional generally leads the debriefing. Only those actively involved in the critical incident can attend the debriefing session. The leader introduces the purpose of the group and assures the participants that everything said in the session will be kept confidential. People are asked to identify who they are and what happened from their perspective, including the role they played in the incident. After preliminary factual data are addressed, the next step is to explore feelings. The leader asks participants to recall the first thing they remember thinking or feeling about the incident. Participants are asked to discuss any stress symptoms they may have related to the incident. The final discussion focuses on the emotional reactions associated with the critical incident. This part of the session is followed by psychoeducational strategies to reduce stress. Any lingering questions are answered, and the leader summarizes the high points of the critical incident debriefing for the group (Rubin, 1990).

Critical incident debriefings is used with families witnessing a tragedy involving a family member, for children and adolescents dealing with the death of a classmate, mass murders, or environmental disasters. A critical incident stress debriefing offers people an opportunity to externalize a traumatic experience through being able to vent feelings, discuss their role in the situation, develop a realistic sense of the big picture, and receive peer support in putting a crisis event in perspective (Curtis, 1995).

Critical Incident Debriefing for Health Care Providers

Research indicates that health care providers who assist or witness critical incidents can vulnerable to experience "secondary traumatization" similar to that experienced by direct survivors of the incident. Principles of critical incident debriefing can also be applied to strengthen the emotional coping skills of staff working in clinical settings on units with frequent or unexpected loss (Dietz, 2009).

Survivors of disaster can experience what Lahad (2000) terms "breaks in continuity." The break in continuity occurs in four spheres:

1. I do not understand what is happening. (*Cognitive continuity*)
2. I do not know myself. (*Historical continuity*)
3. I do not know what to do, how to act here, what it is to be a bereaved, injured, or wounded person. (*Role continuity*)
4. Where is everyone? I am so alone. Where are my loved ones? (*Social continuity*)

The experience of trauma from a disaster or terrorist event varies in intensity and impact for survivors. Each survivor brings to the experience a unique personal history, interpersonal strengths, and deficits, which affects interpretation of the catastrophe and can leave the survivor more vulnerable in future traumatic situations (Maguen et al., 2008). Having limited resources, lack of social support, or mental illness increases trauma stress. Another variable in disaster management is culture, influencing interpretation and dictating behavior. Culture plays a role in how a crisis situation is interpreted and the best means by which people and communities can be helped (Dykeman, 2005).

COMMUNITY RESPONSE PATTERNS

The Joint Commission (2003) explicitly portrays disaster management and emergency preparedness as a community responsibility. When disaster strikes, the existence and function of the community are significantly impaired and even in danger of extinction. Initially people are confused and stunned. Emotions vary as the extent of the impact is realized. The closer the person is to the crisis event, the more intense the impact (Myer and Moore, 2006). The immediate concern is protection of self and those closest to them. The community response to disaster characteristically consists of four phases:

1. Heroic
2. Honeymoon
3. Disillusionment
4. Reconstruction

The shock of the disaster pulls people together. Emergency medical teams, neighbors, and friends rally around the survivors, offering emotional support and tangible supplies needed for recovery. The *honeymoon phase* occurs when the "community pulls together and outside resources are brought in" after an initial search and recovery phase (Bowenkamp, 2000, p. 159). This phase typically lasts up to 6 months after the disaster. The focus of intervention is to ensure victim safety. Establishing an infrastructure to support the immediate needs of the population related to water, sanitation, food supplies, and insect and rodent control are essential services (Campos-Outcalt, 2006). Sharing the experience of the trauma with others and having tangible evidence of continuing support are crucial components of effective response.

The *disillusionment phase* usually appears as the initial emergency response starts to subside. The "shared community" feeling starts to leave as people begin to realize the extent of their losses and the limitations of external support. Survivors can experience anger, resentment, and bitterness at the loss of support, particularly if it is sudden and complete. Kaplan and colleagues (2000) suggest that opportunities for psychological debriefing sessions should continue for a period well beyond the initial disaster experience for victims of extreme stress.

The final *reconstruction phase* occurs when the survivors begin to take the primary responsibility for rebuilding their lives. This period can last for several years after a disaster. Ongoing support is required as survivors learn to cope with new roles and responsibilities and to develop new alternatives to living a full life after trauma. Although the disaster experience recedes in memory, it is never lost, and the person may never again fully trust in the continuity of life and being in control of one's destiny. Kaminsky and colleagues (2007) describe recovery from the clinical distress, impairment, and dysfunction associated with terrorism and mass disaster as evidenced in the ability to adaptively function psychologically and behaviorally.

DISASTER MANAGEMENT IN HEALTH CARE SETTINGS

All hospitals are required to form disaster committees composed of key departments within the hospital, including nursing. Nurses interested in emergency volunteer activities should become aware of credentialing requirements to ensure their participation as part of a national emergency volunteer system for health professionals. Hospital and community disaster planning must be coordinated so that all phases of the disaster cycle are covered. Designated hospital personnel must receive training to carry out triage at the emergency department entrance. Protocols should contain the capability to relocate staff and clients to another facility if necessary, and a plan must be in place detailing mechanisms for equipment resupply. Policies regarding notification, maintenance of accurate records and establishment of a facility control center are required.

Citizen Responders

Unsolicited responders play a large role in sudden onset, large-scale disasters. Auf der Heide (2006) suggests that emergency plans should anticipate the presence of unsolicited responders and have an infrastructure for coordinating their efforts. Public education related to the citizen role in disaster management is essential.

Citizen Corps Programs, developed by FEMA, is a grassroots crisis intervention strategy that can provide community volunteers with a program to develop emergency preparedness and first-aid skills. The web site (www.ready.gov/citizen-corps) provides training and tool kits to help improve the on-site care of disaster victims. It also provides links to information for families interested in developing emergency preparedness around the following issues:

- Providing children and family members with family work and cell phone numbers; name and number of neighbor, friend, or relative; emergency 911, fire, poison control, and police number (these should be posted in a conspicuous place).
- Choosing an out-of-town contact and instructions on how to make contact.
- Choosing a place to meet with other family members in case of emergency.
- Planning for pets, as they are not allowed in emergency shelters. Family emergency preparedness plans should be updated annually.

HELPING CHILDREN COPE WITH TRAUMA

Children do not have the same resources when coping with traumatic events as adults do. Preexisting exposure to traumatic events and lack of social support increases vulnerability. It is not unusual for children to demonstrate regressive behaviors as a reaction to crisis. Knapp (2010) suggests that using rituals and memorials for children experiencing loss of peers at school is helpful in mitigating trauma impact. Having a place where children can bring flowers and other mementos commemorating their peer's death is important.

Children will look for cues from key adults in their lives and tend to mirror their adult caregivers, so it is essential to communicate calm and confidence. More than anything else, children need reassurance that they and the people who are important to them are safe. Encourage the family to maintain regular routines. Parents need to provide children with opportunities both to talk about crisis and to ask questions. Repetitive questions are to be expected. Often they reflect the child's need for reassurance. Offering factual information helps dispel misperceptions.

HELPING OLDER ADULTS COPE WITH TRAUMA

Reducing anxiety is especially important for the older adult disaster victim. Even the most capable older adult can appear confused and vulnerable in a disaster situation. Actions nurses can take include the following:

- Initiate contact and take the older adult to as safe a place as possible.
- Speak calmly and provide concrete information about what is happening and what you need the older adult to do in simple terms.
- Assess for mobility and provide assistance where needed.
- Older adults may need warmer clothing because of compromised temperature regulation.

Functional limitations associated with compromised physical mobility, diminished sensory awareness, and preexisting health conditions create special issues for older clients impacted by a disaster. Older adults have more injury and greater disaster-related deaths than adults in other age groups (Fernandez et al., 2002). Within the older population, special attention should focus on those who require medical or nursing care and those receiving services, care, or food from health, social, or volunteer agencies. Disaster management for older adults needs to be proactive. The following core actions can make a difference in helping older adults weather a disaster event successfully. Proactive planning includes working with clients:

- Identify a support network that can be used in an emergency situation. Facilitate connections with social support systems and community support structures. Have this information readily available for use in an emergency situation.
- Older adults with a disability should wear tags or a bracelet to identify their disability. Keeping extra eyeglasses and hearing aid batteries

on hand and identifying any assistive devices is essential.

- Identify the closest special needs evacuation center.
- Develop a written list of all medications, with any special directions, for example, crushing pills, hours of administration, and dietary restrictions.
- Identify physicians and social support contacts, including someone apart from people in the local area who can be contacted.

Other actions, such as ensuring the safety, meeting mobility needs, and medication administration, need special attention during the course of actual disaster management.

SUMMARY

Crisis is defined as an unexpected, sudden turn of events or set of circumstances requiring an immediate human response. People experience a crisis as overwhelming, traumatic, and personally intrusive. It is an unexpected life event challenging a person's sense of self and his or her place in the world. The most common types of crisis are situational and developmental crises. Most health crises are situational. Crisis can be private, involving one person, or public, involving large numbers of people.

Theoretical frameworks guiding crisis intervention include Lindemann's (1944) model of grieving and Caplan's (1964) model, based on preventive psychiatry concepts. Aguilera's nursing model (1998) explores the role of balancing factors in defusing the impact of a crisis state. Erikson's (1982) model of psychosocial development provides a framework for exploring developmental crises.

Crisis intervention is a time-limited treatment, which focuses on the immediate crisis and its resolution. Roberts' (2005) seven-stage model, used to guide nursing interventions, consists of assessing lethality, establishing rapport, dealing with feelings, defining the problem, exploring alternative options, formulating a plan, and follow-up measures. The goal of crisis intervention is to return the client to his or her pre-crisis level of functioning.

Mental health emergencies require immediate assessment interventions and close supervision. The most common types are violence, suicide, and a psychotic break. Guidelines for communication with clients experiencing mental health emergencies (e.g.,

violence and suicide) focus on safety and rapid stabilization of the client's behavior. CITs represent a new model of collaboration between local law enforcement and mental health services designed to treat rather than punish individuals experiencing mental health emergencies in the community (Davis, 2014; Watson and Fulambarker, 2012).

As the world becomes more dynamically unstable, nurses will need to understand the dimensions of disaster management and develop the skills to respond effectively in disaster situations. Disaster management is a special kind of crisis intervention applied to large groups of people. The Joint Commission (2003) requires hospitals to develop and exercise disaster management plans at regular intervals. Critical incident debriefing is a crisis intervention strategy designed to help those closely involved with disasters process critical incidents in health care, thereby reducing the possibility of symptoms occurring.

ETHICAL DILEMMA   What Would You Do?

Sara Murdano is only 20 years old when she arrives at the mobile intensive care unit (MICU), but this is not her first hospital admission. She has been treated for depression previously. She states she is determined to kill herself because she has nothing to live for and that it is her right to do so because she is no longer a minor. As she describes her life to date, you cannot help but think that she really does not have a lot to live for. How would you respond to this client from an ethical perspective?

DISCUSSION QUESTIONS

1. What would you identify as the essential knowledge, skills, and attitudes required of a nurse confronted with an out-of-control patient?
2. How would you apply The Joint Commission safety standards in the emergency department?
3. How would you explain the meaning of the crisis as a danger and an opportunity?

REFERENCES

Aguilera D: *Crisis intervention: theory and methodology*, ed 7, St Louis, 1998, Mosby.
American Psychiatric Association: *Practice guidelines for the assessment and treatment of patients with suicidal behaviors*, Arlington, VA, 2003, Author.

Auf der Heide E: The importance of evidence-based disaster planning, *Ann Emerg Med* 47(1):34–49, 2006.

Bostwick J, Rackley S: Completed suicide in medical/surgical patients: who is at risk? *Curr Psychiatry Rep* 9:242–246, 2007.

Bowenkamp C: Coordination of mental health and community agencies in disaster, *Int J Emerg Ment Health* 2:159–165, 2000.

Bluhm J: Helping families in crisis hold on, *Nursing* 17(10):44–46, 1987.

Callahan J: Crisis theory and crisis intervention in emergencies. Kleespies PM Emergencies in mental health practice: Evaluation and Management, New York, NY, 1998, Guilford press. 22–40.

Campos-Outcalt D: Disaster medical response: maximizing your effectiveness, *Fam Pract* 55(2):113–115, 2006.

Caplan G: *Principles of preventive psychiatry*, New York, 1964, Basic Books.

Captain C: Is your patient a suicide risk? *Nursing* 36(8):43–47, 2006.

Curtis J: Elements of critical incident debriefing, *Psychol Rep* 77(1):91–96, 1995.

Dass-Brailsford P: *Crisis and disaster counseling: lessons learned from Hurricane Katrina and other disasters*, Thousand Oaks, CA, 2010, Sage Publications.

Davis S: *De-escalation tips in crisis situations. Montgomery County*, Rockville, MD, 2010b, MD Police Department.

Davis S: *Field expedient tool to assess dangerousness in self and others. Montgomery County*, Rockville, MD, 2010a, MD Police Department.

Davis S. (2014) CIT Teams: Unpublished manuscript.

Deeny P, McFetridge B: The impact of disaster on culture, self, and identity: increased awareness by health care professionals is needed, *Nurs Clin North Am* 40(3):431–444, 2005.

Dietz D: Debriefing to help perinatal nurses cope with a maternal loss, *MCN Am J Matern Child Nurs* 34(4):243–248, 2009.

Dykeman BF: Cultural implications of crisis intervention, *J Instr Psychol* 32(1):45–48, 2005.

Erikson E: *The life cycle completed*, Norton, 1982, New York.

Everly G: Five principles of crisis intervention: Reducing the risk of premature crisis intervention, *Int J Emerg Ment Health* 2(1):1–4, 2000.

Everly G, Flynn B: Principles and practical procedures for acute first aid training for personnel without mental health experience, *Int J Emerg Ment Health* 8(2):93–100, 2006.

Fernandez LS, Byard D, Lin C, Benson S, Barbera J: Frail elderly as disaster victims: Emergency management strategies, *Prehospital Disaster Med* 17(2):67–74, 2002.

Flannery Jr R, Everly Jr G: Crisis intervention: a review, *Int J Emerg Ment Health* 2(2):119–125, 2000.

Greene G, Lee M, R. Trask R, J. Rheinscheld J: How to work with strengths in crisis intervention: a solution focused approach. In Roberts AR, editor: *Crisis intervention handbook*, New York, 2005, Oxford University Press.

Hendriks K, Bassi S: Emergency preparedness from the ground floor up: a local agency perspective, *Home Health Care Manag Pract* 21(5):346–352, 2009.

Hoff L: People in crisis: cultural and diversity perspectives. *Routledge*, ed 6, New York, 2009, Taylor & Francis Group.

Butler AS, Panzer AM, Goldfrank LR: *Preparing for the psychological consequences of terrorism: a public health strategy*, Washington, DC, 2003, National Academies Press.

Jacobs D: *Screening for mental health: a resource guide for implementing the Joint Commission on Accreditation of Health Care Organizations (CAHO) 2007 patient safety goals on suicide Screening for Mental Health Inc*, Wellesley Hills, 2007.

James R, Gilliland B: *Crisis intervention strategies*, 7th ed, Belmont CA, 2013, Thomson Brooks/Cole.

James R: *Crisis Intervention Strategies*, 6th ed., Belmont CA, 2008, Thompson Brooks/Cole.

Jose MM: Cultural, ethical, and spiritual competencies of health care providers responding to a catastrophic event, *Crit Care Nurs Clin N Am* 22:455–464, 2010.

The Joint Commission, 2003. Health care at the crossroads: strategies for creating and sustaining community-wide emergency preparedness systems Joint Commission on Accreditation of Health Care Organizations: Oakbrook Terrace, IL

The Joint Commission: A follow-up report on preventing suicide: focus on medical surgical/nursing and the emergency department, *Sentinel event alert* Issue 46, 2010. Available at http://www.jointcommission.org/senti nel_event_alert_issue_46_a_follow-up_report_on_preventing_suicide_focus_on_medicalsurgical_units_and_the_emergency_department/.

Kaminsky M, McCabe O, Langlieb A, Everly G: An evidence-informed model of human resistance, resilience, and recovery: the Johns Hopkins' outcome-driven paradigm for disaster mental health services, *Brief Treat Crisis Interv* 7(1):1–11, 2007.

Kaplan Z, Iancu I, Bodner E: A review of psychological debriefing after extreme stress, *Psychiatr Serv* 52(6):824–827, 2000.

Kavan M, Guck T, Barone E: A practical guide to crisis management, *Am Fam Physician* 74(7):1159–1164, 2006.

Keely B: Recognition and prevention of hospital violence, *Dimens Crit Care Nurs* 21(6):236–241, 2002.

Kleeman K: Families in crisis due to multiple trauma, *Crit Care Nurs Clin North Am* 1(1):25, 1989.

Kleespies PM: *An evidence based resource for evaluating and managing risk of suicide, violence, and victimization. Washington DC*, American Psychological Association, 2009.

Knapp K: Children and crises. In Dass-Brailsford P, editor: *Crisis and disaster counseling: lessons learned from Hurricane Katrina and other disasters*, Thousand Oaks, CA, 2010, Sage Publications, pp 83–97.

Lahad M: Darkness over the abyss: supervising crisis intervention teams following disaster, *Traumatology* 6(4):273–293, 2000.

Lindemann E: Symptomatology and management of acute grief, *Am J Psychiatry* 101:141–148, 1944.

Luck L, Jackson D, Usher K: STAMP: components of observable behaviour that indicate potential for patient violence in emergency departments, *J Adv Nurs* 59(1):11–19, 2007.

Maguen S, Papa A, Litz B: Coping with the threat of terrorism: a review, *Anxiety Stress Coping* 21(1):15–35, 2008.

Merin O, Ash N, Levy G, et al. The Israeli field hospital in Haiti—ethical dilemmas in early disaster response, *N Engl J Med* 362(11):e38, 2010.

Michalopoulos H, Michalopoulos A: Crisis counseling: be prepared to intervene, *Nursing* 39(9):47–50, 2009.

Miller L: On-scene crisis intervention: Psychological guidelines and communication strategies for first responders, *Int J Emerg Ment Health* 12(1):11–19, 2010.

Myer R, Conte C: Assessment for crisis intervention, *J Clin Psychol* 62(8):959–970, 2006.

Myer RA, Moore HB: Crisis in context theory: an ecological model, *J Couns Dev* 84(spring):139–147, 2006.

Office of the Surgeon General (US): *National Action Alliance for Suicide Prevention (US)*, US Department of Health & Human Services (US), 2012, Washington (DC). 2012 Sep.

Perry J, Jagger J: Reducing risks from combative patients, *Nursing* 33(10):28, 2003.

Powley E: Reclaiming resilience and safety: resilience in the critical period of crisis, *Hum Relat* 62(9):1289–1326, 2009.

Ralph M: The impact of crisis intervention team programs: Fostering collaborative relationships, *J Emerg Nurs* 36(1):60–62, 2010.

Rittenmeyer L: Assessment of risk for in-hospital suicide and aggression in high dependency care environments, *Crit Care Nurs Clin North Am.* 24:41–51, 2012.

Roberts A: *Crisis intervention handbook: assessment, treatment and research*, New York, 2005, Oxford University Press.

Roberts A, Yeager K: *Pocket guide to crisis intervention*, New York, 2009, Oxford University Press.

Roberts A, Monferrari I, Yeager K: Avoiding malpractice lawsuits by following risk assessment and suicide prevention guidelines, *Brief Treat Crisis Interv* 8:5–14, 2008.

Rodgers P. Suicide Prevention Resource Center. Understanding risk and protective factors for suicide: a primer for preventing suicide. Available at www.sprc.org/library_resources/ items/understanding-risk-and-protective-factors-suicide-primer-preventing- suicide. Accessed, Aug 22, 2014.

Rubin J: Critical incident stress debriefing: helping the helpers, *J Emerg Nurs* 16(4):255–258, 1990.

Ruzek JI, Brymer MJ, Jacobes AK, et al.: Psychological first aid, *J Ment Health Counsel* 29:17–49, 2007.

Spurlock W, Brown S, Rami J: Disaster care: delivering primary health care to hurricane evacuees, *Am J Nurs* 109(8):50–53, 2009.

Stellrecht N, Gordon K, Van Orden K, et al.: Clinical applications of the interpersonal-psychological theory of attempted and completed suicide, *J Clin Psychol* 62(2):211–222, 2006. II.

Struble LM: Psychiatric disorders impacting critical illness, *Crit Care Nurs Clin North Am* 26(1):115–138, 2014.

Vannoy S: Suicide inquiry in primary care: Creating context, inquiring and following up, *Ann Fam Med* 8(1):33–39, 2010.

Vroomen JM, Bosmans JE, van Hout HP, de Rooij SE: Reviewing the definition of crisis in dementia care, *BMC Geriatr* 13:10, 2013, http://dx.doi.org/10.1186/1471-2318-13-10.

Watson A, Fulambarker A: The crisis intervention team model of police response to mental health crises: A primer for mental health practitioners, *Best Pract Ment Health* 8(2):71–77, 2012.

Webb NB, editor: *Mass trauma and violence: helping families and children cope*, New York, 2004, Guilford Press.

Communicating with Clients and Families at End of Life

Elizabeth C. Arnold

OBJECTIVES

At the end of the chapter, the reader will be able to:
1. Describe the concept of loss.
2. Identify theory-based concepts of grief and grieving
3. Discuss the nature of grief and grieving
4. Describe the nurse's role in palliative care.
5. Discuss key issues and approaches in end-of-life (EOL) care.
6. Identify cultural and spiritual needs in EOL care.
7. Describe supportive strategies for children.
8. Discuss strategies to help clients achieve a good death.
9. Identify stress issues for nurses in EOL care.

The purpose of Chapter 21 is to introduce fundamental elements of palliative care approaches that nurses can use as a context for effectively communicating with clients and families. The chapter identifies selected theoretical frameworks related to loss, stages of dying, and the process of grief and grieving. The "Application" section highlights communication and care issues with clients and their families that nurses face in providing palliative care. Helping clinicians recognize and cope with the high stress of providing quality end-of-life (EOL) care is also addressed.

BASIC CONCEPTS

LOSS

Corless (2010) defines loss as "a generic term that signifies absence of an object, position, ability or attribute" (p. 598). The term is also applied to the death of a person or animal. Important losses occur as part of everyone's personal experience. Anything or anyone in whom we invest time, energy, or a part of ourselves creates a sense of loss when it is no longer available to us. When people *suffer the loss of* someone or something important to them, there is a loss of their sense

of "wholeness" and a break in the person's expected life story (Attig, 2004). The passage of time never fully erases the sense of loss.

The feelings associated with each loss differ only in the intensity with which one experiences them. Mark Twain noted: "Nothing that grieves us can be called little; by the eternal laws of proportion a child's loss of a doll and a king's loss of a crown are events of the same size" (*Mark Twain Quotations*, n.d.). Only the person experiencing the loss can appreciate the unique void and strength of feelings that each loss entails. Exercise 21-1 is designed to help you understand the dimensions of personal loss. Some losses are gradual; others occur concurrently or sequentially. One loss can precipitate connected losses. For example, a client with Alzheimer disease does not simply lose memory. Accompanying cognitive loss are profound losses of role, communication, independence, and loss of identity. Progressive profound emotional and lifestyle changes are required to accommodate for the cognitive loss.

MULTIPLE LOSSES

Acknowledging differences between single and multiple loss helps clients put the enormity of multiple

EXERCISE 21-1	The Meaning of Loss

Purpose: To consider personal meaning of losses.

Procedure

Consider your answers to the following questions:
- What losses have I experienced in my life?
- How did I feel when I lost something or someone important to me?
- How was my behavior affected by my loss?
- What helped me the most in resolving my feelings of loss?
- How has my experience with loss prepared me to deal with further losses?
- How has my experience with loss prepared me to help others deal with loss?

Discussion
1. In the larger group, discuss what gives a loss its meaning.
2. What common themes emerged from the group discussion about successful strategies in coping with loss?
3. How does the impact of necessary losses differ from that of unexpected, unnecessary losses?
4. How can you use in your clinical work what you have learned from doing this exercise?

losses into perspective (Mercer and Evans, 2006). Older adults may experience the deaths of friends and family members with greater frequency, related to age. Others lose family and friends to acquired immunodeficiency syndrome (AIDS), military action, and natural or human-made disasters. A car accident can wipe out an entire family or group of friends. Multiple losses intensify the grief experience and leave clients feeling overwhelmed. These clients usually require more time to resolve grief feelings. Encourage clients to focus on one relationship at a time instead of trying to address the losses together. Patience with oneself is critical to successful working through difficult emotions associated with multiple losses. It takes time, and no one should rush the process.

DEATH: THE FINAL LOSS

Death represents a tangible loss in that the physical presence of the lost person can never be replaced. More than a biological event, death has spiritual, social, and cultural features that help people make sense of its meaning. Regardless of primary medical diagnosis, clients experience many different emotions, ranging from anger or sadness, to a sense of peace about a life well lived with few regrets as they approach death. Silveira and Schneider (2004) suggest that "planning for the end of life is planning for the unknown" (p. 349). Death occurs only once in each person's life. No one can actually tell you how it will be for you based on his or her experience. Pashby (2014), an expert hospice nurse, states that most clients identify fear of pain and dying alone as their two principal fears. Nurses are an important resource in providing practical support and offering meaningful presence to clients and families coping with the dying process.

THEORETICAL FRAMEWORKS

The five-stage model of Elisabeth Kübler-Ross (1969) provides an evidence-based framework for the study of death and dying (Keegan and Drick, 2011).

DENIAL

Kübler-Ross (1969) characterizes the denial stage as the "No, not me" stage. Nurses should be sensitive to the client's need for denial. Some people remain in the denial stage throughout their illness; their right to do so should be respected.

ANGER

Anger is characterized as the "Why me?" stage. This stage can produce feelings about the unfairness of life or anger with God. Feelings often get projected on those closest to the client. Family members need support to recognize that the anger is not a personal attack (although it feels that way to the family member).

BARGAINING

Kübler-Ross (1969) refers to the bargaining stage as the "Yes, me, but...I need just a little more time." Bargaining is not a futile exercise. Sometimes the extra energy a person gets by focusing on living long enough to attend a graduation, birth, or wedding is meaningful to all involved in making it happen. By supporting hope and avoiding challenges to the client's reality, the nurse facilitates the process of living while dying.

DEPRESSION

The "Yes, me" stage of dying is expressed through depressive feelings and mood swings. You can help family members understand that this is a "normal" response to anticipating loss. Review of significant life events and relationships helps clients consider unfinished business that could be reworked. Serving as an empathetic listening witness to the pain that clients and families experience in this stage helps them work through this stage.

ACCEPTANCE

The acceptance stage is characterized by an acknowledgment of an inevitable end to physical life. There is a gradual detachment from the world. The client experiences being almost "void of feeling" (Kübler-Ross, 1969, p. 124). Ideally clients experience a personal sense of peace and letting go. To outsiders the client is straddling between two world realities: the organic and the existential. Not every person experiences each stage.

LINDEMANN'S GRIEF WORK

Eric Lindemann (1944/1994) pioneered the concept of grief work based on interviews with bereaved persons suffering a sudden tragic loss. He described patterns of grief and identified physical and emotional changes associated with significant loss. Lindemann observed that grief can occur immediately after a loss, or it can be delayed. He summarized three components of support: (a) open, empathetic communication; (b) honesty; and (c) tolerance of emotional expression as being important in grieving. When the symptoms of grief are exaggerated or absent, it is considered pathologic or complicated grief. People experiencing complicated grief may require psychological treatment to resolve their grief and move into life again.

ENGEL'S CONTRIBUTIONS

George Engel's (1964) concepts built on Lindemann's work. He described three sequential phases of grief work: (a) shock and disbelief, (b) developing awareness, and (c) restitution.

In the shock and disbelief phase, a newly bereaved person may feel alienated or detached from normal—"literally numb with shock; no tears, no feelings, just absolute numbness" (Lendrum and Syme, 1992, pp. 24-25). Seeing or hearing the lost person or sensing his or her presence is a temporary altered sensory experience related to the loss, which should not be confused with psychotic hallucinations.

The developing awareness phase occurs slowly as the void created by the loss fully enters consciousness. Clients experience a loss of energy, not the kind that requires sleep, but rather recognizing that one lacks the functional energy to engage fully in normal everyday responsibilities.

Case Example

"Throughout the year following my mother's death, I was aware of a persistent feeling of heaviness—not physical heaviness, but emotional and spiritual. It was as if a dark cloud hung over my heart and soul. I tired easily, with little energy to do anything but the most essential activities, and even those frequently received perfunctory attention. My usual pattern of 'sleeping like a log' was disrupted, and in its place I experienced uneasy rest that left me feeling as if I had never closed my eyes." —Anonymous

Listening, identifying feelings, and having an empathetic willingness to repeatedly hear the client's story without needing to give advice or interpretation offer presence without demands.

The *restitution phase* is characterized by adaptation to a new life without the deceased. There is a resurgence of hope and a renewed energy to fashion a new life. With successful grieving, the loss is not forgotten, but the pain diminishes and is replaced with memories that enrich and give energy to life.

CONTEMPORARY MODELS

Contemporary authors (Florczak (2008), Neimeyer (2001) and Attig (2001) emphasize meaning construction as a central issue in grief work. The past is not forgotten but neither does the survivor remain engaged with only past memories. Instead, there is a continuous spiritual connection with the deceased, which illuminates different features of self and offers possibilities for fuller engagement with life. Features of past experiences with the loved one are transformed and rewoven into the fabric of a person's life in a new form.

THE NATURE OF GRIEF AND GRIEVING

The concept of **grief** describes a holistic, adaptive process that a person goes through following a significant loss. The journey through grief is different for each person (Jeffreys, 2011). Grief is a dynamic process, with an ebb and flow to the intense feelings that a death or significant loss usually stimulates in those who remain. More than sadness, an acute awareness of the void a loss creates recurring, wavelike feelings of memories, and desolation. People describe it as "feeling unexpectedly punched in the gut." Intense feelings are likely to surface when the griever is alone, for example, while driving. Certain situations, holidays, and anniversaries, particularly during the first few years, allow grief feelings to resurface.

Case Example

"I would think I was doing okay, that I had a handle on my grief. Then without warning, a scent, a scene on television, an innocuous conversation would flip a switch in my mind, and I would be flooded with memories of my mother. My eyes would fill up with tears as my fragile composure dissolved. My grief lay right under the surface of my awareness and ambushed me at times and in places not of my choosing." —Anonymous

Over time, grief feelings diminish in intensity for most people, but there is no magic time frame. Grief over the loss of a child can be particularly pervasive, sometimes lasting a lifetime. Variables affecting the intensity and timeframe for the grieving process following a death include:

- "Cultural beliefs and rituals
- Nature of relationship with the deceased
- Previous losses
- Spiritual and religious background
- Support system available" (Keegan and Drick, 2011, p. 113).

As people work through their grief, they are more open to the spiritual continuance of a relationship with the deceased, occurring as cherished memories or supportive remembrances of "what the deceased person might say, or do in the situation." These shared moments provide an affirming spiritual union with the deceased and a personal knowing of self in relationship. They offer a unique legacy, which will continue to influence the behaviors of future generations.

John Thomas (2010, 2011) describes his sense of successfully making the journey through grief with a stronger sense of self. He states,

"I want to be known as one who

- Is identified with life and love rather than loss and grief.

- Walks with the stride of renewal rather than the shuffle of grief.
- Still embraces life knowing that the pain of loss is intense.
- Has one foot planted firmly in this life and is developing an equally firm footing in the spiritual realm.
- Is confident about the future without needing a tangible GPS.
- Can be alone without being lonely.
- Has vigor, and is seen as a man younger than his chronological age.
- Faced grief head-on, and reached a deeper core of self, faith, and spirituality.
- Has much to give in many arenas living a life that honors my past, and shares the blessings derived from it"… (Thomas, 2010; 2011, pp. 202-203).

PATTERNS OF GRIEVING

ACUTE GRIEF

Acute grief occurs as "somatic distress that occurs in waves with feelings of tightness in the throat, shortness of breath, an empty feeling in the abdomen, a sense of heaviness and lack of muscular power, and intense mental pain" (Lindemann, 1994, p. 155). Acute grief is intense, and the emotional pain can be beyond imagination. It lasts a short time, and gradually subsides, as the bereaved person begins to reengage in meaningful activities (Zisook et al., 2010).

Violent death can create a higher psychological impact and is linked with poorer psychological outcomes in surviving family members (Lichetenthal et al, 2013). Family survivors of suicide victims are at a particular disadvantage, made worse by their reluctance to discuss death details because of shame, a sense of guilt about not being able to prevent the suicide or perceived stigma. Survivors usually need more support; often they get less because people are uncomfortable about suicide or do not know how to talk about it with those most intimately involved (*Harvard Women's Health Watch*, 2009). Suicide survivor support groups can offer the specialized help that many survivors need after a suicide (Feigelman and Feigelman, 2008).

ANTICIPATORY GRIEF

Anticipatory grief is an emotional response that occurs before the actual death around a family member with a degenerative or terminal disorder. A person thinking about his or her own death also can experience anticipatory grief. These grief symptoms are similar to those experienced after death, but are often accompanied by colored by ambivalent feelings.

Case Example

Marge's husband, Albert, was diagnosed with Alzheimer disease 5 years ago. Albert is in a nursing home, unable to care for himself. Marge grieves the impending loss of Albert as her mate. At the same time, she would like a life of her own. Her "other feelings" of wishing it could all be over cause her to feel guilty. Exercise 21-2 helps you explore grief from a personal perspective.

CHRONIC SORROW

Chronic sorrow differs from anticipatory grief. It is defined as "a normal grief response associated with an ongoing living loss that is permanent, progressive, recurring, and cyclic in nature" (Gordon, 2009, p. 115). Many parents of children with a physical, developmental, emotional, or chronic disorder experience will chronic sorrow. Families need nurses to affirm their coping efforts and acknowledge the legitimacy of their sadness. Providing timely support for families when there is an exacerbation of symptoms can make the situation more manageable.

COMPLICATED GRIEVING

Complicated grieving represents an intense expression of grief, which is significantly longer in duration and emotionally incapacitating. A history of depression, substance abuse, death of a parent or sibling during childhood, prolonged conflict or dependence on the deceased person, or a succession of deaths within a short period predispose a person to complicated grief. Statements such as "I never recovered from my son's death," or "I feel like my life ended when my husband died" can alert to the nurse to potential complicated grief.

Complicated grief sometimes presents as an absence of grief in situations where it would be expected, for example, a marine who displays no emotion over the deaths of war comrades. When deaths and important losses are not mourned, the feelings do not just disappear; they reappear in unexpected ways sometimes years later. Exercise 21-3 provides a personal opportunity to reflect on the relevance of memories making in significant relationships.

Developing an Evidence-Based Practice

Adams J, Anderson R, Docherty S, Tulsky J, Steinhauser K, Bailey D: Nursing strategies to support family members of ICU patients at high risk of dying, *Heart Lung* pii:S0147-9563(14)00047-8, 2014.

This qualitative descriptive study was designed to explore family perceptions of nursing strategies that are helpful to them when a family with a member at high risk for dying is in the intensive care unit (ICU). A purposive sample of family members with a family member at high risk for dying were asked to identify specific strategies nurses used to support their decision making.

Results: Study narratives identified four nursing approaches as being helpful to the family: demonstrating concern, demonstrating professionalism, providing factual information, and supporting their decision-making. These strategies helped the family to have more confidence in their decision-making skills and to better prepare for and accept the impending death of their relative.

Implications for clinical practice: Knowledge of therapeutic approaches important to family members and most likely to improve their ability to make decisions and their well-being in end-of-life care lays a foundation for choosing therapeutic interventions.

EXERCISE 21-2	A Personal Grief Inventory

Purpose: To provide a close examination of one's history with grief.

Procedure

Complete each sentence and reflect on your answers:
   The first significant experience with grief that I can remember in my life was _____.
   The circumstances were _____.
   My age was _____.

The feelings I had at the time were _____.
The thing I remember most about that experience was _____.
I coped with the loss by _____.
The primary sources of support during this period were _____.
What helped most was _____.
The most difficult death for me to face would be _____.

Adapted from Carson VB, Arnold EN: *Mental health nursing: the nurse-client journey*, Philadelphia, 1996, WB Saunders, p. 666.

| EXERCISE 21-3 | Reflections on Memory Making in Significant Relationships |

Purpose: To provide students with an opportunity to see the value of memory making as a strategy for facilitating the grieving process.

With a partner, each student should share his or her story without interruption. When the student finishes his or her story, the listener can ask questions for further understanding.

Procedure
1. Write a letter to someone who has died or is no longer in your life. Before writing the letter, reflect on the meaning this person had for you and the person you have become.
2. In the letter, tell the person what they meant to you and why it is that you miss them.
3. Tell the person what you remember most about your relationship.
4. Tell the person anything you wished you had said but did not when the person was in your life.

Discussion
1. What was it like to write a letter to someone who had meaning in your life and is no longer available to you?
2. Were there any common themes?
3. In what ways was each story unique?
4. How could you use this exercise in your care of clients who are grieving?

APPLICATIONS

PALLIATIVE CARE

Fox (2014) defines *palliative* care as " a comprehensive philosophy of care aimed at primarily relieving symptoms associated with the treatment, as well as providing support for seriously ill patients and their families" (p. 93). Palliative care focuses primary attention on symptom management and relieving suffering. As a form of therapeutic care, palliative interventions supply the supportive physical, psychosocial, practical, and spiritual support services, and assistance people need when faced with a life-limiting illness or injury. Palliative care models emphasize "the totality of the client's experience in the context of their illness and/or dying" (Bruera and Yennurajalingam, 2011, p. 254).

Palliative care is unique in that it considers care for the client and family as an integrated care unit. As a client's life-limiting condition progresses, palliative care supports "living while dying" as comfortably as is possible. Symptom management for the client and practical support for the family as they negotiate the last stage of life becomes the priority. Unlike hospice, clients admitted to palliative care services can still receive active treatment for their disease process to control symptoms and improve quality of life (McIlfatrick, 2007). There are no regulatory requirements limiting admission to palliative care related to life expectancy. By contrast, medicare requirements call for a life expectancy of 6 months or less for admission to hospice. Hospice emphasizes a natural death, pain control and comfort measures to enhance

quality of life for the dying client. A similar interdisciplinary approach is evidenced in both palliative and hospice care. The World Health Organization (WHO) identifies dimensions of palliative care as presented in Box 21-1.

The overarching goal of palliative care is to help clients and their families achieve the highest quality of life possible regardless of stage of disease or the presence of other treatments and to prevent or relieve suffering. Palliative care strategies are designed to help critically ill clients and their families understand the dying process as a part of life and to maximize life options in the time left to them. The basic axiom for palliative care is to follow what clients actually want for themselves (Silveira and Schneider, 2004). After a client's death, palliative care offers grief support for family members.

NURSING INITIATIVES

Nurses have been in the forefront of developing guidelines for quality EOL care for many years beginning with the original work of Dame Cicely Saunders, Florence Wald, and others. The most recent guidelines published by the National Consensus Project (2013) provide a framework for providing quality palliative care. Nationally recognized nursing experts, funded by the American Association of Colleges of Nursing (AACN) and the City of Hope, also developed the End-of-Life Nursing Education Consortium (ELNEC), a national education initiative to improve EOL care in the United States. To date, more than 17,500 nurses have received training through these

BOX 21-1	Dimensions of Palliative Care

- Provides relief from pain and other distressing symptoms
- Affirms life and regards dying as a normal process
- Intends neither to hasten nor postpone death
- Integrates the psychological and spiritual aspects of client care
- Offers a support system to help clients live as actively as possible until death
- Offers a support system to help the family cope during the clients illness and in their own bereavement
- Uses a team approach to address the needs of clients and their families, including bereavement counseling, if indicated
- Will enhance quality of life and may also positively influence the course of illness
- Is applicable early in the course of illness, in conjunction with other therapies that are intended to prolong life, such as chemotherapy or radiation therapy, and includes those investigations needed to better understand and manage distressing clinical complications

From World Health Organization: *WHO Definition of Palliative Care.* nd. Available online: http://www.who.int/cancer/palliative/definition/en/. Accessed August 24, 2014.

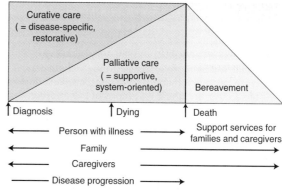

Figure 21-1   Model of curative and palliative care for progressive illness.

national courses (AACN, 2014). Specific EOL training allows nurses to teach others and to enter into the lives of many more people facing EOL as skilled, compassionate professionals with specialized care tools (Malloy et al., 2008).

NURSING ROLES IN PALLIATIVE CARE

Palliative care can be used concurrently with disease-modifying care. The level of comfort care increases according to client need (Savory and Marco, 2009). Palliative care operates as a 24-hour resource, providing comprehensive, holistic services to clients and families in hospitals, people's homes, nursing homes, and community settings. Services should reflect a client's identified cultural, social, and economic circumstances.

Palliative care delivery is best accomplished through skilled interdisciplinary team work. According to Bruera and Yennurajalingam (2012) "the role of the *palliative care team* is to assess and manage patients' and families' care needs in the physical, psychological, social, spiritual, and information domains" (p. 268). An interdisciplinary palliative care team usually consists of nurses, physicians, social workers, psychologists, and

clergy specially trained in palliative care. In addition to practical and supportive care for clients and families, team members provide education and consultation about EOL care for hospital staff.

The treatment focus of palliative care is on pain control, physical symptom management, and easing the secondary psychosocial and spiritual distress experienced by clients with a terminal illness. Nurses play a pivotal role as professional coordinators, direct providers of care, and advocates for client autonomy and control in EOL care. They are in a key position to help families maintain family integrity, to support their efforts in managing the process of living until death, and in preparing families for the death of their loved one. Quality indicators for EOL care are displayed in Figure 21-1.

KEY ISSUES AND APPROACHES IN END-OF-LIFE CARE
Self-Awareness

Self-awareness is a critical foundation for effective palliative nursing practice. Nurses are not immune to fears of being alone at time of death or of feeling stress when helping clients cope with unrelenting pain. Nurses must be aware of their personal feelings about death and influences from previous EOL experiences, including attitudes, expectations, and feelings about death and the process of dying. Otherwise, it may prove difficult for nurses to maintain a balance between personal sensitivity to a client's death and providing the empathy and support needed by clients and families. Self-awareness about death and dying issues is critical in palliative care. Miller (2001) notes, "As you become more clear about who you are and why

BOX 21-2	Principles Guiding End-of-Life Care Decision Making

- Discussions of medical futility with clients and family will be more effective if they include concrete information about treatment, its likelihood of success, and the implications of the intervention and nonintervention decisions.
- Effective decision making at the end of life can be improved with the use of advance directives and surrogate decision makers.
- Ethnic and cultural traditions and practices influence the use of advance directives and health care decision-making surrogates.
- Taking the time to explore the client's perceptions about quality of life at the end of life is a core component of clinical assessment and is essential to ensuring optimal outcomes.
- The cost of failing to offer clients and families a full range of end-of-life care options, services, and settings is an incalculable toll in terms of quality of life and utilization of appropriate health care resources at the end of life.

Modified from Bookbinder M, Rutledge DN, Donaldson NE, et al.: End-of-life care series: part I: principles, *Online J Clin Innovat* 4(4):1-30, 2001, by permission. © 2001, CINAHL Information Systems.

you do what you do, you will become more receptive to whomever you are with" (p. 23).

End-of-Life Decision Making

Thelan (2005) defines **EOL decision making** as "the process that healthcare providers, patients and patients' families go through when considering what treatments will or will not be used to treat a life threatening illness" (p. 29). Clients and families face difficult, irreversible decisions in the last phase of life. Preference decisions related to discontinuation of fluids, antibiotics, blood transfusions, and ventilator support require a clear understanding of a complex care situation. These are emotional issues for families, so that more than simple clinical explanations are needed. Box 21-2 presents principles guiding decisions about EOL care.

EOL decisions should be transparent, meaning that all parties involved in the decision should fully understand the implications of their decision. For example, to make an informed decision about use of life supports for terminal clients, clients and families need to know whether further treatments will enhance or diminish quality of life, their potential impact on life expectancy, and whether the treatment is known to be effective or is an investigative treatment.

Family members need to understand what types of adverse effects the client is likely to experience with each potential option. Financial considerations are important, as keeping clients in a permanent unconscious condition alive on a ventilator can be harmful to the client—and family. Futile "curative" treatments can cause needless pain and physical symptoms, noteworthy quality of life issues, and unnecessary anxiety.

Client preferences can change over time. Care directives may have to be revisited, especially if there is a change in prognosis and the potential for quality of life diminishes significantly (Guido, 2010).

Advance Directives

Ideally, EOL care choices should be made before a life-threatening illness occurs or as early as possible after diagnosis (Kirchhoff, 2002). In 1990, the *Patient Self-Determination Act* was passed into law. This law requires that adult clients be given information about advance directives, and their right to participate in and direct personal health care decisions, including do not resuscitate (DNR) directives—and that this data be documented. An advance directive is not permanently binding and the client has the right to revoke the document. Tulsky (2005) refers to advance planning as a communication "process by which patient, together with their families and health care practitioners consider their values goals and articulate their preferences for future care" (p. 360). Studies of family use of advance directives demonstrate significantly lower stress in families using them (Davis et al., 2005). In the hospital, advance directives should be kept in the front of the client's chart.

The nurse's role is to provide the client with full information about risks and benefits of prolonging life and to serve as client advocate in support of the person's right to make decisions about treatment and care (Erlen, 2005). When clients are decisionally competent, they should be key decision makers. When clients are not competent or cannot speak for themselves, a responsible family member or significant person should assume the responsibility of surrogate spokesperson. Formal family meetings with the palliative care team offer the most effective context for ensuring full disclosure, with opportunities to ask questions. It is important to encourage full family attendance and

BOX 21-3	Talking with Families about Care Options

If neither durable power of attorney nor written directive is in effect:

- Determine who should be approached to make the decisions about care options.
- Determine whether any key members are absent. (Try to keep those who know the client best in the center of decision making.)
- Find a quiet place to meet where each family member can be seated comfortably.
- Sit down and establish rapport with each person present. Ask about the relationship each person has with the client and how each person feels about the client's current condition.
- Try to achieve a consensus about the client's clinical situation, especially prognosis.
- Provide a professional observation about the client's status and expected quality of life—survival versus quality of life. Ask what each person thinks the client would want.
- Should the family choose comfort measures only, assure the family of the attention to client comfort and dignity that will occur.
- Seek verbal confirmation of understanding and agreement.
- Attention to the family's emotional responses is appropriate and appreciated.

Adapted from Lang F, Quill T: Making decisions with families at the end of life, *Am Fam Physician* 70(4):720, 2004.

participation, or at a minimum, those who will be involved in care decisions. If an essential family member cannot be physically present, having that member available by phone is advantageous. While this may be time consuming to arrange, it increases family satisfaction and cuts down on later problems.

Durable Power of Attorney for Health Care

As with advance directives, competent adults can choose to appoint a surrogate decision maker for them in the event that they cannot make important health decisions on their own behalf. This contingency gives clients the most flexibility in having decisions enacted, as they would wish, including the surrogate's authority to accept or refuse treatment on the client's behalf. Some clients have neither power of attorney for health nor advance directives. Box 21-3 provides guidelines for talking with families about care options at EOL when an advance directive or durable power of attorney is not in effect.

PAIN MANAGEMENT

Pain management is an essential component of quality palliative care. Standards for pain management established by The Joint Commission (2010) require that every inpatient be routinely assessed for pain, with documentation of appropriate monitoring and pain management. The American Pain Society (APS), The Joint Commission, and Veteran's Administration identify pain as the fifth vital sign to be assessed with standard vital signs (temperature, pulse, respiration, and blood pressure). Pain can negatively affect quality of life related to well-being and and compromises a client's capacity to perform daily functions, sleep, and engage in social relationships.

ASSESSING FOR PAIN

Pain is a complex phenomenon with sensory, emotional, cognitive, and behavioral dimensions (Wilkie and Ezenwa, 2012). Pain is an unpleasant subjective experience, assessed verbally with the client and/or observed in client behavior. Nurses perform screenings for pain, focused on

- Onset and duration of pain
- Location of the pain
- Character of the pain (sharp, dull, burning, persistent, changes with movement, direct or referred pain)
- Intensity—using a 0 to 10 numerical rating scale, with 0 being no pain and 10 being unbearable pain (use the Wong–Baker FACES Pain Rating Scale for children and people with limited health literacy)
- History of substance dependence (crossover tolerance)
- Aggravating factors such as difficulty breathing or turning
- Relief factors such as distraction with visitors, food or fluids, reassurance

Small children usually cannot meaningfully measure their pain level. Instead, look for behavioral indicators of pain in children such as abrupt changes in activity, crying, inability to be consoled, listlessness or unwillingness to move, rubbing a body part, wincing, or facial grimacing (Atkinson et al., 2009).

Estimates of older adults having significant pain range from upwards of 40%. Some are able to evaluate their pain, using the preceding suggestions. Those with cognitive changes may not be able to do so accurately

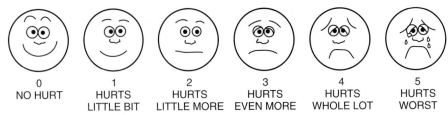

Figure 21-2   Wong–Baker FACES Pain Rating Scale. *(From Hockenberry MJ, Wilson D: Wong's essentials of pediatric nursing, ed. 8. St. Louis, 2009, Mosby. Used with permission. Copyright Mosby.)*

particularly if they are agitated. Chronic pain related to cancer, diabetic neuropathy, osteoporosis, or arthritis may not readily respond to pain medication. Changes in behavior and agitation can indicate pain in cognitively impaired clients. Observation of behavioral distress indicators is particularly important with older adults with even mild cognitive changes.

Clients needing palliative care often experience moderate to severe levels of pain. Having appropriate pain control for moderate-to-severe pain usually requires the use of opioids. Misperceptions about pain-relieving opioids can create major, unnecessary barrier to adequate pain control. Guido (2010) maintains that pain in older clients can be undertreated when it is assumed that they cannot tolerate strong pain medications, or that their pain is due to chronic, persistent conditions. Misperceptions about addiction and medication strength can result in inadequate pain management for children and mentally ill clients.

According to Pashby (2014), nurses need to educate clients and families about pain control, including the differences between disease progression and adverse effects related to opioids. For example, some clients do not want to take opioids for fear of feeling "weird" or not being able to think clearly. A second barrier is fear of addiction (Clary and Lawson, 2009). All clients, including addicts, are entitled to appropriate and adequate pain management of severe pain. People do not become addicted from taking legally prescribed opioid medications for pain associated with terminal illness. There is a fundamental difference between taking essential medication for pain control on a pre-scribed scheduled basis and addictive use. Addicted clients may require larger doses of pain medication because of cross-tolerance. Other barriers include a belief that suffering should be tolerated (stoicism) or is an unavoidable part of the dying process. Limited capacities to accurately describe pain intensity or seeing pain as a weakness also represent obstacles.

Families sometimes attribute signs and symptoms of approaching death such as increased lethargy, confusion, and declining appetite to side effects of opioids. This is not usually true. With or without pain medication, actively dying clients become less responsive as death approaches. Although clients may experience drowsiness with initial dosing, this side effect quickly disappears. Once clients and families understand the mechanisms and goals of pain control and are assured that the client will not die or become addicted from appropriate pain control, most will support its use in palliative care. Clients approaching death can experience *"breakthrough" pain*, which occurs episodically as severe pain spikes. When breakthrough pain occurs, rescue medications, which are faster acting, can be used. Touch and light massage are helpful adjuncts for pain relief. *The bottom line is that no client should suffer from preventable pain.*

COMMUNICATION IN END-OF-LIFE CARE

Curtis (2004) suggests that communication skill is equal to or supersedes clinical skill in EOL care. Everyone experiences a death differently; it is the uniqueness of each person's experience that the nurse attempts to tap into and facilitate discussion through conversation. Conversations with clients and families provide nurses with insights about personal values and preferences regarding EOL care and provide a forum to answer difficult questions in a supportive environment. Clients may alter their preferences and expectations during the course of palliative care treatment. Glass and colleagues (2010) note cancer client reports of "a roller-coaster ride" in which the hopeful points in remission are often followed by crises with relapse or disease progression" (p. 88). Since many cancers today demonstrate this type of pattern, frequent discussions become relevant. When clinicians take the time to discuss client preferences and document them appropriately, client wishes are more likely to be fulfilled (Cox et al., 2011; Moghaddam, Almack, et al, 2011)).

The quality of the relationship between nurse, client, and family members is a key factor in how the last phase of life is experienced and negotiated (Mok and Chiu, 2004). End of life care discussions are not easy. It takes courage to look at the reality of death (Callahan and colleagues, 2003). Clients benefit from talking about their fears and concerns. As they put words to the things that occur to them during this phase of their life journey, the issues, feelings and fears become less frightening. Words place boundaries on difficult experiences, which make them more manageable.

EOL interactions help people find meaning, achieve emotional closure, and provide the best means for helping clients and families make complex life decisions. Listening and responding to clients as they cope with difficult issues around dying is easier said than done (Larson and Tobin, 2000). The challenge for nurses is to remain in a relationship with clients and families even when one feels inadequate to the task.

Schim and Raspa (2007) believe that the process of dying is a narrative: "Life-altering happenings are expressed through stories" (p. 202). Personal reflections are critical sources of assessment data. Once rapport is established, Pashby (2014) suggests nurses can ask clients how they learned of their diagnosis. She notes that a terminal diagnosis is usually a "Technicolor Moment" that the person remembers vividly and appreciates talking about. Other questions such as "What has changed for you since the diagnosis?" or "What is it like for you now?" provide additional data. Giving voice to the experience helps clients discover its personal meaning and this information provides the nurse with a more complete picture of each person's distinctive concerns and goals.

Although most palliative care clients know when their time is growing short, the exact time frame is not known. It is not unusual for a client to ask in the course of conversation, "Am I going to die, or "how much longer do you think I have?" Before answering, find out more about the origin of the question. A useful listening response is, "What is your sense of it?" Box 21-4 provides guidelines for communicating with palliative care clients.

Morgan (2001) suggests using a basic social process between nurse and client in palliative care, which she labeled protective coping and adjustment.

BOX 21-4   Guidelines for Communicating with Clients

- Avoid automatic responses and trite reassurances.
- Each death is a unique, deeply personal experience for the client and should be treated as such.
- Avoid destroying hope. Reframe hope to what can happen in the here and now.
- Let the client lead the discussion about the future. Be comfortable with focusing on the here and now. (This discussion is not a one-time event; openings for discussion should be encouraged as the client's condition worsens.)
- Relate on a human level. Show humor, as well as sorrow.
- Use your mind, eyes, and ears to hear what is said, as well as what is not said.
- Respect the individual's pattern of communication and ways of dealing with stress. Support the client's desire for control of his or her life to whatever extent is possible.
- Maintain a sense of calm. Use eye contact, touch, and comfort measures to communicate.
- Do not force the client to talk. Respect the client's need for privacy and be sensitive to the client's readiness to talk, and let him or her know that you will be available to listen.
- Humility and honesty are essential. Be willing to admit when you do not know the answer.
- Be willing to allow the client to see some of your fears and vulnerabilities. It is much easier to open up to someone who is "human and vulnerable" than to someone who appears to have all the answers.

The *protective coping* process in palliative care involves nursing interactions that protect, maintain, and safeguard the integrity of clients, while simultaneously helping them to determine and act on actions that are in their own best interests. For example, an older adult with multiple comorbidities or beginning dementia may not want aggressive treatment for a heart condition, even though it might extend his or her life.

COMMUNICATING WITH FAMILIES

Family members have different levels of readiness to engage in discussions about the dying process. It is "normal" for an impending death to have a different impact on each family member, because each has had a unique relationship with the dying person. Conversations with families need not be long in duration, but regularity is important.

Common concerns include discontinuing life support; conflicts among family members about care; tensions between the client, family, and/or physician and family about treatment; where death should occur (home, hospital, hospice); if and/or when hospice should be engaged; and other concerns. Other unstated concerns revolve around historical patterns of conflictual relations, role expectations about family member responsibility and post death decisions about services.

CREATING FAMILY MEMORIES

Clients and families need to talk about things other than the disease process and treatments. Nurses can help make this happen. There are spiritual stories, cultural stories, funny stories, developmental stories, narratives of advocacy, and family stories. Each reinforces the bonds and affirms the depth of meaning a family holds with a dying person. The moments of laughter, foibles, and shared experiences are connections that are remembered.

Case Example

Evelyn was an 83-year-old woman diagnosed with terminal lung cancer. During a guided imagery exercise, the nurse asked her to recall a time when she felt relaxed and happy. Evelyn described in vivid detail being with her family at a picnic near a lake many years ago. When her family came to visit that night, Evelyn related the story again, and the entire family talked about their parts in the remembered event. It was one of their last conversations; one that reinforced family bonds in the initial telling and later as her family remembered Evelyn after her death. Later, her daughter made a special point of letting the nurse know how important sharing this story was to the client and family.

Providing Information

Nurses are key informants about client status and changes in the client's condition. There are fundamental differences in the level of information an individual or family will desire. The response of the client should determine the content and pace of sharing information. Talking with families about care details should happen often, but even more frequently when the client's health status begins to decline or show a change. Keep discussions simple and practical.

Ideally, one nurse serves as the primary contact for the client and family and acts as a liaison between providers and clients. This nurse keeps other health team members informed of new issues and shares their input into planning and evaluation of care with the family. Using precise language, giving full and truthful information about the client's condition, and admitting to uncertainty, when it exists, are important dimensions of EOL information giving.

Family EOL Conferences

Family conferences are interdisciplinary communication tools used to alleviate family anxiety about the dying process, reduce unnecessary conflict between family members, and assist family members with important decision-making processes. Proactive family meetings are particularly beneficial in ICU settings (Fox, 2014). A coordinated approach prevents fragmentary and inconsistent sharing of information.

Family conferences should include all legal decision makers, key health professionals, involved family members and the client if he or she is decisionally competent. Before meeting with the family, it is helpful to clarify family conference goals in your mind (Ambuel and Weissman, 2005). It is important to ask yourself what is it that you hope to achieve in the conference and to discuss key objectives with the health team so that everyone is on the same page. If the issues are complex, consider having a follow up meeting. Curtis (2004) recommends that there be a higher ratio of family member–to–health care provider speaking time, with follow-up communication.

Although a physician commonly leads the discussion, nurses often present relevant data and answer questions. Following introductions and identifying Start with questions designed to determine what the family already understands about the client's condition. Asking each family member for their thoughts often provides interesting and different perceptions. When presenting information about current status and treatment options, the data sharing should be compassionate, accurate, and presented in language understandable to the family. Contradictory recommendations and incomplete information add to a family's confusion and cause unnecessary distress (Wright et al., 2009).

Gavrin (2007) notes, "the analog of informed consent is informed refusal" (p. S86). This concept becomes important to clients and families as a component of decision making related to withdrawing or withholding life support in EOL care. Helping clients and families understand the importance of advance directives and DNR orders can prevent later conflicts when tensions arise near the time of death (Boyle et al., 2005). Nurses are invaluable resources in clarifying meanings with clients or individual family members after the conference.

ADDRESSING CULTURAL AND SPIRITUAL NEEDS

INCORPORATING CULTURAL DIFFERENCES

Different cultures have distinctive communication and care standards for clients with life-threatening conditions (Searight and Gafford, 2005). Box 21-5 presents cross-cultural variations found in palliative and EOL care. Cultural distinctions focus on (a) type of care that provides comfort to the dying person; (b) understanding of the causes of illness and death; (c) appropriate care of the body and burial rites; and (d) expression of grief responses (Doolen and York, 2007; LaVera et al., 2002).

As with other aspects of cultural beliefs, there is significant variation within the culture as well as between cultures in EOL care preferences. When cultural differences are considered, it is important to avoid stereotyping, as each person's interpretation of their culture is unique. Once cultural needs are identified, every

---

BOX 21-5	Cross-Cultural Variations in End-of-Life Care

- Emphasis on autonomy versus collectivism
- Attitudes toward advance directives
- Decisions making about life support, code status guidelines
- Preference for direct versus indirect disclosure of information
- Individual versus family-based decision making about treatment
- Disclosure of life-threatening diagnoses
- Provider's choice of words in verbal exchanges
- Reliance on physician as the ultimate authority
- Specific rituals or practices performed at time of death
- Role of religion and spirituality in coping and afterlife
- Views about suffering

Adapted from Searight H, Gafford J: Cultural diversity at the end of life: issues and guidelines for family physicians, *Am Fam Physician* 71(3):515-522, 2005.

effort should be taken to honor their meaning to clients and families by incorporating them in care (see also Chapter 7).

A simple question such as "Can you tell me about how your family/culture/spiritual beliefs views serious illness or treatment?" provides a framework for discussion. Nurses should provide factual information with attention paid to cultural values and emotions (Davies et. al, 2010).

According to Sherman (2010) admitting a person to hospice or engaging in advance directives planning may be a culturally based problem for African American clients. They depend predominantly on family and their church community for major support and assistance. The Chinese culture believes that end of life care should be geared to creating a calm environment for the client. Family members feel a cultural obligation to care for the dying person; hospice is not considered as an option. There is a conspiracy of silence about terminal illness because of a belief that discussing EOL issues leads to hopelessness. In the Latino or Hispanic culture, there is a similar belief that the client who is dying should be protected from any discussion of the terminal condition. In each of these cultures, involvement of the family as a unit is central to providing quality EOL care to clients.

ATTENDING TO SPIRITUAL NEEDS

Glass and colleagues (2010) note, "The transition from life to death is as sacred as the transition experienced at birth" (p. 101). The dying process, grief, and death itself herald a spiritual crisis—a crisis of faith, hope, and meaning for many people. Spiritual pain occurs when a person's sense of purpose is challenged or one's existence is threatened (Millspaugh, 2005).

Spirituality becomes a priority for many people at EOL (Williams, 2006). It is not unusual for clients who have previously declined spiritual interventions to desire them as they move into the final phase of life. Spiritual beliefs and religious rituals provide a tangible vehicle for individuals and families to express and experience meaning and purpose. Religious practices and rituals relevant to EOL can be important to clients even if the person no longer formally practices the religion. Facilitating these practices touches the client's inner core and helps the person move toward a peaceful death (Bryson, 2004).

Most people welcome an inquiry about their spiritual well-being (Morrison and Meier, 2004).

People having a strong relationship with God and/or religious beliefs will usually indicate this connection. To elicit more information about its nature, an appropriate question is: "Is there anything I should know about your spiritual or religious views?" The answer can tell you what is important related to their current circumstances. Steinhauser and colleagues (2006) suggest using the probe "Are you at peace?" as a useful way to ask the client about spiritual concerns without being intrusive. Nurses can ask the client and/or family if they would like a visit from an appropriate clergy or hospital chaplain, facilitate the initial contact if the answer is yes, and provide essential information about the client's condition and/or family concerns (Barclay and Lie, 2007).

Not all people attach their concept of spirituality to a particular belief system. Instead, they define their spirituality from an existential perspective. Attig (2001) describes this sense of spirituality as follows:

> That within us that reaches beyond present circumstances, soars in extraordinary experiences, strives for excellence and a better life, struggles to overcome adversity, and searches for meaning and transcendent understanding. (p. 37)

When individuals frame their spirituality from an existential perspective, it is appropriate to explore spirituality sources in terms of meaningful relationships. Asking a question such as "Can you tell me about the relationship you had with someone whom you loved who has died?" helps start the conversation. A follow-up question relates to how the client feels about the person now. The value of this intervention is that it emphasizes that the person's life held meaning for this other person. This line of questioning indirectly tells the person that they too will be remembered after death (Pashby, 2014).

People benefit from telling stories about how they view their life and validate its meaning. A life review helps people consider the deeper values and purpose of their lives, the experience of joy and sorrow. As one person stated, "I lived my life as best I could. I have no regrets." A follow-up listening response to help the person put into words what he or she reflect on the meaning of a life well lived might be: "Tell me more about this."

Whatever form spiritual distress takes, it is essential for the nurse to address it. Spiritual issues that trouble clients relate to forgiveness, unresolved guilt issues, expressions of love, saying good-bye to important people, and existential questions about the meaning of life, the hereafter, and concern for their family.

Clary and Lawson (2009) suggest that the EOL offers a final opportunity for people to experience spiritual growth. The most important intervention nurses can provide is to actively and respectfully listen to each client's search for clarity about their spirituality with compassion and a desire to understand. Helping clients think through spiritual preferences and assisting them to identify resources that can give them strength, courage, purpose, and encouragement to cope with their situation is highly valued. Providing explicit attention to inclusion of appropriate spiritual advisors, prayer, and scripture reading can be helpful to faith-based clients and families coping with a terminal condition.

Nurses need to take an honest look at their own spirituality. Self-awareness allows nurses to explore their client's worldview from an authentic position, without imposing personal values and beliefs.

PALLIATIVE CARE FOR CHILDREN

It is not the natural order of things for a child to die. People are supposed to live into adulthood. When a child is diagnosed with a life-limiting condition, the effect on parents is devastating. It influences role functioning, friendships, and treatment of siblings (Hinds et al., 2005). Children are such an integral part of their parent's identity that issues of parental protectiveness, guilt, responsible caregiving, balancing family demands, and helplessness parents feel should be part of the discussion. In addition to providing appropriate symptom management medications to make the child more comfortable, the following interventions are supportive to children with a life-limiting illness.

1. Encourage visits from family and friends.
2. Involve and inform the child of everything that is going on with *developmentally* appropriate language and content.
3. Encourage the family to keep the child's life as normal as possible.
4. Suggest ways to enhance family functioning with attention paid to making special time for siblings and involving them in care discussions.

5. Arrange respite for parents and encourage special parent times.
6. Encourage families to maintain or adapt cultural, family, and religious traditions.
7. Encourage families to seek emotional support: support groups, extended family, friends (Field and Behrman, 2002).

Parents serve as a major anchoring force for children. They need to be recognized as the expert and a primary advocate for their child. Here are some ways that nurses can help. Take the time to explore with the parents how they conceptualize quality of life for their child and what is important for the nurse to know about the child's preferences. Nurses can identify situations in which there is a mismatch between a child's condition and a parent's understanding of that condition (Field and Behrman, 2002). This is important information, which needs to be shared with the palliative care team. By observing the child, you also can begin to note preferences. Children value being asked about their likes and dislikes. There should be no surprises. You need to talk with the child and the parents about each procedure in language they can understand. Giving a child a sense that you and the parents are on the same page provides security, and comfort. Critical to parent satisfaction is the knowledge that everything possible was done for their child; that they received accurate, timely information and support; and that preventable suffering was not permitted.

HELPING CHILDREN UNDERSTAND DEATH

Nurses can help parents talk with their children about the impending death of a significant person in their lives. Encourage parents to explain what is happening in a concrete, direct way, using clear, concrete words suitable to the child's developmental level. Questions should be answered directly and honestly at the child's developmental level of comprehension, free of medical jargon. This type of discussion should *not* be a one-time event, and parents may need to be proactive in initiating the conversation.

The family may want to exclude young children from contact with or knowledge about a person who is likely to die soon. Sometimes it is a judgment call as to whether visitation is a good idea. Drawing a picture or sending a note card is another way for a child to connect with a critically ill relative if visitation is not an option.

Death of a significant persons is difficult for children because they have neither the cognitive development nor the life experiences to fully process its meaning. A child younger than 5 years of age has no clear concept of what death means.

Case Example
A short time after 5-year-old Aidan's grandfather died, he asked his grandmother where his grandfather had gone. His grandmother told him that grandpa had died, and was in heaven, to which Aidan said, "Oh no, grandma, he's in that brown box in the ground."

Until children reach the formal operations stage of cognitive development, they can have fantasies about the circumstances surrounding the death and their part in it. With preparation, adolescents can benefit from being allowed to visit with the terminally ill significant people in their lives.

Case Example
Brendan and his grandfather had a close relationship. Earlier in life, they would stroke each other's thumbs as part of a "special handshake." Now, at 15, his grandfather was close to death and unresponsive. As Brendan sat next to him, stroking his thumb in the remembered way, he felt sure that his grandfather had squeezed his hand more than once. This was a meaningful connection for Brendan.

CHILDREN'S GRIEF

Children do not express their grief in the same way as adults. Unpredictable acting out behaviors, withdrawal, anger, fear, and crying are common responses. One minute the child may be playing, the next the child is angry or withdrawn. Preschoolers may repeatedly ask when someone close to them will be coming home even if parents tell them the person has died. Developmentally they do not understand the permanence of death. Elementary school children accept the permanence of death, but view it in a concrete manner. They may have all sorts of fantasies about gravely ill significant people in their lives or those who die suddenly. Grace's interpretation of her role in her grandmother's death actually happened; this is not an uncommon occurrence. Unfortunately, children do not always share their concerns with their caregivers and suffer unnecessarily with misinterpretations about a loved one's death.

Case Example

Grace was nine years old when her beloved grandmother suffered a massive heart attack and died in her sleep. In Grace's eyes, her grandmother was more of a mother to her than her natural mother. The day before her death, Grace had talked back to her grandmother. This was something she rarely did and in her mind, she felt that maybe "this is what killed my grandmother." She never discussed her thoughts with anyone but neither did she ever forget her perception that she had caused her grandmother's death. Even as an adult, the memory persisted.

The National Cancer Institute (2010) identifies three key concerns children may have about the death of someone important to them:

1. Did I cause the death to happen?
2. Is it going to happen to me?
3. Who is going to take care of me?

Parents should anticipate that these concerns may be issues for children and *create* opportunities for children to ask questions. Maintaining daily routines in the child's life after the death of a parent or primary caregiver is critical. Children need to know that they are safe and will be taken care of by the surviving adults in their life. If changes are needed, children should have ample time to make the adjustment rather than have a sudden move thrust on them without discussion.

Children in adolescence are particularly vulnerable to unresolved grief. They are often expected to act grown up and model the grieving process for younger siblings. Adults expect adolescents to grieve a death more as an adult than as a child, but they lack the life experience to do so.

Many adolescents do not openly ask questions because they do not want to increase parental grief. Surviving parents may be unable to fully connect with their daughter or son's grief because they are processing their own grief. Expectations that an adolescent will step up to the plate and perform household chores or child care is common. Without a place to talk about their feelings, the adolescent may bury feelings that are necessary to process. Adolescents need physical contact, reassurance, and benefit from relevant discussions about the person who has died. If parents are unable to provide the level of communication an adolescent needs, nurses can help them with appropriate referrals.

HELPING CLIENTS ACHIEVE A GOOD DEATH

The Institute of Medicine (Field and Cassel, 1997) defines a **good death** as "one that is free from unavoidable distress and suffering for clients, families and caregivers; in general accord with clients' and families' wishes; and reasonably consistent with clinical, cultural, and ethical standards" (p. 82). Death is a deeply personal experience. Pain and symptom relief, transparent decision making, and preparation for what to expect have been identified in research studies as components of a good death experience for terminally ill clients. Comfort and quality of life are key goals. The act of bearing witness to the client's journey as a person of unquestioned worth and honoring the client's truth as the basis for decision making and care during the last segment of human life is perhaps the most significant role the nurse enacts in palliative and hospice care (Perrin, et al, 2012). Also important to dying clients is achieving a sense of completion (Steinhauser et al., 2000). In the following example, a nurse helps a terminally ill client achieve a sense of spiritual completion.

Case Example

George was in the last stages of his end-of-life journey. He had repeatedly refused to have spiritual visits, and no desire for the sacrament of the living (a religious rite in the Roman Catholic Church). His nurse said the priest was on the floor, and asked him if he would like to receive communion. He said yes, but nothing else. The priest gave him communion, following which George asked him to hear his confession and requested the last rites. After the priest left, George told his nurse "You always seem to know what to do, and when to do it; thank you."

A good death requires skilled, *collaborative interdisciplinary team care* with activities "ranging from the simplest needs, such as positioning and communication to advanced medical therapies" (Jevon, 2010, p. 3). Maintaining a sense of control over what happens during the dying process and who is present at the end, having access to spiritual, emotional, and knowledgeable supports, and being afforded hope, dignity, and privacy are also client and family values associated with a good death (Côté and Peplar, 2005; Kirchhoff, 2002; Smith, 2000). Exercise 21-4 provides you with the opportunity to personally think about what constitutes a good death.

EXERCISE 21-4	What Makes for a Good Death

Purpose: To help students focus on defining the characteristics of a good death.

Procedure
1. In pairs or small groups, think about, write down, and then share briefly examples of a "good" and a "not-so-good" death that you have witnessed in your personal life or clinical setting.

2. What were the elements that you thought contributed to its being a "good" or "not-so-good" death?

Discussion
Were there any common themes found in the stories as to what constitutes a "good" death? How could you use the findings of this exercise in helping clients achieve a "good" death?

SIGNS OF APPROACHING DEATH

There usually are usually observable changes in the client's condition when death is immanent. Pain symptoms may intensify. Fatigue, breathlessness, and drowsiness increase. The client may become delirious, anxious and agitated, or somnolent. Constipation can be a problem. Clients lose their appetite and gradually stop eating. With some clients changes are progressive and swift. With others there is gradual downward spiral. Common symptoms include long periods of sleeping or coma, decreased urinary output (dark urine), changes in vital signs, disorientation, restlessness and agitation, severe dyspnea (breathlessness) and Cheyne stokes breathing. Picking at bed clothes, and skin temperature and color changes occur. Dying clients experience profound weakness such that they cannot independently complete even basic hygiene. The American Cancer Society web site offers an excellent description of typical changes in the client when death is near and a clear outline of what caregivers can do to provide comfort to the client.

Family members feel increasingly helpless in being able to properly meet client needs. They need anticipatory guidance about what to expect and concrete suggestions about ways to connect with their loved one. A good way to start the conversation is to ask, "what would be the most helpful issue for us to talk about today?" Direct *comfort care* is essential. Practical suggestions for care and the availability of the nurse to family as well as client are critical components of care as clients approach death. Nurses can recommend simple care measures such as positioning, mouth and hygiene care, and so forth, to support family member efforts. They can provide immediate assessment data and explain its meaning. Nurses can encourage out-of-town family to visit, refer caregivers to support groups, and offer resource referrals for respite care. Most important, nurses can listen and offer empathetic presence.

Creating a care environment in which the dying person feels valued, comforted, and treated as a unique individual (Volker and Limerick, 2007) is vital, even when the client no longer is aware of what is happening. The client's loss of appetite and interest in food often frightens family members. Explaining that this is a natural process, which occurs as the body begins to shut down in preparation for death helps with family understanding (Reid et al., 2009). Clients become increasingly unresponsive to voice and stimulus. Hearing is the last sense to go, so talking with the dying person in a soft voice, playing calming music, and using gentle touch can also soothe the client in a meaningful way.

Flexibility in allowing family and/or significant others open access to the client reduces family anxiety and can be comforting for all concerned. At the same time, as clients weaken, it becomes an effort to respond to family and friends. Nurses act as gatekeepers, family supports and client advocates during this critical time period.

CARE OF THE IMMINENTLY DYING CLIENT

The process of watching someone die is frightening to families. Particularly upsetting is the client's inability to control oral pharyngeal secretions, sometimes referred to as the "death rattle" (Freeman, 2013). The use of morphine can help diminish the client's air hunger and Ativan reduces the restless agitation. Use of these drugs sometimes alarms families who fear that they hasten death. The reality is that both are given in small doses and are beneficial in helping clients breathe more easily and lessen nonproductive restlessness.

As death approaches, communication becomes more challenging. Family members become emotionally and physically exhausted. Grief may be intense. Family members look to the nurse for information about the dying process and for emotional support

BOX 21-6	Imminent Death: Family Communication Needs

- Honest and complete answers to questions; repetition and further explanation if needed.
- Updates about the client's condition and changes as they occur.
- Clear, understandable explanations, delivered with empathy and respect.
- Frequent opportunities to express concerns and feelings in a supportive, unhurried environment.
- Information about what to expect—physical, emotional, spiritual—as death approaches.
- Discussion of whom to call, legal issues, memorial or funeral planning.
- Conversation about cultural and/or religious rituals at time of, and after death.
- Appreciation of the conflicts that families experience when the illness dictates that few options exist; for example, a frequent dilemma at end of life is whether life support measures are extending life or prolonging the dying phase.
- Short private times to be present and/or minister to the client.
- Permission to leave the dying client for short periods with the knowledge that the nurse will contact the family member if there is a change in status.

(Wittenberg-Lyles et al., 2013). A calming presence is perhaps the most important form of communication and emotional support for dying clients and families. Box 21-6 identifies family communication needs when death is imminent.

Family members often find it difficult to leave a dying client, even when it would be in their best interest to take a short respite. Assuring family members that the nurse will check on the client frequently and will call the family immediately if change occurs, gives families permission to take a brief respite from the client.

CARING OF THE CLIENT AFTER DEATH

Respect for the dignity of the client continues after death. If the family is present at time of death, allowing uninterrupted private time with the client before initiating postmortem care is important. If the family is not present, all excess equipment and trash should be removed from the room. You can offer presence and emotional support as you escort the family into the room. Some families will want privacy; others will appreciate having the presence of the nurse or

chaplain. Family preference should be honored. You can acknowledge the impact of the death with a simple statement such as, "I can only imagine how difficult this must be for you." How you say it—speaking from the heart as well as the head—is as important as what you say. The case example below demonstrates the type of connection that is helpful to family members.

Case Example

"I remember standing next to my mom's bed. We had gone to her room to pay our last respects. A young nurse stood near to me and reached out gently and touched my shoulder. Softly she said, 'I'll just stay here with you in case you need something.' When I looked at her I saw eyes brimming with tears and a profound sadness on her face. Her presence meant so much; I was grateful for her open expression of sorrow. It confirmed the pain we were all experiencing."—Anonymous

If the family is not immediately present, the client's belongings should be placed in a bag and given to the family after the visitation. Provide soft lighting, chairs for the family, and tissues. The client's head should be elevated at a 30-degree angle, in a natural position. Hair should be combed, exposed body parts cleaned, and dentures replaced, if possible. The tone of the room and the positioning of the client should "give a sense of peace for the family" (Marthaler, 2005, p. 217). It is important for the nurse to allow the family as much time as they need with the client. The nurse can obtain signatures to release the client to the funeral home *after* the family has spent some time with the client.

STRESS ISSUES FOR NURSES IN PALLIATIVE CARE SETTINGS

Nurses deeply invest themselves in the care and comfort of clients and families facing death. They too can experience grief when the client dies. **Disenfranchised grieving** is a term applied to the grief nurses can experience after the death of a client with whom they have had an important relationship (Brosche, 2007; Rushton et al., 2006). Unacknowledged grieving in professional nurses can be cumulative. Unlike their clients, who live through one loss at a time, nurses can experience several losses a week while caring for terminally ill clients and their families (Brunelli, 2005).

Nurses can experience **compassion fatigue**, a syndrome associated with serious spiritual, physical, and emotional depletion related to caring for clients that can affect the nurse's ability to care for other clients (Worley, 2005). This term is used interchangeably with secondary traumatic stress and as a unique form of burnout related to exposure to the intense suffering of a client and characterized by emotional exhaustion and depersonalization. Compassion fatigue is a common finding with nurses working in oncology and palliative care (Day and Anderson, 2011). Unrelieved compassion fatigue can result in burnout and a nurse's decision to leave nursing.

Case Example

Barbara was a new graduate selected as a nursing intern on a research oncology unit, providing care for seriously ill pediatric oncology clients. She had a degree in another field and an excellent job, but always wanted to pursue nursing. Her original preceptor left the hospital and was replaced by an efficient nurse little empathy who gave her minimal support. The stress of weekly deaths, severe symptomatology, and lack of empathetic support led Barbara to leave nursing entirely after less than a year and return to her former job.

Nurses working in palliative care need to actively pursue ways to experience self-compassion. Self-compassion encourages nurses to balance the care they give others others, with care for self. Reflecting on the meaning of connections with dying clients, becoming aware not only of your personal strengths, but also your limitations are essential forms of the self-awareness needed for self-compassion. Regular self-reflection allows you to know yourself and gives you more options in relating to clients, families, and other members of the health care team (Wittenberg-Lyles et al., 2013). Support groups in which nurses can successfully address and resolve the secondary stress of continuously caring for terminally ill clients and some of the ethical issues involved with that care are helpful to nurses. See also the strategies presented in Chapter 16 related to burnout prevention.

SUMMARY

This chapter describes the stages of death and dying and theory frameworks of Eric Lindeman and George Engel for understanding grief and grieving. Palliative care is discussed as a philosophy of care and an emerging discipline focused on making EOL care a quality

life experience. A good death is defined as a peaceful death experienced with dignity and respect; one that wholly honors the client's values and wishes at the EOL. Nurses can offer compassionate communication, presence, and anticipatory guidance to ease the grief of loss.

Nursing strategies are designed to help clients cope with the secondary psychological and spiritual aspects of having a terminal illness such that they achieve the best quality of life in the time left to them. Talking with clients about advance directives is a professional responsibility of the nurse, and it reduces unnecessary conflict among family members at this critical time in a person's life. Talking with children about terminal illness and death in a relative, or in coping with a terminal diagnosis themselves, should take into consideration the child's developmental level. Questions should be answered honestly and empathetically.

As death approaches, nurses can help families understand the physiological changes signaling the body's natural shutdown of systems and provide emotional support. Providing support for clinicians is considered a quality indicator in EOL care. When not addressed, the disenfranchised grief that nurses experience with providing EOL care to multiple clients can lead to compassion fatigue, burnout, and moral distress.

ETHICAL DILEMMA　What Would You Do?

Francis Dillon has been on a ventilator for the past 3 weeks, He is not decisionally competent and he is not able to communicate. Although he has virtually no chance of recovery, his family refuses to take him off the ventilator because "there is always the chance that he might wake up." What do you see as the ethical issues and how would you, as the nurse, address this problem?

DISCUSSION QUESTIONS

1. What is meant by the statement, "there is potential for healing and meaning even in the face of impending death"?
2. What was your most challenging EOL experience and how did you cope with it?
3. Think of a relevant example of family disagreement related to a client's deteriorating condition. What strategies could be used to turn this EOL conversation into a productive discussion?
4. What does the concept quality of life mean in EOL care?

REFERENCES

Ambuel B, Weissman DE. (2005) Moderating an end-of-life family conference. 2d ed. Fast Facts and Concepts, No. 016. End of Life/Palliative Education Resource Center, Medical College of Wisconsin. http://www.eperc.mcw.edu/EPERC/FastFactsIndex/ff_016.htm. Accessed August 24, 2014.

American Association of Colleges of Nursing. 2014. *End-of-Life Nursing Education Consortium (ELNEC) fact sheet, updated March 2014.* Available online: http://www.aacn.nche.edu/ELNEC/about. htm. Accessed March 29, 2014.

Atkinson P, Chesters A, Heinz P: Pain management and sedation for children in the emergency department, *BMJ* 339:b4234, 2009.

Attig T: Relearning the world: making and finding meanings. In Neimeyer R, editor: *Meaning reconstruction and the experience of loss,* Washington, DC, 2001, American Psychological Association, pp 33–53.

Attig T: Meanings of death seen through the lens of grieving, *Death Stud* 28:341–360, 2004.

Barclay L, Lie D: New guidelines issued for family support in client-centered ICU, *Crit Care Med* 37:605–622, 2007.

Boyle D, Miller P, Forbes-Thompson S: Communication and end-of-life care in the intensive care unit, *Crit Care Nurs Q* 28(4):302–316, 2005.

Brosche T: A grief team within a healthcare system, *Dimens Crit Care Nurs* 26(1):21–28, 2007.

Bruera E, Yennurajalingam S: *Oxford American handbook of hospice and palliative medicine,* New York, 2011, Oxford University Press.

Bruera E, Yennurajalingam S: Palliative care in advanced cancer patients: How and when? *Oncologist* 17:267–273, 2012.

Brunelli T: A concept analysis: the grieving process for nurses, *Nurs Forum* 40(4):123–128, 2005.

Bryson KA: Spirituality, meaning, and transcendence, *Palliat Support Care* 2(3):321–328, 2004.

Callahan K, Maldonado N, Efinger J: Bridge over troubled waters: End-of-life (EOL) decisions, a qualitative case study, *TQR* 8(1):32–56, 2003.

Clary P, Lawson P: Pharmacologic pearls for end of life care, *Am Fam Physician* 79(12):1059–1065, 2009.

Corless I: Chapter 30: Bereavement. In Ferrell B, Coyle N, editors: *Oxford Textbook of palliative nursing,* New York, 2010, Oxford University Press, pp 597–612.

Côté J, C. Peplar C: A focus for nursing intervention: realistic acceptance or helping illusions, *Int J Nurs Pract* 11:39–43, 2005.

Cox K, Moghaddam N, Almack K, Pollock K, Seymour J: Is it recorded in the notes? Documentation of end-of-life care and preferred place to die discussions in the final weeks of life, *BMC Palliat Care* 10(81), 2011.

Curtis JR: Communicating about end-of-life care with clients and families in the intensive care unit, *Crit Care Clin* 20:363–380, 2004.

Davies B, Contro N, Larson J, Widger K: Culturally sensitive information sharing in pediatric palliative care, *PediatricsPediatrics* 4:e859–e865, 2010.

Davis B, Burns J, Rezac D, et al.: Family stress and advance directives: a comparative study, *Am J Hosp Palliat Care* 7(4):219–229, 2005.

Day J, Anderson R: Compassion fatigue: an application of the concept to informal caregivers of family members with dementia, *Nurs Res Prac* Vol. 2011:1–10, 2011.

Doolen J, York N: Cultural differences with end of life care in the critical care unit, *Dimens Crit Care Nurs* 26(5):194–198, 2007.

Engel G: Grief and grieving, *Am J Nurs* 64(7):93–96, 1964.

Erlen J: When clients and families disagree, *Orthop Nurs* 24(4):279–282, 2005.

Feigelman B, Feigelman W: Surviving after suicide loss: the healing potential of suicide survivor support groups, *Illness Crisis Loss* 16(4):285–304, 2008.

Field M, Behrman R: *When children die: improving palliative and end-of-life care for children and their families,* Washington, DC, 2002, The National Academies Press.

Florczak K: The persistent yet everchanging nature of grieving a loss, *Nurs Sci Q* 21(1):7–11, 2008.

Fox M: Improving communication with patients and families in the intensive care unit: Palliative care strategies for the intensive care unit nurse, *J Hospice Palliat Nurs* 16(2):93–98, 2014.

Freeman B: CARES: An acronym organized tool for the care of the dying, *J Hosp Palliative Nurs* 13(3):147–153, 2013.

Glass E, Cluxton D, Rancour P: Principles of patient and family assessment. In Ferrell B, Coyle N, editors: *Oxford Textbook of palliative nursing,* New York, 2010, Oxford University Press, pp 87–106.

Gavrin J: Ethical considerations at the end of life in the intensive care unit, *Crit Care Med* 35(2):S85–S94, 2007.

Gordon J: An evidence-based approach for supporting parents experiencing chronic sorrow, *Pediatr Nurs* 35(20):115–119, 2009.

Guido G: *Nursing Care at the End of Life,* Pearson, 2010, Upper Saddle River NJ.

Harvard Women's Health Watch. July 2009. Left behind after suicide. Available at: www.health.harvard.edu.

Hinds P, Schum L, Baker J, et al.: Key factors affecting dying children and their families, *J Palliat Med* 8(Suppl 1):S70–S78, 2005.

Field MJ, Cassel CK, editors: *Approaching death: improving care at the end of life,* Washington: DC, 1997, National Academy Press.

Jeffreys J: *Helping grieving people—when tears are not enough: a handbook for care providers,* ed 2, New York, 2011, *NY*: Brunner-Routledge.

Jevon P: *Caring of the Dying and Deceased Patient: A Practical Guide for Nurses,* Oxford UK, 2010, Wiley-Blackwell.

The Joint Commission: *The Approaches to pain management: an essential guide for clinical leaders,* ed 2, Oakbrook Terrace, IL, 2010, Joint Commission Resources.

Keegan L, Drick C: *End of Life: Nursing Solutions for Death with Dignity,* New York, 2011, Springer.

Kirchhoff KT: Promoting a peaceful death in the ICU, *Crit Care Clin North Am* 14:201–206, 2002.

Kübler-Ross E: *On death and dying: What the dying have to teach doctors, nurses, clergy, and their own families,* New York, 1969, Scribner.

Lang F, Quill T: Making decisions with families at the end of life, *Am Fam Physician* 70(4):719–723, 2004.

Larson DG, Tobin DR: End-of-Life Conversations; Evolving practice and Theory, *JAMA* 284(12):1573–1583, 2000.

LaVera M, Crawley M, Marshall P, et al.: Strategies for culturally effective end of life care, *Ann Intern Med* 136(9):673–677, 2002.

Lendrum S, Syme G: *Gift of tears: a practice approach to loss and bereavement counseling,* London, 1992, Routledge.

Lichetenthal W, Neimeyer R, Currier J, Roberts K, Jordan N: Cause of death and the quest for meaning in the loss of a child, *Death Studies* 37(4):311–342, 2013.

Lindemann E: Symptomatology and management of acute grief, *Am J Psychiatry* 151(6 sesquicentennial Suppl):155–160, 1994 (Originally published in 1944).

Malloy P, Paice J, Virani R, et al.: End of life-nursing education consortium: 5 years of educating graduate nursing faculty in excellent palliative care, *J Prof Nurs* 24(6):352–357, 2008.

Mark Twain Quotations, Newspaper Collections, & Related Resources. n.d. Available online: www.twainquotes.com.

Marthaler MT: End of life care: practical tips, *Dimens Crit Care Nurs* 24(5):215–218, 2005.

McIlfatrick S: Assessing palliative care needs: views of clients, informal carers and healthcare professionals, *J Adv Nurs* 57(1):77–86, 2007.

Mercer D, Evans J: The impact of multiple losses on the grieving process: an exploratory study, *J Loss Trauma* 11:219–227, 2006.

Miller J: *The art of being a healing presence*, Ft. Wayne, IN, 2001, Willowgreen.

Millspaugh D: Assessment and response to spiritual pain: part I, *J Palliat Med* 8(5):919–923, 2005.

Mok E, Chiu P: Nurse-client relationships in palliative care, *J Adv Nurs* 48(5):475–483, 2004.

Morgan A: A grounded theory of nurse-client interactions in palliative care nursing, *J Clin Nurs* 10(4):583–584, 2001.

Morrison S, Meier D: Palliative care, *N Engl J Med* 350:2582–2590, 2004.

National Cancer Institute. 2010. Children and grief. Available online: http://www.cancer.gov/cancertopics/pdq/supportivecare/bereavement/Client/page9.

Neimeyer RA, editor: *Meaning reconstruction and the experience of loss*, Washington, DC, 2001, American Psychological Association.

Pashby N, 2014: Personal Communication, Odenton, MD, March 2014.

Perrin K: Chapter 4, Ethical responsibilities and issues in palliative care. In Perrin K, Sheehan C, Potter M, Kazanowski M, editors: *Palliative Care Nursing: Caring for Suffering Patients*, Sudbury MA, 2012, Jones & Bartlett.

Reid J, McKenna H, Fitsimons D, et al.: Fighting over food: client and family understanding of cancer cachexia, *Oncol Nurs Forum* 36(4):439–445, 2009.

Rushton CH, Reder E, Hall B, et al.: Interdisciplinary interventions to improve pediatric palliative care and reduce health care professional suffering, *J Palliat Med* 9:922–933, 2006.

Savory E, Marco C: End of life issues in the acute and critically ill client, *Scand J Trauma Resuscitation Emerg Med* 17:21, 2009.

Schim S, Raspa R: Cross disciplinary boundaries in end-of-life education, *J Prof Nurs* 23(4):201–207, 2007.

Searight H, Gafford J: Cultural diversity at the end of life: issues and guidelines for family physicians, *Am Fam Physician* 71(3):515–522, 2005.

Sherman DW: Culture and spirituality as domains of quality palliative care. In Matzo M, Sherman DW, editors: *Palliative Care Nursing: Quality care at the end of life*, ed 3, New York, 2010, Springer, pp 3–52.

Silveira M, Schneider C: Common sense and compassion: planning for the end of life, *Clinics Family Practice* 6(2):349–368, 2004.

Smith R: A good death: An important aim for health services and for us all, *BMJ* 320:129–130, 2000.

Steinhauser KE, Clipp E, McNeilly M, et al.: In search of a good death: observations of patients, families, and providers, *Ann Intern Med* 132(10):825–832, 2000.

Steinhauser K, Voils C, Clipp E, et al.: Are you at peace?: one item to probe spiritual concerns at the end of life, *Arch Intern Med* 166(1):101–105, 2006.

Thelan M: End of life decision making in intensive care, *Crit Care Nurse* 25(6):28–37, 2005.

Thomas J: *My Saints Alive: A Journey of Life, Loss, and Love Unpublished Manuscript*, Charlottesville, VA, 2010, September.

Thomas J: *My Saints Alive: Reflections on a Journey of Love, Loss and Life*, Charlottesville VA, 2011, CreateSpace Independent Publishing Platform.

Tulsky J: Beyond advance directives: The importance of communication skills at the end of life, *JAMA* 293(3):359–365, 2005.

Volker D, Limerick M: What constitutes a dignified death? The voice of oncology advanced practice nurses, *Clin Nurse Spec* 21(5):241–247, 2007.

Wilkie D, Ezenwa M: Pain and symptom management in palliative care and at end of life, *Nurs Outlook* 60(6):357–364, 2012.

Williams AL: Perspectives on spirituality at the end of life: a meta-summary, *Palliat Support Care* 4:407–417, 2006.

Wittenberg-Lyles E, Goldsmith J, Ferrell B, Ragan S: *Communication in Palliative Nursing*, New York, 2013, Oxford University Press.

World Health Organization, nd. *WHO definition of palliative care* Available online: http://www.who.int/cancer/palliative/definition/en/ Accessed August 24, 2014

Worley CA: The art of caring: compassion fatigue, *Dermatol Nurs* 17(6):416, 2005.

Wright B, Wurr K, Tomlinson H, et al.: Clinical dilemmas in children with life-limiting illnesses: decision making and the law, *Palliat Med* 23:238–247, 2009.

Zisook S, Simon N, Reynolds C, et al.: Bereavement, complicated grief and DSM, part 2: complicated grief, *J Clin Psychiatry* 71(8): 1097–1098, 2010.

ADDITIONAL WEB RESOURCES

American Academy of Hospice and Palliative Medicine: www.aahpm.org.

Center to Advance Palliative Care: www.capc.org.

Canadian Virtual Hospice: www.virtualhospice.ca.

Children's Hospice & Palliative Care Coalition: www.chpcc.org

Hospice and Palliative Nurses Association: www.hpna.org

National Hospice and Palliative Care Organization: www.nhpco.org

National Cancer Institute: *Grief, bereavement, and coping with loss*, Retrieved from Bethesda, MD, 2011, Author. http://cancer.gov/cancertopics/pdq/supportivecare/bereavement/HealthProfessional.

National Consensus Project for Quality Palliative Care. (2013) *Clinical Practice Guidelines for Quality Palliative Care*. ed 3. accessed March 25, 2014. http://www.nationalconsensusproject.org/NCP_Clinical_Practice_Guidelines_3rd_Edition.pdf

CHAPTER 22

Role Relationships and Interprofessional Communication

Elizabeth C. Arnold

OBJECTIVES

At the end of the chapter, the reader will be able to:

1. Define professional role relationships in health care.
2. Distinguish among the professional roles of the nurse.
3. Describe the components of professional role socialization in nursing.
4. Describe what interprofessional education is and is not.
5. Cite key elements of professional role development for a registered nurse.
6. Identify factors that support work environments for nurses.
7. Discuss professional role relationship behaviors with colleagues.
8. Describe professional role behaviors that support nurse-client relationships.
9. Discuss the advocacy role in nurse-client relationships.

Chapter 22 presents an overview of the historical roots, current perspectives, and future directions of role relationships in professional nursing and their implications for professional communication, education and practice. Being clear about one's professional role is essential for meaningful functional relationships with physicians, pharmacists, social workers, physical therapists, and other members of the health care team. Applications address the process of professional socialization and role development in nursing. Leadership competencies, and collaborative team role development with other health disciplines are discussed.

BASIC CONCEPTS

ROLE

Role is a multidimensional psychosocial concept defined as a traditional pattern of behavior and self-expression, performed by or expected of an individual within a given society. People develop social, work and professional roles throughout life. Some roles are conferred at birth (ascribed roles) and some are attained

through circumstance during a lifetime (acquired roles). Personal ascribed role performance standards reflect social, cultural, gender, and family expectations. For example, consider the performance standards held for Prince George in England versus those of most other babies of his generation.

Personal, professional and work relationships have distinctive expectations for role performance, which differentially influence communication content and style of presentation. Work relationships have tangible and intangible structural elements that define communication. For example, nurses will communicate differently with their peers, immediate supervisor and their direct reports. Institutional norms also have an effect on the enactment of professional roles and vary according to the characteristics of the work environment. The ability to accurately interpret and negotiate role relationships in a work setting helps nurses respond more effectively to different people and situations in their work environment.

Role expectations in health care tend to mirror differentiated practice roles and are recognizable through differences in work responsibilities, cooperative activities, education, and social affiliations. Stronger personal and professional role expectations are held for those in public trust roles, such as elected political and religious leaders, health care professionals, and teachers. Exercise 22-1 examines general role relations.

PROFESSIONAL ROLES

Professional nurses comprise the largest professional group of health care providers (Goodman, 2014). They spend more sustained professional time with clients and families than any other hospital care professional. Yet nursing is a young profession compared to medicine, law, and dentistry. Since the time of Florence Nightingale, professional nursing roles have steadily evolved from being that of being a functional "handmaiden of the physician" to current national expectations for nurses to assume leadership roles and to act as first-line providers in implementing health care reform initiatives. Nurses are no longer the instruments of another profession's intent. McBride (2011) states, "our task now is to harness our field's competence in service to quality health care that is both accessible and affordable."

EXPANDED PROFESSIONAL ROLES

Advanced practice and leadership roles for nurses are the wave of the future. Contemporary nurses are expected to take leadership roles, working with physicians, pharmacists, and other health professionals on an equal playing field to meet the challenges of health care reform. Transformational differences in health care delivery emphasize a stronger focus on primary care, meaningful use of technology, empowered shared

leadership, and interdisciplinary collaboration competencies. For example, technology has improved the diagnosis, available treatments and quality of life for many people in ways that were not possible even a decade ago. Nursing's time has arrived with unprecedented changes in the health care environment, but only if the profession seizes the moment. Nurses must develop a unified advocacy role in putting forth the value of nurses as skilled health care providers. Evolved scope of practice and professional standards serve as the foundation for practice accountability and decision authority in contemporary nursing practice (O'Rourke, 2003).

In 2010, the economics of health care and diminishing numbers of health care providers led to legislative passage of the Patient Protection and Affordable Care Act (PPACA). With passage comes a mandate to provide quality health care to a greater number of people at a lower cost, at a time when there is a growing shortage of nurses and physicians. The shortage is expected to increase dramatically over the next decade. This contradiction in resource/demand creates an urgent need to restructure the current health care delivery system. There is a corresponding pre-requisite need to overhaul fundamental health education structures to support the development and sustainability of collaborative team based care delivery.

Advanced Practice Nurses (APRN)

An advanced practice nurse (APRN) is a licensed skilled practitioner holding a minimum of a masters degree in a clinical specialty with the expert knowledge base, complex decision-making skills and clinical

---

EXERCISE 22-1 **Understanding Life Roles**

Purpose: To expand students' awareness of the responsibilities, stressors, and rewards of different life roles.

Procedure
1. Think of all the roles you assume in life.
2. Write a description of the specific responsibilities, stressors, and rewards related to each role.
3. Share some of your roles and their descriptions. (Share only what you feel comfortable revealing.)

Discussion
As a group, discuss how these different aspects of life roles affect a person's overall functioning.
1. How can this help you to understand your clients better?
2. Discuss what would happen with these roles if you were incapacitated?
3. How might such a situation affect your coping ability?
4. How might it affect others?
5. What roles do you hold in common with other participants in this exercise?
6. What does this exercise suggest about possible role overload or conflict?

competencies required for expanded specialty practice (NCSBN, 2008). Box 22-1 identifies the four core categories of advanced practice nursing found in contemporary health care. Specialized training allows APRNs to diagnose and independently manage care including prescriptive authority and medication management. In addition to clinical roles, advanced practice nurses function in research, educational, and administrative roles. Advanced practice roles build upon basic nursing practice competencies. A significant issue yet to be completely resolved is a lack of consistency that has lessened but still exists surrounding role responsibilities and scope of practice of APRNs (Lowe et al, 2012). Clarity is particularly relevant for standardization of nurse practitioner scope of practice in the context of interdisciplinary team role relations.

Contemporary professional nursing roles reflect the increasing complexities of health care, globalization, changing client demographic characteristics and diversity, and the exponential growth of health information technology (Hegarty et al., 2009). A strengthened focus on health promotion/disease prevention and self-management of chronic disorders also echoes new economic realities and provider availability.

Figure 22-1 identifies the core professional role competencies required of contemporary nurses, identified by the Institute of Medicine (IOM, 2003). Teamwork and collaboration with designated providers and clients are considered modern hallmarks of clinical role competence. Clinical communication and relational skills related to health promotion, risk reduction, and self-management of chronic disorders are expected role competencies (Rogers, 2014).

The scope of practice for professional nurses has expanded to include reimbursable health screening and promotion, risk reduction, and disease prevention strategies to improve the health and quality of life for clients and families. Nursing roles are being adapted for practice in prisons, schools, home care, shopping malls, and faith-based settings. Nurses increasingly provide care as part of interprofessional health care teams in hospitals and the community. Nurses hold walk in clinic hours in shopping centers and senior centers. They serve with the military, during disasters, and in the juvenile justice system. They work in the fields with migrant workers, in the home with the homebound, and in clinics for the uninsured.

Contemporary nurses are expected to advocate for health care transformation and to take a leadership role in addressing environmental, social, and economic determinants of health (Wallis, 2012). Nurses are assuming public advocacy roles to inform policy makers, educators, and other health care providers about health-related issues. By serving on advisory committees in the community, nurses help secure and protect the service funding needed to increase accessibility and availability of quality health services. Nurses also provide leadership and coordination in health care improvement through education and participation in research. Exercise 22-2 is designed to help you look at the different role responsibilities of practicing nurses.

CARING LEADERSHIP AND TECHNOLOGY

(This section was developed by Dr. Bonnie DeSimone, 2014). While advances in technology have changed the landscape of nursing practice and nursing leadership in many positive ways, nurses do the business of

---

| **BOX 22-1** | **Advanced Practice Roles** |

Nurse practitioners (NPs) provide first-line health care services across the health-illness continuum in primary and acute care settings. NPs have prescriptive authority; they diagnose and treat common medical conditions and injuries, conduct physical examinations, provide preventive care, and medically manage common chronic health problems in the community. Acute care and specialty NPs (such as neonatal, pediatric, psychiatric, and geriatric NPs) provide skilled care to special populations with specialized health care needs.

Certified nurse-midwives provide a wide variety of first-line and clinical management of prenatal and gynecologic care to normal, healthy women. They perform uncomplicated delivery of babies in hospitals, private homes, and birthing centers, and continue with follow-up postpartum care. Certified nurse-midwives also have prescriptive authority under a mandated agreement with a designated collaborating physician, approved by the state Board of Nursing.

Clinical nurse specialists provide skilled care and consultation in a specialty area, such as cardiac, oncology, neonatal, pediatric, obstetric/gynecologic, medical-surgical, or psychiatric nursing. Clinical nurse specialists also perform indirect clinical nursing roles such as staff development, nursing education, administration, and informatics.

Certified registered nurse anesthetists administer anesthesia and conscious sedation in more than one-third of the hospitals in the United States.

nursing with a new 'elephant in the room' - a PDA, a computer, even a video camera. Digital technology has become the predominant means of monitoring, communicating, and interacting with patients (Porter-O'Grady & Malloch, 2013, p. 540). Contemporary nurse leaders are distancing themselves from the once-prized personal ownership of their day-to-day work activities, to engage in the more global impacts of the technological devices they use (Porter-O'Grady & Malloch, 2013, p. 82). Yet, while technology permits swift transactions, universal access, and levels of portability unanticipated 20 years ago, the defining aspects of caring and patient communication are at risk. Despite new technologies

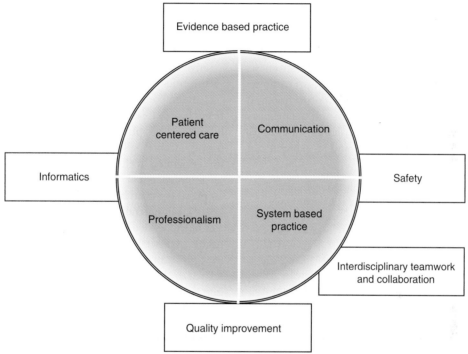

Figure 22-1 Professional nursing role: core competencies for health professionals. *(Adapted from Institute of Medicine [IOM]: Health professions education: a bridge to quality. Washington, DC, 2003, National Academies Press, pp. 45-46.)*

EXERCISE 22-2 | **Professional Nursing Roles**

Procedure: Ask an RN that you admire if you can have a 20-minute interview related to his or her role development as a registered nurse in clinical practice. Ask the following questions:

1. What are the different responsibilities involved in his or her job?
2. What training and credentials are required for the nurse's position?
3. What is the type of client population encountered?
4. What are the most difficult and rewarding aspects of the job?
5. Why did the nurse choose a particular area or role in nursing?

6. What opportunities does the nurse see for the future of nursing?

You are also encouraged to create your own explorative questions.

Discussion

1. Were you surprised by any of your interviewee's answers? If so, in what ways?
2. What similarities and differences do you see in the results of your interview compared with those of your classmates?
3. In what ways can you use what you learned from doing this exercise in your future professional life?

that can improve patient care outcomes, nurses must be mindful that such devices "support", not "drive" their work (Bell, 2010). They must remain cognizant that decisions are made by humans, likely from data generated by technology, but not totally derived from "computer applications" (Bell, 2010). Hence, contemporary nurse leaders are more responsible than ever to devise communication strategies that preserve the caring aspects of nursing, the very pillars of the nurse-patient relationship (Porter-O'Grady & Malloch, 2011, 2013). Nurses must understand that communication supported, not led, by technology is what generates new levels of leadership effectiveness. When nurses integrate the caring aspects of communication with the emerging landscape of technology, they keep the essence of nursing alive and their capacity for leadership effectiveness flourishing. Hesburgh's (1971) description of leadership, and its relationship to caring, still holds true:

> The mystique of leadership, be it educational, political, religious, commercial or whatever, is next to impossible to describe, but wherever it exists, morale flourishes, people pull together toward common goals, spirits soar, order is maintained, not as an end in itself, but as a means to move forward together. Such leadership always has a moral as well as intellectual dimension; it requires courage as well as wisdom; it does not simply know, it cares (p. 764).

PROFESSIONAL ROLE CLARITY

Professional role clarity is an essential quality of effective leadership. If nurses are not clear about their professional roles, it is difficult for them to communicate their value as health care providers to other professionals. Role clarity about professional competencies is necessary to support client safety initiatives that lead to improved client outcomes (O'Rourke and White, 2011). Influencing change and making difficult decisions becomes easier when nurses have a clear vision of their professional role because they are better able to stimulate confidence in others.

NURSING EDUCATION AND PROFESSIONAL ROLE DEVELOPMENT

Transformation of the health care system calls for a fundamental restructuring of discipline specific professional education to meet the global complex demands of health care reform (Yoder and Terhorst, 2012).

A system approach to practice based education underscores the interdependence between health and education. Three structural shifts in health care education are required to accomplish this task. Frenk et al (2010) note, transformative learning environments need to move *from*:

- fact memorization to searching, analysis, and synthesis of information for decision making;
- seeking professional credentials to achieving core competencies for effective teamwork in health systems; and
- non-critical adoption of educational models to creative adaptation of global resources to address local priorities", (p. 6).

Contemporary nursing curriculums are competency based. **Competency** is defined as "a set of capabilities, skills, aptitude, and experience" (Rick, 2014, p. 64) Additionally, there are explicit expectations for integrated technology proficiency and inclusion of interdependent education formats or concepts, emphasizing team based communication skills. Bianco (2014) recommends that leadership related competencies be embedded at all education levels and across all health care settings. Educational methodologies will need to incorporate meaningful learning experiences related to clinical and population-based decision making in predominantly primary care settings (Frenk et al, 2010).

NEW DIFFERENTIATED PRACTICE ROLES

The IOM (2010) mandate to increase the number of professional nurses in advanced practice roles makes a strong statement about public recognition of professional nursing's leadership role in implementing health care reform. Two new nursing models have emerged in the last decade designed to strengthen professional leadership roles. The clinical nurse leader (CNL) model offers a competency based curriculum, which prepares nurses for leadership roles in clinical nursing practice at the unit level (ANCC, 2013). Emphasizing leadership at the unit level, the CNL "designs, implements, and evaluates client care by coordinating, delegating and supervising the care provided by the health care team, including licensed nurses, technicians, and other health professionals" (AACN, 2003, paragraph 2).

The CNL curriculum prepares students with a baccalaureate degree in another field to become an advanced generalist nurse, with a master's degree in nursing and eligibility for licensure as a registered nurse. Courses combine baccalaureate and master's level content, emphasizing clinical leadership skills and training in health care systems management at the clinical unit level. Graduates passing the National Council Licensure Examination (NCLEX) professional nursing licensing examination and CNL certification exam are eligible for American Nurses Credentialing Center (ANCC) certification as CNLs. To practice as an advanced practice nurse in a *clinical specialty*, the CNL must complete further master's-level preparation in either a selected advanced practice specialty or as part of the doctorate of nursing practice (DNP) program.

In 2004 AACN introduced the Doctor of Nursing Practice (DNP) as a *terminal practice* degree for professional nurses. The complexity of the nation's health care environment served as a major impetus for promoting transitions to practice doctorates as did the need to position nursing professionally on a par with other major health professions, all of which offer practice-focused doctorates. Ten years later, more than 14,000 nurses hold a practice doctorate in nursing (Kirschling, 2014). The curriculum combines advanced nursing practice skill proficiency with a solid foundation in the clinical sciences, evidence-based practice methods, system leadership, information technology, health policy, and interdisciplinary collaboration (AACN, 2004).

Interprofessional Education

O'Grady (2014) notes that the enactment of PPACA, with its emphasis on providing access to services across the health continuum, strongly supports the need to develop "different roles and relationships in the delivery of health service" (p. 66). Nursing, medicine, dentistry, pharmacy, social work, and other health care providers represent distinct health disciplines. Historically, each discipline prepared clinicians to assume different practice roles using discipline-specific practice standards with associated values and behavioral expectations. New to advanced skilled health care preparation is the push for interprofessional education to become an essential component of professional health care curriculums. Contemporary nursing graduates are increasingly expected to be "competent in their own discipline and a collaborative team member in the workplace" (Hood et al., 2014, p. 109).

In its landmark report, *Health Professions Education: A Bridge to Quality*, IOM (2003) identifies "working in

interdisciplinary teams" as core competencies needed in today's health care delivery. The Pew Health Professions Commission (1993) recommended revision of health professions curricula to include shared interprofessional learning in academic settings, and the AACN (2008) more recently has identified "interprofessional communication and collaboration for improving patient health outcomes" (p. 3) as an essential outcome expected of nursing graduates. The Joint Commission further suggests that safe, effective clinical care requires an interdisciplinary collaborative team approach (Walsh et al., 2005).

Interprofessional education is defined as "occasions when two or more professions learn from and about each other to improve collaboration and the quality of care" (Oandasan and Reeves, 2005, p. 24). Its competency-based goal is to provide students with the knowledge, skills, and attitudes needed to effectively collaborate and improve the quality of health care through interdisciplinary problem solving. Skills to enhance teamwork and to clarify roles in providing client-centered care are important in both discipline-specific *and* interprofessional learning (Pecukonis et al., 2008).

Interprofessional education is not intended to replace discipline specific education because interprofessional health care roles and skills are not interchangeable. Rather it is the combined effect of skillful health professionals from different disciplines collaboratively working together that defines interprofessional quality in health care delivery. Yoder and Terhorst (2012) identify the need to develop synergistic collaborative methods and principles, technology, and professional development as essential methodologies associated with interdisciplinary learning behaviors. Cultivating the natural interdependence between health professionals required for quality care in an era of cost containment is noted as being critical to success in meeting national health goals (IOM, 2003; Interprofessional Education Collaborative Expert Panel, 2011).

Understanding how the different elements of health care fit together and synergistically complement the overall quality of care provision is a new emphasis in health care education. Interprofessional team communication skills *must* become be part of formal nursing education curriculums in developing the broader framework "that will care for the sick and maintain sustainability throughout a future rich with crisis and controversy (Nagel and Andenoro, 2012, p. 25). Since the decision-making process with team approaches is more complex than with single discipline methods, *acknowledging* and *respecting* the unique expected behaviors and skill sets of each health discipline is essential to collaborative team learning. Frequent communication is essential to good results.

Providing shared learning opportunities is essential to the mutual understanding of different disciplinary role expectations and the respectful integration of tasks that need to occur in order to function effectively on interprofessional health care teams. In the process of sharing knowledge and experience, students learn the tools of collaborative problem solving (Fronek et al., 2009). Students gain firsthand understanding of the professional values held by other disciplines. This knowledge helps students collectively identify and work collaboratively to resolve important health care issues.

Interdisciplinary education depends heavily on experiential learning. Functioning side by side with other interprofessional students (e.g., medical, pharmacy, social work, physical therapy and nutrition students) allows nursing students opportunities to work through different elements of a clinical situation using a collaborative approach. When supported with situational collaborative debriefing and reflection, students learn how different professional disciplines *think* about quality care, and what a collaborative understanding means for coordinating effective client- and family-centered care.

Clinical simulation is a preferred learning strategy because it allows interdisciplinary students to give close attention to all aspects of the clinical environment and to actively problem solve solutions from a collaborative team perspective. Students construct and develop "live" understanding of interdisciplinary health team functioning through shared reflection on their actions and interactions with each other in collectively meeting identified client-centered goals.

In preparing courses, Aveyard and colleagues (2005) suggest that course topics need to be "enhanced by an interdisciplinary approach and not hindered by a lack of detailed attention to field-specific content" (p. 64). Interprofessional simulations and problem-based learning scenarios provide innovative opportunities for medical, nursing, and pharmacy students to collaboratively analyze and problem solve creative solutions to complex health problems. Examples of shared interprofessional electives include ethics, death and dying, culture, quality improvement (QI), genomics,

emergency preparedness, gerontology, health policy and legal issues. Clinical simulation courses open to students from multiple health disciplines provide unique opportunities for students in the health care professions to work together in the clinical management of complex disease health conditions.

Introducing interprofessional courses early in the basic nursing curriculum helps students articulate professional nursing roles and actions as they learn to merge their talents in holistically caring for clients and families. Students can better understand how collaboration and teamwork can more effectively resolve complex issues to enhance clinical outcomes (Margalit et al., 2009). Hood and colleagues (2014) suggest that the ideal learning experience would be "the authenticity of an interprofessional clinical placement" (p. 113). Shared clinical experiences amplify the learning experience. Case Example 22-1

Case Example

This fall, a multidisciplinary learning opportunity is being offered in collaboration with the University of Maryland and Montgomery County's Department of Health and Human Services involving nursing, pharmacy and social work students. The students will be engaged in seeing clients and participating in collaborative discussions with faculty preceptorship related to their care at the Mercy Health Clinic. This outpatient clinic serves those without medical insurance and has a large culturally diverse clientele. The goals of the project are 1. to expose students to interprofessional collaborative practice in a community setting with diverse client values and needs and 2. to enhance the quality of care for clients with complex medical, cross-cultural and social issues through interdisciplinary collaboration.

Interprofessional TEAM Roles

Collaborative professional teams represent a coordinated form of care delivery. Each team member pools his or her expertise with that of other team members to achieve common agreed-on treatment outcomes. The precise role and involvement of each discipline specific team member depends on team member expertise and individualized client needs. The setting, professional, and system resources enable or hinder team functioning. For example, in the intensive care unit (ICU), care will focus on the life-threatening nature of the client's condition, requiring the concentrated assistance of specialists. In rehabilitation and home care settings,

Developing an Evidence-Based Practice

Muller-Juge V, Cullati S, Blondon KS, et al: Interprofessional collaboration between residents and nurses in general internal medicine: a qualitative study on behaviors enhancing teamwork quality, *PLoS One* 9(4):e9610, 2014.

This qualitative study used a volunteer purposive sample of 14 pairs of residents and nurses in internal medicine. Each pair was asked to clinically manage one urgent and one nonurgent clinical case simulation. Following the simulation, participants reviewed a videotape of the simulation and explained their actions and perceptions related to quality of team work, efficiency of client management, and the presence of team spirit and shared management goals.

Results: The majority of resident nurse pairs functioned with residents taking the leadership role, and nurses assuming roles consistent with nursing, such as executing medical prescriptions and providing clinical supervision and care for the client. Openness to exchanging suggestions, sharing of responsibilities, and positive team building were present in the research finding.

Application to clinical practice: Study results affirm the need for addressing communication in interprofessional education at undergraduate and graduate levels. Formative development of interdisciplinary roles are more easily learned when they are a foundational component of the profession education process.

the composition of team members would be different. However, similar overarching goals of achieving health outcomes and improving a client's quality of life underscore clinical team efforts.

APPLICATIONS

PROFESSIONAL ROLE SOCIALIZATION AND IDENTITY FORMATION

Professional role socialization is an educational process through which student nurses acquire the norms, values and attitudes associated with the nursing profession. Key elements of the professional nursing role include the acquisition, development, and integration of health-related psychomotor, social, cognitive and critical competencies, related to health care.

Identity formation as a professional nurse begins when a student enters a nursing program. Initially, nursing students are absorbed in learning the basic knowledge required of the professional role. They depend on textbooks and their instructors to help them find the right solution to health care problems.

As students become comfortable with foundational nursing knowledge and expected competencies, they begin to consider multiple options based on textbook information *and* clinical experience. They are able to apply scientific knowledge to practice in a realistic manner and "to relate new material to their previous knowledge base" (Cohen, 1981, p. 18). Students begin to trust their professional reasoning in making clinical judgments. Each experience helps the student to develop comfort as a professional nurse operating within an ethical, competency-based framework.

The next phase involves internalizing the *profession's culture*, which refers to the values, standards, and role behaviors associated with professional nursing. Pecukonis and colleagues (2008) note, "each discipline possesses its own professional culture that shapes the educational experience; determines curriculum content, core values, dress, salience of symbols" (p. 417). As students begin to try out new professional behaviors they receive feedback and support for their efforts from clinical staff, faculty and clients. Positive feedback empowers students by acknowledging their clinical judgments and encourages them to perform successfully. In addition to developing a professional role identity, nurses have to acquire an inteprofessional identity consistent with team based collaborative care initiatives. (Khalili, et al, 2013).

SOCIALIZING AGENTS

Nursing faculty, clinical preceptors, and nursing mentors serve as important socializing agents, helping students learn the values, traditions, norms, and competencies of the nursing profession. A *clinical preceptor* is an experienced nurse, chosen for clinical competence and charged with supporting, guiding, and participating in the evaluation of student clinical competence (Paton et al., 2009). A clinical preceptor models professional behaviors, gives constructive feedback, and promotes clinical thinking in the novice nurse or nursing student. The attitudes, actions, and directed support of the preceptor encourages students to adopt clinically appropriate professional behaviors (Boyer, 2008). Clients and families, mentors, and peers serve as informal socializing agents. They promote a student's understanding of the professional nursing role from a consumer perspective.

PROFESSIONAL SKILL ACQUISITION AND ROLE DEVELOPMENT

Patricia Benner (2001) describes five developmental stages of formative role development in professional nursing. Based on the Dreyfus model (1980) of skill acquisition, each developmental stage demonstrates increasing proficiency in implementing the professional nursing role: novice, advanced beginner, competence, proficiency, and expert.

The first stage is referred to as the *novice stage.* Initially students have limited or no nursing experience to perform required nursing tasks. Novice nurses need structure and exposure to the objective foundations upon which to base their nursing practice. They tend to compare clinical findings with the textbook picture because they lack the practice experience to do otherwise. Theoretical knowledge and confidence in the expertise of more practiced nurses and faculty serve as guides to practice. Veteran nurses can re-experience the novice stage any time that nurse makes a career change and enters a new clinical area or specialty, never having had experience with a particular client population (Thomas, 2003).

In the *advanced beginner* stage, nurses understand the basic elements of practice and can organize and prioritize clinical tasks. Although clinical analysis of health care situations occurs at a higher level than strict association with the textbook picture, the advanced beginner is only able to partially grasp the unique complexity of each client's situation. Mentors and preceptors help nurses at this stage to hone their nursing skills. Preceptors can make a difference in helping new nurses cope with the uncertainty of new clinical situations. They act as a "guide by the side" in helping new nurses gain nursing proficiency (Dracuup et al, 2004) The new nurse's clients are also an important resource Clients can help students develop a greater appreciation for the complexity of social, psychological, and physical aspects of chronic disease as a result of their interactions. By paying close attention to their clients, and what seems to work best, advanced beginner nurses learn the art of nursing.

The *competence stage* occurs 1 to 2 years into nursing practice. The competent nurse is able to easily "manage the many contingencies of clinical nursing" (Benner, 2001 p. 27). Nurses begin to practice the "art" of nursing. They view the clinical picture from a broader perspective and are more confident about their roles in health care.

The *proficiency stage* occurs 3 to 5 years into practice. Nurses in this stage are self-confident about their clinical skills and perform them with competence, speed, and flexibility. The proficient nurse sees the clinical situation as a whole, has well-developed psychosocial skills, and knows from experience what needs to be modified in response to a given situation (Benner, 1984).

The *expert stage* is marked with a high level of clinical skill and the capacity to respond authentically and creatively to client needs and concerns. Expert nurses "have confidence in their own ability and rarely panic in the face of a breakdown" (Benner, 2001, p. 115). They can recognize the unexpected and work creatively with complex clinical situations. Expert nurses demonstrate mastery of technology, sensitivity in interpersonal relationships, and specialized nursing skills in all aspects of their caregiving. Being an expert nurse is not an end point; nurses have the professional and ethical responsibility to continuously upgrade and refine their clinical skills through professional development and clinical skill training. Table 22-1 identifies behaviors associated with different levels of Benner's model (Norman, 2008).

PROFESSIONALISM

In 1915, Abraham Flexner presented a seminal paper at a national conference in which he identified criteria for determining whether an occupation was a profession. Box 22-2 offers an adaptation of Flexner's criteria for professional status.

A century later, nursing has emerged as a legitimate profession with expectation that nurses will take a major leadership role in moving health agendas forward. As health professionals seriously embrace the goals of health care reform, professionalism becomes a curriculum matter. Wear and Castellani (2000) propose that professionalism requires significant, integrated experiences and exposure to "relevant tools for professional development that can be provided only by particular knowledge, methods, and skills outside bioscience domains" (p. 603).

McBride 2011 notes, "You have to look and act professional to be taken seriously"…and know "how to behave appropriately in an array of social situations" (p. 127). In the public's eye, a nurse's personal and professional self is merged. You are "one" nurse, but to the larger community system, *you* represent the nursing profession. In addition to how nurses dress, and present themselves to the public, nurses are judged by

TABLE 22-1	Benner's Stages of Clinical Competence
Nurse Competency Level	**Description of Behaviors**
Advanced beginner	• Enters clinical situations with some apprehension • Sees task requirements as central to the clinical context, whereas other aspects of the situation are seen as background • Requires knowledge application to meet clinical realities • Perceives each clinical situation as a personal challenge • Are typically dependent on standards of care, unit procedures
Competent	• Focuses more on clinical issues in contrast to tasks • Can handle familiar situations • Expects certain clinical trajectories on the basis of the experience with particular patients • Searches for broader explanations of clinical situations • Has enhanced organizational ability, technical skills • Focuses on managing patients' conditions
Proficient	• Responds to particulars of clinical situations in a broader way • Requires an experiential base with past patient populations • Understands patient transitions over time • Learns to gauge involvement with patients and families to promote appropriate caring
Expert	• Has increased intuition regarding what are important clinical factors and how to respond to these • Engages in practical reasoning • Anticipates and prepares for situations while remaining open to changes • Performs care in a "fluid, almost seamless" manner • Bonds emotionally with patients and families depending on their needs • Sees the big picture, including the unexpected • Works both with and through others

From Norman V: Uncovering and recognizing nurse caring from clinical narratives, *Holis Nurs Pract* 22(6):324, 2008, by permission.

BOX 22-2	Flexner's Criteria

• Members share a common identity, values, attitudes, and behaviors.
• A distinctive specialized substantial body of knowledge exists.
• Education is extensive, with both theory and practice components.
• Unique service contributions are made to society.
• Acceptance of personal responsibility in discharging services to the public.
• Governance and autonomy over policies that govern activities of profession members.
• A code of ethics that members acknowledge and incorporate in their actions.

how they act toward others in their profession, communicate with their clients, attend to the dynamics of interdisciplinary communication, and communicate with ancillary personnel. It is important to act professionally with everyone in the health care environment from the administrative assistant to the manager

(Larson, 2006). Clients look at the "whole of their health experience" not just one segment unless that segment has been particularly traumatic or inspirational. They will note your interactions with housekeeping, dietary workers etc. as well as how you relate to physicians, and other therapists involved in the client's care. In some ways, you are always on stage as a professional nurse as you work with clients, families, and other health professionals.

Principled ethical behavior in every facet of the nurse's work life is a critical dimension of professionalism (Crigger, 2011). Individual nurses identify moral integrity, purpose, and commitment as key components of professionalism. Laabs' (2011) research describes the professional nurse as being "honest, trustworthy, consistently doing the right thing and standing up for what is right despite the consequences" (p. 433). Professionalism represents authentic attitudes and intrinsic values. Professionalism in the context of health care expertise is evidenced through critical reflection and the ability to make decisions in the presence of complex dilemmas (Consorti et al., 2012). Nurses demonstrate professionalism through accountability for the care they provide, using recognized professional practice standards and operating within ethical and regulatory professional frameworks. As Malloch and Porter O'Grady (2013) observe.

> Being a member of a profession is not just a different way of doing work: it is a different way of being, an expression of the role and its relationship to the world, representing a social contract and reflecting high expectations for its exercise from those who will depend on it. (p. 2)

CONTINUING EDUCATION

Professional development represents a lifelong commitment to excellence in nursing and requires regular upgrading of skills. Standard means of continued professional development include relevant continuing education presentations, staff development, conference attendance, academic education, specialized training, and research activities. Professional development also occurs through informal means such as consultation, professional reading, experiential learning, giving presentations, and self-directed activities. At advanced practice levels, nurses are required to complete a certain level of continuing education activities within designated time frames to maintain APRN certification. Continuing education and professional conferences offer professional nurses unique opportunities to network, share expertise, and learn different perspectives from others in the field.

Continuing education and career planning are complementary professional development behaviors, each enriching the other. Continuing education provides opportunities to connect with people having similar interests and allows participants to develop new knowledge and skills. Rodts and Lamb (2008) stress the importance of career planning as being essential to achieving future career goals and provides a sample resume and curriculum vitae (CV). They suggest that nurses ask themselves the question: "Where do I go from here and what is it that I want most out of my career?"(p.126), as they begin strategic career planning. Serious career plans should reflect careful appraisal of values, skills, interests and different career possibilities. Mentors can be helpful in acting as a sounding board for career option discussions, and for providing guidance in looking at the whole picture. A sometimes forgotten consideration is the need to examine how the nurse's career plans will fit with other life responsibilities and commitments. Knowing as much as possible about job requirements is useful in making the best career choices as well as for interview preparation.

INTERPROFESSIONAL ROLE RELATIONSHIPS

Petri (2010) identifies interprofessional education, role awareness, communication and interpersonal relationship skills as essential to the development of effective interprofessional role relationships. Mandates in health care reform emphasize development of self-management care models, integrated team approaches to deliver quality client-centered treatment and coordinated care provided across the health care continuum. An interdisciplinary professional practice model offers the best options for decision-making and accountability given the broad complexity of clinical practice (O'Rourke, 2003). Practice models address issues of accountability, define professional identity, and clarify overlapping scopes of practice across the spectrum of team based clinical care delivery (Mathews and Lankshear, 2003).

The 2011 IOM report on the future of nursing calls for nurses to become equal partners with physicians and other health care providers in the redesign of health care systems, stating: "The future of health care rests solidly with the strength nursing brings in holistic care, ability to collaborate and innovate from the bedside to the community and the ability to adapt to the changing environment." Box 22-3 presents key recommendations from this report.

Box 22-3	Key Messages of the Institute of Medicine Report: *The Future of Nursing: Leading Change, Advancing Health*

- Nurses should practice to the full extent of their education and training.
- Nurses should achieve higher levels of education and training through an improved education that promotes seamless academic progression.
- Nurses should be full partners, with physicians and other health professionals, in redesigning health care in the United States.
- Effective workforce planning and policy making require better data collection and an improved information infrastructure.

NEW EXPECTATIONS FOR INTERPROFESSIONAL ROLE RELATIONSHIPS

Developing productive interdisciplinary role relationships with other professionals does not just happen. To achieve the goals set forward in the IOM reports related to interdisciplinary education and practice, nurses must commit to:

- Developing new partnerships with community, business, and health care institutions
- Educating themselves to their fullest potential, with availability of seamless progression to advanced levels of education
- Promoting inclusion of nurses on local, state, and national health care advisory and policy committees
- Developing care models that cross disciplines and foster collaboration
- Adapting education and curriculum to the new century demands and advocating for the education and health policies to support those innovations

Masters (2005) asserts that if nurses are to engage in interprofessional work relationships, they must be able to clearly articulate professional nursing values. Leadership skills include an optimistic attitude and an ability to effectively take a stand when needed. Clear communication, altruism, caring, and professional ethics are essential components of interprofessional professionalism. Professional role behaviors and strong relationships with other professional colleagues include accountability for one's fair share of the workload. Maintaining zero tolerance for gossip and criticism helps establish you as a professional with ethical integrity, worthy of trust.

Developing productive interprofessional role relationships within the nursing profession are essential to quality nursing care (Lubbe and Roets, 2014). Development of supportive, dependable relationships with coworkers—with those you dislike as well as with those you can work with easily—is also an essential competency. Respecting the views of other disciplines and communicating in an organized, thoughtful manner has an effect on how practitioners from other disciplines perceive nurses as competent health care professionals. Use critical thinking to focus your discussion on essential points, even in informal discussions. Using considerate approaches that respect the other person's viewpoints and acting in a confident flexible manner with professional collaborators and colleagues is just as important as it is with clients and their families. How nurses formally present their ideas verbally and in writing is critical to effective communication. If you use e-mails to communicate, remember that your e-mail is a reflection of you as a professional person. Use complete, well-thought-out sentences. Check punctuation, grammar, and spelling. Voice-mail messages should be professional in content and delivery.

COLLABORATIVE TEAMWORK AND COMMUNICATION

Overall treatment goals should function as the primary guiding force in team conversations. It is important to remain sensitive to the tasks at hand and to develop an understanding of how the work of each different discipline affects the nurse's work and vice versa.

Interdisciplinary team functioning is both role-focused and task-based, with skill sets focused on developing mutual trust, shared decision-making and integrated functionality. In addition to having different skill sets relevant to client needs, each health care team consists of individuals with unique personalities, egos and idiosyncrasies. Yet, each care team must function as a coordinated single unit.

Creating an esprit de corps among team members provides a different form of synergy. It takes time to function effectively as a team. Playing to each team member's strengths enhances understanding, as there is more positive energy available than will be the case if the message is defensively received. Collaboration in joint decision-making and coordination of care with colleagues requires knowing when to hold and when to let go of ideas and opinions. Most of the time, decisions are not either/or processes, but in a heated discussion, it is easy to lose sight of alternative options. Disagreements and hard feelings often arise from misunderstandings about the "whole" rather than direct positional conflicts about an aspect of care. Respect for the dignity and integrity of each team member facilitates understanding without judgment. Placing issues in order of priority is a useful organizing strategy for assessing, defining, and clarifying problems. Persistence and a good sense of humor are essential characteristics of honest interpersonal communication in relationships with professional peers.

Simultaneous communication to multiple team members can be a challenge. E-mail or memos can provide quick routine or follow-up information. Face-to-face interactions are preferred for communication about complex or emotional issues that could be misinterpreted. Serving as an informed resource to other providers helps build rapport and encourages others to work with you to achieve relevant treatment and organizational goals.

SELF-AWARENESS

Malloch and Porter-O'Grady (2005) assert "knowing from the internal self what needs to be done and living those beliefs and values in the real world marks the leader's journey" (p. 101). Self-awareness is defined as the capacity to accurately recognize emotional reactions as they happen and to understand your responses to different people and situations. Self-awareness helps nurses work from their strengths and cope more effectively to minimize personal weaknesses in interactions with others. Developing self-awareness allows nurses

to make higher quality decisions because decisions are more likely to be based on facts than personal feelings.

It is not always easy to be completely honest about one's personal weaknesses, values, and beliefs. Yet this level of self-awareness is a crucial component of effective professional leadership development. Self-awareness directly affects self-management and how we professionally respond to others. Professional self-awareness promotes recognition of the need for continuing education, the acceptance of accountability for one's own actions, the capacity to be assertive with professional colleagues, and the capability of serving as a client advocate when the situation warrants it, even if it is uncomfortable to do so. Exercises 22-3 asks you to describe your personal role development and Exercises 22-4 is designed to help you explore

---

EXERCISE 22-3	Looking at My Development as a Professional Nurse

Purpose: To help students focus on their self-development as professional nurses.

Procedure
Write the story of how you chose to become a nurse in a one- or two-page essay (may be done as a homework assignment). There are no right or wrong answers; this is simply *your* story. You may use the following questions as guides in developing your story.
  1. What are your reasons for choosing nursing as a profession?
  2. What factors influenced your decision (e.g., people, circumstances, or situations)?
  3. What does being a nurse mean to you?
  4. What fears do you have about your ability to function as a professional nurse?

  5. How do you think being a nurse will affect your personal life?
  6. What type of nursing do you want to pursue?

Discussion
1. In what ways is your story similar to or different from those of your classmates?
2. As you wrote your story, were you surprised by any of the data or feelings?
3. Students can discuss some of the realistic difficulties encountered as nursing students, both professionally and personally, and ways to handle them. Through discussion, explore the following:
   a. The practices nursing students will need to follow to achieve their vision
   b. The types of supports nurses need to foster their ongoing professional development

---

EXERCISE 22-4	Incorporating Personal Strengths in Role Development

Purpose: To help highlight the use of personal strengths as skills or assets in role development.

Procedure
1. Pair up with another student.
2. Share a personal strength that you have observed about your assigned partner related to implementation of the professional nursing role and describe the behavior that supports your assessment. (Examples might be persistence, sense of humor, balanced approach, energetic, thoughtful, caring, inquisitive, take charge, laid-back, etc.)

Discussion
1. Discuss how personal strengths can be used to enhance the professional role.
2. Compare and contrast what different students envisioned as personal strengths.
3. Did doing this exercise help you to learn something about the value of personal strengths?
4. Did anything surprise you about doing this exercise?
5. How can you use this information in your own role development?

the use of personal strengths in professional role development.

Nurses have rights, as well as significant responsibilities, in professional relationships with colleagues and clients. Box 22-4 lists the American Nurses Association (ANA, 2002) Bill of Rights for Registered Nurses. Rights carry with them corresponding responsibilities.

Think about your professional collegial relationships and your dual professional commitment to self and others. How can you balance your legitimate responsibilities to self and your responsibilities to clients and coworkers?

CREATING SUPPORTIVE WORK ENVIRONMENTS

Improving work environments in health care shapes *both* nursing and client outcomes (Bianco et al, 2014). A responsive work environment that values nurses and is committed to quality client-centered care attracts nurses and improves clinical outcomes

---

BOX 22-4	The American Nurses Association's Bill of Rights for Registered Nurses

- Nurses have the right to practice in a manner that fulfills their obligations to society and to those who receive nursing care.
- Nurses have the right to practice in environments that allow them to act in accordance with professional standards and legally authorized scopes of practice.
- Nurses have the right to a work environment that supports and facilitates ethical practice, in accordance with the Code of Ethics for Nurses and its interpretive statements.
- Nurses have the right to freely and openly advocate for themselves and their patients, without fear of retribution.
- Nurses have the right to fair compensation for their work, consistent with their knowledge, experience, and professional responsibilities.
- Nurses have the right to a work environment that is safe for themselves and their patients.
- Nurses have the right to negotiate the conditions of their employment, either as individuals or collectively, in all practice settings.

Reprinted from American Nurses Association: Know your rights: ANA's Bill of Rights arms nurses with critical information, *Am Nurs* 34(6):16, 2002, by permission.

---

for clients. Likewise, nurses who are enthusiastic, competent, dependable, adaptable, and responsible are key variables in creating a satisfying, quality work environment. In a study of what types of environmental support create the most satisfaction for professional nurses, the majority surveyed identified the following factors:

- Working with other nurses who are clinically competent
- Good nurse-physician relationships and communication
- Nurse autonomy and accountability
- Supportive nurse manager-supervisor
- Control over nursing practice and practice environment
- Support for education (in-service, continuing education, etc.)
- Adequate nurse staffing
- Paramount concern for the patient (Kramer and Schmalenberg, 2002)

MAGNET HOSPITALS AND THE FORCES OF MAGNETISM

In an effort to develop and support quality work environments favorable to nurses, the ANA through its credentialing center developed the Magnet Recognition Program in 1993. The magnet recognition program recognizes nursing excellence in health care institutions and agencies. Over the years magnet recognition has become "the global standard for excellence in nursing practice" (Morgan, 2009, p. 105). Hospitals must meet stringent requirements for excellence in nursing care. Characteristics of a magnet culture include:

- Active support of education
- Clinically competent nurses
- Positive interdisciplinary professional relationships
- Control over and autonomy in nursing practice
- Client-centered care for clients and families
- Adequate staffing and nurse-manager support (ANCC, 2006)

Magnet work environments are designed to act as a draw for nurses who choose to work there because of their high standards of excellence (ANCC, 2014b; Hughes, 2008). Fourteen forces of magnetism related to such characteristics as nursing leadership, policy and programs, autonomy, interdisciplinary relationships, and professional development serve as benchmark foundations for the magnet appraisal process (ANCC, 2014 a). Five interactive dimensions of magnetism originally described in Donabedian's model are essential components of the magnet model (Donabedian, 1980; Rogers, 2014). These dimensions are presented in Figure 22-2.

- Transformational leadership
- Structural empowerment
- Exemplary professional practice
- New knowledge, innovation and improvements
- Empirical quality outcomes

Transformational Leadership

Leadership plays a pivotal role in setting expectations regarding scope of practice, collaboration, optimal interdisciplinary teamwork, and empowered knowledge partnerships in professional nursing practice. Transformational leadership requires engaging the hearts as well as the minds of those engaged in the work. Leaders have passion, and they care about whom they work with and for. Alvarado (2013) states: "The transformational leader is self-actualized, stays focused on group processes, influences, inspires trust, challenges the status quo, and empowers others" (p. 51). Exercise 22-6 provides an opportunity to examine nurse leadership behaviors.

Demonstration of transformational leadership is required for magnet status designation (Schwartz et al., 2011). Transformational leadership qualities include a clear vision and commitment to excellence, with a willingness to take reasonable risks, consult with others, and persistent dedication to task completion Transformational nursing leaders work within an organizational system to develop a vision, commit to it, and when

needed to, let go of past models that no longer work. They understand leadership as a communication process, not an event or position. Transformational leaders are energetic, positive thinkers, who act as visible role models in helping other nurses develop leadership skills (Rolfe, 2011). Transformational leaders do feel discouraged and tired at times—even confused. When these feelings occur, the secret of successful leadership performance is to have the determination and resilience to regroup, seek support, and push forward in the face of obstacles. Creative persistence is a relevant quality of effective transformational leadership.

Structural Empowerment

Structural empowerment is a concept, which describes the organizational commitments and configurations, which give informational and supportive power to health care workers to accomplish their work effectively in significant ways. Examples include access to information and support, essential resources to complete required tasks, sufficient time allotments to accomplish organizational goals and opportunities for learning and growth (Laschinger and colleagues, 2014). Empowered work environments have a direct effect on nurse work output, level of satisfaction and quality of care.

Shared governance is identified as a fundamental component of structural empowerment in the magnet model (Clavelle et al., 2013). Evidence-based best practices coupled with systems thinking form a foundation for the concepts of change and risk required of a

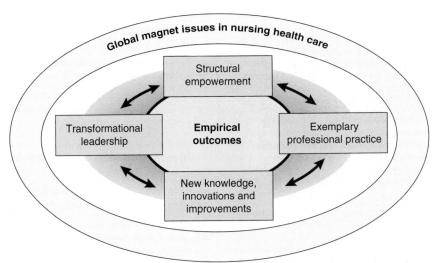

Figure 22-2   Magnet model components. *(Developed from Morgan S: The magnet (TM) model as a framework for excellence, J Nurs Care Qual 24(2):106, 2009.)*

transformed health care system. Involving nurses in decision making at all levels that influence their practice is an essential characteristic of organizations (Rogers, 2014).

Complex health care issues require different types and levels of expertise. *Synergy* refers to the process of two or more people combining efforts and working together to achieve an outcome or effect that is greater than the sum of their individual efforts. Shared governance models allow nurses to have a collective influential voice as active participants in shaping new realities and responding effectively to present and future health care demands.

Exemplary Professional Practice

A magnet health care facility is characterized as one in which nurses have a high level of job satisfaction and lower staff nurse turnover, exemplary professional practice, and demonstrate commitment at every nursing level to effective, efficient, quality care (ANCC, 2014b). Nurses working in a magnet work environment are valued. They have a strong voice in decision making about care delivery. They are encouraged and rewarded for involvement in shaping research-based nursing practice. Staffing ratios in magnet hospitals are viewed as appropriate, and the hospital demonstrates excellent treatment outcomes and client satisfaction. Communication among health professionals is open, and there is an appropriate mix of health care personnel to ensure quality care. Exercise 22-5 can help you think about how you would see yourself in the professional nursing role in the future.

EXERCISE 22-5	Developing Fulfilling Career Goals

Purpose: To help students think about the nursing role they would like to aspire to in the future. Envisioning the future helps nurses to develop focused career goals.

Procedure
1. Envision your career 3 to 5 years after graduation.
2. Write a detailed narrative of what you would be doing and what your career would be like as you might describe it to a classmate at your 5-year reunion.
3. Have one student take the role of the storyteller and the other the role of the classmate at the

reunion. The person taking the role of the classmate should ask questions to clarify any aspects of the speaker's career vision that are not clear.
4. Reverse positions and repeat.

Discussion
1. How difficult was it for you to think about what you want to do in the future?
2. What steps will you have to take to achieve your goal?
3. How will you go about finding out more about the career path you would like to take?

EXERCISE 22-6	Characteristics of Exemplary Nurse Leaders

Purpose: To help students distinguish leadership characteristics in exemplary leaders and managers encountered in everyday nursing practice. Identifying leadership characteristics helps students become aware of professional behaviors associated with achieving the mission of professional nursing.

Procedure
This exercise is most effective when the reflections take place prior to class time and findings are discussed in small groups of 4 to 6 students.
1. Reflect on the professional characteristics and behaviors of a professional nurse you admire as a leader in your work or educational setting.
2. Write down what stood out for you about this person that a leader in your mind. What specific characteristics framed this person as a leader? How did this person relate to other health professionals including students?

3. Share and discuss your findings with your small group. Have one student act as a scribe Identify commonalities and differences in student perceptions.
4. Share small group findings with your larger class group.

Discussion
1. How similar or different were student group small perceptions of leadership qualities or characteristics?
2. What specific behaviors are associated with effective leadership?
3. In what ways is nursing leadership a dynamic, interactive process?
4. What are some of the ways nurses can demonstrate leadership in contemporary health care?

New Knowledge, Innovations, and Improvements

The ANCC states, "Magnet organizations have an ethical and professional responsibility to contribute to patient care, the organization, and the profession in terms of new knowledge, innovations, and improvements" (ANCC, 2014a). This leadership responsibility is closely related to quality improvement in professional nursing and health care delivery. To achieve innovative quality nursing care, effective work units must build a pattern of relationships (social capital) designed to enhance the extent of reciprocal interactions required for shared understanding among all team members involved with a client's care. (Laschinger and colleagues, 2014).

DEVELOPING LEADERSHIP SKILL SETS

NETWORKING ROLES

Networking is an essential component of professional role development, and ultimately of advancing the status of professional nursing roles in health care delivery systems. Professional networking is defined as "establishing and using contacts for information, support, and other assistance in order to achieve career goals" (Puetz, 2007, p. 577). Nurses can use networking when they are in the market for a new job, need a referral, want to receive or share information about an area of interest, or need assistance with making a career choice. For example, if you want to write an article, you might want to discuss your ideas and get guidance from someone who is published.

Networking is a two-way interactive process. As a form of communication, networking offers valuable professional opportunities for developing new ideas and receiving feedback that might not otherwise be available. Contacts can be with peers, with people you meet at a professional conference, or in informal conversations in the course of your work. Participating in activities of nursing organizations or continuing education events provides fertile opportunities for networking. Networking with health professionals from other disciplines is also important. Having business cards with you and following up with a thank-you e-mail or note is helpful.

Nurses can communicate their own expertise and share ideas while gathering information from their contacts. Sharing information is often the bridge to developing or strengthening collaborative relationships with others in the field. For example, extensive networking among oncology nurses was the impetus for the formation of the Oncology Nursing Society. Networking is closely associated with coordination and collaboration activities and is destined to become increasingly important in determining the future impact of advanced practice nursing.

MENTORING ROLES

Mentoring describes a long-term commitment to help all nurses become the best professionals they can be. ***Mentoring*** represents a special type of professional relationship in which an experienced nurse or clinician (mentor) assumes a role responsibility for guiding the professional growth and advancement of a less-experienced person (protégé). Hawkins and Fontenot (2010) refer to mentorship as "the heart and soul of health care leadership" (p. 31). Most effective nursing leaders have had mentors and view it as a professional responsibility to act as mentors for those aspiring to become leaders.

The mentor relationship is broader and more personal than a preceptor relationship, although a good preceptor also offers advice and suggestions similar to those provided by a mentor. Mentors provide new nurses with valuable information about career options and also provide contacts. They act as an experienced sounding board for nurses to help them sort out different options and take reasoned risks in pursuit of excellence in decision making (Dracup et al. 2004).

Desirable mentor characteristics include a high level of competence, self confidence and a strong commitment to the development of potential nurse leaders (McCloughen et al, 2009). Mentees most likely to benefit from mentorship are those who are committed to the profession with the initiative to view mentorship as an important commitment and to fully engage in the process. A mentoring relationship can last over several months or years, whereas an assigned relationship between a preceptor and less experienced nurse is a short-term relationship, with a defined end date focused on clinical teaching; a preceptor is expected to provide input into a student's evaluation. The relationship serves to nurture nurses and improve retention.

Mentorship does not include a formal evaluation (Yonge et al., 2007). Mentors share values and tips for success as they come up in formal and informal nursing situations. They provide support and guidance to the mentee or protégé and often facilitate contacts with significant people related to career development. Mentorship can also develop within interprofessional relationships. Hoffman and colleagues (2008) suggest that mentoring of students in interprofessional education should contain the following elements:

- "Engagement in students' own values
- Guidance reflecting principles of self-directed learning
- Creation of awareness for opportunities that facilitate self-discovery and maturation" (p. 103)

Some hospitals provide incentives for experienced nurses to become mentors for new nurses (Tinkham, 2013. Often these relationships happen spontaneously through networking and chance opportunities. Each mentoring experience is unique because of the people and situations involved. Benefits to the mentor include satisfaction in seeing the achievements of the mentee and expansion of clinical excellence.

CLIENT ADVOCACY ROLES

Merriam-Webster Online (n.d.) defines **advocate** as "one that pleads the cause of another; one that supports or promotes the interests of another." Nurses are advocates for clients every time they protect, defend, and support a client's rights, and/or intervene on behalf of clients who cannot do so for themselves. The ANA (2001) affirms advocacy as an essential role in its Code of Ethics for Nurses, stating, "The nurse promotes, advocates for, and strives to protect the health, safety and rights of the patient."

Clients who benefit from advocacy fall into two categories: those who need advocacy because of vulnerability caused by their illness, and those who have trouble successfully navigating the health care system. Nursing actions that constitute client advocacy include facilitating access to essential health care services for clients, ensuring quality care, protecting client rights, and acting as a liaison between clients and the health care system to procure quality care.

Advocacy is a strategy nurses use to facilitate care and support for clients and families to improve health and reduce health deviations. Nurses at the front line of care advocate for their clients through education and providing health promotion opportunities for their clients (Fardellone and Click, 2013). Skill sets associated with client advocacy are identified in Box 22-5.

The goal of client advocacy support is to empower clients and to help them attain the services they need for self-management of health issues. Examples of individuals needing advocacy include survivors of

---

BOX 22-5	Knowledge Base Needed for Client Advocacy

- Client values, beliefs, and preferences
- Alignment with treatment goals
- Informed consent procedures, client's third-party insurance
- Nurse's personal, professional, and cultural biases
- Print materials, and online resources relevant to client needs
- Organizational system variables related to service delivery
- Current laws, service delivery policies, and regulations
- Community resources including referral processes, eligibility and access requirements
- Effective communication strategies related to consultation and collaboration
- Understanding of required documentation, management, and interpretation of client records

---

domestic violence, chronically mentally ill clients, pregnant teenagers, the homeless, frail elders—in fact, virtually anyone unable to act cogently on their own behalf. As health care services in the public sector become scarcer because of economic considerations, advocacy becomes an even greater emphasis. Several authors (Mahlin, 2010; Welchman and Griener, 2005) argue that nursing's professional organizations need to take up the gauntlet to collectively advocate for resolution of systemic client care issues in health care settings. For more information on nurse involvement in community-based advocacy, see Chapter 24.

Advocacy should support client autonomy. Clients need to be in control of their own destiny, even when the decision reached is not what you as the nurse would recommend for the client's health and well-being. Effective advocacy efforts for clients reflect client-identified needs, beliefs and values, and preferences. Questions you can ask to ensure the relevance of advocacy efforts for a particular client might include the following: (a) What do clients believe is their most pressing problem? (b) What supports (e.g., family, minister, rabbi, social services) are in place? (c) What health or social services is the client familiar with or resistant to considering? A client's sense of powerlessness can decrease when the answers to these questions become the starting points for developing realistic solutions to difficult problems. Referrals to community resources should be chosen, based on compatibility with the client's expressed need, financial resources, accessibility (time as well as place), and ease of access.

Client advocacy sometimes provides a connective link between ethics and the law. Nurses must be willing and able to take a stand in situations involving poor medical management of a client. This is not easy, when risk to employment or possibility of censure is associated with this form of client advocacy. Conversely, being too cautious or having misplaced loyalties to colleagues that interfere with appropriate protective advocacy for clients can become a legal and an ethical issue. Sometimes, the only person willing to defend or promote the cause of the client is the nurse.

Sometimes the nurse serves as dual advocate for both client and family members. For example, in a child abuse situation, nurses act as an advocate of the child by taking the steps necessary to provide a protective and safe environment for the child, including reporting abuse situations. The same nurse can be an advocate for the parents by referring them to appropriate community resources and helping them develop more productive methods for coping with situational stressors.

ROLE RELATIONSHIPS WITH CLIENTS

Professional performance behaviors in the nurse-client relationship include much more than simple caring; they require a sound knowledge base, as well as specific technical and interpersonal competencies. On a daily basis, nurses must collect and process multiple, often indistinct pieces of behavioral data. They work creatively with clients and families to problem solve and come up with workable solutions that are realistic and in tune with the client's beliefs, values, and preferences. Through words and behaviors in relationship with other health care providers and agencies, nurses consistently serve clients and family members; they also act as advocates not only for clients, but for the profession as well.

Today's nurse functions in a high-tech, managed health care environment in which the human caring aspects of nursing are easier to overlook. Unique challenges to the nurse-client relationship in clinical practice include shorter client contacts, technology, and lower levels of trust in relation to these factors. Yet, the nurse-client relationship will become increasingly important in helping clients feel cared for in a health care environment that sometimes neglects the psychosocial needs of clients in favor of cost-effectiveness and efficient use of time.

In today's health care environment, clients are expected to take an active role in self-management of their condition to whatever extent is possible. The relational expectation is for an equal partnership, with clients having shared power and authority as joint decision makers in their health care. With a client-centered model of health care delivery, the client's thoughts, concerns, and questions are welcomed and encouraged. Every decision related to the client's diagnosis and treatment should be a shared determination made with the medical team based on combined input and joint responsibility for implementing the recommendations. This use of the client's self-knowledge and inner resources allows nurses to more effectively respond to client needs. Electronic client data management and integration of technology into usual nursing practice activities requires a high level of technology competence. Developing mastery of communication integration and documentation technology for complex clients requires a new level of communication competencies for professional nurses. Malloch and Porter-O'Grady (2005) suggest that we are living in an information-based societal infrastructure that is primarily relational.

Becoming Key Players in a Global Health Care Arena

A transformed health care system is designed to function horizontally in a global world without boundaries. Professional nursing requires an expanded set of skill competencies in the twenty-first century, as presented in Table 22-2.

TABLE 22-2	Old versus New Skill Sets for Professional Nurses in the Twenty-First Century	
Employee	**Knowledge Worker**
Functional Analysis	Conceptual Synthesis
Manual Dexterity	Competent Integrated Care
Fixed Skill Set	Multiple Intelligences
Process Value-Based Practice	Outcome Based Practice
Individual Unilateral Performance	Interdisciplinary Team Performance

Modified from Porter-O'Grady T, Malloch K: A new vessel for leadership: new rules for a new age. In *The quantum leader: applications for the new world of work*, 3rd Ed. Sudbury, MA, 2011, Jones & Bartlett, p.3.

In addition to redefining professional nursing roles, nurses need to project a positive activist image of the professional nursing role within their communities by:

- Developing partnerships with clients, health care professionals, policy makers, and community agencies in the care of vulnerable populations
- Reflecting on and documenting what nurses do and the broad scope of services they provide for the public
- Participating as members of interdisciplinary teams and multidisciplinary groups with defined expertise as nurses to address significant health care issues from a nursing perspective
- Maintaining competence and acting in a professional manner
- Advocating for systems of care that provide adequate accessible health care for all people
- Developing and participating in continuing education programs to ensure continued competence as a professional nurse
- Promoting the public and professional understanding of the professional nursing role
- Contributing to ethical discussions that support principled practices in clinical settings

SUMMARY

How nurses perceive their professional role and how they function as a nurse in that role has a sizable effect on the success of interpersonal communication in the nurse-client relationship. The professional nursing role should be evidenced in every aspect of nursing care, but nowhere more fully than in the nurse-client relationship. A professional nurse's first role responsibility is to the client. Because hospitals no longer are the primary settings for nursing practice, nurse practice roles take place in nontraditional and traditional community-based health care settings. Advanced practice roles include the nurse practitioner, clinical nurse specialist, certified nurse-midwife, and nurse anesthetist. Two new roles, the CNL and the DNP, introduced in 2003 are flourishing. A new concept in nursing education is interdisciplinary course sharing.

Nurses learn professional role behaviors through the process of professional role socialization. Benner's five developmental stages of increasing proficiency describe the nurse's progression from novice to expert. Professional development as a nurse is a lifelong commitment. Mentorship and continuing education

assist nurses in maintaining their competency and professional role development. Interdisciplinary collaboration and health care teams have stimulated the development of shared elective classes involving two or more disciplines, for example, nursing and medicine or pharmacy.

ETHICAL DILEMMA | What Would You Do?

As a new nurse on the unit, you witness diminished client care quality due to poor interdisciplinary team communication and lack of provider continuity. If you raise the issue in a team meeting, you fear your opinion will not be taken seriously because the others have been working together for a much longer time. You also feel it is important to have the team's acceptance before raising possible controversial issues. What should you do?

DISCUSSION QUESTIONS

1. What skills do you consider the most important in developing a collaborative team approach to clinical care?
2. What would you identify as critical indicators of professionalism in professional nursing?
3. What does the statement, "Every nurse should be a leader," mean and how might this ideal be realized in contemporary health care?
4. What do you see as the distinct and collaborative contributions of different professional roles to client care and health care delivery?

REFERENCES

Alvarado LV: The golden hour for nursing, *Nurse Leader* 11(4):50–53, 2013.

American Association of Colleges of Nursing (AACN): *Competencies and Curricular Expectations for Clinical Nurse Leader Education and Practice*, Available online. Accessed August 9, 2014. http://www.aacn.nche.edu/publications/white-papers/cnl, 2013.

American Association of Colleges of Nursing (AACN): *AACN position statement on the practice doctorate in nursing*, American Association of Colleges of Nursing Washington, 2004, DC. Available online. Accessed March 28, 2014. http://www.aacn.nche.edu/DNP/DNP PositionStatement.htm.

American Association of Colleges of Nursing (AACN): *The essentials of baccalaureate education for professional nursing practice*, Washington, DC, 2008, Author.

American Nurses Association (ANA): Know your rights: ANA's Bill of Rights arms nurses with critical information, *Am Nurse* 34(6):16, 2002.

American Nurses Credentialing Center (ANCC): 2014a *Forces of Magnetism*. http://www.nursecredentialing.org/Magnet/ProgramOverview/HistoryoftheMagnetProgram/ForcesofMagnetism.aspx.

American Nurses Credentialing Center (ANCC): 2014b *Magnet Application manual*, Silver Spring, MD, Author.

American Nurses Credentialing Center (ANCC): 2014c *Magnet Recognition Program Model*. accessed June 21, 2014 http://www.nursecredentialing.org/magnet/programoverview/new-magnet-model, .

Edwards H, West S: Core topics of health care ethics: the identification of core topics for interprofessional education, *J Interprof Care* 19(1):63–69, 2005.

Bally JM: The role of nursing leadership in creating a mentoring culture in acute care environments, *Nurs Econ* 25(3):143–148, 2007. Quiz 149.

Bell K: Will the internet destroy us? *Harvard Business Review* 88(11):138–139, 2010.

Benner P: *From Novice to Expert: Excellence and Power in Clinical Nursing Practice*, New York, 2001, Commemorative ed Prentice Hall.

Benner P: Using the Dreyfus model of skill acquisition to describe and interpret skill acquisition and clinical judgment in nursing practice and education, *Bull Sci Tech Soc* 24(3):188–199, 2005.

Bianco C, Dudkiewicz P, Linette D: Building nurse leader relationships, *Nurs Manag* 42–48, 2014.

Boyer S: Competence and innovation in preceptor development: Updating our programs, *J Nurses Staff Dev* 24(2):E1–E6, 2008.

Dreher M, Clinton P, Sperhac A: Can the institute of medicine trump the dominant logic of nursing? Leading change in advanced practice education, *J Prof Nurs* 30:104–109, 2014.

Clavelle JT, Porter-O'Grady T, Drenkard K: Structural Empowerment and the Nursing Practice Environment in Magnet Organizations, *J Nurs Admin* 43(11):566–573, 2013.

Cohen H: *The nurse's quest for a professional identity*, Menlo Park, CA, 1981, Addison-Wesley.

Consorti F, Notarangelo M, Potasso L, Toscano E: Developing professionalism in medical students: an educational framework, *Adv Med Educ Pract* 3:55–60, 2012.

Crigger N, Geofrey N: *The Making of Nurse Professionals*, Sudbury, MA, 2011, Jones & Bartlett.

DeSimone B. (2014a) Unpublished manuscript.

Donabedian A: Methods for driving criteria for assessing the quality of medical care, *Med Care Rev* 37:653–698, 1980.

Dracup K, Bryan-Brown CW: From novice to expert to mentor: Shaping the future, *Am J Crit Care* 13:448–450, 2004.

Dreyfus SE, Dreyfus HL: A Five-Stage Model of the Mental Activities Involved in Directed Skill Acquisition. Berkeley, CA, 1980, University of California at Berkeley. Contract Unpublished report supported by the Air Force Office of Scientific Research, USAF (contract F49620-79-C0063).

Fardellone C, Click E: Self-perceived leadership behaviors of clinical ladder nurses, *Nurse Leader* 51–53, 2013.

Flexner A: Is social work a profession?, New York (paper presented at the National Conference on Charities and Correction, 1915) *Proceedings of the National Conference on Social Work* 581:584–588, 590 1915.

Frenk J, Chen L, Bhutta ZA, Cohen J, Crisp N, Evans T, Zurayk H: Health professionals for a new century: Transforming education to strengthen health systems in an interdependent world, *Lancet* 376:1923–1958, 2010.

Fronek P, Kendall M, Ungerer G, J. Malt J, Eugard E, Geraghty T: Towards healthy professional-client relationships: the value of an interprofessional training course, *J Interprof Care* 23(1):16–29, 2009.

Goodman T: The future of nursing: an opportunity for advocacy, *AORN* 99(6):668–671, 2014.

Hawkins J, Fontenot H: Mentorship: the heart and soul of health care leadership, *J Health Care Leadersh* 2:31–34, 2010.

Hegarty J, Condon C, Walsh E, Sweeney J: The undergraduate education of nurses: looking to the future, *Int J Nurs Educ Scholarsh* 6(1, Article 17):1–11, 2009.

Hesburgh T: Presidential leadership, *Journal of Higher Education* Vol. 42(9):763–765, 1971.

Hoffman S, Harris A, Rosenfield D: Why mentorship matters: students, staff and sustainability in interprofessional education, *J Interprof Care* 22(1):103–105, 2008.

Hood K, Cant R, Leech M, Baulch J, Gilbee A: Trying on the professional self: nursing students' perception of learning about roles, identity and teamwork in an interprofessional clinical placement, *Appl Nurs Res* 27:109–114, 2014.

Institute of Medicine (IOM): *Health professions education: a bridge to quality*, Washington, DC, 2003, National Academies Press.

Institute of Medicine (IOM): *The Future of Nursing: Leading Change, Advancing Health*, Washington DC, 2011, Author.

Khalili H, Orchard C, Health K, Laschinger S, Farah R: An interprofessional socialization framework for developing an interprofessional identity among health professions students, *Journal of Interprofessional Care* 27(6):448–453, 2013.

Kirschling JM: *Reflections on the future of doctoral programs in nursing*, Naples FL, 2014, AACN Doctoral Education Conference. January 30, 2014.

Kramer M, Schmalenberg C: Staff nurses identify essentials of magnetism. In McClure M, Hinshaw AS, editors: *Magnet hospitals revisited: attraction and retention of professional nurses*, Washington, DC, 2002, American Nurses Publication. (25-59.)

Laabs C: Perceptions of moral integrity: Contradictions in need of explanation, *Nurs Ethics* 18(3):431–440, 2011.

Larson S: Create a good impression: Professionalism in nursing, *NSNA Imprint* 50–52, 2006.

Laschinger H, Read E, Wilk P, Finegan J: The influence of nursing unit empowerment and social capital on unified effectiveness and nurse perceptions of patient care quality, *JONA* 44(6):347–352, 2014.

Lowe G, Plummer V, O'Brien A, Boyd L: Time to clarify-the value of advanced practice nursing roles in health care, *J Adv Nurs* 68(3):677–685, 2012.

Lubbe JC, Roets L: Nurses'scope of practice and the implication for quality nursing care, *J Nurs Scholarship* 46(1):58–64, 2014.

Lundmark V: Chapter 46 Magnet environments for professional nursing practice. In Hughes RG, editor: *Patient Safety and Quality: An Evidence-Based Handbook for Nursing*, Rockville, MD, 2008, Agency for Healthcare Research and Quality (US).

Mahlin M: Individual patient advocacy, collective responsibility and activism within professional organizations, *Nurs Ethics* 17(2):247–254, 2010.

Malloch K, Porter-O'Grady T: *The quantum leader: applications for the new world of work*, Sudbury, MA, 2005, Jones & Bartlett.

Malloch K, Porter-O'Grady P: *Leadership in Nursing Practice: Changing the Landscape of Health Care*, Burlington MA, 2013, Jones & Bartlett.

Margalit R, Thompson S, Visovsky C, et al.: From professional silos to interprofessional education: campuswide focus on quality of care, *Qual Manag Health Care* 18(3):165–173, 2009.

Masters K: *Role development in professional nursing practice*, Sudbury, MA, 2005, Jones & Bartlett.

Mathews S, Lankshear S: Describing the essential elements of a professional practice structure, *Nurs Leadersh* 16(2):63–71, 2003.

McBride A: *The Growth and development of Nurse Leaders*, New York, NY, 2011, Springer Publishing Company LLC.

McCloughen A, O'Brien L, Jackson D: Esteemed connection: Creating a mentoring relationship for nurse leadership, *Nurs Inq* 16(4): 326–336, 2009.

Merriam-Webster. Online. s.v. "advocate." Available online: Accessed December 30, 2009. http://www.merriam-webster.com/dictionary/advocate.

Morgan S: The magnet (TM) model as a framework for excellence, *J Nurs Care Qual* 24(2):105–108, 2009.

Muller-Juge V, Cullati S, Blondon KS, et al.: Interprofessional collaboration between residents and nurses in general internal medicine: A qualitative study on behaviors enhancing teamwork quality, *PLoS One* 9(4):e9610, 2014.

Nagel C, Andenoro A: Healing leadership: the serving leader's impact on patient outcomes in a clinical environment, *J Healthc Leadersh* 4:25–31, 2012.

Oandasan I, Reeves S: Key elements for interprofessional education. Part I: The learner, the educator and the learning context, *J Interprof Care* 19:21–38, 2005.

O'Rourke M, White A: Professional role clarity and competency in health care staffing—the missing pieces, *Nurs Econ* 29(4):183–188, 2011.

O'Rourke M: Rebuilding a professional practice model. The return of role-based practice accountability, *Nurs Adm Q* 27(2):95–105, 2003.

Paton B, Thompson-Isherwood R, Thirsk L: Preceptors matter: an evolving framework, *J Nurs Educ* 48(4):213–216, 2009.

Petri L: Concept analysis of interdisciplinary collaboration, *Nurs Forum* 45(2):73–82, 2010.

Pecukonis E, Doyle O, Bliss D: Reducing barriers to interprofessional training: Promoting interprofessional cultural competence, *J Interprof Care* 22(4I):417–428, 2008.

Pew Health Professions Commission: *Health professions education for the future: schools in service to the nation*, San Francisco, 1993, Pew Commission.

Porter-O'Grady T, & Malloch, K. (2011). Quantum leadership: Advancing innovation, transforming health care, p. 205. Jones & Bartlett Learning.

Porter-O'Grady T, & Malloch, K. (2013). Leadership in nursing practice, pp. 65 & 540. Jones & Bartlett Learning.

Porter O'Grady T: From tradition to transformation: Revolutionary movement for nursing in the age of reform, *Nurse Leader*.65–69, 2014.

Puetz B: Networking, *Public Health Nurs* 24(6):577–579, 2007.

Rick C: Competence in executive nursing leadership for the 21st century, *NL* 64–66, 2014.

Rolfe P: Transformational leadership theory: What every leader needs to know, *Nurse Leader* 54–57, 2011.

Rodts M, Lamb K: Transforming your professional self: encouraging lifelong personal and professional growth, *Orthop Nurs* 27(2):125–131, 2008.

Rogers J: Reinventing shared leadership to support nursing's evolving role in health care, *Nurse Leader* 29–43, 2014.

Schwartz D, Spencer T, Wilson B, Wood K: Transformational leadership: Implications for nursing leaders in facilities seeking magnet status, *AORN J* 93(6):737–748, 2011.

Thomas J: Changing career paths: from expert to novice, *Orthop Nurs* 22(5):332–334, 2003.

Tinkham M: The road to magnet: Encouraging transformational leadership, *AORN J* 98(2):186–188, 2013.

Wallis L: Canadian commission calls on nurses to be a force for change, *Am J Nurs* 112(9):17, 2012.

Walsh C, Gordon MF, Marshall M, Wilson F, Hunt T: Interprofessional capability: a developing framework for interprofessional education, *Nurse Educ Pract* 5:230–237, 2005.

Wear D, Castellani B: The development of professionalism: Curriculum matters, *Academic Medicine* 75(6):602–611, 2000.

Welchman J, Griener G: Patient advocacy and professional associationsd individual and collective responsibilities, *Nurs Ethics* 12(3):296–304, 2005.

Willis D, P.J. Grace P, Roy C: A central unifying focus for the discipline: facilitating humanization, meaning, choice, quality of life, and healing in living and dying, *Adv Nurs Sci* 31(1), E28–E40. 2008.

World Health Organization(WHO, 2010): *Framework for Action on Interprofessional Education and Collaborative Practice*, Geneva Switzerland, 2010, WHO.

Yoder SL, Terhorst R: "Beam me up, Scotty": designing the future of nursing professional development, *J Contin Educ Nurs* 43:456–462, 2012.

Yonge O, Billay D, Myrick F, Luhanga F: Preceptorship and mentorship: not merely a matter of semantics, *Int J Nurs Educ Scholarsh* 4(1, Article 19):1–13, 2007.

CHAPTER 23

Communicating with Other Health Professionals

Kathleen Underman Boggs

OBJECTIVES

At the end of the chapter, the reader will be able to:

1. Identify standards for effective teamwork and collaboration in the health care environment.
2. Identify communication barriers in professional relationships, including disruptive behaviors.
3. Describe methods to handle conflict through interpersonal negotiation when it occurs.
4. Discuss methods for communicating effectively with others in organizational settings (QSEN Competency).
5. Discuss application of research to evidence-based clinical communication, including the Team Strategies and Tools to Enhance Performance and Patient Safety (TeamSTEPPS) approach.

To be effective as a nursing professional, it is not enough to be deeply committed to the client. You need proficient communication skills to function as a member of an interprofessional team to effectively provide quality client care. To create and maintain an effective team, each member needs to foster open communication, demonstrate mutual respect, and share in decision making (QSEN n.d.) Pre-licensure Competency, www.QSEN.org). An essential communication skill is the ability to adapt your own communication style to meet the needs of team members and to mesh with changing situations. This chapter will focus on principles of communication with other professionals. Strategies will be suggested that you can use to help deal with other professionals and to function more effectively as an interdisciplinary team member and leader. Specific bridges to communication with other health professionals are described to help you remove communication barriers. Collaboration in health care teams will also be discussed in Chapter 24.

BASIC CONCEPTS

Every expert cites **effective communication** as a bedrock principle of quality care. Effective communication is timely, accurate, complete, unambiguous, and understood by the recipient. Communication breakdowns affect client care. For example, the literature shows that the greatest determinant of intensive care death rates is how smoothly nurses and physicians work together in planning and providing client care.

STANDARDS FOR A HEALTHY WORK ENVIRONMENT

A culture of collegiality is essential for a work environment that is to provide high-quality client care. The interprofessional team depends on an effective blending of the collective competencies of each provider to deliver quality health care. **Collaboration** begins with communicating an awareness of each other's knowledge and skills and continues with the development of shared values. If team members do not **trust** and **respect** each other and communicate in an open and respectful manner, they are more likely to make mistakes (Herlehy, 2011). Reflect on the following case example, Conflict on a Surgical Unit.

Case Example: Conflict on a Surgical Unit

Two nursing teams work the day shift on a busy surgical unit. As nurse manager, Ms. Libby notices that both teams are arguing over use of the computer, have become unwilling to help cover the other team's client, and are taking longer to complete assigned work, and so on. To achieve a more harmonious work environment, she arranges a staff meeting to get the teams communicating. Rather than just issues about sharing the computer, these multiple problems suggest inadequate time management and overload. Ms. Libby listens actively, responds with empathy, and provides positive regard and feedback for solutions proposed by the group. She asks the group to decide on two prioritized solutions. Recognizing that her staff feel unappreciated and knowing that compromise is a strategy that produces behavior change, she resolves to offer more frequent performance feedback. She herself assumes responsibility for requesting an immediate second computer purchase under her unit budget's emergency funding allocation. A team member who is on the employee relations committee assumes responsibility for requesting that the human services department schedule an in-service training on time management and stress reduction within the next month. The group agrees to meet in 6 weeks to evaluate.

Even with recent emphasis on the importance of collegiality, when TJC surveyed nurses, more than 90% reported witnessing disruptive behavior; more than half reported they themselves had been subjected to verbal abuse (TJC, 2008). In another survey, 30% of health care team members admitted to having acted rudely to other members on occasion. The American Association of Critical Care Nurses (AACCN, 2004) has issued six *standards* characteristic of a healthy workplace (www.aacn.org):

1. Nurses must be as efficient in communication skills as they are in clinical skills.
2. Nurses must be relentless in pursuing and fostering true collaboration.
3. Nurses must be valued and committed partners in making policy, directing and evaluating clinical care, and leading organizational operations.
4. Staffing must ensure the effective match between patient needs and nurse competencies.
5. Nurses must be recognized and recognize others for the value each brings to the work of the organization.
6. Nurse leaders must fully embrace the imperative of a healthy work environment, authentically live it, and engage others in its achievement.

Other professional nursing organizations have identified the following *elements* of a healthy workplace environment:

- Collaborative culture with respectful communication and behavior
- Communication-rich culture that emphasizes trust and respect
- Clearly defined role expectations with accountability
- Adequate workforce
- Competent leadership
- Shared decision making
- Employee development
- Recognition of workers' contributions

CODE OF BEHAVIOR

The goal of collaboration is to communicate effectively with team members to provide the best care. As part of creating a culture of teamwork where staff is valued, a standard across organizations should be zero tolerance for disruptive or bullying behaviors. To accomplish this, each organization needs one well-defined code of behavior applied consistently to all staff. TJC mandates that each health care organization has a code of conduct defining acceptable and unacceptable behaviors, as well as an agency process for reporting and handling disruptive behaviors, discrimination or disrespectful treatment (TJC, 2008, 2010).

DEFINITION OF DISRUPTIVE BEHAVIORS

Conflict was defined in Chapter 13 as a hostile encounter. The nursing literature uses a variety of terms to refer to persistent uncivil behaviors in the workplace: bullying; verbal abuse; horizontal violence; lateral violence; "eating your young"; in-fighting; mobbing, harassment, or scapegoating. For discussion purposes in this textbook, we use the term **disruptive behavior,** defined as situations in which lack of civility or lack of respect occurs within a professional relationship as frequently as weekly and is repeated over time.

Disruptive behaviors are prolonged and may include overt behaviors: rudeness, verbal abuse, intimidation, put-downs; angry outbursts, yelling, blaming, or criticizing team members in front of others; sexual harassment; or even threatening physical confrontations. Other disruptive behaviors are more covert: passive-aggressively withholding need-to-know information, withholding help, assigning excessively heavy workloads, refusing to perform an assigned task, being impatient or reluctance to answer questions, not returning telephone calls or pages, and speaking in a condescending tone (O'Reilly, 2008). These behaviors threaten the well-being of nurses and the safety of clients (Wachs, 2009).

INCIDENCE

Disruptive behavior is fairly common in large organizations, especially hospitals. Although it is estimated that only a minority of staff exhibit disruptive behaviors, this is enough to affect client outcomes. In one study, 17% of professionals surveyed reported a disruptive behavior that resulted in a specific adverse client outcome; 86% of nurses reported witnessing disrespect or harassment from physicians; and 72% reported receiving disrespectful behavior from other nurses (O'Daniel and Rosenstein, 2008). Others have found that nurse-to-nurse disruptive behaviors occur more frequently than disruptive physician-nurse interactions and tend to occur more often in high-stress areas such as surgical suites or emergency departments (Agency for Healthcare Research and Quality [AHRQ] PSNet, n.d.; Woelfle and McCaffrey, 2007). At least one in six nurses reports bullying from peers (Blair, 2013). Weaver (2013) describes a particularly distressing type of bullying in which experienced nurses exhibit these behaviors against inexperienced new graduates, perhaps perceiving them as less competent.

OUTCOMES OF DISRUPTIVE BEHAVIOR

AHRQ specifically states that disruptive behaviors impede the delivery of patient care (PSNet, n.d.). Refer to Box 23-1 for some sources of interpersonal workplace conflict.

As described earlier, failures in collaboration and communication among health team members are among the most common factors cited for nurse dissatisfaction, job abandonment, lost productivity, absenteeism, task avoidance, poor morale, and effects on nurses' physical and mental health. Costs to agency are related to increases in care errors, decreases in care quality, more adverse client outcomes, and increases in staff turnover, and even legal action (Olender-Russo, 2009; Spence-Laschinger et al., 2009).

CREATING A COLLABORATIVE CULTURE OF REGARD TO ELIMINATE DISRUPTIVE BEHAVIOR

Corporate climate changes are gradually shifting to a collaborative, patient-centered care model in which the hierarchical power model is replaced by a model

---

BOX 23-1	Interpersonal Sources of Conflict in the Workplace: Barriers to Collaboration and Communication

1. Different expectations
   - Being asked to do something you know would be irresponsible or unsafe
   - Having your feelings or opinions ridiculed or discounted
   - Getting pressure to give more time or attention than you are able to give
   - Being asked to give more information than you feel comfortable sharing
   - Differences in language
2. Threats to self
   - Maintaining a sense of self in the face of hostility or sexual harassment
   - Being asked to do something to a client that is in conflict with your personal or professional moral values
3. Differences in role hierarchy
   - Differences in education or experience
   - Differences in responsibility and rewards (payment)
4. Clinical situation constraints
   - Emphasis on rapid decision making
   - Complexity of care interventions

---

in which all team members are valued. Collaboration is broadly defined as working with all the members of the health care team to achieve maximum health outcomes for our mutual client. Organizational support is essential if this model of care is to be successful.

1. Common goal: Developing a **collaborative culture** in which all team members keep the delivery of safe, high-quality client care foremost in mind, requires that we trust and respect the decision making of all team members. Different professionals were educated to hold differing beliefs and styles of communication. We need to develop an understanding of these various perspectives, not so we can change them, but so that we can utilize them.
2. Open communication: Creating a communication-rich environment requires that all team members value open communication. We combine assertiveness (speaking up, giving and receiving feedback) with cooperation.
3. Mutual respect and shared decision making: The Institute of Medicine (IOM) (2003) says nurses should be full partners with physicians and other health team members. Leadership is required to

avoid duplication of tasks and to ensure that all tasks are completed.

4. Role clarity: Members of a team that has been working together smoothly generally have developed complementary roles. We know our scope of practice and recognize when we need to call on the expertise of others. An important part of working together is developing mutual trust; you trust coworkers to "have your back."

Collaboration is a dynamic process benefiting from ongoing practice and evaluation. In the past, some organizations tolerated disruptive workplace behaviors. Pressures on nurses exist to increase productivity and cost-effectiveness. Accrediting agencies now require agency-wide, published behavior codes and a process for reporting disruptive behaviors. Agencies are encouraged to hold interdisciplinary discussions on this topic and practice zero tolerance of these behaviors. Individually, we need to become aware of how to discourage disruptive behaviors as we work to develop a healthy, collaborative workplace atmosphere to ensure high-quality client care (TJC, 2009). A hallmark of a professional is acceptance of accountability for one's own behavior. Preventing conflicts is accomplished by avoiding public criticism, cultivating a willingness to help attitude, and willingness to do one's fair share.

RESPECT

Feeling respected or not respected is an integral part of how nurses rate the quality of their work environment. Three key factors are a positive climate of professional practice, a supportive manager, and positive relationships with other staff.

Nurses say they feel respected and appreciated if their opinions are listened to attentively and they receive feedback from authority figures as to the value of their work competence. When their opinions are discounted or ridiculed, they feel disrespected, angry, and frustrated. Feelings of powerlessness decrease self-esteem and increase anger. In an unhealthy atmosphere in which a staff member feels intimidated by authority and unable to change disruptive behaviors, they may direct anger toward peers. Respect is a natural extension of the practice of nursing, as identified in the American Nurses Association's Code of Ethics (ANA, 2001). Typically, nurses describe behaviors indicating lack of respect to include demeaning verbal comments; nonverbal actions such as eye rolling;

not paying attention to their opinions; interrupting; not responding to telephone or e-mail; and physical or sexual harassment.

FACTORS THAT AFFECT NURSE BEHAVIOR TOWARD OTHER TEAM MEMBERS
Gender

The relationship between physicians and nurses remains an evolving process. Traditional culture proscribed gender role communication. Because physicians were predominantly male and nurses female, this greatly affected communication patterns. Also because health care authority was vested in a hierarchical structure, control rested with the physician. Changes in the physician-nurse communication process are occurring as nurses become more empowered, more assertive, and better educated. Team training has been instituted to educate all team members to work in a collaborative manner.

Contemporary society is redefining traditional gender role behavior, negating some of the traditional gender stereotypical behaviors. Most nurses occasionally encounter problems in the physician-nurse relationship. The differences in power, perspective, education, pay, status, class, and sometimes gender are contributing factors. If you encounter a conflict situation at work, reflect on whether gender is a factor or whether the problem is due to differences in communication style.

GENERATIONAL DIVERSITY

Members of older and younger generations differ in their preferred communication styles. In fact, generational and cultural differences among nurses is cited as a main barrier to smooth communication. According to the U.S. Department of Health and Human Services, today's nursing workforce members now span four generations. As might be expected, members of different generations hold differing work values and attitudes and have differing communication preferences. Generational differences are a big source of conflict today. Differences exist not only in communication styles, but also in work ethic, attitudes, style of interacting with authority figures, and in learning styles (QSEN Institute Teamwork and Collaboration, n.d.). In studies of generational differences in learning, findings indicate younger nurses might prefer digital communication (via texting, etc.), while nurses from an older generation might prefer face-to-face communication. A study by Robinson and colleagues (2012) finds younger nurses more likely to be abstract learners, using inductive reasoning, while older nurses are more concrete, and rely more on intuitive, experienced-based strategies. They suggest that nurses need to plan to use different methods to communicate based on the recipient's age.

OUTCOMES OF SUCCESSFUL TEAM TRAINING IN COMMUNICATION

In a metaanalysis of several studies on effects of team training, Weaver and Rosen (2013) say evidence is strong in showing improved efficiency and increased client safety. Changing the organizational climate requires administrative support and resources, but also local unit buy-in to using the Team Strategies and Tools to Enhance Performance and Patient Safety (TeamSTEPPS) strategies. Each nurse team member needs to participate and be accountable for facilitating team communication.

APPLICATIONS

As nurses, we can help to establish and sustain a healthy workplace. This requires continuous assessment of our own and others' current communication practices and implementation of "best practices" to prevent and deal with conflict. Communication and conflict-resolution strategies can be learned but require continued reinforcement through ongoing communication training.

CONFLICT RESOLUTION

Whenever people work together, conflicts will inevitably arise. As nurses, we each have a responsibility to practice collaboratively. Aside from the nurse-client-family conflicts described in Chapter 13, the more distressing workplace conflicts occur between nurses rather than between the nurse and authority figures, such as managers or physicians. In addition, conflict may arise from agency employee policies. Internal employee-management disputes detract from the agency's health care mission and from its financial bottom line.

TEAMSTEPPS: A TRAINING PROGRAM TO IMPROVE TEAMWORK

Communication skills are crucial to effective health care team function. Effective communication skills convey accurate information and provide awareness of your role responsibilities. Teamwork and collaboration are a major focus of both TeamSTEPPS and QSEN. Each team member shares a clear vision of expected outcomes for each client. As a team member, you communicate to keep all others informed. Miscommunication is often cited as a major factor in unsafe care. AHRQ (TeamSTEPPS, n.d.), in conjunction with the Department of Defense, has developed a TeamSTEPPS training program to create a transformed health care model. The acronym stands for *Team Strategies and Tools to Enhance Performance and Patient Safety*. Since its release in 2006, TeamSTEPPS has provided public domain resources and team training programs that when applied at each agency, improves client care. This includes standardized goals and skills to improve team performance through use of team structure tools. This program provides tools and strategies for developing better communication knowledge, skills, and attitudes. One goal of TeamSTEPPS is to improve team function by increasing communication clarity. Content teaches team members, including nurses, how to increase their competencies in leadership, situation monitoring, mutual support, and communication. Examples of leadership competency are clarifying team goals and roles. Competencies for situation monitoring include use of decision making skills in emergent situations and providing corrective feedback. Mutual support skills include assisting others and using tools such as "the two-challenge rule" (stating your concerns at least two times) to make sure all team members are aware of risk situations. Communication tools include SBAR (which stands for situation, background, assessment, recommendation), teach-backs or check-backs (to verify that your communication message is understood accurately), and call-outs, as well as use of conflict resolution strategies. TeamSTEPPS encourages the use of standardized communication tools, especially during emergency situations.

Communication strategies as described in Chapter 4 include use of briefs and debriefs, huddles, call-outs, check-backs, and other team behaviors discussed at the AHRQ web site. Outcomes include development of a shared mental model of team care, increased trust among team members, and the major goal of safer client care. Table 23-1 lists their standards of effective communication.

TABLE 23-1	TeamSTEPPS: Using a Team Training Program Improves Team Communication	
Essentials of Communication	**Sending Technique**	**Receiving Technique**
Clear	Common language/terminology used	Validate: use feedback or "talk back" to confirm understanding
Brief	Communicate only information essential for this situation	Clarify any nonverbal information
Timely	Verify message is received; respond quickly to requests for additional information; provide updates	Verify receipt of information
Complete	Give all relevant information; use standardized communication tools	Document: essential information validated, understood, and recorded

Adapted from Agency for Healthcare Research and Quality (AHRQ): *Curriculum/Instructors Guide*. http://www.ahrq.gov/professionals/education/curriculum-tools/teamstepps/instructor/fundamentals/module6/igltccommunication.pdf. Accessed August 8,2014.

CONFLICT RESOLUTION

Many of the same strategies for conflict resolution discussed for conflicts between client and nurse can be applied to conflicts between the nurse and other health team members. Review the principles of conflict management in Figure 13-1 in Chapter 13. As mentioned, conflict is not necessarily detrimental to productivity and job satisfaction. Successful resolution often has a positive outcome. Instead of picturing a straight line of either you win or I win, envision the outcome of conflict resolution as a triangle with an outcome of mutual resolution as a peak, where you both have built something greater together.

IDENTIFY SOURCES OF CONFLICT

Conflict often stems from miscommunication. You need to think through the possible causes of the conflict. Conflict also stems from overly defensive responses to a situation. So you need to identify your own feelings about it and respond appropriately, even if the response is a deliberate choice not to respond verbally. But interpersonal conflicts that are not dealt with leave residual feelings that reappear in future interactions.

SET GOALS

Your primary goal in dealing with workplace conflict is to find a high-quality, mutually acceptable solution: a win-win strategy. Remembering that we all share the ultimate goal of delivering high-quality patient-centered care may help us work together even if we personally do not like each other. In many instances, a better collaborative relationship can be developed through the use of the following conflict management communication techniques (Johansen, 2012). To reframe a clinical situation as a cooperative process in which the health goals and not the status of the providers becomes the focus:

- *Assume responsibility* for one's own behaviors and for maintaining a "blame-free" work environment.
- *Identify your goal.* A clear idea of the outcome you wish to achieve is a necessary first step in the process. Remember the issue is the conflict, not your coworker.
- *Obtain factual data.* It is important to do your homework by obtaining all relevant information about the specific issues involved—and about the individual's behavioral responses to a health care issue—before engaging in negotiation.
- *Intervene early.* Be assertive. The best time to resolve problems is before they escalate to a conflict. Create a forum for two-way communication, preferably meeting periodically. Structured formats have been developed for you to use in conflict resolution, especially in team meetings. Nielsen and Mann (2008) mention the format of *DESC:*
  D = describe the behavior (the problem)
  E = express your concern
  S = specify a course of action
  C = obtain consensus
- *Avoid negative comments that can affect the self-esteem of the receiver.* Even when the critical statements are valid (e.g., "You do…" or "You make me feel…"), they should be replaced with "I" statements that define the sender's position. Otherwise, needless hostility is created and the meaning of the communication is lost.

BOX 23-2	Strategies to Turn Conflict into Collaboration

1. Recognize and confront disruptive behaviors.
   - Use conflict-resolution strategies.
   - Take the initiative to discuss problems.
   - Use active listening skills (refrain from simultaneous activities that interrupt communication).
   - Present documented data relevant to the issue.
   - Propose resolutions.
   - Use a brief summary to provide feedback.
   - Record all decisions in writing.
2. Create a climate in which participants view negotiation as a collaborative effort.
   - Develop agency behavior policies with stated zero tolerance for disruptive or bullying behaviors.
   - Model communicating with staff in a respectful, courteous manner.
   - Participate in organizational interdisciplinary groups.
   - Solicit and give feedback on a regular, periodic basis.
   - Clarify role expectations.

- *Consider the other's viewpoint.* Having some idea of what issues might be relevant from the other person's perspective provides important information about the best interpersonal approach to use. In addition to dealing with your own feelings, you need an ability to deal with the feelings of the others. Be cooperative, acknowledging the team's interdependence and mutual goals.

COMMUNICATE TO PROMOTE EFFECTIVE COLLABORATION: AVOID BARRIERS TO RESOLUTION

Refer to Box 23-2 for tips on how to turn conflict into collaboration.

Individual behaviors such as avoiding the use of negative or inflammatory, anger-provoking words, or avoiding phrases that imply coercion have been described. Examples include: "We must insist that…" or "You claim that…" Most individuals react to anger directed at them with a fight-or-flight response. Anyone can have a moment of rudeness, but monitor your own communications to avoid any pattern of abusive behaviors, including blaming or criticizing staff to others. When nurse supervisors become aware of how their behavior affects their nurses, they can increase the nurses' performance, increase their job involvement, and increase organizational identification. Participating

in mentoring newly hired nurses, even helping sustain internship programs for novice nurses, may help avert conflict (Weaver, 2013).

PHYSICIAN-NURSE CONFLICT RESOLUTION

The history of nurse-physician communication is described by Seago (2008) as a "game" in which nurses made treatment recommendations without appearing to do so and physicians asked for recommendations without appearing to do so, with both parties striving to avoid open disagreements. She notes that the literature indicates that communication between doctor and nurse is still often contentious. Remarkable increases in safety in airline and space programs were achieved by creating a climate in which junior team members were free to question decisions of more senior, powerful team members. It is recommended that health care adopt a similar philosophy. The American Medical Association (AMA, 2008) has specifically stated that codes of conduct define appropriate behavior as including a right to appropriately express a concern you have about client care and safety. While this is being set forth as a medical code of conduct for physicians, should it also apply to nurses?

Nurses influence physician-client communication. Nurses assess what physicians tell clients, encourage clients to seek clarification, and support our client's right to ask questions. This is an important aspect of our belief that the client is a valued member of our health team. Nurses have a responsibility to foster good physician-client communication. This is especially true when it becomes obvious to you from content, tone, or body language that antagonism is developing. Do you think it is ever appropriate for a nurse to criticize a physician's actions to a client? A common underlying factor in at least 25% of all malpractice suits is an inadvertent or deliberate critical comment by another health care professional concerning a colleague's actions.

Better collaboration and better communication are associated with safer care and better client care outcomes. In a meta-analysis of existing research, Seago (2008) found these factors to be associated with reduced drug errors, reduced client mortality, improved client satisfaction, and somewhat with shorter hospital stays. Methods to improve safe communication are discussed in Chapter 4.

There will be occasions when you have collaboration difficulties. One major factor related to job satisfaction and job retention is *"disruptive" communication* between other professionals, especially physician-nurse interactions. Case law defines disruptive physician behavior as conduct that disrupts the operation of the hospital, affects the ability of others to get their jobs done, and creates a hostile work environment.

Some doctors are reluctant to be challenged; some nurses are quick to feel slighted. Some physician-nurse relationships are marked with conflict, mistrust, and disrespect. Although these feelings are changing, it is slow, and some physicians still regard themselves as the only legitimate authority in health care, seeing the professional nurse as an accessory. An attitude that excludes the nurse as a professional partner in health care promotion benefits no one and is increasingly challenged as being costly to professionals and clients alike.

It is important to remain flexible yet not to yield on important, essential dimensions of the issue. Sometimes it is difficult to listen carefully to the other person's position without automatically formulating your next point or response, but it is important to keep an open mind and to examine the issue from a number of perspectives before selecting alternative options. The communication process should not be prematurely concluded. You can apply the same principles of conflict resolution discussed in Chapter 13 when dealing with a physician-nurse conflict.

MAKE A COMMITMENT TO OPEN DIALOGUE

Listening should constitute at least half of a communication interaction. Foster a feeling of collegiality. Use strategies from that chapter to defuse anger. During your negotiation, discussion should begin with a statement of either the commonalities of purpose or the points of agreement about the issue (e.g., "I thoroughly agree Mr. Smith will do much better at home. However, we need to contact social services and make a home care referral before we actually discharge him; otherwise, he will be right back in the hospital again."). Points of disagreement should always follow rather than precede points of agreement. Empathy and a genuine desire to understand the issues from the other's perspective enhance communication and the likelihood of a successful resolution.

Solutions that take into consideration the needs and human dignity of all parties are more likely to be considered as viable alternatives. Backing another health professional into a psychological corner by using intimidation, coercion, or blame is simply counterproductive. More often than not, solutions developed through such tactics never get implemented. Usually there are a number of reasons for this, but the basic issues have to do with how the problem was originally defined and the control issues that were never actually dealt with in the problem-solving discussion. The final solution derived through fair negotiation is often better than the one arrived at alone.

NURSE-TO-NURSE CONFLICT RESOLUTION

Although it is inevitable that you will encounter some communication problems with nurse colleagues, remember that, if managed appropriately, these conflicts can lead to innovative solutions and improved relationships.

Negotiating with Nursing Authority Figures

Negotiating can be even more threatening with a nursing supervisor or an instructor who has direct authority, because these people have some control over your future as a staff nurse or student. Supervision implies a shared responsibility in the overall professional goal of providing high-quality nursing care to clients. The wise supervisor is able to promote a nonthreatening environment in which all of the aspects of professionalism are allowed to emerge and prosper. In a supervisor-nurse relationship, conflict may arise when expectations for performance are unclear or when the nurse is unable to perform at the desired level. Communication of expectations often occurs after the fact, within the context of an employee performance evaluation. To effectively manage requires that performance expectations are known from the beginning. The supervisor needs to advise you about the need for improvement as part of an ongoing, constructive, interpersonal relationship. When the supervisor gives constructive criticism, it is in a nonthreatening and genuinely caring manner. In studying approaches to authority figures, you are encouraged to analyze your overall personal responses to authority, as in Exercise 23-1.

Managing Problems Among Nursing Staff

Improving how nurses deal with conflict is an investment in coworkers, our organization, and ultimately in improved client outcomes. Nurse managers have learned that ignoring conflict among staff does not solve problems. Avoidance perpetuates the status quo or leads to an escalation. When managed

EXERCISE 23-1	Feelings about Authority

Purpose: To have students recognize their feelings about authority.

Procedure
1. Lean back in your chair, close your eyes, and think of the word *authority*.
2. Who is the first person that comes to mind when thinking of that word?
3. Describe how this person signifies authority to you. Next, think of an incident in which this person exerted authority and how you reacted to it.
4. After you have visualized the memory, answer the following questions:
   a. What were your feelings about the incident after it was over?

b. What changes of feelings occurred from the start of the incident until it was over?
c. Was there anything about the authority figure that reminded you of yourself?
d. Was there anything about the authority figure that reminded you of someone else with whom you once had a strong relationship (if the memory viewed is not mother or father)?
e. How could you have handled the incident more assertively?
f. Can you see any patterns in yourself that might help you handle interactions with authority figures?
g. What about those patterns are not assertive?
h. How could those patterns be improved to be more assertive?

Adapted from Levy R: *Self-revelation through relationships*, Englewood Cliffs, NJ, 1972, Prentice Hall.

appropriately, you reduce time wasted by staff in griping, defending, and so on, as illustrated in the following case.

Case Example: Confusing Mr. Santos

"Jane, we seem to disagree about the best way to teach Mr. Santos about his…He seems to be getting confused about our two different approaches. Let's talk about how we might be able to work more effectively together. What is the most important point you want to teach him?"

Use active listening skills to really pay attention to what Jane says. Do a self-inventory to eliminate any nonverbal behavior that is triggering Jane's reaction and eliminate it. Ask yourself, "Do I want to win, or do I want to fix this problem?" Then state your expectations in a calm tone.

COLLABORATING WITH PEERS

The nurse-client relationship occurs within the larger context of the professional relationship with other health disciplines. How the nurse relates to other members of the health team will affect the level and nature of the interactions that transpire between nurse and client. Interpersonal conflict between health team members periodically is concealed from awareness and projected onto client behaviors.

Issues arise now and again when there is no input from different work shifts in developing a comprehensive care plan. The shift staff may not agree with specific interventions, but instead of talking the discrepancy

through in regularly scheduled staff conferences, they may act it out, unconsciously undoing the work of the other shifts.

Occasionally you may have to work with a peer with whom you develop a "personality conflict." Stop and consider what led up to the current situation. Generally it is due to an accumulation of small annoyances that occurred over time. The best method to avoid such situations is to verbalize occurrences rather than ignoring them until they become a major problem. Avoid the "blame game" and discuss in a private, calm moment what you *both* can do to make things better. Modeling positive interactions may assist in resolution of conflict. Holding "an intervention" or a "crucial conversation" discussion is needed. Blair (2013) suggests using the mnemonic CRIB to guide the conversation:

C = Commit to seeking a mutual purpose (to move toward resolution of the conflict).
R = Recognize the purpose (use a mentor to help).
I = Invent a mutual purpose (agree to a win-win purpose).
B = Brainstorm new strategies (agree to work together differently to move forward).

Whenever there is covert conflict among nursing staff or between members of different health disciplines, it is the client who ultimately suffers the repercussions. The level of trust the client may have established in the professional relationship is compromised until the staff conflict can be resolved.

DELEGATION OR SUPERVISION OF UNLICENSED PERSONNEL

Delegation is defined as the transfer of responsibility for the performance of an activity from one individual to another while retaining accountability for the outcome. Whether delegating to a peer or unlicensed assistive personnel (UAP), the nurse is only transferring the responsibility for the performance of the activity, not the professional accountability for the overall care (ANA, 1994). Delegation can free a nurse for attending to more complex care needs (ANA, 2005). In earlier times delegating and trusting went hand in hand, because the nurse was transferring responsibility to a peer and had some assurance of the skills and knowledge of that peer. The present health care environment poses a much different reality in which some UAPs possess minimal experience, skills, or knowledge.

We face the challenges of maintaining professional integrity and providing care efficiently, while dealing with increased workloads. Effective and appropriate use of delegation can facilitate your ability to meet these challenges. But more often than not, novice nurses are inadequately prepared for the demands of delegating much of their nursing tasks to UAPs while retaining responsibility for interpreting patient outcomes. Reflect on the following case example of Monica Lewis, RN.

Case Example: Monica Lewis, RN

After receiving the report on her client assignments, Monica Lewis, RN, assigns a newly hired unlicensed assistive personnel (UAP) to provide routine care (e.g., morning care, assistance with meals, vital signs, finger sticks for glucose, and reporting of any changes) to Mrs. Jones, who was recently admitted for exacerbation of her type 2 diabetes. While on routine rounds during lunch, Monica finds Mrs. Jones unresponsive, with cold, clammy skin, a heart rate of 110 beats per minute, and a finger stick reading of 60 mg/dL, which the UAP had obtained. Thinking Mrs. Jones was experiencing hypoglycemia, Monica requested the UAP to obtain another blood glucose reading. While administering high-glucose intravenous solutions to raise Mrs. Jones's blood sugar, Monica observed the UAP violate a number of basic principles in obtaining an accurate blood glucose level. On further questioning, the UAP admitted never having been taught the proper procedure and thought reading the directions was sufficient. Monica had wrongly assumed all UAPs underwent training on the principles of obtaining blood glucose finger sticks.

Inherent in effective delegation is an adequate understanding of the skills and knowledge of UAPs, as well as of the Nurse Practice Act of the state in which you are practicing. Within each state's Nurse Practice Act are specific guidelines describing what nursing actions can and cannot be delegated, and to what type of personnel these actions can be delegated. In addition to knowing nurse practice guidelines and the skills and knowledge level of UAPs, the nurse must educate and reinforce the UAP's knowledge base, assess the UAP's readiness for delegation, delegate appropriately, oversee the task, and evaluate and record the outcomes. A helpful resource is the National Council of State Boards of Nursing. The appropriate implementation of these principles (e.g., educating, assessing, overseeing, and evaluating) is a costly process both in time and energy. Practice Exercise 23-2 to facilitate your understanding of the principles of delegation.

STRATEGIES A NURSE CAN USE TO COMMUNICATE AND HELP CREATE A BETTER WORK ENVIRONMENT

Agency administrators have tried various strategies to promote a healthier work environment, such as redesigning rooms so nurses do not have to walk so far. Communication-friendly devices are offered in some agencies, such as the hands-free devices described in Chapter 26 to allow nurses to locate each other. What are individual nurses able to do?

Try Exercise 23-3 to help develop your communication skills.

ADVOCACY

Nursing organizations have identified trends toward increased use of unlicensed workers in agencies wishing to reduce costs. Such organizations speak out about the burden this places on registered nurses. Becoming active in your state nurses' association or professional specialty organization allows you to add your voice to this debate. Obtain a copy of your state's Nurse Practice Act. Usually these can be downloaded from your state Board of Nursing's web site. This document will spell out what you, as a registered nurse, can delegate and to whom.

Even as a beginning staff nurse you will be expected to delegate some client care duties to others. You are responsible for the completeness, quality, and accuracy

EXERCISE 23-2	Applying Principles of Delegation

Purpose: To help students differentiate between delegating nursing tasks and evaluating client outcomes.

Procedure

Divide the class into two groups: A and B. The following case study is a typical day for a charge nurse in an extended-care facility. After reading the case study, Group A is to describe the nursing tasks they would delegate and instructions they would give the nursing assistants and certified medicine aides (CMAs). Group B is to describe the professional nursing responsibilities related to the delegated tasks. The two groups then share their reports.

Situation

Anne Marie Roache is the day-shift charge nurse on one of the units at Shadyside Nursing and Rehabilitation Facility. On this particular day, her census is 24, and her staff includes four nursing assistants and two CMAs who are allowed to administer all oral and topical medications. Her nursing assistants are qualified to perform morning care: assist with feedings;

obtain and record vital signs, fluid intake and output, and blood glucose finger sticks; turn and position residents; assist with ambulation; and perform decubitus dressing changes. Of the residents, 12 are bedridden, requiring complete bed baths and some degree of assistance with feeding. The remaining 12 require varying degrees of assistance with their morning baths and assistance to the dining rooms for their meals. Nine of the residents are diabetics requiring premeal blood glucose finger sticks; seven are recovering from cerebrovascular accidents and display varying degrees of right- or left-sided weakness; three require care of their sacral decubiti; and all of the residents are at risk for falling because of varying degrees of confusion, disorientation, or general weakness. The night shift reported that all the residents' conditions were stable and they had slept well. Ms. Roache is ready to assign her staff.

Discussion

Entire class can identify client goals.

EXERCISE 23-3	Communication to Promote a Healthy Work Environment

Suggestions include negotiating with nurse administrators to avoid being assigned to multiple shifts or allowing small breaks every few hours to recharge; texting or posting affirmation (positive) messages for all the staff to read; saying or texting a message of "good job" or "thank you" to a team member; using humor; putting a smile on your face.

Purpose: To brainstorm ideas about communicating with team members and administration to facilitate a healthier workplace.

Directions

Gather in small groups to compile a list of ways to communicate which might help promote a pleasant, healthy work environment. Compare lists.

of this care. To avoid conflicts in delegating client care, clearly state your expectations. It is your responsibility to ensure that care was given correctly.

STRATEGIES TO REMOVE BARRIERS TO COMMUNICATION WITH OTHER PROFESSIONALS

Generally, conflict increases anxiety. When interaction with a certain peer or peer group stimulates anxious or angry feelings, the presence of conflict should be considered. Once it is determined that conflict is present, look for the basis of the conflict and label it as personal or professional. If it is personal in nature, it may not be appropriate to seek peer negotiation. It might be better to go back through the self-awareness exercises

presented in previous chapters and locate the nature of the conflict through self-examination.

Sharing feelings about a conflict with others helps to reduce its intensity. It is confusing, for example, when nursing students first enter a nursing program or clinical rotation, but this confusion does not get discussed, and students commonly believe they should not feel confused or uncertain. As a nursing student, you face complex interpersonal situations. These situations may lead you to experience loneliness or self-doubt about your nursing skills compared with those of your peers. These feelings are universal at the beginning of any new experience. By sharing them with one or two peers, you usually find that others have had parallel experiences. In reviewing Exercise 23-4, think of a conflict or problem that has implications for your

EXERCISE 23-4	Applying Principles of Confrontation

Purpose: To help students understand the importance of using specific principles of confrontation to resolve a conflict.

Procedure
1. Divide the class into two groups: Group A is the day shift (7 a.m. to 7 p.m.) and Group B is the night shift (7 p.m. to 7 a.m.).
2. The following case study is an example of some problems between the night and day shifts resulting in mistrust and general tension between the two groups. After reading the case study, each group is to use three principles as identified in the text (i.e., identify concerns, clarify assumptions, and identify real issue). The two groups then share their concerns, assumptions, and what they believe to be the real issue. Finally, both groups are to apply the fourth principle, collaboratively identifying a solution or solutions that satisfy both groups.

Situation
The night shift's (Group B) responsibilities include completing as many bed baths as possible and the taping report as close to the shift change (7 a.m.) as possible. The day shift (Group A) finds that few, if any, of the bed baths are completed and that the taped report is usually done at about 5 a.m., reflecting few of the client changes that occurred between 5 a.m. and 7 a.m. The day shift is angry with the night shift, feeling they are not assuming their fair share of the workload. The night shift feels the day shift does not understand their responsibilities; they believe they are contributing more than their fair share of work.

Discussion
Instructor might role-play the part of the nurse manager who acts to facilitate resolution of this conflict.

practice of nursing, one you would be willing to share with your peers.

STEPS WE CAN TAKE AS INDIVIDUALS TO DEAL WITH WORKPLACE CONFLICTS

Consider using the behaviors listed in Table 23-2 when directly dealing with conflict in the workplace yourself. Discussion of these behaviors may give you some ideas about how to implement them.

MODEL BEHAVIORS THAT CONVEY RESPECT

Prevent conflict by behaving with respect. Just as you treat clients with respect, you have an ethical responsibility to treat coworkers with respect. In a survey by Costello and colleagues (2011), 30% of surgical team respondents admitted to having treated coworkers with disrespect. Nurses need to be appreciated, recognized, and respected as professionals for the work they do. Unsupportive and uncivil coworkers and workplace conflicts negatively influence retention of nursing staff. Unprofessional communication can range from rudeness or gossip to overt hostile comments. Communication can become distorted rather than open when you are concerned about offending a more powerful individual. Strategies for dealing with disrespectful or disruptive behaviors include establishing common communication expectations and skills, teaching conflict resolution skills, and creating a culture of mutual

respect within the health care system. Ideally, the system has ongoing education, leadership and team collaboration support, and policies to evaluate behavior violations.

MENTOR NEW NURSES

Can it really be true that 50% of newly hired nurses leave within the first 3 years? A number of these transfer to other places, but some actually abandon the nursing profession entirely. Orientation of novice nurses is expensive for the institution. QSEN and IOM encourage agencies to establish internships or mentoring programs for the first 1 to 2 years of each novice nurse's employment.

CLARIFY COMMUNICATIONS

You can use the tools taught in Chapter 4 and the skills taught throughout this textbook to improve both the clarity of message content and the emotional tone of interactions. Communication problems lead to a large percentage of disruptive behaviors, especially telephone communication. Message clarity is enhanced when standardized formats such as SBAR, discussed in Chapter 4, are used: The nurse identifies self by name and position, the client by name, diagnosis, the problem (include current problem, vital signs, new symptoms, etc.), and clearly states his or her request.

TABLE 23-2	Examples of Unclear Communication Processes That Block the Development of Cooperation Reframed to Develop Shared Client-Centered Care Goals

Situation	Cognitive Processes	Reframed to Improve Communication
Low self-disclosure	No one knows my real thoughts, feelings, and needs. *Consequently:* I think no one cares about me or recognizes my needs. Others see me as self-sufficient and are unaware that I have a problem. *Consequently:* Others are unable to respond to my needs.	Attitude: • Respect • Value working with others • Willingness to collaborate Use skills: • Open communication—I verbalize aloud my needs clearly so others can have an opportunity to respond, to speak up. • Conflict-resolution strategies
Reluctance to delegate tasks	Other people think I do not believe that they can do the job as well as I can. *Consequently:* The others work at a minimum level. I do not expect or ask others to be involved. *Consequently:* Other people do not volunteer to help me. *Consequently:* I feel resentful, and others feel undervalued and dispensable.	Attitude: • Cooperate—I am part of a team. • Trust—I need to assign team members to do the tasks they can complete competently. Use skills: • Interdisciplinary communication
Making unnecessary demands	I expect more from others than they think is reasonable. *Consequently:* I feel the others are lazy and uncommitted and I must push harder. Others see me as manipulative and dehumanizing. *Consequently:* Others assume a low profile and do not contribute their ideas. *Consequently:* Work production is mediocre. Morale is low. Everyone, including me, feels disempowered.	Attitude: • Shared mental team model—accept team model and shared decision making • Willingness to listen • Acknowledge shared accountability—relinquish some autonomy Use skills: • Interdisciplinary communication strategies • Role clarity—I need to clearly define my expectations and capabilities; I need to set clear work goals and deadlines. • Develop situational awareness—crosscheck and offer assistance when needed. • Validation—I need to give feedback.
Using communication styles unfamiliar to other disciplines	*Consequently:* communication is unclear to others	Attitude: • Willingness to reflect on personal communication style • Willingness to participate in conflict resolution Use skills: • Adapt own style to the needs of others on the health care team. • Use standardized communication tools especially during emergent situations.

EXERCISE 23-5	Barriers to Interprofessional Communication

Purpose: To help students understand the basic concepts of client advocacy, communication barriers, and peer negotiation in simulated nursing situations.

Procedure

1. The following situation is an example of situations in which interprofessional communication barriers exist. Refamiliarize yourself with the concepts of professionalism, client advocacy, communication barriers, and peer negotiation.
2. Formulate a response.
3. Compare your responses with those of your classmates, and discuss the implications of common and disparate answers. Sometimes dissimilar answers provide another important dimension of a problem situation.

Situation

Dr. Tanlow interrupts Ms. Serf, RN, as she is preparing pain medication for 68-year-old Mrs. Gould. It is already 15 minutes late. Dr. Tanlow says he needs Ms. Serf immediately in Room 20C to assist with a drainage and dressing change. Knowing that Mrs. Gould, a diabetic, will respond to prolonged pain with vomiting, Ms. Serf replies that she will be available to help Dr. Tanlow in 10 minutes (during which time she will have administered Mrs. Gould's pain medication). Dr. Tanlow, already on his way to Room 20C, whirls around, stating loudly, "When I say I need assistance, I mean now. I am a busy man, in case you hadn't noticed."

If you were Ms. Serf, what would be an appropriate response?

Discussion

This situation could be discussed in class, assigned as a paper, or used as an essay exam.

USE CONFLICT-RESOLUTION STRATEGIES

Self-reflection. Self-awareness is beneficial in assessing the meaning of a professional conflict. The strategies for handling angry clients, as described in Chapter 13, can be applied when disrespect or anger is directed toward you from colleagues. First take a moment to reflect on your own behaviors. Have you inadvertently triggered inappropriate behavior in others? Take responsibility for how you communicate both verbally and nonverbally. Understand your own role. Do you value the role of other team members? Do you treat each of them in a courteous manner? Try Exercise 23-5 to practice new skills.

Take stress-reduction measures. Because we know that you are at higher risk for conflict if you are highly stressed, take whatever steps are needed to reduce personal stress.

Commit to a collaborative resolution process. Just as the agency should have a code of conduct defining respectful behavior, there should also be an established process for direct resolution of conflict issues, with support and even "coaches" who help staff resolve conflicts constructively (Box 23-3).

Process for responding to put-downs. In addition, you need to develop a strategy to respond to unwarranted put-downs and destructive criticisms. Generally, the person delivering them has but one intent: to decrease your status and enhance the status of the person delivering the put-down. The put-down or criticism may be handed out because the speaker is feeling inadequate or threatened. Often it has little to do with the actual behavior of the nurse to whom it is delivered. Other times the criticism may be valid, but the time and place of delivery are grossly inappropriate (e.g., in the middle of the nurses' station or in the client's presence). In either case, the automatic response of many nurses is to become defensive and embarrassed, and in some way actually begin to feel inadequate, thus allowing the speaker to project unwarranted feelings onto the nurse.

Recognizing a put-down or unwarranted criticism is the first step toward dealing effectively with it. If a comment from a coworker or authority figure generates defensiveness or embarrassment, it is likely that the comment represents more than just factual information about performance. If the comment made by the speaker contains legitimate information to help improve one's skill and is delivered in a private and constructive manner, it represents a learning response and cannot be considered a put-down. Learning to differentiate between the two types of communication helps the nurse to "separate the wheat from the chaff." Consider the following case example of this Student Nurse.

BOX 23-3	Steps to Promote Conflict Resolution among Health Care Team Members

1. Set the stage for collaborative communication.
   - Self-reflection: Assume responsibility for own behavior.
   - Privacy: Meet in an appropriate venue, bringing together all involved groups.
   - Acknowledge the conflict problem using clear communication.
   - Allow sufficient time for discussion and resolution process.
2. Attitude: Maintain a respectful, nonpunitive atmosphere.
   - Solicit the perspectives of each.
   - Define the problem issue and objectives clearly.
   - Stay focused while respecting the values and dignity of all parties.
   - Group members can be assertive but not manipulative.
   - Remember to criticize ideas, not people.
3. Be proactive: Initiate early discussion:
   - Use communication skills.
   - Identify the conflict's key points.
   - Have an objective or a goal clearly in mind.
   - Seek mutual solutions.
   - Have group members propose a solution: Identify the merits and drawbacks of each solution.
   - Be open to alternative solutions in which all parties can meet essential needs.
   - Depersonalize conflict situations.
4. Decide to implement the best solution.
   - Specify persons responsible for implementation (role clarity).
   - Establish timeline.
   - Decide on the evaluation method.
   - Emphasize common goal is our shared value of quality client care.
   - Emphasize shared responsibility for team success.

Case Example: Student Nurse

You examine a crying child's inner ears and note that the tympanic membranes (eardrums) are red. You report to your supervisor that the child may have an ear infection.

A. *Response:* When a child is crying, the drums often swell and redden. How about checking again when the child is calm? *(Learning response)*

Or

B. *Response:* Of course they are red when the child is crying. Didn't you learn that in nursing school? I haven't got time to answer such basic questions! *(Put-down response)*

Which response would you prefer to receive? Why?

Whereas the first response allows the nurse to learn useful information to incorporate into practice, the second response serves to antagonize, and it is doubtful much learning takes place. What will happen is that the nurse will be more hesitant about approaching the supervisor again for clinical information. Again, it is the client who ultimately suffers.

Once a put-down is recognized as such, you need to respond verbally in an assertive manner as soon as possible after the incident has taken place. Waiting an appreciable length of time is likely to cause resentment and loss of self-respect. It may be more difficult later for the other person to remember the details of the incident. At the same time, if your anger, not the problem behavior, is likely to dominate the response, it is better to wait a few minutes for the anger to cool a little and then to present the message in a reasoned manner. You can respond to put-downs in the following way:

- *Address the objectionable or disrespectful behaviors first.* Briefly state the behavior and its impact on you. *Emphasize the specifics of the put-down behavior.* Once the put-down has been dealt with, you can discuss any criticism of your behavior on its own merits. Refer only to the behaviors identified.
- *Prepare a few standard responses.* Because put-downs often catch one by surprise, it is useful to have a standard set of opening replies ready. Examples might include the following:
  - "I found your comments very disturbing and insulting."
  - "I feel what you said as an attack. That wasn't called for by my actions."

CRITICIZE CONSTRUCTIVELY

Giving constructive criticism and receiving criticism is difficult for most people. Refer to Box 23-4. When a supervisor gives constructive criticism, some type of response from the person receiving it is indicated. Initially, it is crucial that the conflict problem be clearly defined and acknowledged. To help handle constructive criticism, nurses can do the following:

- Schedule a time when you are calm.
- Request that supervisory meetings be in a place that allows privacy.
- Defuse personal anxiety.
- Listen carefully to the criticism and then paraphrase it.

| BOX 23-4 | Constructive Criticism |

Steps in Giving

1. Express sympathy. *Sample statement:* "I understand that things are difficult at home."
2. Describe the behavior. *Sample statement:* "But I see that you have been late coming to work three times during this pay period."
3. State expectations. *Sample statement:* "It is necessary for you to be here on time from now on."
4. List consequences. *Sample statement:* "If you get here on time, we'll all start off the shift better. If you are late again, I will have to report you to the personnel department."

Steps in Receiving

1. Listen and paraphrase. If unclear, ask for specific examples. *Sample reply:* "You are saying being late is not acceptable."
2. Acknowledge you are taking suggestions seriously. *Sample comment:* "I hear what you are saying."
3. Give your side by stating supportive facts, without being defensive. *Sample comment:* "My car would not start."
4. Develop a plan for the future. *Sample plan:* "With this paycheck I will repair my car. Until then I'll ask Mary for a ride."

- Acknowledge that you take suggestions for improvement seriously.
- Discuss the facts of the situation but avoid becoming defensive.
- Develop a plan for dealing with similar situations; become proactive rather than reactive.
- Maintain open dialogue.

As students, you will encounter situations in which the behavior of a colleague causes a variety of unexpressed differences or disagreement because the colleague's interpretation of a situation or meaning of behavior is so different from yours. The conflict behaviors can occur as a result of age differences, differences in values, philosophical approaches to life, ways of handling problems, lifestyles, definitions of a problem, goals, or strategies to resolve a problem. These differences cause friction and turn relationships from collaborative to competitive. Resolve to communicate in a respectful but open, honest and positive manner.

DOCUMENT AND REPORT DISRUPTIVE BEHAVIORS

A crucial aspect of sustaining quality care is the ability to confront a team member whose behaviors violate accepted norms. Studies show that reporting a colleague to an authority figure without talking the objectionable behavior over with him or her is not effective in restoring harmony. Yet surveys show that the vast majority of physicians and nurses are reluctant to either confront or report. Amer (2013) and other experts say that nurses should hold other nurses and team members accountable for behavior that follows the standards and policy of the agency. If your attempts to directly discuss behavior with the involved person fail to achieve behavior change, then you need to follow the agency's process and report the problem. In handling disruptive behavior occurrences, documentation is a key step. Hopefully the agency has a no-blame process, but remember when pushed, many people will retaliate. Be aware!

Some agencies may hold "communication training sessions" after the offenses have been documented.

DEVELOP A SUPPORT SYSTEM

Collegial relationships are an important determinant of success as professional men and women entering nursing practice. Although there is no substitute for outcomes that demonstrate professional competence, interpersonal strategies can facilitate the process. Integrity, respect for others, dependability, a good sense of humor, and an openness to sharing with others are communication qualities people look for in developing a support system.

Form a reliable support system at work. Mutual support networks that share information, ideas, and strategies with colleagues add a collective strength to personal efforts and minimize the possibility of misunderstanding. With problem or conflict situations, getting ideas from trusted colleagues beforehand enhances the probability of accomplishing outcomes more effectively. Support lowers job-related stress and increases job satisfaction. Professional organizations do not usually have the primary purpose of providing emotional support; however, small subgroups within professional organizations may be used for personal support. A professional support group composed of individuals with similar work experience can be comforting. Often, family and friends have a limited understanding of the emotional impact of your experiences.

POSITIVE REINFORCEMENT

Everyone likes to be recognized for their efforts. Simple steps such as saying "thank you" or texting a "job well done" message to colleagues is appreciated. In organizations that have integrated team training and safety initiatives, participation in team activities is integrated into job evaluations. Positive evaluations are tied to bonuses. Other organizations hold formal and informal affairs to recognize efforts to improve communication and client safety. Individuals or units that identify problems and develop interventions are nominated for recognition at annual "Safety Fairs."

ORGANIZATIONAL STRATEGIES FOR CONFLICT PREVENTION AND RESOLUTION: WORK TOWARD AN ORGANIZATIONAL CLIMATE OF MUTUAL RESPECT

Some organizational strategies that affect safe care are discussed in Chapter 4. Other strategies within the organization could include understanding the organizational system. The corporate climate needs to be one that conveys respect for all workers.

SEEK OPPORTUNITIES FOR INTERDISCIPLINARY COMMUNICATION

Creating opportunities for interdisciplinary groups to get together is a highly effective strategy for enhancing collaboration and communication. Ideas include collaborative rounds, huddles, team briefings and debriefings, and committees to discuss problems. Some studies associate daily team rounds and joint decision making with shorter hospital stay and lower hospital charges.

UNDERSTAND THE ORGANIZATIONAL SYSTEM

Whenever you work in an organization, you automatically become a part of a system that has norms for acceptable behavior. Each organizational system defines its own chain of command and rules about social processes in professional communication. Even though your idea may be excellent, failure to understand the chain of command or an unwillingness to form the positive alliances needed to accomplish your objective dilutes the impact. For example, if your instructor has been defined as your first line of contact, then it is not in your best interest to seek out staff personnel or other students without also checking with the instructor.

Although sidestepping the identified chain of command and going to a higher or more tangential resource in the hierarchy may appear less threatening initially, the benefits of such action may not resolve the difficulty. Furthermore, the trust needed for serious discussion becomes limited. Some of the reasons for avoiding positive interactions stem from an internal circular process of faulty thinking. Because communication is viewed as part of a process, the sender and receiver act on the information received, which may or may not represent the reality of the situation.

SEEK TO ESTABLISH CLEAR POLICIES

As mentioned earlier, TJC is requiring all health care organizations to have written codes of behavior and to establish internal processes to handle disruptive behaviors.

Ongoing continuing education prevention strategies might include participation in assertiveness training in-services or the TeamSTEPPS program. Educational interventions that increase staff awareness are extremely effective, as are simulations similar to the exercises in this book. It is not enough to offer an educational intervention once. Team training is necessary. Literature recommends periodic reassessment of need and offering reviews of communication skills and conflict management strategies.

DEBRIEFING

Following resolution of a conflict situation, administrators or nurse managers should implement a debriefing. The intent is to help develop insight, understanding, and make changes to hopefully prevent a similar incident.

SUMMARY

In this chapter the same principles of communication used in the nurse-client relationship are broadened to examine the nature of communication among health professionals on the health care team. Most nurses will experience conflicts with coworkers at some time during their careers. The same elements of thoughtful purpose, authenticity, empathy, active listening, and respect for the dignity of others that underscore successful nurse-client relationships are needed in relations with other health professionals. Building bridges to professional communication with colleagues involves concepts of collaboration, coordination, and networking. Modification of barriers to professional communication includes negotiation and conflict resolution. Learning is a lifelong process, not only for nursing care skills but for communication skills. These will develop as you continue to gain experience working as part of an interdisciplinary health care team.

You are working a 12-hour shift on a labor and delivery unit. Today, Mrs. Kalim is one of your assigned clients. She is fully dilated and effaced, but contractions are still 2 minutes apart after 10 hours of labor. Mrs. Kalim, her obstetrician, Dr. Mary, and you have agreed on her plan to have a fully natural delivery without medication. However, her obstetrician's partner is handling day shift today, and Dr. Mary goes home. This new obstetrician orders you to administer several medications to Mrs. Kalim to strengthen contractions and speed up delivery, because he has another patient across town to deliver. Your unit adheres to an empowering model of practice that believes in client advocacy. How will you handle this potential physician conflict? Is this a true moral dilemma?

DISCUSSION QUESTIONS

1. Reflect on a time someone tried to intimidate or bully you. How did you feel? In hindsight, what are some productive strategies for responding in this situation?

2. What strategies seem to work best when communicating with team members from outside nursing to facilitate a collaborative environment?

Developing an Evidence-Based Practice

Laschinger HK, Wong C, Regan S: Workplace incivility and new graduate nurses' mental health: the protective role of resiliency, *J Nurs Admin* 43(7-8), 415-421, 2013.

Purpose: A survey of 272 new graduate nurses in Ontario was done to examine the relationship between workplace incivility and new graduate nurses' mental health, and the protective role of personal resilience.

Results: New graduates are experiencing incivility from a variety of workplace sources, which leads to increased stress and frustration. A regression analysis demonstrated that all types of incivility were related to higher levels of mental health symptomology including anger, fear, and sadness. The authors' findings suggest that personal resilience may protect some nurses from the negative effects of incivility. They concluded that incivility from coworkers is particularly damaging.

For fun, access some of the many videos on the Internet, such as www.bing.com/videos/browse (type in "communication of hospitals").

Application to Your Clinical Practice: Incivility is a violation of workplace norms for mutual respect. As a new graduate, you need to recognize disruptive behaviors; use confrontation communication strategies as well as unit-based civility interventions. If behavior continues, be aware of and use the reporting process in your agency. Each of us as nurses should make an effort to convey positive behaviors to make our colleagues feel respected.

REFERENCES

Agency for Healthcare Research and Quality (AHRQ). (n.d.) PSNet: patient safety network.

Patient Safety Primers. Disruptive and unprofessional behavior. Accessed December 11, 2013. http://psnet.ahrq.gov/primerHome. aspx.

Agency for Healthcare Research and Quality (AHRQ). (n.d.). /

Agency for Healthcare Research and Quality: *TeamSTEPPS 2.0: Instructor Manual:Table of Contents. March, 2014*, Rockville, Md, 2014, Agency for Healthcare Research and Quality. [Module 6: Mutual Support].

Amer KS: *Quality and Safety for Transformational Nursing: Core Competencies*, Upper Saddle River, NJ, 2013, Prentice Hall.

American Association of Critical Care Nurses (AACCN): *Zero tolerance for abuse position statement* 2004. Accessed December 11, 2013. www.aacn.org/WD/Practice/Docs/Zero_Tolerance_for_ Abuse.pdf.

American Medical Association (AMA): *Opinion 9.045 Physicians with Disruptive Behavior*, 2008. Available online. Accessed August 11, 2014. www.ama-assn.org/ama/pub/physician-resources/medical-ethics/code-medical-ethics/opinion9045.pageabout-ama/our-people, 2008. or www.ama-assn.org/go/omss.

American Nurses Association (ANA): *Code of Ethics for nurses with interpretative statements*, Washington, DC, 2001, Author.

American Nurses Association (ANA): *Position Statements; Delegation*, 2005. www.nursingworld.org/MainMenuCategories/Pol icy-Advocacy/Positions-and-Resolutions/ANAPositionStatements/ Position-Statements-Alphabetically/Joint-Statement-on-Delegation-American-Nurses-Association-and-NationalCouncil-of-State-Boards.html.

American Nurses Association (ANA): *Registered professional nurses and unlicensed assistive personnel*, Washington, DC, 1994, Author.

Bing.com. Bing videos. [type in "communication in hospitals"].

Blair PL: Lateral violence in nursing, *J Emerg Nurs* 38(5):1–4, 2013.

Costello J, Clarke C, Gravely G, D'Agostino-Rose D, et al.: Working together to build a respectful workplace: Transforming OR culture, *AORN J* 93(1):1–11, 2011.

Farahani MA, Sahragard R, Carroll JK, Mohammadi E: Communication barriers to patient education in cardiac inpatient care: A qualitative study of multiple perspectives, *Int J Nurs Pract* 17:322–328, 2011.

Herlehy AM: Influencing safe perioperative practice through collaboration, *AORN J* 94(3):1–2, 2011.

Institute of Medicine (IOM): *Health Professions Education: A Bridge to Quality*, Washington DC, 2003, National Academies Press.

Johansen ML: Keeping the peace: Conflict management strategies for nurse managers, *Nurs Manag* 43(2):50–54, 2012.

Johnson SL, Rea RE: Workplace bullying: concerns for nurse leaders, *J Nurs Admin* 39(2):84–90, 2009.

The Joint Commission (TJC): Behaviors that undermine a culture of safety, *Sentinel Event Alert No. 40,* July 9, 2008. Accessed December 12, 2013. http://www.jointcommission.org/assets/1/18/SEA_40.pdf.

The Joint Commission (TJC): Preventing Violence in the health care setting, *Sentinel Event Alert No. 45,* 2010. June 3. http://www.joint commission.org/assets/1/18/sea_45.pdf.

The Joint Commission (TJC): Appendix A: Checklists to Advance effective communication, cultural competence, and patient- and family-centered care for the lesbian, gay, bisexual, and transgender (LGBT) community. In *Advancing Effective Communication, Cultural Competence, and Patient- and Family-Centered Care for the Lesbian, lesbian, gay, bisexual, and transgender (LGBT) community,* A Field Guide, 2011, p 35. http://www.jointcommission.org/assets/1/18/LGBTFieldGuide.pdf.

The Joint Commission (TJC): *Advancing Effective Communication, cultural competence, and patient- and family-centered care,* 2010. http://www.jointcommission.org/Advancing_Effective_Communication/.

Levy R: *Self-revelation through relationships,* Englewood Cliffs, NJ, 1972, Prentice Hall.

Nielsen P, Mann S: Team function in obstetrics to reduce errors and improve outcomes, *Obstet Gynecol Clin* 35(1):61–65, 2008.

O'Daniel M, Rosenstein AH: Professional communication and team collaboration. In Hughes RG, editor: *Patient safety and quality: an evidence-based handbook for nurses* Agency for Research and Quality, Rockville, MD, 2008, pp . [AHRQ Pub no 08–0043].

Olender-Russo L: Creating a culture of regard: an antidote for workplace bullying, *Creat Nurs* 15(2):75–81, 2009.

O'Reilly KB: *AMA meeting: disruptive behavior standard draws fire. amednews.com,* 2008. Available online www.ama-assn.org/amednews/2008/12/01/prse1201.htm.

QSEN Institute. (n.d.). Pre-licensure KSAS. http://qsen.org/competencies/pre-licensure-ksas/.

QSEN Institute. (n.d.). Teamwork and Collaboration QSEN Learning Module. www.qsen.org/. Accessed June 1, 13.

Robinson J, Scollan-Koliopoulos M, Kamienski M, Burke K: Generational differences and learning style preferences in nurses from a large metropolitan medical center, *J Nurses Staff Dev* 28(4):166–172, 2012.

Seago JA: Professional communication. In Hughes RG, editor: *Patient safety and quality: an evidence-based handbook for nurses,* Rockville, MD, 2008, Agency for Healthcare Research and Quality. [AHRQ Publication no. 08–0043].

Spence-Laschinger HK, Leiter M, Day A, et al.: Workplace empowerment, incivility and burnout: impact on staff nurse recruitment and retention outcomes, *J Nurs Manag* 17:302–311, 2009.

Wachs J: Workplace incivility, bullying, and mobbing, *AAOHN J* 57(2):88, 2009.

Weaver KB: The effects of horizontal violence and bullying on new nurse retention, *J Nurses Prof Dev* 29(3):138–142, 2013.

Weaver SJ, Rosen MA: Chapter 40: Team-Training in Health Care, *Brief update review* 472–479, 2013. AHRQ: Making health care safer II: an updated critical analysis of the evidence for patient safety, Evidence Reports/technology assessments, No.211, report no.13-E001-EF, Rockville, MD, 2013, Author. ahrq.gov/research/findings/evidence-basedreports/patientsftyupdate/ptsafetyIIchap40.pdf.

Woelfle CY, McCaffrey R: Nurse on nurse, *Nurs Forum* 42(3):123–131, 2007.

CHAPTER 24

Communicating for Continuity of Care

Elizabeth C. Arnold

OBJECTIVES

At the end of the chapter, the reader will be able to:

1. Explain the concept of continuity of care (COC) and its operational role in health care.
2. Describe current challenges in the health care system, related to COC.
3. Discuss applications of relational continuity in client-centered care and interdisciplinary team collaboration.
4. Apply informational continuity concepts in transitional and discharge planning processes.
5. Discuss applications of management continuity related to case management, care coordination, and navigation of the health care system.

Addressing the role of communication in continuity of care is essential to ensuring quality, safety and client satisfaction in contemporary health care systems. Chapter 24 describes the concept of continuity of care (COC) as the linchpin in collaborative health team functionality, central to its structure, and operations in contemporary health care systems. Three key features: relational, informational, and management continuity provide a conceptual framework for study and application of COC strategies (Haggerty et al., 2003).

BASIC CONCEPTS

CURRENT CHALLENGES IN HEALTH CARE DELIVERY

Health care systems organized around acute, episodic care no longer suffice as a primary service model. The complexity of contemporary health care requires a different care process to match new health realities (Mitchell et al., 2012). There are several reasons: demographics of the population with greater ethnic and racial diversity, longer life spans, serious economic challenges, health disparities associated with social determinants of health, globalization and significant skilled provider shortages, and most notably, physicians and nurses. Clients are discharged earlier and sicker, often with complex medication and treatment regimens to be followed in the community in primary care settings.

Technology advances in diagnosis and treatment, discovery of novel medications and workable treatments have eradicated the incidence of premature death from previous health conditions. People now self-manage previously untreatable cancers and other conditions as chronic health conditions with a good quality of life for longer periods of time as the rule rather than the exception. Thus attention has turned to chronic disease management, early detection and interventions to enhance lifestyle health behaviors within a shared care process.

It is estimated that worldwide, chronic diseases account for 60% of deaths (Paquette-Warren et al. 2014) nb. Effective treatment approaches for people with chronic diseases is increasingly recognized as a priority for health care delivery. Technical and scientific advances have revolutionized the prevention, diagnosis, and treatment of acute illness. As people live longer, however, there is a higher incidence of chronic conditions requiring an array of supportive health care services. For these reasons, and more, focus on care provision has shifted from the hospital to the community and a public health focus (Cooke et al., 2008; Institute of Medicine [IOM], 2003).

The 2010 passage of the Patient Protection and Affordable Care Act (PPACA) provides a new urgency for development of coordinated community based COC health initiatives. Not only does this act dramatically increase the number of individuals eligible for affordable care; it enlarges the scope of reimbursable health promotion and disease prevention activities available to people and provides new consumer protections. An unprecedented number of people will now be eligible for care. require a tighter understanding and implementation of care continuity in the community. Using an integrated service framework based in the community capable of providing a continuum of aggregated services offers the most comprehensive option for care of clients with chronic physical and mental conditions (Stan et al, 2013; Porter O'Grady, 2014).

CONTINUITY OF CARE CONCEPTS

Continuity of care **(COC)**, a term first used by Haggerty (2003) describes a multidimensional longitudinal construct in health care, which emphasizes seamless provision and coordination of client-centered quality care across clinical settings. COC operates across three dimensions: relational, informational, and management continuity. These dimensions are interdependent essential components of client care (Haggerty, 2003; Schultz, 2009).

Haggerty and colleagues (2008) define **relational continuity** as "a therapeutic relationship with a practitioner that spans more than one episode of care and leads, in the practitioner, to a sense of clinical responsibility and an accumulated knowledge of the client's personal and medical circumstances" (p. 118). Frequent team communication about all aspects of care helps ensure relational continuity among treatment teams. **Informational continuity** refers to the use of data to tailor current treatment and care to each client's evidenced needs. The concept includes accurate record sharing and technology to allow real time communication exchanges between providers

and with clients in remote sites. It is a primary communication vehicle during care transitions and is used to help clients and families make quality client care decisions. **Management continuity** refers to a consistent, coherent care management approach, which can be flexibly adjusted, as client needs change. Care coordination and case management have emerged as significant methodologies associated with management continuity.

COC links acute care with primary care approaches for clients through coordinated, acute, and community-based health services. Sparbel and Anderson (2000) explain the COC construct as "a series of connected client-care events both within a health care institution and among multiple settings" (p. 17). Continuity of care exemplifies the shift in emphasis from acute care to long-term self-management of chronic illness in the community. The COC process is concerned with the safety and quality of care as well as a seamless coordination of services. The overarching goal of COC is to ensure reliable coordinated transition of clients from one health care setting to another, such that care in each setting continues to provide a secure health safety net for individuals and families that they can rely on for support and information.

Haggerty (2003) suggests that COC contributes to the development of

- Increased accessibility to coordinated health care services with a smoother flow of care from one service area to another
- Personalization of care to meet a client's changing needs across delivery systems
- Informational data sharing of various elements of personal and medical data electronically over time and place, which contribute to appropriate care delivery
- Health services provided in an organized, logical, and timely manner, using a shared management plan.

Sparbel and Anderson (2000) explain the COC construct as "a series of connected client-care events both within a health care institution and among multiple settings" (p. 17). The processes of collaboration and coordination in COC are concerned with the safety and quality of care as well as a seamless coordination of services for clients and families. Prescribed communication in COC acts as a bonding agent to help the treatment process across multiple settings run smoothly.

COC decreases the potential for service duplication, conflicting assessments, gaps in service, and reduces the use of preventable acute care services. Improved continuity lessens medication and treatment errors, provides timely follow-up, and can ease transitions between care settings. For chronically ill and elderly clients, COC means that they are more likely to have health care providers familiar with their overall history, who can notice subtle changes in health status (von Bultzingslowen et al., 2006).

COC: TREATMENT PATHWAY OF CHOICE FOR CHRONIC CONDITIONS

COC is the treatment model of choice for chronic health conditions in primary care. The World Health Organization (WHO) (2002) defines **chronic health conditions** as "health problems that require ongoing management over a period of years or decades" (p. 11). Examples include asthma, fibromyalgia, cancer, multiple sclerosis, diabetes, serious persistent mental disorders, chronic obstructive pulmonary disease (COPD), and congestive heart failure. Chronic illness is a major cause of death and disability nationally and globally. The Agency for Healthcare Research and Quality (AHRQ, 2013) estimates that up to a third of all adults and 80% of older adults suffer from at least two comorbid chronic conditions, which negatively impact health status, functional capacity, or quality of life, and require health treatment. Chronic disorders typically have periods of exacerbations and remissions. They share a requirement for ongoing health support and self-care management (Wagner, 2001). Chronic disorders disrupt a person's personal life in multiple unexpected ways.

Kleinman (1988) explains,

> The undercurrent of chronic illness is like the volcano: it does not go away, it menaces. It erupts. It is out of control...confronting crises is only one part of the total picture. The rest is coming to grips with the mundaneness of worries...Chronic illness also means the loss of confidence in one's health and normal bodily processes. (pp. 44-45)

The COC construct is based on an expanded version of the Chronic Care Model, originally developed by Wagner and associates (2001). The model is designed to foster productive interactions between informed clients and families and prepared proactive practice teams leading to improved clinical outcomes. Application of the chronic care model within the primary health care system functions as a safety net and support through productive interactions and with the community supports needed to achieve improved clinical outcomes. Empowering individuals and families to assume primary responsibility for self-management of chronic illness in partnership with ongoing professional support is a critical means of community based care. It is a key component of care which helps bridge the gap gap between diminishing financial support for chronic care and multifaceted care demands that can last for years. Relevant primary care strategies focus on "client centered care, collaborative goal setting, problem solving, and coordinated follow up" (Glasgow and Goldstein, 2008, p. 129).

RELEVANCE OF CONTINUITY OF CARE IN PRIMARY CARE

Primary care, described as the hub of community-based care, provides a wide range of integrated health care services delivered in a single community-based setting. Medical homes in primary care are the first point of entry and serve as central resources for chronic disorders. Primary care practices offer diagnosis and treatment of common undifferentiated illness. Services also include health promotion education, preventive screenings, and health maintenance care. Community resource support, integrated decision backing, and information technology work together to strengthen client-centered relationships and improve health outcomes (Coleman et al., 2009).

Clients are considered active agents in a dynamic health care delivery process. The expectation is that most clients will be able to self-manage the care of their chronic health conditions in the community with coordinated, readily accessible health care network supports available in primary care settings. Key features of primary care include

- *Person centeredness*, with sustained continuity of relationships between provider and client
- Functions as a *first contact point* with easy access to services for common health care problems
- *Comprehensive care*, which can meet many client needs without referral
- A highly *personalized form of care* related to a stronger knowledge about individual health care needs and responses over time (IOM, 2012; Starfield and Horder, 2007).

Developing an Evidence-Based Practice

Cramm J, Nieboer A: Professional views on interprofessional stroke team functioning, *Int J Integr Care* 11(25):1-8, 2011.

Background: The purpose of this research study was to explore interdisciplinary health provider perspectives on factors that contribute to successful stroke team functioning as perceived by team members functioning in this capacity.

Methods: A purposive sample was used to elicit factors contributing to successful team functioning on two levels: individual and team. Questionnaires were completed by 558 respondents representing different professional disciplines serving on 34 different integrated stroke care teams. Data was analyzed, using a hierarchical random-effects model.

Study results: Analyses showed that personal development, social well-being, interprofessional education, communication, and role understanding significantly contributed to stroke team functioning on an individual level. Team-level constructs significantly affecting interprofessional stroke team functioning were communication and role understanding. No significant relationships were found with individual-level personal autonomy and team level cohesion. Findings suggest that developing professional interpersonal communication skills and role clarity through interprofessional education and interventions to improve team members' social well-being, communication, and role understanding will improve teams' performance.

Implications for practice: Clear role understandings and communication competencies skills are relevant skills at both individual and team levels. Question: If nurses are to fulfill key roles on interdisciplinary collaborative teams, what would be important for you to understand about your discipline role as a professional nurse on an interprofessional health care team?

APPLICATIONS

Ferrer and Gill (2013) contend "A common trap in primary care is to consider problems in isolation, failing to respect its multidimensional and longitudinal nature (p. 301) Continuity of care (COC) recognizes the importance of structured collaborative efforts in creating workable solutions for clients across clinical settings. Coping with chronic conditions is always considered within the context of the larger life patterns and availability of health related resources. COC should be intentionally designed to safeguard care stability and to provide a secure health safety net for individuals and families that they can rely on for support and information. Each dimension of COC: relational, informational, and management continuity should work together to set directions and implement coordinated interventions throughout the health care system. Guilliford and colleagues (2006) advocate viewing COC from both client and provider perspectives. This makes sense given the level of partnership needed to ensure continuity.

RELATIONAL CONTINUITY

Relational continuity refers to the interpersonal elements of the COC model across time and care settings. The term applies to nurse–client and family relationships, team relationships, and relationships between health system providers and community-based supports. The stronger the relationships, the greater are the potential for quality-coordinated care. Respect for client and family values, beliefs, knowledge, cultural background, and preferences are fundamental aspects of client-centered relational continuity. Trusting relationships with a primary provider, or "medical home" health care team gives clients confidence that their care needs will be consistently met.

The goal of relational COC is to develop sustained client-provider relationships in which informed, motivated clients interact with prepared, proactive professional health care teams to achieve identified health goals for chronic health conditions. New Joint Commission patient-centered communication standards include data on communication with physicians and nurses, responsiveness of staff, communication about medications, pain management, and discharge planning as measurable outcomes (The Joint Commission, 2013). Increasing the level of collaboration among health care professionals is identified as a primary strategy for improving the level of continuity needed for successful health care outcomes (San Martin-Rodriguez et al., 2008; van Servellen et al., 2006).

NEW ROLES IN CONTINUITY OF CARE

Health care reform has led to the development of new professional relational roles and service delivery approaches to better address the nation's health needs. Innovative roles include the hospitalist, the medical home, and collaborative interdisciplinary team-based care delivery.

Hospitalist

A new professional role designed to improve COC in acute care settings is that of the "hospitalist" (Amin and Owen, 2006). The hospitalist may be a physician or nurse practitioner employed by the hospital to clinically manage a client's medical care. The hospitalist specializes in medical care of hospitalized clients and assumes *full* responsibility for coordinating care, ordering, and integrating diagnostic test results, making decisions, presenting options to the client and family, and communicating with other professionals who may be, or will become involved in the client's care after discharge. The specific dimensions of the hospitalist role are determined by the care site rather than clinical specialty (Schneller and Epstein, 2006). Specialty physicians function as consultants.

Nurses play an important communication role with hospitalists. They function as key informants, skilled practitioners, client advocates, and supporters of coordinated care in hospital settings. Clients do not have a prior relationship with the hospitalist prior to hospitalization and vice versa. As the client's nurse, you are responsible for carrying out the hospitalist's orders. Nurses should be proactive by talking informally with hospitalists about their clients and presenting information formally in collaborative team meetings.

As a client's condition changes, the hospitalist meets with the family to discuss changes, treatment options, and family concerns. Even in the best of circumstances, client and family meetings with the hospitalist and/or health care team to discuss sensitive health issues such as discontinuing life support or transfer of clients can be intimidating. Nurses can help clients and families by continuing conversations after the hospitalist or health care team leaves, answering questions and providing support.

Medical Home

The **medical home** is a concept as well as a "place" in primary care. As a concept, it has particular relevance for increasing access to primary care in the public sector (Crabtree et al., 2010). A medical home accepts responsibility for providing regular, accessible, comprehensive primary care services for designated clients and families within a single familiar setting. It serves as a central first point of contact in primary care through which the majority of client health needs are met (Grumbach and Bodenheimer, 2002; Keeling and Lewenson, 2013).

Clients depend on their medical home as a first-line treatment resource. Physicians, nurse practitioners, physician's assistants, nurses, social workers, dentists, and other health care providers can provide better quality care because they have ongoing knowledge of the client's medical and lifestyle issues. Subtle changes in the client's situation or health status are recognized in subsequent care visits.

External coordination of health care services with specialists and community agencies expand the capabilities of the medical home. Referrals are accomplished efficiently, and information passes swiftly and accurately between providers. There is less chance of duplicative or unnecessary medical appointments because care is coordinated through the client's medical home. Of course a critical element is that recipients of client data have to carefully read the reports. Quality and safety are essential characteristics of primary care medical homes (see Chapter 4 for general principles associated with safety).

Team-Based Care

A third role change is a move away from single provider care delivery to service delivery through collaborative care teams. Katzenbach and Smith (1999) define **collaborative teams** as "a small number of people with complementary skills who are committed to a common purpose, performance goals, and approach for which they are mutually accountable" (p. 45).

Relational continuity on collaborative health teams describes an active, ongoing alliance between health care professionals from different disciplines who work together in complementary, synergistic roles to provide health care services. Each team member brings skills to address different aspects of a client's illness experience as an integrated unit. Some functions overlap; others are complementary; all are coordinated by the treatment team. Team meetings allow skilled professionals to develop mutual understandings developed about common problems as a foundation for generating stronger innovative solutions. Professional health care team collaboration is an important contributor to total quality management, and is identified as a nursing QSEN competency (see Chapter 2).

Team composition, purpose, and activities to ensure COC take many forms and are linked with targeted client-centered needs. Examples include disaster response teams, acute care hospital teams, medical home–based and home care teams, mental health emergency teams, and palliative care teams (Mitchell et al., 2012). Collaborative health care teams are broadly classified as multidisciplinary, interdisciplinary, and transdisciplinary teams with the expectation that care will be provided through the combined collaborative efforts of two or more skilled clinical practitioners.

Team communication takes place informally and in structured formal team meetings. Interdisciplinary team relationships should take into account diverse standards and behaviors associated with each clinical discipline, while emphasizing a common mission of working together to resolve complex clinical problems (Clark et al., 2007; D'Amour and Oandasan, 2005). Acknowledgment of separate and combined spheres of responsibility is essential to smoother working relationships. Members need to value and respect diversity in the personal, cultural, experiential backgrounds, and organizational responsibilities of team members, all of which affect communication and priorities.

In formal meetings team members should take responsibility for effective group communication focused on moving health goals forward. Setting a direction, prioritizing care activities, and establishing realistic boundaries are as important as content

contributions. Members monitor potential relationship safety issues such as status differences and receptiveness to taking interpersonal risks when others disagree. When interdisciplinary health care teams deal with relational group process issues successfully, members experience higher levels of learning and satisfaction with team care outcomes.

ESSENTIAL ELEMENTS OF RELATIONAL CONTINUITY

Development of therapeutic relationships with known providers offers a consistent fundamental communication channel clients can use to secure better health care services, tailored to their specific health needs. The interpersonal process relations required for continuity of care involve the three C's: client centeredness, collaboration, and coordination in a shared enterprise of therapeutic care delivery across multiple systems (Stans et al, 2013) .

CLIENT CENTERED CARE

Figure 24-1 presents components of client-centered care. Clients should be key informants, active negotiators, final decision makers, and engaged participants in evaluating treatment outcomes (Engebretson et al., 2008). They need to be actively involved in defining and updating realistic .treatment goals. Client centeredness is evidenced in a partnership characterized

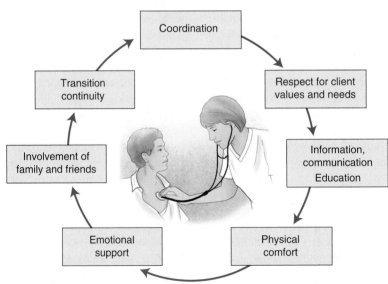

Figure 24-1   Dimensions of client-centered care in continuity of care (COC).

by mutual valuing and safeguarding of the legitimate interests of the provider and the client in creating and managing health care decisions.

Joint decision-making is a key element. The decision-making process starts with providing each client with sufficient information tailored to his or her unique circumstances to make an *informed* decision. Equally important, the information must be easily understandable to the client. Information should be relevant to each client's diagnosis, treatments, and treatment options. The first question to consider is: "What essential information does this client need to have in order to make an informed decision?" Some clients value knowing as much as possible; others want just the basic facts. Another may need to have essential information developed in steps and spread over several encounters to allow for better processing and formulation of related questions. Cultural norms can dictate levels of information and to whom the information should be given (see Chapter 7).

A second query is what level of information does the client *desire at this point in time*? For example, a client with newly diagnosed terminal ovarian cancer focuses on a long trip she wants to take in the future and suggests several times that she is going to make it

and not die from her cancer. Empathetic acceptance of the client as she is in processing her diagnosis is more helpful than presenting her with "facts" that she is not willing to accept in the current moment.

To ensure that care decisions respect client values, needs, and preferences, you need to observe and listen carefully to the client description of the health experience. This data becomes the basis for providing clients and families with the tailored education and support they need to make reasoned health care decisions. Relevant information includes:

- Detailed information on diagnosis
- Options for treatment and what to expect
- Risks and benefits of each treatment approach
- Anticipated clinical outcomes
- Treatment and care processes required to achieve desired clinical outcomes

Consistency of personnel over time allows clients and the professional team to share a stronger investment in achieving personalized quality health outcomes. Providers and clients learn to know, value, and respect each other. Box 24-1 identifies essential competencies for effective collaborative communication in team meetings.

| **BOX 24-1** | **Essential Competencies for Effective Collaboration in Team Meetings** |

- Self-awareness of professional strengths and limitations, values, assumptions, biases, and expectations of self and others.
- Appreciate and accommodate for individual and professional diversity among team members, including gender-related communication style, different professional cultures, and differential professional perspectives.
- Develop professional tact and constructive conflict resolution skills to cope with contested professional barriers in delivery of collaborative care.
- Develop a synthesis of perspectives through negotiation and work toward a creative integration of ideas acceptable to all interdisciplinary team members.
- Deliberately develop a sense of shared power to create win-win situations. Invite less verbal participants to express their opinion. Emphasize mutual exchange of ideas as the best way to develop shared power.
- Cultivate clinical competence, self-confidence, and assertiveness as professional attributes underlying your professional contributions. Seize all opportunities to present expertise as a way of building trust.

- Demonstrate knowledge of multiple interconnections associated with systems thinking and group dynamics. Develop the ability to view each clinical situation, and collaborative processes within the larger organization, and health care system.
- Be prepared, and present (physically and mentally) throughout structured team meetings. Become aware of conflicting agendas, and the diverse values of team members, so you can advocate effectively for clients.
- Become knowledgeable about timing and group development through group processes (see Chapter 7).
- Legitimize and incorporate opportunities for spontaneous collaborative conversations into more formal discussions.
- Respect the balance between autonomy and unity present in collaborative discussions.
- Remember that there is no "perfect" solution and that the client is usually the final decision maker.
- Differentiate between problems requiring simple decisions and complex challenging clinical situations, requiring a collaborative, integrative solution. Collaboration is not required for all decisions.

Adapted from Gardner D: Ten lessons in collaboration, *Online J Issues Nurs* 10(1):2, 2005.

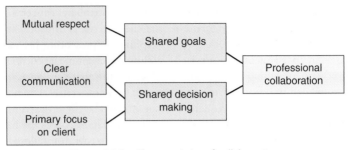

Figure 24-2   Characteristics of collaboration.

COLLABORATION

The second C is collaboration. A goal of interprofessional relational collaboration is to produce "a synthesis of the information such that the outcomes are more than additive" (Muir, 2008, p. 5). Clients need an integrated consistent flow of informed communication among providers and community agencies about their treatment and care.

Interdisciplinary collaboration enables practitioners to learn new skills and approaches and encourages synergistic creativity among professionals (Sievers, 2006). As different disciplines work closely together, they build new understandings about each other's expertise and trust in each other to develop consensus about the best approaches to each client's unique health care situation. Each discipline member is cognizant of unique and shared spheres of responsibility with team members from other disciplines. Structured team collaboration decreases fragmentation and duplication of effort and promotes safe quality care (See Chapter 4). Figure 24-2 presents desired characteristics of relational interprofessional collaboration.

The level of collaborative team communication between clients and providers and between providers affects treatment outcomes and client satisfaction. Receiving care within an ongoing therapeutic relationship with the same group of providers over time, with care that follows the client across primary and secondary care setting enhances the client's confidence. Mitchell and colleagues (2012) identifies five principles of collaborative team effectiveness: "shared goals, clear roles, mutual trust, effective communication, and measurable processes and outcomes" (p. 6). Setting forward measurable process and outcome benchmarks from the outset of care planning helps all involved participants keep an eye on the goal with formative evaluations along the way to correct for error.

COORDINATION

The third C of relational COC is coordination. Effective coordination depends on the development of dynamic relationships among involved professionals. Relationships are as important to success as content. Shared goals and basic knowledge regarding each provider's work such that each provider knows how that work fits together as a whole is key to understanding coordination and its role in facilitating positive clinical outcomes. Havens et al, (2010) suggests that relational understanding is particularly important as "participants from different disciplines often reside in different 'thought worlds' because of differences in training, socialization and expertise (p. 928). The other knowledge requirement for active coordination relates to client factors—preferences, financial resources, access to care, support systems, etc, as any of these can result in an unintended misalliance. Developing shared goals allows for effective coordination for treatment of chronic conditions.

Shared Goals

Shared goals are an essential product of effective team collaboration and coordination. The client and family should be critical team members in determining, refining, and updating goals. Their inclusion as a collaborative team member allows for a more realistic assessment of a client's needs, preferences, resources, and personal goals. They can provide important input into how things are going and can sensitize providers to realistic needs and priorities.

Clients and families are unique members of the care team. Usually they lack formal training in health care and may not always understand the medical language used in team meetings. While the same team members interact with each other on a regular basis informally in the care of clients, this is not true of client members. Nurses are an essential resource in helping to orient and introduce client team members to the roles and expectations of collaborative teamwork and to adapt medical language so that it is easily understood (Mitchell et al., 2012).

Discussion at team meetings should focus on shared goals developed by the client and professional team members. Carefully defining the client's health problem and identifying possible contributing factors is an essential first step before moving on to brainstorming potential solutions. Unrelated data, or an initial focus on past, rather than on current information is discouraged because this can compromise the concentration of the team on key client and family needs and solutions. Problem-solving communication should be respectful, accurate, timely, and frequent. Aim for developing share meanings, rather than simple information exchanges. Mutual trust and respect for differences offer powerful reinforcement for open dialogue. Once agreement is reached, the entire team, including the client needs to take full responsibility for implementing it.

Clear Roles

Role clarity is an essential prerequisite for successful collaboration on interdisciplinary health care and community-based family care teams. Effective relational participation requires a clear understanding of one's own discipline's values and expected level of skill and scope of practice, *plus* a knowledge of and mutual respect for other team member discipline's roles, professional responsibilities, and expertise (Lidskog et al., 2007).

Team members function both as an individual professional representing a distinct discipline *and* as a collaborative health care team member. Mosser and Begun (2014) note, "the roles, education and values of different health professions give each profession a distinctive character on teams" (p. 55). Each discipline has its own set of behavioral norms and professional ethics. While they may be similar, they are neither identical in scope nor in implementation of care. Studies of provider perspectives on effective team functioning identify role understanding, and interpersonal communication as being the most important variables affecting role functioning on interdisciplinary teams (Cramm and Nieboer, 2011).

Even when core personal and professional values, attitudes, and practices are not at odds with each other, professional training and interpretations of standards can shape how professional values are prioritized (D'Amour and Oandasan, 2005; Hall, 2005). Team role confusion, fueled by professional rivalries, territoriality, and lack of clarification about job responsibilities, is identified as a potential barrier to effective team communication (Sparbel and Anderson, 2000). Exercise 24-1, Learning about Other Health Professions, offers an opportunity to understand roles of different health professions.

Mutual Trust

In time health professionals from different disciplines learn to trust and rely on each other's competence and it becomes easier to support each other's efforts (Guilliford et al., 2006). This is unlikely to

---

EXERCISE 24-1	Learning about Other Health Professions

Purpose: To familiarize students to differences and similarities in education and skill sets of key interdisciplinary health team members.

Procedure
1. Break the class into teams of four to six students. Assign each student group a professional role to explore by describing the educational preparation and expected skill set of one of the following professional disciplines: physician, pharmacist, social worker, nurse practitioner.
2. (Initial research can be done as an out of class assignment.) Write a concise description about your assigned discipline, which can be easily explained to your team members.

3. Identify and agree upon 10 to 12 key descriptors related to your findings and the dominant features of the profession within your team group.
4. Each discipline team group should present its findings to the larger class group.

Discussion
1. Compare and contrast similarities and differences in education and expected skill sets identified by each team.
2. In what ways might the skill sets of each discipline complement each other in client-centered clinical care and decision making?
3. How could you use what you learned in this exercise to create better communication with other health care professionals?

happen without regularly scheduled interdisciplinary team meetings. Unless there is a formal time and place for collaborative dialogue, the necessary professional connectivity for interdisciplinary collaboration will not take place in a meaningful way. Team meetings allow different disciplinary professionals to get to know each other. They also provide a forum for discussion of potential conflicts. Clients can sense when their care team is having conflicts. This tends to make the team's comments less credible, leading to potential confusion and adverse outcomes. Consistent consultations offer a scheduled opportunity to develop team-working processes, discuss potential conflicts, and reinforce commitment to delivering quality collaborative health care.

Effective Communication

Team communication skills are similar to those you would employ in any professional group interaction. Start with introducing yourself to other members of the team. Identify your professional role on the team and issues/plans with respect to the target client situation. Seek specific feedback from other team members (Zwarenstein, et. al., 2007).

Interdisciplinary team meeting communication differs from other forms of work group communication, although similar group development processes occur (see Chapter 8). The focus of team group meetings is always on the immediate care issues of the client. Each team member, including the client, is personally accountable for sharing relevant client information, listening to the comments of others, and actively participating in focused problem solving and decision discussions. In team group meetings, it is important to respect the diversity, professional values, and ideas of each team member even when you do not agree with them. It is important to respect and consider the input of other team members who may approach the same situation from a very different perspective.

Here are some simple tips you can use in team meetings to enhance communication in team and task groups:

- *Listen before you speak.* Attentive listening is one of the strongest collaborative communication skills. When you take a measured listening stance, you show respect for the speaker. As you hear the other person's words, visually attend to the attitudes and nonverbal behaviors of the speaker and other team members. These are important information-transmitting factors, which can influence understanding, so that you can respond appropriately.

- *Know what you are talking about.* When you share clinical observations and professional opinions in team meetings, be as informed, authentic, specific, and descriptive as possible. Honest feedback and genuine sharing builds trust and strengthens professional relationships, even when ideas are being challenged. Evidence-based data provides an underpinning for interdisciplinary discussions. Nurses can communicate a critical appraisal of a client's presenting issues, health needs, preferences, values, and personal responses. This is your forte. Nurses spend the most time with clients and have the most "talking and observing" sustained contact with them.

- *Use your voice wisely.* Nurses' active participation in formal team meetings is essential. You do not have to comment on everything, but your input is unique and critical to the discussion. Information about the client as a person and human responses to illness and treatment represents data nurses are best positioned to share.

- *Be open to different ideas.* A strong advantage of team communication is that it allows more than one viewpoint to bear on a health situation. Exploration of different ideas and perspectives enriches the problem-solving approaches needed to develop a coordinated consistent and workable approach to difficult client issues. Have knowledge of the differences in role responsibilities and common values of other disciplines so you can better frame messages and can understand their perspective. Recognize your limitations as well as your strengths and how you might be able to incorporate the expertise of other disciplines in total client care.

- *Ask for feedback.* Encourage other team members with whom you interact to provide relevant feedback, for example, "I'd like to hear what you think about this." Analyze the information you receive and ask relevant open-ended questions. Brainstorming and problem solving processes are indispensable to developing the most workable solutions. Interdisciplinary team decisions should be negotiated, not dictated, with all members being mindful of working though their individual differences in a respectful manner. Consensus solutions work best and are more easily implemented.

- *Work within the system.* Whereas clients are the core focus of care, health care centers are part of much larger health care management systems, which influence team functions and outcomes (Ginter et al., 2013). System factors beyond the control of the client and the direct care team will influence what is and is not possible in a given health care situation. Valuable time is saved when team members are knowledgeable about the constraints and opportunities available within their delivery system.

CONTENT VERSUS COMMUNICATION PROCESSES IN TEAM MEETINGS

Content and process are interwoven in effective team meetings. Content should be focused, with each team member as fully prepared as possible. This means that you need to understand what you do know and what you do not know about the client's situation. Scheduled team meetings should have clear agendas, with the time to be spent on each item identified. Structure keeps people on track. The agenda can be brief. Additional critical items can be added at the beginning of the meeting, if needed. Minutes taken at each meeting should highlight decisions made, identify action items to be completed, and specify individual team member responsibilities for tasks when indicated. Rotation of leadership and scribe roles help team members share the workload and build a sense of collaborative team responsibility. Clarifying roles and expectations and identifying the scope of functional activities helps direct attention to what is important and meaningful; it also helps save time.

Sharing ideas with professional tact is an art. Skills can be learned. If someone makes a point that is particularly relevant, acknowledge its merit. If members have reservations about an idea, they should be encouraged to speak up. Presenting a concern, or an alternative with a rationale is different from judging the rightness or wrongness of another team member's ideas and it is easier to hear. Explain your rationale in neutral terms about the issue, not about the person. Learning to deal with conflict is as essential to team building as it is to individual professional collaborative conversations (see Chapter 23).

Smoothly run collaborative care meetings are those in which each team member understands and agrees to support the team mission of quality coordination of care. Time is a precious commodity for busy health care providers; team meetings should begin and end on time. An agenda keeps all team members focused on the business at hand. Exercise 24-2 provides an opportunity for students to understand collaboration skills in team decision making.

INFORMATIONAL CONTINUITY

Informational continuity refers to data exchanges among providers and provider systems and between providers and clients for the purpose of providing continuously coordinated quality care. Instant electronic transmission of data "links provider to provider, and health care event to health care event" (Pontin and Lewis, 2008, p. 1199). Ideally there is an uninterrupted flow of data and clinical impressions between health

EXERCISE 24-2	Collaborative Decision Making

Purpose: To help students discover how they can work together to achieve consensus about an uncertain situation.

Procedure
Break up the class into groups of three to four students. Identify one student for each group to act as scribe.
1. Each group member should present a real-time clinical scenario related to a client with complex medical needs in one or two paragraphs.
2. Each student should present his or her scenario for group consideration. Other group members can ask questions.
3. The group must select one of the scenarios and provide a rationale for its choice.

Discussion
How did each group reach their decision?
What was it like to know you had to make a team decision about an issue for which there is no perfect answer?
What factors made collaborative discussion and decision making easier or harder?
What did you learn from doing this exercise about how people function as a team in making a difficult decision within a short time frame?

care providers and agencies, with clients and their families, over time and space. Specific information follows the client from primary to secondary care settings, and vice versa. The same client information is available to providers throughout the health care system (Agarwal and Crooks, 2008). Data about possible medication interactions, start and stop dates, and personal responses to specific medications is easily accessible.

Informational continuity is critical to providing safe, quality care. Gaps can occur as a result of misplaced clinical records, inadequate discharge planning or referral data, deficient or delayed authorization for treatment, and a lack of understanding by the client about their illness, treatment, or self-management. Lack of information at time of transfer can result in treatment delays, which increases client and family's anxiety unnecessarily. Information continuity provides a safety net for clients who often become overwhelmed with the number of procedures, appointments, and providers involved with their care. The capacity to communicate directly with various providers, and treatment centers—and feeling comfortable that everyone involved in their care has the same information is one less thing clients and providers have to worry about.

Immediate forms of informational continuity within hospital units include interdisciplinary team meetings, huddles, comfort rounds, and progress notes. Handovers, discharge plans, referral contacts, and client summaries are used for client transfers from one care setting to another.

In the community, informational continuity can empower clients through appointment reminders and call-back checks, careful instruction about diagnosis and care options, and accurate electronic health records (EHRs) shared with clients and providers. The goal for informational continuity is to help ensure that everyone involved in the care of a client is on the same page. Sharing health and treatment information with clients and families should be consistent, complete, accurate, value neutral, and delivered in an easily understandable and supportive manner. Knowing what to expect, with contingency plans in place increases client security (Haggerty et al., 2013). Notifying the family of changes in the client's condition or treatment recommendations is an essential part of ensuring informational continuity, particularly if the family is not in close contact with the client. Informational COC facilitates effective and efficient transition of care from one clinical setting to another. Receiving consistent information from different providers bolsters client confidence and is more likely to be believed.

TRANSITION AND DISCHARGE PLANNING IN CONTINUITY OF CARE

Rhudy et al (2010) identify improving the quality of client transitions across health care settings as a national priority. Clients with complex chronic conditions typically experience multiple care transitions in their health experience. Unfortunately, changeovers between care settings are associated with a larger number of "avoidable adverse events" and "near misses" (Mitchell et al., 2012). Accurate recording of information and sharing it between the giving and receiving institutions is part of information continuity, but there is a relational aspect too.

In addition to time constraints imposed by insurance regulations, a transfer from one care setting to another often is precipitated by a change in health, functional status, or change in the complexity client needs rather than client choice. Care transition, whether from the hospital to home, or to a rehabilitation center, assisted living, or skilled care setting, or from a community setting to a hospital is an emotional as well as a physical event for clients and families. It is a vulnerable time. Clients and families caring for them are anxious because they do not know what to expect. Carr (2008) notes, "care transitions shouldn't be an abrupt end of care previously provided, but rather considered to be a coordinated changeover for the client to a new team of involved caregivers" (p. 26).

NURSING ROLE IN TRANSITIONAL CARE

The Case Management Society of America (CMSA, 2008) makes a distinction between transitional care and care transitions. Transition of care refers to managing movement of clients between different levels of care, and between health care locations or providers as client care needs change. American Geriatrics Society (2007) defines *transitional care* as "a set of actions designed to ensure the coordination and continuity of health care as patients transfer between different locations or different levels of care within the same location" (p. 30). Transitional care begins in the hospital and represents an expansion of the nurse's traditional role in hospital care. Successful transitions consider the combined needs of the client and family, which are paired with the resources of an agency or health

TABLE 24-1	Key Elements in Planning for Care Transitions
SUMMARY OF CARE ELEMENTS	
Activity	**Components**
Needs assessment	Medical and functional status, cognitive, emotional and behavioral support needs, nature, and level of support system
Choose best next care setting	Nursing home
	Inpatient rehabilitation
	Assisted living
	Home, with home health care aide
	Home, with family or alone
Arrange services	Identify suitable agency(ies) and verify financial or insurance coverage
Clinical summary	Course (diagnosis and treatment)
	Key data (laboratory, radiographs, other)
	Care plan's main elements (how to care for the client)
Medication reconciliation	Current medication list
	What was stopped and why
	What was started and why
Follow-up medical care	Appointments (names, times, dates, phone numbers)

Adapted from Boling P: Care transitions and home health care, *Clin Geriatri Med* 25:135-148, 2009.

care provider to realistically identify and meet identified care needs (Naylor, 2012). Table 24-1 identifies key elements in effective transitional care.

Acute care hospitals are intended for short-term stays. When clients require skilled medical and nursing care beyond a designated time period, they may be transferred to a long-term care hospital. Clients and families need to know what parameters will be used for discharge as soon as this is known (The Joint Commission, 2013). Usually, the hospital has a care coordinator, but nurses are often involved in arranging for this person to see the client and for working with follow-up concerns. It is not unusual for a family to think their family member is being arbitrarily moved to a long-term acute care hospital or nursing home, rather than because of external regulatory parameters. All recommendations for transfer should be thoroughly discussed with the client and family and included in the client's treatment plan.

Nurses play a crucial role in planning transitions between care settings. Early planning for transition to a different care setting gives clients and significant caregivers the best chance to develop a realistic plan consistent with the client's care needs, strengths, preferences, and financial means. Even the most basic transition plan should involve respect for client autonomy and choice (Birmingham, 2009). Workable follow up plans are better negotiated if people have sufficient time to consider all aspects and thought them through to their satisfaction. There are more options and fewer surprises; everyone involved has a clear picture of what to expect. Transition planning conversations allow nurses to uncover hidden client issues such as fears of being abandoned, or receiving substandard care in the new setting, home responsibilities, safety, financial concerns, social supports, fears about competence or outcome, and need for additional support such as respite care, and environmental safety needs. If a client is unable to participate in transitional care planning or decisions, the process can be initiated with the designated family or responsible caregiver. Exercise 24-2 provides an opportunity to collaboratively develop a transition plan for a client with complex care needs.

All communications in care transitions need to be secure and compliant with HIPAA requirements. The sender needs to include a contact person and relevant phone number for questions or concerns (Snow et al, 2009). Transitions between different care settings provide opportunities for unintentional information gaps (Coleman and Berenson, 2004; Greenwald et al., 2007). Guidelines for sending and receiving team functions during transfers are presented in Box 24-2. The sending team should pay extra attention to the completeness and accuracy of transferred information. Receiving teams need to carefully review transition reports and to ask as many questions as needed to ensure understanding.

DISCHARGE PLANNING

Successful discharge planning involves a significant component of informational continuity, which occurs at a critical transition point in a client's treatment process (Lees, 2013). The goal of discharge planning is to provide clients and their families with the level and kinds of information they need to secure their recovery and/or maintain health status during the immediate post-hospital period. Routine discharges with people able to handle post-hospitalization self-care on their own are relatively straightforward and easily implemented. Even with routine discharges, relevant client education about a client's situation with medication reconciliation, specific instructions for post discharge care, and contact numbers should be fully discussed with clients and families. Offering choices about about available and appropriate post acute providers represents a unique form of advocacy for clients and families (Birmingham, 2009).

Nonroutine discharges in which the client needs a postdischarge rehabilitative or subacute placement, additional health support services, and/or equipment at home requires a more complex discharge planning process for optimum results. A complex discharge planning process begins with a careful review of initial admission data and continues as a thread with each subsequent review. Starting early in the hospitalization allows time for clients and families to become physically and emotionally prepared for transition

and to have needed supports available post discharge. Informal discussions can be introduced during routine care. Other times client education can be offered in a more concentrated way with teach-back and return demonstrations. Frequent checks with clients and families encourage them to ask questions and express concerns in a supportive environment. Box 24-3 presents nursing actions associated with complex discharges. Exercise 24-3 provides practice with discharge planning processes.

The goal of discharge planning is to provide clients and their families with the level and kind of information they need to secure their recovery and/or maintain health status during the immediate post-hospital period. Research shows that having discharge plans tailored to individual client needs seems to have an effect on reduced hospital stay and readmission rates and increases client satisfaction (Shepperd et al., 2013).

| **BOX 24-2** | Core Functions for Transitional Sending and Receiving Teams |

Both the **sending** and **receiving** care teams are expected to:
- Shift their perspective from the concept of a client discharge to that of a client transfer with continuous management expectations.
- Begin planning for a transfer to the next care setting on or before a client's admission.
- Elicit the preferences of clients and caregivers and incorporate these preferences into the care plan, where appropriate.
- Identify a client's system of social support and baseline level of function (i.e., How will this client care for himself or herself after discharge?).
- Communicate and collaborate with practitioners across settings to formulate and execute a common care plan.
- Use the preferred mode of communication (i.e., telephone, fax, e-mail) of collaborators in other settings.

The **sending** health care team is expected to ensure that:
- The client is stable enough to be transferred to the next care setting.
- The client and caregiver understand the purpose of the transfer.
- The receiving institution is capable of and prepared to meet the client's needs.
- All relevant sections of the transfer information form are complete.

- The care plan, orders, and a clinical summary precede the client's arrival to the next care setting. The discharge summary should include the client's baseline functional status (both physical and cognitive) and recommendations from other professionals involved with the client's care, including social workers, occupational therapists, and physical therapists.
- The client has a timely follow-up appointment with an appropriate health care professional.
- A member of the sending health care team is available to the client, caregiver, and receiving health care team for 72 hours after the transfer to discuss any concerns regarding the care plan.
- The client and family understand their health care insurance benefits and coverage as they pertain to the transfer.

The **receiving** health care team is expected to ensure that:
- The transfer forms, clinical summary, discharge summary, and physician's orders are reviewed before or on the client's arrival.
- The client's goals and preferences are incorporated into the care plan.
- Discrepancies or confusion regarding the care plan, the client's status, or the client's medications are clarified with the sending health care team.

From HMO Work Group on Care Management: *One client, many places: managing health care transitions*, Washington, DC, 2004, AAHP-HIAA Foundation, p. 7.

Medication reconciliation is an important dimension of admission and discharge planning. The Joint Commission specifically identifies it as National Patient Safety Goal No. 8. Clients may come into a care setting on a wide variety of medications. Some

---

- Assess clients' understanding of the discharge plan by asking them to explain it in their own words.
- Advise clients and family of any tests completed at the hospital with pending results at time of discharge. Also notify appropriate clinicians of this contingency.
- Schedule follow-up appointments or tests after discharge, if needed. Provide relevant contact numbers.
- Provide information about home or health care services if needed, or not initiated prior to discharge.
- Confirm the medication plan and ensuring that the client and family understands any changes (e.g., medication in the hospital not available or accessible in the community).
- Review written summary care instructions with the client and family and go over in detail what to do if a problem develops.
- Identify the responsible caregiver in the home and transportation arrangements.
- Expedite transmission of the discharge summary to health care providers and case managers accepting responsibility for the client.

---

medications may be changed or discontinued. Others may be added. When the client is being discharged, a medication reconciliation, including the name of the medication, generic and prescribed name, dosage, frequency, and the time each medication was last taken should be entered into the EHR, with a computer-generated or written list given to the client. Go over the list with the client, and designated caregiver if applicable. Medication reconciliation also should be done periodically with the client in primary care settings especially if the client is seeing more than one provider.

A crucial question is who in the client's close support system is available to help the client in the immediate postdischarge period, and what arrangements are in place if additional care support is required. It is important to ask open-ended questions about the home environment and the support the client is able to muster. This information needs to be precise. Just because a client has family in the area does not mean that they would be available to the client for direct support. You will need to identify the name of a primary support person and/or specific post hospital arrangements in the client's EHR. Very important is asking clients about their concerns and expectations after discharge. Clients discharged to home and their caregivers need specific instruction to successfully self-manage recovery and chronic health problems at home, not just once, but several times. Written instructions should be verbally explained and given to each client. Arrangements and/or referrals for essential support or training needs should be in place before discharge.

| EXERCISE 24-3 | Using a Discharge Planning Process |

Purpose: To provide an opportunity for students to develop an experiential understanding of a discharge planning process.

Procedure
Using the guideline data, develop a simple discharge planning report for a newly admitted client on your unit or use the case study below.

Jeff O'Connor is a 66-year-old man originally admitted to the emergency department with severe chest pain, shortness of breath, dizziness, and intermittent palpitations. He was diagnosed with a myocardial infarction and admitted to the coronary care unit. He was placed on oxygen and remained there for several days because his serum markers continued to rise. He received morphine for pain and sedatives to

keep him comfortable. He is currently stabilized with digoxin, demonstrates a normal sinus rhythm, and is being transferred to the step-down unit this afternoon. His wife and daughter have visited him several times each day. His wife states she is exhausted but glad he is being transferred. Jeff has long-standing coronary artery disease and a family history of cardiac events. This is his first heart attack.

Discussion
If this is the only information you have on Jeff, what other data might you need to develop a full transitional report using the SBAR (situation, background, assessment, recommendation) format described in Chapter 4?

Note: This exercise can be completed using a current client transfer.

Discharge Summary

The Joint Commission (2013) mandates that discharge summaries be completed within 30 days of hospital discharge. A discharge summary should communicate diagnostic findings, hospital management, and plans for follow-up at the end of a client's hospitalization (Kripalani et al., 2007). Content mandated for each client's written discharge summary includes

- Reason for hospitalization
- Significant findings
- Procedures and treatment provided
- The client's condition at discharge
- Client and family instructions (as appropriate)
- Attending physician's signature

Nurses are accountable for verbally reviewing discharge summaries with the client and/or caregiver, providing written instructions, and completing discharge documentation in the chart. Clients and/or their significant caregiver should be given a copy of the discharge summary and encouraged to keep it in a safe place. Clients should bring their discharge summary to initial follow-up appointments. Although the physician is responsible for initiating and signing discharge summaries and orders, nurses play a critical role in the discharge of clients.

Discharge instructions are not the same as discharge orders or discharge summaries. Specific *written* discharge instructions should include a basic follow-up plan identifying diet, activity level, weight monitoring, what to do if symptoms develop or worsen, and the contact numbers of relevant hospital, and primary care providers. Written instructions should be simple and concrete—for example, "Call the doctor if you gain more than 2 pounds in 1 week." A written list of all medications prescribed at discharge, including prescription, over-the-counter medications, vitamins and herbals, should be given to the client and caregiver. Use teach-back methods (see Chapter 15) to ensure that your discharge home management instructions are understood.

Subheadings help organize and highlight pertinent information for follow-up care (Kripalani et al., 2007). Discharge documentation in the client's chart should include the client's condition or functional status at time of discharge, followed by a summarization of the treatment and nursing care provided and discharge instructions given to the client/family and the client's responses. Clearly identify the intermediate placement (nursing home, rehabilitation center) or home.

You need to document that the client and/or caregiver was physically given a copy of the discharge instructions.

MANAGEMENT CONTINUITY

The triple aim of transformational approaches required to overhaul the U.S. healthcare system is designed to improve client care experiences improving patient experiences of care (including quality and satisfaction), cultivate overall population health and reduce the per capita cost of healthcare (Berwick et al 2008; Brandt et al, 2014).

Strong system-based management continuity facilitates self-care management. *Management continuity* is defined as "A consistent and coherent approach to the management of a health condition that is responsive to a patient's changing needs" (Al-Azri, 2008, p. 147). As a longitudinal approach to the clinical management of chronic disorders in the community, management continuity involves aligning client needs with community supports through care coordination and case management. Care coordination is the term used to describe "management of interdependencies among tasks" (Yang and Meiners, 2014, p. 96).

CARE COORDINATION, AND CLIENT SYSTEM NAVIGATION*

The basic goals of care coordination and client system navigation are to proactively guide patients through the barriers in complex health systems, decrease fragmentation, coordinate services, and improve health outcomes. Care coordinators are responsible for ensuring that the plan of care developed by the provider is carried out in partnership with the client. This process begins with developing a nonjudgmental collaborative relationship with a patient to identify health goals and any barriers that could impede success. Care coordinators are responsible for identifying an individual's health goals and coordinating services and providers to meet those goals. They must learn to be adept at navigating complex systems and communicating with patients, families, and professionals involved with the patient's care. Coordination activities include the following:

- Establishing relationships based on trust
- Communicating with patients, families, providers, and community resources that lead to shared expectations for communication and care

*This section was developed by Mary Joseph, RN, BC, CPHQ 2014.

- Providing health education
- Assessing strengths, challenges, needs, and goals
- Implementing a proactive plan of care
- Monitoring progress and assisting with follow-up
- Supporting self-management goals
- Facilitating informed choice, consent, and decision-making
- Facilitating transitions in care
- Linking patients to community resources
- Aligning resources to meet the patient's needs
- Developing connectivity that provides pathways that encourage timely and effective information flow between all entities involved including the patient

Effectively establishing and maintaining professional boundaries is essential when working with patients and families to coordinate care. Boundaries provide the limits that enable care coordinators to maintain professionalism and to secure an environment where both patient and care coordinator are mutually respected. Listed below are some important tips on maintaining boundaries.

- Always work within the treatment recommendations of the client's provider. The care coordinator should never give any recommendations contrary to the recommendations of the provider.
- The care coordinator is in a position of influence and the patient is in a vulnerable position. Over involvement with a patient can be draining on the care coordinator and can interfere with the important tasks of the job.
- Assess your cultural ideas and prejudices. Know your community.

The success of care coordination depends to a large extent on the strength of the interpersonal relationships between individual clinicians and community support organization. Without familiarity and shared objectives, the administrative transfer of information will not occur or be sustained. Ongoing use of the broad stakeholder group (the medical neighborhood) and joint review of performance data at care coordination meetings can help foster a community of continuous quality improvement among multiple providers. Routine performance measurement and reporting about the effectiveness and quality of care coordination are critical to understand if clients' needs are being met.

CASE MANAGEMENT

The Case Management Society of America defines **case management** as "a collaborative process of assessment, planning, facilitation and advocacy for options and services to meet an individual's health needs through communication and available resources to promote quality cost-effective outcomes." Whether one works in the hospital or primary care setting, all nurses should have knowledge of how case management works and how it fits into COC.

Case management is a professional support intervention, which assists clients to self-manage their health (Nazareth et al., 2008; Saultz and Albedaiwi, 2004). AHRQ (2013) advocates care coordination, team-based approaches, integration of behavioral and mental health with primary care, and stronger linkages with the community as the best means of improving the quality of health care delivery in the community. The goal of case management strategies is to help clients function at their highest possible level in the least restrictive environment. Case management strategies are designed with the following purposes:

- To enhance the client's quality of life
- To decrease fragmentation and duplication of health delivery processes
- To contain unnecessary health care costs (Gallagher et al., 2009)

Case management allows clients with multiple or serious physical and mental chronic conditions to stay in their homes and function in the community (Ploeg et al., 2008). Clients need a case manager when they are unable to safely establish or maintain self-management of a chronic health condition in a consistent manner without external supports. Included in the population group served by case managers are frail elders, clients with mental illness or dementia, and clients with chronic mental illness or chronic physical disabilities affecting activities of daily living.

Carter (2009) notes, "Case management is a core component of what is needed to improve health care quality overall, while reducing costs" (p. 166). Knowledge of community resources to facilitate health care delivery in primary care settings allows case managers to consistently deliver the right care at the right time to the right client and family. Standards of practice for case management related to quality of care, collaboration, and resource utilization are consistent with National Patient Safety goals developed by the Joint Commission (Amin and Owen, 2006).

Case Example

Ray Bolton is a 48-year-old man with severe chronic Crohn's disease. He has a permanent ileostomy, is on multiple medications, and suffers from periodic exacerbations in his condition, resulting in hospitalization. Ray has Social Security Disability Insurance (SSDI) as his only source of income. He has neurologic issues affecting his balance and gait and causing him significant pain. He cannot sleep and is socially isolated. He lives by himself with his cat. Apart from his 80-year-old mother who lives in another state, Ray has no support system except his physicians. He was referred for case management, following his latest hospitalization. Exercise 24-4 provides an opportunity to assess and plan for client care using a case management approach.

CASE MANAGEMENT PRINCIPLES AND STRATEGIES

Case management strategies are designed to coordinate and manage client care across a wide continuum of health care services and community supports. Case management models follow the nursing process as a structural framework. Strategies incorporate COC concepts related to communication, team building, and data sharing with all members of the multidisciplinary care team, including the client and family caregivers.

Case finding is a proactive case management strategy to identify individuals at high risk for potential health problems (Thomas, 2009). The manner in which you approach the client will determine the completeness of information you receive.

An intake assessment should include the names, addresses, and phone numbers of the client's health care providers, social service representatives, school or work contacts, if applicable, and health insurance information. Availability of social supports and religious affiliations, previous hospitalizations, and history of treatment, current medications and allergies, advance directives and do not resuscitate (DNR) status, cognitive and mental status, mobility status, and functional assessment of activities of daily living are other pieces of case management assessment data. Identifying potential barriers to treatment adherence, including the impact that the client's diagnosis has on family members and coworkers is important. Case managers interact directly with all members of the collaborative health team, clients, and families on a regular basis. The case manager works with an assigned client to identify the individual needs and health goals. Operationalizing client self management of chronic conditions requires special attention to empowering clients related to role and emotional self management as well as the client's medical or behavioral management needs (McAlister et al, 2012). Case management treatment strategies are customized for each client, based on personal needs, values, and preferences, using a rehabilitative strength-based focus. Because case management represents a longitudinal treatment management process, care plans will likely need adjustment from time to time to reflect changes in the client's situation. Decisionally competent clients should have final responsibility for decision-making.

| EXERCISE 24-4 | Planning Care for Ray Bolton: Case Management Approaches |

Purpose: To provide practice with assessing and planning care for Ray Bolton using a case management approach.

Procedure
(Initial consideration of Ray's issues can be completed as an out-of-class assignment.) In groups of four to five students, consider the case example of Ray Bolton in this chapter.
  Each group should identify:
  • Relevant assessment data
  • The best ways to address Ray's complex health needs and why
  • What kinds of resources Ray will need to effectively self-manage his multiple chronic health problems

After 15 to 20 minutes, have each student group share with the rest of the students what their plan would be, the resources they will need to accomplish the task, and why.

Discussion
1. What was your experience of doing this exercise?
2. What were the commonalities and differences developed by different student teams?
3. Were you surprised by anything in doing this exercise?
4. What are the implications for your future practice?

Case managers help clients to coordinate services, overcome barriers, and provide clients with needed support to assume as much responsibility as possible in self-management of their health issues. They meet with clients at scheduled intervals to monitor client status and make changes as needed. When single agency resources are insufficient to meet complex health needs, case managers help clients and families identify and coordinate services with other agencies. Networking and communication with other health professionals involved with the client help prevent or minimize emergence of full-blown health problems. Strategies include guidance or referrals to social supports such as legal aid, social security benefits and disability, safe affordable housing, social services, and/or mental health and addiction services. To be effective, case managers need a strong understanding of community resources' strengths and weaknesses, including accessibility, availability, affordability, and how systems work.

Case managers have an advocacy role; they may educate people in the community who work with disabled or chronically ill clients about the social aspects of disability to facilitate understanding and acceptance of the client's problems. Goodman (2014) suggests that the opportunities for nursing advocacy are boundless, depending on a nurse's personal interests and skills. For example, nurses often speak before legislative and other funding sources to advocate for essential services. Their testimony is believable because of their close relationship in caring for vulnerable populations. Case managers also frequently negotiate on a client's behalf with insurance companies and equipment suppliers as a supportive adjunct when a client is unable to do so.

Case management outcomes are described in terms of client satisfaction, clinical outcomes, and cost. Quality improvement variances related to achievement of actual clinical outcomes are analyzed with recommendations for treatment planning, related to observed changes in the client's situation, health condition, or in health care resources. Documentation from external providers and agencies needs to be included in the client's case management record, as do variances from the treatment plan, reasons for the variance, and plans for modification in care plans.

MANAGEMENT CONTINUITY RESOURCE FOR FAMILY CAREGIVERS

Case managers provide ongoing support and encouragement for family caregivers. Cott and colleagues (2008) describe the medical home as "a unique clinical setting, different from acute care or institutional environments" (p. 19). Living with chronic illness increasingly is a home care responsibility, with family members as informal caregivers providing most of the care. Family caregiving is neither a career choice, nor a role for which one can prepare. The caregiver has

---

EXERCISE 24-5	Understanding the Role of a Family Caregiver

Purpose: To help students understand the caregiver role from the perspective of family caregivers.

Procedure
1. Interview the family caregiver of a client with a long-standing chronic illness or mental disability, and write a summary of the caregiver's responses.
2. Use the following questions to obtain your data.
   a. Can you tell me why and how you assumed responsibility for caregiving?
   b. In what ways has your life changed since you became a caregiver for your parent, spouse, disabled child or adult, or mentally ill family member?
   c. What do you find most challenging about the caregiving role?
   d. What do you find rewarding about the caregiving role?
   e. How do you balance caring for your ill or disabled family member with caring for yourself?
   f. What advice would you give someone who is about to assume the caregiving role for a chronically ill or disabled family member?

Discussion
- What was it like to get a picture of the caregiver role?
- Were you surprised by any of the caregiver's responses?
- What were the similarities and differences in caregiver responses?
- What are some of the reasons for any of the variants between student reports?
- How could you incorporate what you learned doing this exercise in your clinical practice?

no "care map to lead the way," states Wright and colleagues (2009, p. 209). Exercise 24-5 offers insights into the role of family caregivers from the caregiver perspective.

Caring for clients with significant disability at home has positive and negative aspects. Being cared for at home offers stronger COC management as home is associated with personal identity, security, and relationships with people who genuinely care about the client. Variation exists in a family member's capacity to be supportive, especially if the caregiver's health is not optimal, the care is labor intensive and time consuming, or the relationship with the client is conflictual (Weinberg et al., 2007). Case managers can fill in essential information gaps for family caregivers through careful questioning, observation, validation about feelings and observations, and consultation about emerging health issues. Working with families should include providing educational information on medications, signs and symptoms of impending problems and potential adverse reactions and when to call a health care provider. Names, locations and phone numbers of primary care and follow up providers should be discussed and the information provided in written form to the caregiver.

CASE MANAGEMENT FOR CHRONICALLY MENTALLY ILL CLIENTS

COC is essential for effectively in caring for chronically mentally ill clients in the community (Wierdsma et al., 2009). These clients find fulfilling even basic needs for shelter, food, clothing, and transportation to be quality-of-life issues. Chronically mentally ill and substance-dependent clients often function at a marginal level because of their symptoms. Many are homeless and in poor physical health. These clients often do not seek out help proactively. Yet, as A. C. Benson (n.d.) notes, "People seldom refuse help, if one offers it in the right way."

Case management for the chronically mentally ill is key to providing quality health care, particularly for youths and seniors in the public sector (Trachtenberg, 2010). Case managers provide mentally ill individuals with mentoring, coaching, and referrals for job training services. They help clients avert crisis relapses that precipitate rehospitalization. Case managers use recovery principles of care, such as linking clients with counseling and alternative treatment services, social services, and community networks.

COC for mentally ill and dually diagnosed clients includes formal wraparound support services for mentally ill children and families and case management for adults and children. Wraparound services use a strengths-based format, which involves the family, community, school, and service providers in the child's environment. Professionals work with the family and other social providers to promote adaptive functioning. Strengthening family ties to supportive people within the family's social environment are deliberately included in wrap around services help to strengthen social support (Walker and Schutte, 2004).

SUMMARY

COC is a dynamic, multidimensional concept, consisting of relational, informational, and management continuity and focused on assisting individuals and families with the resources they need to manage chronic illness within and across clinical settings. The goal of COC is to ensure a seamless continuum of quality care for clients, provided through coordinated, community-based health services. COC-integrated delivery systems focus on what really matters to a client and family and have the capacity to provide services to meet the client's needs.

Relational continuity embraces collaborative relationships and shared decision making between health care providers and clients. Successful outcomes also depend on interdisciplinary collaboration and interprofessional team communication caring for the client, who can be defined as an individual, family, or community in need of care.

Informational COC allows for an uninterrupted flow of data and clinical impressions between health care providers and agencies, with clients and their families, in a care experience that is connected and coherent over time. Informational COC is a critical component in effective transition and discharge planning.

Case management is a major vehicle in ensuring management continuity for individuals, who otherwise might not be able to function independently in the community because of physical or mental disability. Care coordination and service navigation in public sector health care helps clients and families get the support they need when multiple service providers are involved.

ETHICAL DILEMMA | What Would You Do?

Paul is ready to be discharged from the hospital, but it is clear that he can no longer live independently by himself. He has had several heart attacks in the past with significant heart damage and currently suffers from serious chronic obstructive pulmonary disease (COPD). His recent hospitalization was for uncontrolled diabetes. Paul has difficulty complying with diet restrictions and his need to take daily insulin. He is not an easy person to live with, but Paul is sure that his daughter will welcome him into her home because he is "family."

Although his daughter agrees to assume care for her father, she does so reluctantly. She has her own life and does not have a positive relationship with her father. She resents that he just assumes that she will take care of him. Without her support, Paul cannot live independently in the community. What would you do as the nurse in this situation to help them resolve this dilemma? What are the implications of this situation as an ethical dilemma?

DISCUSSION QUESTIONS

1. What do you see as facilitators and barriers for continuity of care in your current care setting?
2. In what ways do different interdisciplinary roles influence and complement each other in complex clinical care situations?
3. In what ways does COC support the triple aim of effective health care? What do you understand better about continuity of care as a result of reading this chapter?

REFERENCES

Agarwal G, Crooks V: The nature of informational continuity in general practice, *Br J Gen Pract* November e1–e8, 2008.

Al-Azri M: Continuity of care and quality of care-inseparable twin, *Oman Med J* 23(3):147–149, 2008.

Amin A, Owen M: Productive interdisciplinary team relationships: the hospitalist and the case manager, *Lippincotts Case Manag* 11(3): 160–164, 2006.

Agency for Healthcare Research and Quality (AHRQ): AHRQ updates on primary care research: Multiple chronic conditions research network, *Ann Fam Med* 485–486, 2013.

Agency for Healthcare Research and Quality (AHRQ): Chapter 2: What is care coordination? In *Care Coordination Measures Atlas*, Rockville, MD, 2011, Agency for Healthcare Research and Quality, pp 6–12.

American Geriatrics Society: Improving the quality of transitional care for persons with complex care needs (American Geriatrics Society (AGS) position statement), *Assisted Living Consult* 30–32, 2007. March/April.

Benson AC. (n.d.). BrainyQuote.com. Retrieved October 27, 2013, from BrainyQuote.com: http://www.brainyquote.com/quotes/quotes/a/acbenson101010.html

Berwick DM, Nolan TW, Whittington J: The triple aim: Care, health, and cost, *Health Affairs* 27:759–769, 2008.

Birmingham J: Patient choice in the discharge planning process, *Prof Case Manag* 14(6):296–309, 2009. quiz, 310-311.

Bodenheimer T, Wagner E, Grumbach K: Improving primary care for clients with chronic illness, *JAMA* 288(14):1775–1779, 2002.

Boling P: Care transitions and home health care, *Clin Geriatr Med* 25:135–148, 2009.

Brandt B, Luftiyya M, King J, Chioresco C: A scoping review of interprofessional collaborative practice and education using the lens of the triple aim, *J Interprof Care* 28(5):393–399, 2014.

Carr D: On the case: effective care transitions, *Nurs Manag* 32(1): 25–31, 2008.

Carter J: Finding our place at the discussion table: case management and heath care reform, *Prof Case Manag* 14(4):165–166, 2009.

Case Management Society of America: *What is a case manager?* Available online, nd. http://www.cmsa.org/Home/CMSA/Whatisa CaseManager/tabid/224/Default.aspx Accessed December 3, 2014.

Clark P, Cott CC, Drinka T, et al.: Theory and practice in interprofessional ethics: a framework for understanding ethical issues in health care teams, *J Interprof Care* 21(6):591–603, 2007.

Coleman E, Berenson R: Lost in transition: challenges and opportunities for improving the quality of transitional care, *Ann Intern Med* 140:533–536, 2004.

Coleman K, Austin BT, Brach C, Wagner EH: Evidence on the Chronic Care Model in the new millennium. Health Aff (Millwood), vol, 28, no 1:75–85, 2009.

Cooke L, Gemmill R, Grant M, et al.: Advance practice nurses core competencies: a framework for developing and testing an advanced practice nurse discharge intervention, *Clin Nurse Spec* 22(5):218–225, 2008.

Cott C, Falter L, Gignac M, et al.: Helping networks in community home care for the elderly: types of team, *Can J Nurs Res* 40(1):18–37, 2008.

Crabtree B, Nutting P, Miller W, Stange K, Stewart E, Jaen CR: Summary of the national demonstration project and recommendations for the patient-centered medical home, *Ann Fam Med* 1:580–590, 2010. 8 no. Suppl.

Cramm J, Nieboer A: Professional views on interprofessional stroke team functioning, *Int J Integr Care* 11(25):1–8, 2011.

D'Amour D, Oandasan I: Interprofessionality as the field of interprofessional practice and interprofessional education: an emerging concept, *J Interprof Care* 19(Suppl 1):8–20, 2005.

Engebretson J, Mahoney J, Carlson E, et al.: Cultural competence in the era of evidence based practice, *J Prof Nurs* 24:172–178, 2008.

Ferrer R, Gill J: Shared decision making, contextualized, *Ann Fam Med* 303–305, 2013. Editorial.

Gallagher L, Truglio-Londrigan R, Levin R, et al.: Partnership for healthy living: an action research project, *Nurse Res* 16(2):7–29, 2009.

Gardner D: Ten Lessons in Collaboration, *Online J Issues in Nurs* 10(1):2, 2005.

Ginter P, Duncan WJ, Swayne L: *Strategic Management of Health Care Organizations*, 7th ed, San Francisco, 2013, Jossey-Bass.

Glasgow R, Goldstein M, Kaplan-Liss E: Chapter 5, Introduction to the principles of health behavior change. Health Promotion and

Disease Prevention. In Woolf S, Jonas S, editors: 2 ed, Philadelphia, PA, 2008, Lippincott Wilkins, pp 129–147.

Goodman T: Guest Editorial: The future of nursing: An opportunity for Advocacy, *AORN* 99(6):668–670, 2014.

Greenwald JL, Denham CR, Jack BW, et al.: The hospital discharge: a review of high risk care transition with highlights of a reengineered discharge process, *J Patient Saf* 3(2):97–106, 2007.

Grumbach K, Bodenheimer T: A primary care home for Americans: putting the house in order, *JAMA* 288(7):889–893, 2002.

Guilliford M, Naithani S, Morgan M: What is "continuity of care"? *J Health Serv Res Policy* 11(4):248–250, 2006.

Haggerty JL, Reid PJ, Freeman GK, et al.: Continuity of care: a multi-disciplinary review, *BMJ* 327:1219–1221, 2003.

Haggerty JL R, Pineault R, Beaulieu M, et al.: Practice features associated with client reported accessibility, continuity, and coordination of primary health care, *Ann Fam Med* 6(2):116–123, 2008.

Haggerty JL, Roberge D, Freeman GK, Beaulieu C: Experienced continuity of care when clients see multiple clinicians: a qualitative metasummary, *Ann Fam Med* 11(3):262–271, 2013.

Hall P: Interprofessional teamwork: professional cultures as barriers, *J Interprof Care* 19(Suppl 1):188–196, 2005.

Havens D, Vasey J, Gittell J, Lin W: Relational coordination among nurses and other providers: impact on the equality of patient care, *Nurs Manag* 18(8):926–937, 2010.

Institute of Medicine (IOM): *The future of the public's health in the 21st century*, Washington, DC, 2003, National Academies Press.

Institute of Medicine (IOM): *Primary care and public health: Exploring integration to improve population health*, Washington DC, 2012, National Academy Press.

Jeffcott SA, Lee: *Conceptual model of handover elements*, 2009 (From Jeffcott SA, et al. Improving measurement in clinical handover. Qual Saf Health Care. 2009;18[4]:272–277.)

Jeffcott SA, Evans SM, Cameron PA, et al.: Improving measurement in clinical handover, *Qual Saf Health Care* 18(4):272–277, 2009.

Joseph MJ: Project Manager: Center for Health Improvement, Primary Care Coalition of Montgomery County, Maryland, *Unpublished manuscript*, 2014. Received, March 2014.

Katzenbach JR, Smith DK: *The Wisdom of Teams: Creating the High-Performance Organization*, New York, 1999, HarperBusiness.

Keeling A, Lewenson S: A nursing historical perspective on the medical home: Impact on health care policy, *Nurs Outlook* 61:360–366, 2013.

Kleinman A:, The illness narratives: suffering, healing, and the human condition Basic Books: 1988 New York.

Kripalani S, LeFevre F, Phillips C, et al.: Deficits in communication and information transfer between hospital-based and primary care physicians: implications for client safety and continuity of care, *JAMA* 297(8):831–841, 2007.

Lidskog M, Lofmark A, Ahlstrom G, et al.: Interprofessional education on a training ward for older people: students conceptions of nurses, occupational therapists and social workers, *J Interprof Care* 21(4):387–399, 2007.

McAllister, et al.: Client empowerment: The need to consider it as a measurable client-reported outcome for chronic conditions, *BMC Health Serv Res* 12:157, 2012.

Mitchell P, Wynia M, Golden R, McNellis B, Okun S, Webb CE, Rohrbach V, Von Kohorn I: *Core principles & values of effective team-based health care. Discussion Paper*, Washington, DC, 2012, Institute of Medicine. www.iom.edu/tbc.

Mosser G, Begun J: *Teamwork in Health Care*, New York, NY, 2014, McGraw Hill.

Muir JC: Team, diversity and building communities, *J Palliat Med* 11(1):5–7, 2008.

Naylor MD: Advancing high value transitional care: Thecentral role of nursing and its leadership, *Nursing AdministrationQuarterly* 36:115126, 2012.

Nazareth I, Jones L, Irving A, et al.: Perceived concepts of care in people with colorectal and breast cancer—a qualitative case study analysis, *Eur J Cancer Care (Engl)* 17:569–577, 2008.

Lees L: The key principles of effective discharge planning. *Nurs Times* 109(3). Accessed October 6, 2013 www.nursingtimes.net/nursing.discharge-planning/5053740.article, 2013.

Porter-O'Grady T: From tradition to transformation: A revolutionary moment for nursing in age of reform, *Nurse Lead* 12(1):65–69, 2014.

Paquette-Warren Roberts E, Fournie M, Tyler M, Brown J, Harris S: Immprovint chronic care through continuing education of interprofessional primary care teams: a process evaluation, *J Interprof Care* 28(3):232–238, 2014.

Ploeg J, Hayward L, Woodward C, et al.: A case study of a Canadian homelessness intervention programme for elderly people, *Health Soc Care Community* 16(6):593–605, 2008.

Pontin D, Lewis M: Maintaining the continuity of care in community children's nursing caseloads in a service for children with life-limiting, life-threatening or chronic health conditions: a qualitative analysis, *J Clin Nurs* 18:1199–1206, 2008.

Rhudy L, Holland D, Bowles K: Illuminating hospital discharge planning: Staff nurse decision making, *Appl Nurs Res* 23(4):198–206, 2010.

San Martin-Rodriguez L, D'Amour D, Leduc N, et al.: Outcomes of interprofessional collaboration of hospitalized cancer client, *Cancer Nurs* 31(2):E18–E27, 2008.

Saultz J, Albedaiwi W: Interpersonal continuity of care and client satisfaction: a critical review, *Ann Fam Med* 2(5):445–451, 2004.

Schneller E, Epstein K: The hospitalist movement in the United States; agency and common agency issues, *Health Care Manag Rev* 31(4):308–316, 2006.

Schultz K: Strategies to enhance teaching about continuity of care, *Can Fam Physician* 56:666–668, 2009.

Shepperd S, Lannin N, Clemson L, McCluskey A, Cameron ID, Barras SL: Discharge planning from hospital to home, *Cochrane Database Syst Rev* 1:CD000313, 2013.

Sievers B, Wolf S: Teams: communication in multidisciplinary care, *Clin Nurse Spec* 20(2):75–80, 2006.

Snow V, Beck D, Budnitz T, Miller D, Potter J, Williams: Transitions of care consensus policy statement: society of general internal medicine, society of hospital medicine, American geriatrics society, American College of Emergency Physicians and Society for Academic Medicine, *Journal of Hospital Medicine* 4:364–370, 2009.

Sparbel K, Anderson MA: Integrated literature review of continuity of care: part 1, conceptual issues, *J Nurs Sch* 32(1):17–24, 2000.

Stans SE, Stevens JA, Beurskens AJ: Interprofessional practice in primary care: development of a tailored process model, *J Multidiscip Health* 6:139–147, 2013.

Starfield B, Horder J: Interpersonal continuity: Old and new perspectives, *Br J Gen Pract* 57(540):527–529, 2007.

The Joint Commission: Comprehensive Accreditation Manual for Hospitals: The Official Handbook (CAMH). Oakbrook Terrace, IL, *Joint Commission on Accreditation of Health Care Organizations*, 2013.

Thomas D: Case management for chronic conditions, *Nurs Manag* 15(10):22–27, 2009.

Trachtenberg D: *County Council Member, Montgomery county Member*, Rockville MD, January 7, 2010, Montgomery county Mental Health Advisory Committee.

Van Servellen G, Fongwa M, Mockus D'Errico E, et al.: Continuity of care and quality care outcomes for people experiencing chronic conditions: a literature review, *Nurs Health Sci* 8:185–195, 2006.

Von Bultzingslowen I, Eliasson G, Sarvimaki A, et al.: Clients' views on interpersonal continuity based on four core foundations, *Fam Pract* 23(2):210–219, 2006.

Wagner E, Austin B, Davis C, Hindmarsh M, Schaerer J, Bonomi A: Improving chronic illness care: Translating evidence into action, *Health Aff* 20(6):64–78, 2001.

Walker JS, Shutte KM: Practice and process in wraparound teamwork, *Journal of Emotional and Behavioral Disorders* 12(3):182–192, 2004.

Weinberg D, Lusenhop RW, Gittell G, et al.: Coordination between formal providers and informal caregivers, *Health Care Manag Rev* 32(2):140–149, 2007.

Wierdsma A, Mulder C, de Vries S, et al.: Reconstructing continuity of care in mental health services: a multilevel conceptual framework, *J Health Serv Res Policy* 14:52–57, 2009.

World Health Organization (WHO): *Innovative care for chronic conditions: building blocks for action Author*, Geneva, 2002, Switzerland.

Wright J, Doherty M, Dumas L, et al.: Caregiver burden: three voices-three realities, *Nurs Clin North Am* 44:209–221, 2009.

Yang YT, Meiners M: Care coordination and the expansion of nursing scopes of practice, *Journal of Law, Medicine & Ethics* 42(1):93–103, 2014.

Zwarenstein M, Reeves S, Russell A, et al.: Structuring communication relationships for interpersonal teamwork (SCRIPT): a cluster randomized controlled trial, *Trials* 8:23–36, 2007.

CHAPTER 25

Documentation in an Electronic Era

Kathleen Underman Boggs

OBJECTIVES

At the end of the chapter, the reader will be able to:

1. Identify five purposes for documentation.
2. Discuss electronic health records (EHRs) and computerized provider order entry (CPOE) systems as part of larger electronic health information technology (HIT) systems, evaluating whether "meaningful use" requirements have improved care quality.
3. Discuss the need for coding and nursing taxonomy in the use of EHRs.
4. Identify how use of electronic care plans, decision support, CPOE, and other aspects of HIT systems improves client outcomes.
5. Identify legal aspects of documenting in client records.

The process of obtaining, organizing, and conveying client health information to others in print or electronic format is referred to as **documentation.** As illustrated in Figure 25-1, documentation serves five purposes: (1) communicates to others care received or not received; (2) conveys pertinent information about the client's condition and response to treatment interventions; (3) substantiates the quality of care by showing adherence to care standards; (4) provides evidence for reimbursement; and (5) serves as source of data, which can be compiled or aggregated and then analyzed to establish "best practice" interventions. This includes electronic data that can be aggregated to monitor outcomes of care processes for quality improvement, a QSEN competency.

The process of interdisciplinary communication has been increasingly integrated into electronic health records. This chapter focuses on **health information technology** (HIT) including **electronic health records** (EHRs) as the method nurses use to document client care. Use of **computerized provider order entry (**CPOE) systems are also described. Your use of EHR technology to communicate and manage client information is a skill specifically cited as part of

QSEN's informatics competency. As a professional, you are expected to know how to use and even manage digital databases. Aspects of EHR use as well as regulatory and ethical implications of documentation will be described. This chapter concludes with a discussion of coding and nursing taxonomies. New technology and devices for medical communication at the point of care, clinical decision support systems (CDSSs), and remote monitoring, secure messaging, and telehealth are discussed in Chapter 26.

BASIC CONCEPTS
COMPUTERIZED HEALTH INFORMATION TECHNOLOGY SYSTEMS

Computers make information more accessible to all who are involved, including your client. The U.S. federal government, the American Nurses Association (ANA), and the Institute of Medicine, among others, believe computerized systems will not only improve the quality of health care, but will also eventually reduce its cost. As stated in *Healthy People 2020*, the goal is to use HIT to improve population

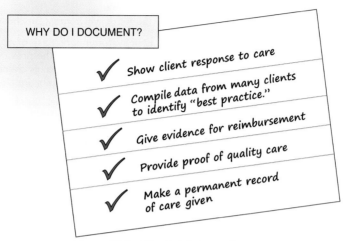

WHY DO I DOCUMENT?

✓ Show client response to care

✓ Compile data from many clients to identify "best practice."

✓ Give evidence for reimbursement

✓ Provide proof of quality care

✓ Make a permanent record of care given

Figure 25-1 Why do I document?

health outcomes and health care quality. Since the Health Information Technology for Economic and Clinical Health (HITECH) Act was passed in 2009, the American government has spent $30 billion to subsidize purchase of HIT by agencies and private care providers. HIT is expected to facilitate achievement of American national priorities: making care safer, engaging clients as partners in their health care, promoting better communication, and increasing use of preventive practices and evidence-based "best practices" (Dolin et al., 2014). Data are just beginning to become available showing better outcomes for client health status (McCullough et al., 2013). This is true internationally, as computerization is accepted as a strategy to improve health care, making it more efficient and effective (Ben-Assuli and Leshno, 2013).

MEANINGFUL USE

Adoption of HIT creates an interactive computerized information and communication system. Far more complex than just putting existing paper documentation on a computer, HIT systems are designed to support the multiple *information needs* required by today's complex client care; provide you and others on the health team with *clinical decision support*; and achieve safer care for your client. Unlike other developed countries, providers in the United States have been amazingly slow to fully adopt integrated computerized health systems.

Under the American Recovery and Reinvestment Act of 2009, the Centers for Medicare and Medicaid Services (CMS) have specified EHR components required for use by providers and agencies who serve their clients. These regulations, known as "meaningful use," spell out what EHR competencies must be phased in by target dates beginning in 2015. Crucial meaningful use information is listed in Table 25-1. In addition to using EHRs, providers must submit electronic client data to government agencies as well as share data across agencies to demonstrate quality and to facilitate care coordination. Under Stage 2 of "meaningful use" requirements, clients will be able to view online and download their records (Heeter, 2013). These regulations are driving major changes in our health care documentation systems and directly impact the way you document.

ELECTRONIC HEALTH RECORDS: IMPROVED INFORMATION FLOW

A comprehensive computer information system changes the way information flows through the health care delivery system. Communication is more rapid. HIT can be used to communicate quickly among doctors, nurses, client, families, and across agency departments. Consider the following case.

TABLE 25-1	Components of an Electronic Health Information Technology System in Our Journey to Consumer-Driven Health Care	

Mandatory (Required by CMS under its "meaningful use" criteria)	Desirable (Some of which must be chosen to be used)
An integrated, accessible electronic repository of client data with easy access by a variety of health care providers for exchange of information. Contains and records changes in: Updated problem list Hx; Dx; VS; PE data Medication list Allergy list (crosschecks for drug-drug-allergy problems and sends alerts to providers) Imaging files with real-time access at the point of care	EHR system needs ease of access, perhaps by use of templates that the provider checks or customizes/modifies, e.g., a box is checked when an ECG was done and results are checked "normal" or "abnormal." Information is accessed before and after each task, with nurse documenting not only care given but also client's progress toward goals. EHR can be remotely accessed by providers who can work from anywhere at any time. HIT system has financial tools, as well as clinical tools, e.g., it is able to generate newest ICD codes, do billing information, schedule appointments, etc. Incorporates accommodations to improve work flow and thus increase productivity. Ease of access allows provider to access many screen files with one login.
Has clinical decision support capabilities. Incorporates standard "evidence-based best practice" protocols that monitor your care and send you prompts if care is not recorded.	Sends alerts to providers
Uses CPOE	
Reports quality outcome measures to the government (CMC); public health agencies; state or local governmental agencies while safeguarding privacy/HIPAA requirements	Each year the percentage of total clients for whom you must submit reportable information increases.
Required use of EHRs also mandates capability to generate written prescriptions to avoid handwriting errors	May electronically send prescriptions to client's preferred pharmacy
On request can provide client with clinical summaries: copies of records, laboratory findings, discharge instructions, educational resources, forms for advanced directives, etc.	Client may not have access to all levels of information. Has online portals for clients to access their information. Sends electronic reminders or alerts to clients
Provides summary of care at each point of transition, and for referrals	
Aggregates data	

Abbreviations: CPOE, computerized physician/provider order entry; Dx, diagnosis; CMS, Center for Medicare and Medicaid Services; ECG, electrocardiogram; EHR, electronic health record; HIPAA, Health Insurance Portability and Accountability Act; HIT, health information technology; Hx, history; ICD, International Statistical Classification of Diseases and Related Health Problems; PE, physical examination; VS, vital signs.

Adapted from multiple sources including HealthIT.gov; Higgins L, Personal interview, January 10, 2014; Keenan GM, Yakel E, Tschannen D, Mandeville M: Chapter 49: documentation and the nurse care planning process. In Hughes RG, editor: *Patient Safety and Quality: An Evidence-Based Handbook for Nurses*, Rockville, MD, 2008, Agency for Healthcare Quality and Research (AHRQ). http://www.ahrq.gov/professionals/clinicians-providers/resources/nursing/resources/nurseshdbk/KeenanG_DNCPP.pdf. Accessed January 4, 2014; Kennedy A: Looking back and moving forward, *J AHIMA* 85(1):10, 2014.

Case Example:

Mary Levin, age 69 years, is admitted via the emergency department (ED) to a medical unit at General Hospital at 11 a.m. with a diagnosis of congestive heart failure. Her ED physician accesses her prior electronic health record (EHR), updates information, and documents his notes and her electrocardiogram (ECG) results in her EHR. The health information technology (HIT) system flags her own physician, who comes in to examine her and enters diagnostic and treatment orders using a computerized provider order entry (CPOE) system. He does not need to repeat the ECG since the system already contains this data. These orders are simultaneously and instantly transmitted to the pharmacy, the laboratory, radiology, as well as to you, the nurse assigned on her unit.

EHRs) are one part of the overall HIT system. The authors use the term *EHR* in this book, although electronic records are also known as electronic clinical records, electronic patient records, person-centered health records, or **electronic medical records** (Figure 25-2). Most of these terms initially applied to computerized records within a provider's office or agency. Currently there are many different versions of electronic systems in use. Unlike electronic medical records, EHRs have portability and can follow your client to other providers or specialists, or other hospitals, nursing homes, and so forth. Technology exists for secure storage on supercomputers in **the "cloud,"** which would allow anytime, anywhere remote access by multiple providers (with client permission).

THREE KEYS TO ELECTRONIC RECORDS

The three keys to electronic records are **interoperability**, **portability**, and **ease of use.**

INTEROPERABILITY (INTERAGENCY ACCESSIBILITY)

Exchanging health information among agencies is critical to smoothly delivering comprehensive

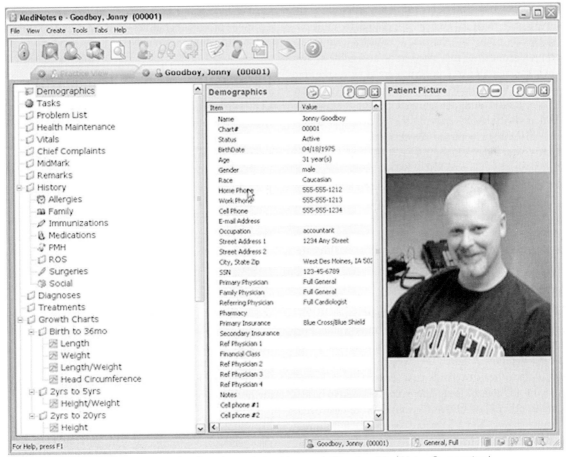

Figure 25-2   Example of an electronic health record. *(Courtesy MediNotes Corporation.)*

patient-centered care. It is essential if we are to reduce costs by eliminating redundancy. For example, when your client's laboratory results or imaging files are available to multiple providers, unnecessary repetition of tests or procedures can be eliminated and costs reduced. However incompatibility of software or privacy regulations can interfere with the communication of information. So we need to aim for interoperability, where differing agency HIT systems can "talk to each other."

Early companies developing EHRs were highly competitive, marketing various and different products to health care providers who had very different needs, content references, and budgets. Vendors created systems whose software was not compatible with competing products. Now government, the health care industry, and the insurance industry are working to enable different systems to exchange information—to "talk" to each other. The U.S. Office of the National Coordinator for HIT created a certification process to harmonize EHR products for better interoperability. Not only must EHRs be integrated in multiple departments such as pharmacy, radiology, physical therapy, and nursing, they need to be accessible across agencies. A number of companies are now marketing software applications to enable interoperability. Some states are transitioning to statewide EHR systems such as Arkansas' SHARE system. The goal is that a client's EHR can be accessed across agencies. So in one example, your client's laboratory results can be directly entered into the client's EHR at his or her primary provider's office by an outside laboratory, then accessed by you from your outpatient clinic. With interoperability, information flows to providers as needed. Transitions in client care become seamless. With interoperability we may realize anytime, anywhere access of health care records using remote devices.

PORTABILITY

Electronic records are more durable than paper charting and are portable. They are easily transferable. For example, during Hurricane Katrina in 2005, the New Orleans Veterans Affairs (VA) was able to send their 50,000 client health records to a secure site in Texas, while untold thousands of paper records stored in basements in other New Orleans hospitals were destroyed by flood waters. The VA record system is fully integrated with the Department of Defense. Therefore, if a soldier is wounded abroad, diagnosed and treated, shipped home, and eventually discharged, his or her record including computed axial tomography (CAT) scans are seamlessly available to VA doctors. Consider another example: You celebrate graduation by traveling across the country on vacation. If you are in a car accident and are admitted to an emergency department (ED) in another state, your records stored "in the cloud" are potentially available to the ED physician via Internet. At the very least, you can carry them with you on a flash drive or CD.

EASE OF ACCESS

Ease of access ideally means access at the point of care or remotely using any type of device. While maintaining record security, clients can give permission for access by multiple caregivers for anytime, anywhere communication. This 24/7 access from remote devices will markedly change the way health care is practiced. Through use of Internet **portals,** clients can also access their health information. Barriers currently exist including incompatible hardware, software, government privacy regulations and most importantly, the great difficulty in keeping stored data secure.

DOCUMENTING CLIENT INFORMATION

CLIENT AS PARTNER IN DOCUMENTING

Studies repeatedly show that when clients are actively involved in decision making about their health, they manage their illnesses better, complying with treatment protocols. In accord with making clients active partners in their health care, new "meaningful use" regulations require that they have access to some areas of their EHRs, allowing them to look at information or even possibly add additional data as needed. For example, Kaiser Permanente's nearly 9 million members can access their immunization records at anytime from anywhere. We have the technology by which the client can communicate home health–monitored data such as blood pressure, glucose level, weight, and so forth, to the primary provider's office electronically. In fact, some systems automatically input this data. Thus the provider is immediately aware of significant changes. Client use of EHRs via use of Internet portals will be further described in Chapter 26.

NURSING DOCUMENTATION

We need to communicate care our client received. Timely and accurate documentation of care given is crucial to providing team members with the information they need to make informed decisions (Byrne, 2012). The primary purpose of documentation is to maintain an exchange of information about the client among all care providers. Documentation in EHRs supports the continuity, quality, and safety of your client's care. Good documentation not only improves communication about the admitting diagnosis but also may increase recognition of comorbid conditions that can then also be treated (Towers, 2013). Standards of documentation must meet the requirements of government, health care agency, professional standards of practice, accreditation standards, third-party payers, and the legal system. Every health care agency has its own version of what constitutes complete clinical documentation. Medicare has published guidelines for primary providers saying documentation should include a client history (a database that often includes a summary list of health problems and needs); physical examination findings; a description of the presenting problem; and rationales for decision making, counseling, and coordination of care in a client-centered care plan. Nursing documentation contains a daily record of client progress and evaluation of outcomes. Daily records may include flow sheets, nursing notes, intake and output forms, and medication records. Some data, such as vital signs, are automatically recorded into the EHR.

CLARITY

Information should flow in an efficient manner so all members of the team have access to current data, so they are able to do ongoing evaluations of treatment outcomes. Such improvements in communication lead to improved outcomes for clients. Try thinking of it this way: Every task sequence you perform requires you to access data before and after completion to maintain continuity. As you chart continually, entering information into the system, communication among the health team is improved.

HIT should enhance communication. In one example, nurses in a study by Nemeth and colleagues (2007) accessed current laboratory test results at the point of care, allowing them to discuss changes in care during home visits. A specific example might be instant access to laboratory results on blood clotting time, allowing you to contact the physician for a change in anticoagulation medication levels while you are still at your client's home.

Clear documentation means using standardized terms that are understood by every member of the health team. Documentation of care must be accurate. For example, you are expected to document the presence on admission of catheters and intravenous lines, as well as facts about the status of any decubiti (bed sores).

Efficiency

Access time to records should be enhanced using HIT systems. For example, when using paper files, it took a lengthy time to do audits for agency quality assurance or by insurance companies verifying reimbursement.

Some literature suggests that nurses feel caught between the demands for meeting all their client care needs and the agency requirements for complete documentation. But the majority of evidence shows that EHRs actually save time, allowing staff nurses more time at the bedside (Keenen et al., 2008; Yee et al., 2012). Evidence shows this is especially true when the agency has terminals or devices for charting at the bedside. The potential impact of EHRs on nursing efficiency is measured by a reduction in the amount of time you spend doing activities other than direct nursing care of your client. Computerization improves the efficiency and quality of charting, by prompting for information needed, while eliminating duplication. For example, instead of re-questioning your client about health history, this information is already available on his or her EHR. Efficiency is increased because providers all across the agency have immediate access to client information. Thompson and colleagues (2009) list HIT benefits that improve nursing efficiency in other "downstream" ways beyond what is apparent in documentation activities, such as medication record resolution, automatic medication calculations, automatic downloading of bedside monitoring records, automated nursing discharge summaries, and so forth. Capability to document your care from your client's bedside or home is known as "point of care" and is described in Chapter 26.

COMPLETENESS

The literature suggests that nurses have ambivalent feelings about their documentation in HIT systems. Is it possible to fully document all nursing care given? Lack of visibility seems to be a recurring theme. Nurses complain that the individualized care they give their clients is not visible in the format demanded by the computer, especially when a checklist format is used for care. Consequently some nurses are said to rely on "informal" communication about their client passed along during change of shift as well as the information on the client's EHR. Records that are inaccurate or incomplete compromise clinical decisions and quality of care reporting (Chtourou, 2013). Communicate your client's current condition and response to treatment in the record.

ENHANCED QUALITY OF CARE
Safety

As discussed in Chapter 4, HIT systems have made care safer. HIT systems force standardization of nursing terminology, eliminate use of inappropriate abbreviations, and avoid problems of illegibility. Errors are prevented because assistance is given with drug calculations, as well as assistance with decision support such as checking drug incompatibility, allergies, and so on. Studies of the medication process show errors or potential errors cut by half (Radley et al., 2013).

Documentation to Demonstrate Quality

A major shift in health care has moved emphasis toward achievement of quality outcome indicators. Financial incentives reward evidence of clinical quality rather than volume (Dolin, 2014). The United States (Agency for Healthcare Quality and Research [AHRQ], n.d.) has adopted a **National Quality Strategy** outlining three aims:

1. Better health care
2. Healthier people
3. More affordable care

Reviews are done to determine the extent to which evidence-based care standards are being met. Ongoing reviews of care are done by internal agency review committees, as well as external audits by entities such as insurance companies or government regulatory bodies, such as those associated with the Centers for Medicare and Medicaid Services (CMS). Assessments as to quality of care are based on what was documented and coded. Data are examined to see whether the care listed is in compliance with quality and safety guidelines and established standards of care. Clear documentation also provides evidence of effective care and client outcomes during accreditation reviews. Evidence is slowly accumulating that shows HIT systems can make health care more client-centered, by engaging clients as partners, promoting better coordination of care, and making communication more effective.

Aggregation of Data

Computerized systems offer ease of access to **aggregate** information from many clients for reports, disease surveillance, and to research "best practice" nursing care.

Health Outcomes. Aggregated information from a number of records can be analyzed to determine client health outcomes. For example, information about the number of postoperative infections that have occurred on your unit can be obtained. Or you may want to find out how many diabetic clients in your primary care practice failed to return for follow-up teaching and then generate a list for call-backs for more education. Keepnews and colleagues (2004) demonstrated that a HIT system could be used to obtain reports about predictors of client outcomes in home health care. For example, you can easily get information identifying the most effective specific nursing interventions to establish "best practice" and identify other interventions that need to be changed.

Evidence for Best Practice

Nurses use HIT systems to identify contributions nurses make to attain better client outcomes. For example, in a study examining nurse adherence to clinical guidelines, results showed significant correlation with improved diabetic foot care (Rolley, 2012). By combining data, nurses identify better treatment methods and evaluate the outcomes of their interventions on groups of clients. Data can be used to compile reports, not just to government agencies, but internally to improve practice within your agency. Many HIT systems have not utilized nursing terminologies and coding, making it more difficult for nursing care to be aggregated to identify best practice.

Timely feedback from data compilation organizations can help you improve your practice. As an example, participation in centralized disease registries can give real-time feedback to providers, and participants in the National Cancer Data System can receive electronic "alerts" if best practice care is not started within a certain time frame.

Epidemiological Data

Combining data from many clients quickly can speed identification of adverse outcomes. For example, public health agencies analyze information to identify disease trends to generate epidemiologic information. One example would be when a government agency such as the Centers for Disease Control analyzes the spread of influenza across the world. In another example, Kaiser Permanente was able to analyze information from 1.3 million clients receiving Vioxx to identify potential harm from this medication, which led to its removal from the market.

USE OF COMPUTERIZED PROVIDER ENTRY SYSTEMS

Computerized provider order entry (CPOE) refers to that part of HIT in which providers such as physicians, physician assistants, nurse practitioners, or sometimes staff nurses directly enter their orders for diagnosis or treatment, which then transmits the order directly to the recipient responsible for carrying out that order, such as the pharmacy, the laboratory, or radiology. At a minimum, this aspect of the system assures that orders are complete, use standard terms, and are available in a legible format. But this system not only processes an order, it cross compares it with data in the client's EHR such as whether the client is allergic to this newly ordered medication, has a potential for a drug-drug adverse interaction, or whether the dose or route ordered exceeds standard guidelines for safety. CPOE may also check for errors of omission. For example, it would give a prompt about a need to also order a laboratory test to verify acceptable blood level of the new medication. CPOE systems are usually paired with computer-assisted **clinical decisional support systems** (CDSS), which are discussed in Chapter 26.

Outcomes for Use of Computerized Provider Entry

Evidence is beginning to suggest that use of these systems improve the appropriateness of orders, positively affect communication, and improve client outcomes, particularly by reducing adverse drug events and even increasing client compliance (AHRQ PSNet; Finkelstein et al., 2012; McKibbon et al., 2011). Computerized provider order entry (CPOE) is one of thirty "safe practices for better health care" recommended by AHRQ and the National Quality Forum. However, there is still some potential for error (Nanji et al., 2011). Nurses still need to employ critical thinking skills to evaluate for safe practice, especially in the area of medication administration.

OTHER FORMATS FOR DOCUMENTING NURSING CARE

Use of structured documentation has been found to be associated with more complete nursing records, better

continuity of care, more meaningful nursing data, and perhaps with better client outcomes. In charting electronically, the nurse can call up a template to record today's data. There is some evidence that use of EHRs that provide reminders or "prompts" results in more complete documentation.

Flow Sheets or Checklists

Electronic charting can use **flow sheets** with predefined client progress parameters based on written standards with preprinted categories of information. They contain daily assessments of normal findings. For example, in assessing lung sounds, the nurse needs to merely indicate "clear" if that information is normal. Deviations from norm must be completely documented. By marking a flow sheet or checklist, you are saying all care was performed according to existing agency protocols.

PLAN OF CARE

Nursing care plans are still valued by nursing instructors as a tool for student learning. However, in the age of electronic records in hospitals, clinics, and long-term care facilities, the traditional nursing care plans for each client are being replaced by electronic **longitudinal plans of care (LPCs).**

A plan of care basically uses the interdisciplinary team to set goals for each client's progress. Using it, the nurse and other team members daily document client progress toward those goals. Plans of care use best evidence standards related to the client's diagnoses and adapts these to meet the client's specific needs. In the hospital or long-term care facility, nurses have the major responsibility to participate in establishing interdisciplinary plans and then to daily document each client's progress toward these goals. Clinical pathways stating daily client goals have mostly either been incorporated into the EHR or been replaced by electronic prompts.

Electronic Longitudinal Plans of Care

CMS, in an effort to reduce regulations for hospitals, has issued a recommendation that nurses coordinate client care through use of interdisciplinary care plans (replacing nursing care plans). U.S. Department of Health and Human Services, the national HIT office, and CMS issued a single plan of care format to assist in communication, coordination, and continuity.

The plan of care needs to be accessible to all providers across all settings (Cipriano et al., 2013). Data from every discipline on the health care team is used to develop a single individualized interdisciplinary plan of care that best addresses a client's needs. Sophisticated electronic plans of care are being developed within HIT to replace the care plans previously used just within a single discipline such as nursing, because these siloed plans were less likely to result in true patient-centered care. According to Cipriano, the plan of care must harmonize data requirements for home care, long-term care, acute and post-acute care; this is the patient-centered LPC.

STANDARDS: ETHICAL, REGULATORY, AND PROFESSIONAL

The use of electronic medical records and storage of personal health information in computer databases has refocused attention on the issues of ethics, security, privacy, and confidentiality that are described earlier in this book. For example, a nurse in one unit of a hospital who accesses the electronic medical record of a client who is in another unit and for whom the nurse has no responsibilities for care is violating confidentiality. Ethical professional practice requires that you do not allow others to use your access log on. Other ethical issues with electronically-generated care plans and standard orders center on how to determine who is responsible for the computer-generated care decisions.

CONFIDENTIALITY AND PRIVACY

The Institute of Medicine defines **confidentiality** as the act of limiting disclosure of private matters appropriately, maintaining the trust that an individual has placed in an agent entrusted with private matters. In the United States, most states have laws that grant the client ownership rights to the information contained in the client's health record. Electronic storage and transmission of medical records have sparked intense scrutiny over privacy protection. More than two-thirds of consumers express concerns that their personal health records stored in an EHR with Internet connections will not remain private. Ethical and legal parameters limit with whom you can share client information. In the future, rules will be expanded to include associated businesses, imposing more rigorous penalties.

When computers are located at the bedside, the screen displays information to anyone who stops by the bedside. You need to be alert to this potential violation of your client's privacy. Violations of confidentiality because of unauthorized access or distribution of sensitive health information can have severe consequences for clients. It may lead to discrimination at the workplace, loss of job opportunities, or disqualification for health insurance. Issues of privacy will dominate how nurses and other health care providers address clinical documentation in the years ahead. Currently, a **personal medical identification number** is used on client records. Hardware safeguards such as workstation security, keyed lock hard drives, and automatic log-offs are used in addition to user identification and passwords to prevent unauthorized access. Some advocate that clients be able to choose how much of their information is shared and be notified when their information is accessed. In the United States, federal law now requires clients be notified in the event of a breach of their EHR. Authorization is not needed in situations concerning the public's health, criminal, or legal matters. Refer to Chapter 2 for federal medical record privacy regulations (Health Insurance Portability and Accountability Act [HIPAA]).

LEGAL ASPECTS OF CHARTING

Management literature emphasizes the need for quicker documentation that still reflects the nursing process. At the same time, documentation must be legally sound. The legal assumption is that the care was not given unless it is documented in the client's record, which is a legal document, even though it is digital. Malpractice settlements have approached the multimillion-dollar mark for individuals whose charts failed to document safe, effective care.

"If it was not charted, it was not done." This statement stems from a legal case (*Kolesar v. Jeffries*) heard before Canada's Supreme Court, in which a nurse failed to document the care of a client on a Stryker frame before he died. Because the purpose of the medical record is to list care given and client outcomes, any information that is clinically significant must be included. Legally, all care must be documented. Aside from issues of legal liability, third-party reimbursement depends on accurate recording of care given. Major insurance companies audit client records and contest any charges that are not documented. Every nurse should anticipate having their clients' records subpoenaed at some time during their nursing career (refer to Box 25-1 for recommendations).

BOX 25-1	Documentation Tips

Content

- Chart promptly, but never ahead of time. Do not wait until end of shift.
- Document complete care reflecting the nursing process.
- Document all noncooperative or bizarre behavior.
- Document all refusals of ordered treatments.
- Document teaching (information you gave the client and/or family).
- When care or medicine is omitted, document action and rationale (who was notified and what was said).
- Document all significant changes in the client's condition and who was notified, as well as your nursing interventions.

Mistakes to Avoid

- Failing to record complete, pertinent health information
- Making "untimely" entries (e.g., charting after the fact, passed the day)
- Failing to record drug administration, route, outcome
- Not recording all nursing actions
- Recording on the wrong chart
- Failing to document a discontinued medication
- Failing to record outcome of an intervention such as a medicine
- Writing about mistakes or incident reports in the client record; incident reports are stored separately.

Developing an Evidence-Based Practice

Hyde E, Murphy B: Computerized clinical pathways (care plans): piloting a strategy to enhance quality patient care, *Clin Nurse Spec* 26(5):277-282, 2012.

The purpose of this study was to provide a basis for transitioning paper clinical pathways into digital, which are part of the client's electronic health record. The pilot used one computerized pathway on a specific medical-surgical unit. Prompts were built in, for example, as alerts to prompt staff to educate the client.

Results: There was a 60% increase in client teaching; a 10% increase in documentation of client medication teaching; a 31% increase in documentation by ancillary staff using the computerized pathway; and a 69% increase in documentation of barriers to client progression and utilization of the problem list. The pilot was so successful the administration decided to develop system-wide computerized pathways.

Application to Your Clinical Practice: The authors conclude that electronic records need to be accessible to all and complement the day-to-day work flow. While you may be writing nursing care plans as a student learning exercise, health care agencies are developing interdisciplinary electronic longitudinal plans of care. How would you respond to electronic prompts, knowing that evidence on your unit showed clients would have improved outcomes?

Any method of documentation that provides comprehensive, factual information is legally acceptable. This includes graphs and checklists. By signing a protocol, check sheet, pathway, and so forth, you are documenting that every step was performed. If a protocol exists in a health care agency, you are legally responsible for carrying it out.

ACCOUNTABILITY

We in health care will increasingly focus on measures that matter. HIT allows us to develop data for multiple levels of accountability, including for individual nurses, units, or agencies. There is a move to make health care outcomes more transparent to consumers. For example, some hospital web sites now post their infection rates. Just as there are web sites that post customer evaluations of individual hotels, there are sites such as CMC's site www.hospitalcompare.com that post client comments about their care and their caregivers by name.

APPLICATIONS

COMPUTER LITERACY

One of the QSEN competencies expected of the new graduate is ability to use **informatics.** To practice nursing in coming years, you will need to continually upgrade your technology skills. As students, you learn skills such as data entry, data transmission, word processing, Internet accessing, spreadsheet entry, and use of standard language and codes describing practice. Voice recognition software may eventually revolutionize clinical documentation, making documentation easier for nurses.

COMMUNICATING MEDICAL ORDERS

WRITTEN ORDERS

Nurses are required to question orders that they do not understand or those that seem to them to be unsafe.

Failure to do so puts the nurse at *legal risk*. "Just following orders" is not an acceptable excuse. Conversely, nurses can be held liable if they arbitrarily decide not to follow a legitimate order, such as choosing to withhold ordered pain medication. Reasons for such a decision would have to be explicitly documented. With computerization, it is possible to have standing orders, such as for administering vaccines. The computer is programmed to recognize the absence of a vaccination and then to automatically write an order for a nurse to administer. What might the legal implications be?

Persons licensed or certified by appropriate government agencies to conduct medical treatment acts include physicians, advance practice nurses, and physician assistants. These providers have their own state prescribing numbers and must abide by government rules and restrictions. To prescribe controlled substances they must also have a Drug Enforcement Agency (DEA) number. Nurse practitioners may choose not to apply for a DEA number. Consult your agency policy regarding who is allowed to write client orders for the nurse to carry out.

FAXED ORDERS

The physician or nurse practitioner may choose to send a faxed order. Because this is a form of written order, it has been shown to decrease the number of errors that occur when transcribing verbal or telephone orders. However, there is the risk for violating client confidentiality when faxing health-related information. See the American Health Information Management Association's general guidelines for faxing medical orders (Hughes, 2001).

VERBAL ORDERS

Often, a change in client condition requires the nurse to telephone the primary physician or hospital staff resident to obtain new orders. Most primary providers work in group practices, so it is necessary to determine who is "on call" or who is covering your client when the primary provider is unavailable. It may be necessary to call for new orders if there is a significant change in the client's physical or mental condition as noted by vital signs, laboratory value reports, treatment or medication reactions, or response failure. Before calling for verbal orders, obtain the chart and familiarize yourself with current vital signs, medications, infusions, and other relevant data. Read Chapter 4 on using the SBAR (situation, background, assessment, recommendation) format to communicate with doctors.

With the growth of unlicensed personnel, there is greater likelihood that a verbal order will be relayed through someone with this status. The legality is vague, but basically, if harm comes to the client through miscommunication of a verbal order, you (the licensed nurse) will be held responsible. Reflect on what you might do differently when Dr. Uganda calls.

Case Example:

Tracy Smith, the secretary on your unit, answers the telephone. Dr. Uganda gives her an order for a medication for a client. Tracy asks him to repeat the order as soon as she gets a registered nurse to take the call. If you cannot answer the telephone immediately, have her tell him you will call back in 5 minutes to verify the order.

CHARTING FOR OTHERS

It is not acceptable to chart for others. Reflect on what you would do in the following case if you were called by Juanita Diaz, RN.

Case Example:

Juanita Diaz worked the day shift. At 6 p.m. she calls you and says she forgot to chart Mr. Reft's preoperative enema. She asks you to chart the procedure and his response to it. Can you just add it to your notes? In court this would be portrayed as an inaccuracy. The correct solution is to chart, "1800: Nurse Juanita Diaz called and reported…"

WORKLOAD AND WORK-AROUNDS

In their review of multiple studies, Ranji and colleagues (2013) suggest that during the initial phase of becoming knowledgeable about using computerized records, some nurses perceive adverse impact on their workload and on their ability to care for their clients. Nurses carry heavy workloads and do not like technology that disrupts or adds to their work flow. For example, "alarm fatigue" was described in Chapter 4. To avoid burden, some nurses create shortcuts to bypass aspects of the computerized system, known as "work-arounds." This raises safety concerns and was also discussed in Chapter 4. Brecher (2014) urges us to report system problems including computer issues as well as reporting our errors so we can work together to create a safer system.

DOCUMENTING ON A CLIENT'S HEALTH RECORD

Documenting electronically requires learning the specific system at your agency. There is a learning curve; that is, initially it may take longer, but as you become familiar with the system, EHRs should increase your nursing efficiency. Electronic charting for nurses usually combines dropdown boxes with forced choice pick lists with free text boxes for narrative information. Keep in mind the need to use standardized terminology and where possible to use checklists. These allow for combining information into large data sets to examine client outcomes for the purpose of establishing "best practices."

You are encouraged to document completely and not to rely on checklists that may not entirely describe changes in your client's status or outcomes of your care. Use Exercise 25-1 to stimulate discussion of appropriate documentation. But remember that free text boxes may have word count limits. Also, narrative comments may provide needed detail, but they may also perpetuate the electronic invisibility of nursing unless information can be captured into categories (Byrne, 2012). Tips for efficient documentation include use of checklists and flow sheets; not repeating any of this information in the narrative; proofreading narrative comments and running spellcheck; checking all numbers to detect transpositions; and avoiding abbreviations.

KEEPING THE INTERPERSONAL WHILE DOING COMPUTERIZED CHARTING

Nurses have also reported reservations about unintended effects on their communication with clients. Though some clients complain, most have adapted to providers who spend time not making eye contact or pausing the dialog because they are busy typing data into the EHR. According to HealthIT, 74% of patients report that EHRs have enhanced their care. How would you manage communication rapport during a client interview, when the HIT system keeps prompting you to obtain data?

Make documenting at the bedside warmer in a human relation sense. If your client seems to be bothered by the lack of interpersonal contact while you are busy typing on the bedside computer, what steps could you take? One suggestion is to face the computer terminal toward the client, so you do not turn your back to him while typing information. Some nurses comment aloud about the general information they are inputting, stopping every minute or so to make eye contact with their client. Asking your client for information and then typing it in may make them realize they are actively contributing to their EHR information. Also explaining about how these entries are keeping the team aware of updated information about the client's condition may help them value this process.

CONFIDENTIALITY

Ethical and legal dilemmas inherent in use of computerized systems require continued vigilance, especially regarding the concern of protecting client privacy. As cases come to court, a body of case law will provide some guidance. As discussed in Chapter 2, HIPAA regulations that mandate right to privacy are the current guidelines. You need to become aware of threats to privacy and your

---

EXERCISE 25-1	Documenting Nursing Diagnoses

Purpose: To help students clarify diagnoses.

Procedure
Discuss in small groups which of the following examples help provide a direction for independent nursing interventions.

Example 1
Incorrect: Inability to communicate related to deafness
   Suggested: Impaired social interaction (00052) related to anatomical (auditory), as evidenced by refusal to interact with others

Discussion
What additional information is provided in the correct diagnosis? Why would the first statement be incorrect? Are all people who are deaf unable to communicate?

Example 2
Incorrect: Acute lymphocytic leukemia
   Suggested: Acute pain (00132) during ambulation related to leukemia disease process, as evidenced by limping, grimacing, and increased pulse

Discussion
Could a nurse make any independent intervention based on the information provided by the diagnosis "acute lymphocytic leukemia"?

Coding Nursing Practice Provides Information:

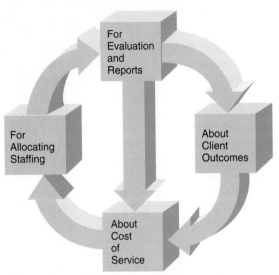

Figure 25-3   Coding in nursing practice.

obligation to protect your clients' privacy where possible. Discuss the ethical dilemma provided.

CODING

As shown in Fig. 25-3, coding allows nursing information to be easily communicated and extracted from EHRs for the purpose of compiling information to make cross comparisons: evaluations, audits, research, or develop standards of care. A prerequisite for this was to move nursing terminology to a standard taxonomy. It is crucial to nursing that nursing terminologies become embedded into EHRs, both to improve communication between nurses, such as at change of shift, and to allow data to be extracted to describe nursing care.

Codes for care, treatments, procedures, medications, and so on are accessed by insurance company employees to verify that items billed for are recorded as care actually delivered before they will reimburse for that care. If a heart medication is given, then data must be recorded documenting the existence of the heart problem.

CLASSIFICATION OF CARE: USE OF STANDARDIZED TERMINOLOGIES AND TAXONOMIES

The nursing profession was very active in developing **coding systems** for the classification of nursing care.

Nursing must classify the care provided and the outcomes of that care, in order to effectively communicate, document, and get reimbursed for its essential role in the health care of the individual, family, and community.

GOAL FOR THE CLASSIFICATION OF NURSING CARE

Problem statements, interventions, and outcomes recorded using a standard language communicate a commonly understood message across a variety of health care settings. These terms are consistent with the scope of nursing practice. When standardized language is used to document practice, we can compare and evaluate effectiveness of our care, regardless of which nurse in which setting is delivering this care. In the past, nursing has been unable to describe the units of care, its effect on client outcome, or to establish a cost for its contributions to client care. Nowhere on a client's hospital bill does the cost of our nursing care appear. It traditionally has been part of the "room charge." The goals of developing standardized terminology and classification codes are to improve communication, to make nursing practice visible within (computerized) health information systems, and to assist in establishing evidence-based nursing practice.

DEVELOPING CLASSIFICATIONS FOR CODING

Use of a standardized nursing classification language clearly describes clients' needs, interventions used, and the outcomes of care. Communication among staff members is improved across the continuum of primary care, acute care, long-term care, and home care practice. The time spent teaching, providing support, and assisting in grieving are the types of nursing activities that nurses spend considerable time doing, yet they rarely show up in the medical record. In home health records, nurses most often document nursing problems or diagnoses related to the medical diagnosis, but some report they actually spend most of their care in client teaching.

TAXONOMIES: STANDARDIZED LANGUAGE TERMINOLOGY IN NURSING

ANA recognizes a number of different taxonomies for describing nursing care, based on specific criteria. Because no one system meets the needs of nurses in all areas of practice, technologic applications are needed to communicate across classification systems.

EXERCISE 25-2   **Application of Nursing Intervention Classification Finding**

Purpose: To make use of Nursing Interventions Classification (NIC) meaningful.

Procedure

Consider the following finding from Dochterman's (2005) study, then answer the questions.

On Day 3 of hospitalization, nurses averaged four intravenous therapy interventions for clients with a diagnosis of hip fracture but averaged only two interventions for (oral) fluid management.

1. How could you use this information to justify the need for skilled nursing care?
2. Suppose data showed that by Day 6, skilled care activities had been cut in half. How might

the nurse manager readjust the client assignment for her nurse aides?

On Day 3, clients with hip fractures received three times as many nursing interventions encouraging proper coughing as were made for clients with congestive heart failure.

1. Speculate about why there was this difference.
2. Suppose hospital units with more nursing interventions to encourage coughing were shown to have greatly decreased rates of clients with pneumonia complications. Could this information be used to justify a better nurse-to-client ratio?

From Dochterman J, Titler M, Wang J, et al.: Describing use of nursing interventions for three groups of patients, *J Nurs Scholarsh* 37(1):57-66, 2005.

Taxonomy is defined as a hierarchical method of classifying a vocabulary of terms according to certain rules. Various taxonomies have been developed to be used in communication and comparisons across health care settings and providers, insurers and payers, and policy makers who set priorities and allocate resources. So far, the international nursing community has not agreed on one common terminology. Evidence suggests that North American Nursing Diagnosis Association International (NANDA-I) is the best researched and most widely implemented nursing classification internationally.

The N3 terminologies (NANDA-I, Nursing Interventions Classification [NIC], and Nursing Outcomes Classification [NOC]), used together to plan and document nursing care, are sometimes referred to as **NNN.** Their use creates a systematic schema for implementing the nursing process.

North American Nursing Diagnosis Association International

NANDA-I uses domains based on Gordon's Functional Health Patterns with diagnoses of actual problems, at-risk for diagnoses, potential problems or syndromes in illness, as well as wellness diagnoses. A nursing diagnosis is a clinical judgment about responses to actual or potential health problems and/or life processes. They provide the basis for your choice of nursing interventions. A nursing diagnosis is not another name for a medical diagnosis; rather, it delineates areas for independent nursing actions.

Nursing Interventions Classification

This classification of nursing interventions was developed as a standardized language that names and defines an intervention you will use to give direct and indirect care. The interventions are actions that nurses perform in settings relevant to illness prevention, illness treatment, and health promotion. Nursing interventions are classified in domains such as physiologic, behavioral, safety, and so forth. Under each domain are classes and under the classes are the specific interventions that you can modify to meet your client's needs. Each nursing intervention has a unique code number and thus can be computerized and potentially could be used to reimburse the nurse. Try exercise 25-2, above.

Nursing Outcomes Classification

NOC provides a standard language to name and define client outcomes attained through nursing actions to communicate among nurses and across settings. NOC complements NANDA-I and NIC and provides a language and coding numbers for evaluating the nursing process. An outcome assesses the client's actual status on specific behaviors (indicators) using a five-point scale, ranging from 1 (severely compromised function) to 5 (function not compromised). Table 25-2 provides an example of the linked use of N3 (Nanda, NIC, NOC).

The Omaha System

Omaha System was initiated to address the needs of community health nurses, managers, and administrators.

| TABLE 25-2 | N3: Example of Linkages of North American Nursing Diagnosis Association, Nursing Interventions Classification, and Nursing Outcomes Classification |

Nursing Diagnosis	Nursing Outcome (rate each indicator on 1-5 scale)	Nursing Intervention
Chronic Pain (Domain: Perceived Health V)	Pain Control—1605	Pain Management
Defining Characteristics:	*Indicators:*	*Nursing Activities:*
• Sudden or slow onset	Recognizes pain onset—160502	Determine impact of pain on quality of life.
• Consistent or reoccurring	Uses analgesics as recommended—160505	Evaluate effectiveness of past pain-control measures.
• Duration >6 months	Uses diary to monitor symptoms over time—160510	Administer analgesics as prescribed.
	Reports symptom changes to provider—160513	Administer or teach client nonpharmacologic measures of pain control (such as massage, biofeedback, heat/cold, guided imagery, music therapy, therapeutic touch).
	Reports pain controlled—160511	Use pain-control measures before pain increases.
		Promote adequate rest.
		Teach client to monitor own pain levels.

Modified from Bulechek GM, Butcher HK, Dochterman J (McCloskey): *Nursing classification (NIC)*, ed 5, St. Louis, 2008, Mosby/Elsevier; Johnson M, Bulechek G, Dochterman JM et al.: *Nursing diagnosis, outcomes, and interventions: NANDA, NOC, and NIC linkages*, St. Louis, 2001, Mosby; Moorhead M, Johnson M, Maas M, Swanson E: *Nursing outcomes classification (NOC)*, ed 4, St. Louis, 2008, Mosby/Elsevier.

The **Omaha System** is a comprehensive practice, documentation, and information management tool.

ADVANTAGES AND DISADVANTAGES OF NURSING CLASSIFICATION SYSTEMS

Nursing classification systems provide a standard and common language for nursing care so that nursing contributions to client care become visible and define professional practice. Standardized terminologies allow nursing research to explore nursing interventions and outcomes for common problems to identify "best practices" (Tseng, 2013). ANA says that standards for terminology are an essential requirement for a computer-based patient record (ANA, 2012).

Standardized nursing languages need to convince the business and medical interests managing health care agencies of the need to incorporate nursing classification codes as part of their information technology systems. The greatest problem has been that nursing classifications have not been thoroughly incorporated into many agency's electronic clinical records.

OTHER CODING SYSTEMS IN HEALTH CARE

The National Library of Medicine maintains a metathesaurus for a unified medical language. Because of the complexity of health care and the variety of providers involved, multiple medical classification systems have emerged. Often providers use several in combination. A major drawback for nursing is that use of computerized documentation systems based on medical code numbers often forces nurses to use classification systems designed to describe medical practice instead of describing nursing assessment and care of clients. In doing so, the richness of the nursing care provided often goes undocumented. Common medical classification and coding systems include tenth revision of the International Statistical Classification of Diseases and Related Health Problems (ICD-10) codes for medical diagnoses by body system; ICD-10-PCS codes for medical procedures; and the fifth edition of the *Diagnostic and Statistical Manual of Mental Disorders* (DSM-5) diagnoses for psychiatric conditions (Kupfer et al., 2013).

THE JOINT COMMISSION COMPUTERIZED DOCUMENTATION GUIDELINES

The Joint Commission has developed standards for uniform data for agencies it accredits. In the past, The Joint Commission required that nurses repeat information recorded by the physician. Now, nursing documentation may consist merely of updating.

OUTCOME AND ASSESSMENT INFORMATION SET

Beginning in 1998, home care agencies phased in a new requirement to complete a functional health assessment on all Medicare clients before they begin care. The results of the assessment feed into a standardized database. The Health Care Financing Administration (HCFA) developed the Outcome and Assessment Information Set (OASIS) assessment for the purpose of describing home care clients, developing outcome benchmarks, and providing feedback regarding quality of care to home health agencies. The OASIS assessment is required for home health agencies to receive reimbursement for the care provided to Medicare recipients.

To learn more, visit HCFA's Medicare web site (www.medicare.gov/).

REFERENCE TERMINOLOGY SYSTEMS THAT EXCHANGE DATA BETWEEN CLASSIFICATION SYSTEMS

ANA recognizes two reference terminologies that can translate the terms between the various classification systems. These allow us to retrieve data even when agencies use several different classification systems. Systematized nomenclature of medical-clinical terms (SNOMED-CT) is the most comprehensive reference of medical terminology from many health care languages. Logical Observation Identifiers Names and Codes (LOINC) provides electronic exchange of data from many classification systems. For example, it includes terms from the Omaha System and the Nursing Management Minimum Data Set.

SUMMARY

This chapter focuses on electronic documentation of care in the nurse-client relationship. Documentation refers to the process of obtaining, organizing, and conveying information to others in the client record. Discussion of HIT, including the nurse's role in using EHRs, emphasized its role in reducing redundancy, improving efficiency, reducing cost, decreasing errors, and improving compliance with standards of practice. Chapter 26 discusses technology that can facilitate communication among health care workers, increase client education, and assist the providers of health care with decision making.

ETHICAL DILEMMA | What Would You Do?

You work in an organization with a computerized clinical documentation system. A coworker mentions that Alice Jarvis, RN, has been admitted to the medical floor for some strange symptoms and that her laboratory results have just been posted, showing she is positive for hepatitis C, among other things.

1. Identify at least two alternative ways to deal with this ethical dilemma. (What response would you make to your coworker who retrieved information from the computerized system? What else might you do?)
2. What ethical principle can you cite to support each answer?

From Sonya R. Hardin, RN, PhD, CCRN.

DISCUSSION QUESTIONS

1. Which of the five reasons to document do you expect to be most concerned with as a novice staff nurse?
2. Discuss why "use of technologies to assist in effective communication in a variety of health care settings" is listed as an expected nurse competency by QSEN and other nursing organizations.

REFERENCES

Keenan GM, Yakel E, Tschannen D, Mandeville M: Chapter 49: Documentation and the Nurse Care Planning Process. In Hughes RG, Rockville MD, editors: *Patient Safety and Quality: An Evidence-Based Handbook for Nurses*, Agency for Healthcare Quality and Research (AHRQ), 2008. Accessed January 4, 2014 http://www.ahrq.gov/professionals/clinicians-providers/resources/nursing/resources/nurseshdbk/KeenanG_DNCPP.pdf.

Agency for Healthcare Quality and Research (AHRQ) (n.d.). About the national quality strategy (NQS). Working for Quality. www.ahrq.gov/workingforquality/about.htm. Accessed January 12, 2014.

American Nurses Association (ANA): *Electronic Personal Health Record: ANA Position Statement*, 2012. Accessed September 20, 2013 http://nursingworld.org/MainMenuCategories/Policy-Advocacy/Positions-and-Resolutions/ANAPositionStatements/.

Ben-Assuli O, Leshno M: Using electronic medical records in admission decisions: A cost effectiveness analysis, *Decision Sci* 44(3):463–481, 2013.

Brecher D: A new year, *J Emerg Nurs* 40(1):1–2, 2014.

Bulechek GM, Butcher HK, Dochterman J: (McCloskey). *Nursing classification (NIC)*, ed 5, St. Louis, 2008, Mosby/Elsevier.

Byrne MD: Write the wrong: Narrative documentation, *J Perianesth Nurs* 27(3):1–4, 2012.

Chtourou H: CDI programs used to improve quality reporting accuracy, *J AHIMA* 84(7):50–51, 2013.

Cipriano PF, Bowles K, Dailey M, Dykes P, et al.: The importance of health information technology in care coordination and transitional care, *Nurs Outlook* 61:475–489, 2013.

CMS. Center for Medicare and Medicaid Services. www.cms.gov/ Accessed August 13, 2014.

Dochterman J, Titler M, Wang J, et al.: Describing use of nursing interventions for three groups of patients, *J Nurs Scholarsh* 37(1):57–66, 2005.

Dolin RH, Goodrich K, Kallem C: Getting the standard: EHR quality reporting rises in prominence due to meaningful use, *J AHIMA* 85(1):42–48, 2014.

Finkelstein J, Knight A, Marinopoulos S, et al.: Enabling patient-centered care through health information technology, *Evid Rep Technol Assess (Full Rep)* 206:1–1531, 2012. Accessed January 4, 2014.

HealthIT. (n.d.). www.HealthIT.gov/providers-professionals/benefits-electronic-health-records-ehrs Accessed August 13, 2014.

U.S. Department of Health and Human Services. (n.d.). Healthy People 2020. Health Communication and Health Information Technology. www.Healthypeople.gov/2020/topicsobjectives2020/overview.aspx?topicid=18/ Accessed August 12, 2014.

Heeter C: EHR progress and future development, *AORN J* 97(3):c7–c8, 2013.

Hughes G: Practice brief: facsimile transmission of health information (updated), *J AHIMA* 72(6):64E–64F, 2001.

Hyde E, Murphy B: Computerized clinical pathways (care plans): piloting a strategy to enhance quality patient care, *Clin Nurse Spec* 26(5):277–282, 2012.

The Joint Commission: Accessed September 17, 2013 www.jointcommission.org/Advancing_Effective_Communiation_Cultural_Competence_and_Patient, 2010.

Johnson M, Bulechek G, Dochterman JM, et al.: *Nursing diagnosis, outcomes, and interventions: NANDA, NOC, and NIC linkages*, St. Louis, 2001, Mosby.

Keepnews D, Capitman JA, Rosati RJ: Measuring patient-level clinical outcomes of home health care, *J Nurs Scholarsh* 35(1):79–85, 2004.

Kennedy A: Looking back and moving forward, *J AHIMA* 85(1):10, 2014. January 14.

Kupfer DJ, Kuhl EA, Regier DA: DSM-5-The future arrived, *JAMA* 309(16):1691–1692, 2013.

McCullough JS, Christianson J, Leerapan B: Do electronic medical records improve diabetes quality in physician practices? *Am J Manag Care* 19(2):144–149, 2013.

McKibbon KA, Lekker C, Handler SM, et al.: *Enabling Medication Management through Health Information Technology. Evidence Report/ Technology Assessment No. 201. Agency for Healthcare Research and Quality*, Rockville, 2011, MD.

Moorhead M, Johnson M, Maas M, Swanson E: *Nursing outcomes classification (NOC)*, ed 4, St. Louis, 2008, Mosby/Elsevier.

NANDA International: *Nursing diagnoses: definitions and classifications 2012–2014*. Philadelphia, 2011, Wiley-Blackwell. www.NANDA.org.

Nanji KC, Rothschild JM, Salzberg C, et al.: Errors associated with outpatient prescribing systems, *J Am Med Inform Assoc* 18:767–773, 2011.

Nemeth LS, Wessell AM, Jenkins RG, et al.: Strategies to accelerate translation of research into primary care with practices using electronic medical records, *J Nurs Care Qual* 22(4):343–349, 2007.

Agency for Healthcare Quality and Research (AHRQ). PSNet: Patient Safety Network. Patient Safety Primer: Computerized Provider Order Entry. http://psnet.ahrq.gov/printviewPrimer.aspx?primerID=6. Accessed September 2, 2013.

QSEN Institute. (n.d.) Quality and Safety Education for Nurses. www.QSEN.org/ Accessed May 21, 2013.

Radley DC, Wasserman MR, Olso L, Shoemaker SJ, et al.: Reduction in medication errors in hospitals due to adoption of computerized provider order entry systems, *J Am Med Inform Assoc* 20:470–476, 2013.

Ranji SR, Rennke S, Watcher RM: Chapter 41: Computerized provider order entry with clinical decision support systems: A brief update review. In Health Care Safer Making, editor: *An Updated Critical Analysis of the Evidence for Patient Safety Practices*, (2013). Evidence Report/Technology Assessment No. 211. Agency for Healthcare Quality and Research (AHRQ): Rockville, MD. Accessed June 29, 2013 II http://www.ahrq.gov/research/findings/evidence-based-reports/services/quality/ptsafetyII-full.pdf.

Rolley JX: Three-year follow-up after introduction of Canadian best practice guidelines for asthma and footcare in diabetes suggests that monitoring of nursing care indicators using electronic documentation system improves sustained implementation, *Evid Based Nurs* 15(1):5–6, 2012.

Thompson D, Johnston P, Spurr C, et al.: The impact of electronic medical records on nursing efficiency, *J Nurs Admin* 39(10):444–451, 2009.

Towers A: Clinical documentation improvement—A physician perspective, *J AHIMA* 84(7):34–43, 2013.

Tseng H: *Exploring nursing diagnoses, interventions, outcomes in oncology specialty units in an acute setting: The impact of the use of electronic standardized terminology*, Prague, 2013, Czech Republic. Paper presented at 24th Sigma Theta Tau, International Nursing Research Congress July 22–26.

Yee T, Needleman J, Pearson M, Parkerton P, et al.: The influences of integrated EMRs and computerized nurses' notes on nurses' time spent in documentation, *Comp Inform Nurs* 30(6):287–292, 2012.

CHAPTER 26

Communication at the Point of Care: Application of e-Health Technologies

Kathleen Underman Boggs

OBJECTIVES

At the end of the chapter, the reader will be able to:

1. Discuss applications available for wireless technologies used with decentralized "point-of-care" nursing communication.
2. Discuss the advantages and disadvantages of various assistive technologies for continual communication at point of care, as well as anytime, anywhere access.
3. Describe nurse advantages in using clinical guidelines and clinical decision support systems with regard to increasing information efficiently for delivery of safe, quality health care.
4. Analyze strengths and weaknesses of various health technologies in improving communications.
5. Distinguish between appropriate and inappropriate use of new technologies, such as texting and posts on social media sites.

Nursing is reliant on health information technology (HIT). Electronic communication is now a standard aspect of health care (Schickedanz et al., 2013). HIT provides remote access to client records in a timely, actionable, and portable fashion (Cipriano et al., 2013). The areas of major transformation changing our communication are:

- Electronic health record (EHR) and accompanying ordering and taxonomy (discussed in Chapter 25), allowing aggregation of data to develop "best practice" information.
- Handheld wireless devices and voice-activated systems, which allow continual **real-time interactive communication** of information, customized clinical decision making, and **decentralized, remote access** to client information at the point of care.
- Enhanced work flow through expanded use of "smart" technology devices, providing automatic data input, providing "alerts" and use of remote communication technology such as telehealth.

- Client engagement in interactive Internet programs enabling client communication for health promotion and self-management of diseases.

Nursing organizations, such as the National League for Nursing, advocate informatics proficiency for student nurses. Nursing students are expected to be capable of accessing real-time information and use EHRs to improve client care (Barnsteiner et al., 2013). Novice nurses are expected to be proficient in uses of digital technologies for communication and for information management (American Academy of Colleges of Nursing [AACN], 2008; Barnsteiner et al., 2013; Institute of Medicine [IOM] competency; QSEN Prelicensure Competency). In addition to the EHR management, technology used in client care management includes client monitoring systems and medication administration systems. All nurses are expected to be skillful in using technology to communicate and to keep abreast as innovations are introduced to help us meet professional standards and to manage care for our clients. *Being open to change* is now nursing's mantra. Broad use of HIT can improve our communication, the quality and safety of our care, and our efficiency. Electronic compilation of client outcome data should lead us to better decision making. An expected outcome of improved communication is decreases in health care costs over the long term. So in many ways HIT is moving beyond mere data storage toward a focus on making health care better (Crawford, 2014).

This chapter focuses on nurse and client use of electronic HIT to enhance **health care communication.** *Healthy People 2020* goals state that health communication strategies and HIT will be used to improve health outcomes and health care quality and to achieve health equality. *Healthy People 2020's* Objective HC/HIT2 says an increased proportion of persons will report that their health care providers have satisfactory communication skills, listening to them carefully and explaining things so they understand them. Is it not probable that new technology will play an increasing role in fostering this goal? This chapter also covers other HIT tools such as computerized clinical decision support systems (CDSSs), secure messaging, telehealth, remote monitoring, use of social media, Internet-based client use for education, support, health promotion, and disease self-management. Also discussed are Internet uses for nurses' professional education and access to clinical practice guidelines. Discussion of these emerging technologies is limited to a focus on their relation to information communication.

BASIC CONCEPTS

Evidence shows that emerging technologies facilitate our communication and teamwork. As noted in Chapter 25, interoperability is crucial. Health care information technologists are ideally working to establish **fully integrated computerized systems** that share information across the entire health care system. This will greatly increase care quality, improve safety, and provide relevant information and reminders to all. Portable electronic devices such as tablets and smartphones with Internet access are small enough to be easily carried. We refer to them in this book as **"handheld" devices.** These devices have Internet access, which we term "wireless." Decentralized access to information and ability to document your care at your client's location are referred to as **"point-of-care"** capability. You can use your handheld device to access nursing information databases to obtain evidence-based clinical

care interventions. You can document care while at your clients' bedsides and in their homes.

Case Example

Sam is a new graduate who is employed by Modern Medical on a medical unit. This hospital is part of a large health care system of primary care offices, clinics, laboratories, nursing homes, and three hospitals, all of which use the fully integrated computer system affectionately termed "Simon." Sam is notified at 0800 that his new client, Mrs. Sulif, is in admissions getting her bar-coded name bracelet with her picture image affixed to it. In admissions she is entering her own history information into "Simon," which has scanned her smart card. Dietary is flagged because she has nut allergies. Preadmission laboratory results are already in her electronic health record (EHR), having been sent there by her hometown lab tech, who notes the system has flagged her low hematocrit results and sent an "alert" to Sam and her admitting physician's office. Sam is also advised as to her need for handicapped accessible equipment. On the unit by 0845, a robot has delivered equipment to the room while Sam has summoned an orderly by text (instant messaging [IM]) to help lift Mrs. Sulif into bed wearing linen stored right in her room (refer to Transforming Care at the Bedside [TCAB]). Sam reviews the reason for admission and enters additional information into Mrs. Sulif's EHR using his handheld device. The intensivist physician examines her and enters his orders into the computerized provider order entry (CPOE) system, which simultaneously notifies the lab and pharmacy. Sam prints out lab tapes bar coded with Mrs. Sulif's identity number, sends off urine for analysis, and then checks the pneumatic tube for her STAT meds, which he administers after scanning her name band and double verifying her name orally.

1. Is the care described so far both safe and efficient?
2. What additional steps could make care more efficient?
3. When it is time for her transfer to the nursing home, what other communication should occur?

Technology is driving a major shift in our nursing practice. Health care is increasingly focused on patient-centered care, promoting greater client control of their own care. In the future, clients will use more and more technology **apps** (application programs) to communicate and to actively participate in their own care. Nursing should align our interventions to increase client engagement (Drenkard, 2014), as greater client involvement should lead to improved health outcomes.

Development of technology is advancing hundreds of times faster than at any previous time in history, although implementation is slower than desired. This chapter describes a few of the current choices. Nurses believe that technology should be designed to reduce the burden associated with work flows in documentation, medication administration, communication, orders, and obtaining equipment and supplies (Bolton et al., 2008). Nurses also say it is essential to have smart, portable, point-of-care devices to document and transmit information. But this technology must be user friendly, function well, and not add to existing workload or nurses will be dissatisfied. For technology to be effective and congruent with nursing expectations, nurses need to seek input into software design (Zadvinskis et al., 2014). If use is cumbersome, nurses will devise workarounds so they can complete their assigned care in a timely manner. Studies show, for example, that when an agency uses a combination of electronic and paper documentation, this impedes work flow. Some workarounds are potentially unsafe, as described in Chapter 4.

Governmental agencies in many countries have been funding use of eHealth technology and giving incentives to providers. Government programs mandate use of aspects of HIT. For example, in the United States, legislation requires that health care providers for some clients must do e-prescribing and must demonstrate "meaningful use" of EHRs by 2015 or face financial penalties (CMS, 2014; HealthIT.gov, 2009).

Statutes address the delivery of information to the point of care to enable more informed decisions about appropriate, more cost-effective medications. Active electronic participation by clients is seen as a way to alleviate demands on staff. Among others, the American Academy of Family Physicians supports the concept of a "medical home," embodying active client participation via e-mail, client use of Internet portals, and transmission of remote monitoring information.

DECENTRALIZED ACCESS: TECHNOLOGY FOR COMMUNICATING AT THE POINT OF CARE

Available electronic technology is revolutionizing our nursing care communication (Figure 26-1). In addition to the EHR discussed in Chapter 25, new handheld devices with Internet capability allow nurses decentralized access to client records, incorporating point-of-care information and documentation. Mobile wireless devices allow continual use of updated client

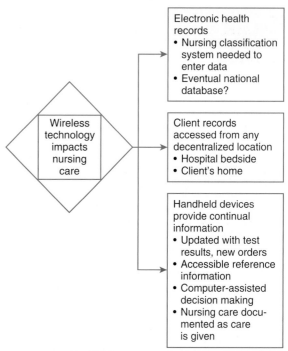

Figure 26-1   Health information technology: wireless technology impacts nursing care.

information and reference material at any client location. Communication in a timely manner is a standard of effective communication. Communication in "real time" is the hallmark of bedside nursing in the age of technology. With fiscal cutbacks, fewer nurses per client, and increased acuity of client situations, use of technology can enhance our **critical thinking**, **clinical decision making**, and **delivery of safe, efficient care** (Carter and Rukholm, 2008; HealthIT.gov(n.d.)).

HANDHELD WIRELESS DEVICES FOR ACCESS AT THE POINT OF CARE

Wireless handheld devices with Internet access are in common use, providing anytime, anywhere communication. Box 26-1 presents a summary of advantages and disadvantages for use of wireless technology by nurses. Nurses in out-patient community sites can have continual access to client records and databases with standards of care. Wireless devices can be used in the client's hospital room, in an outpatient clinic, or in the community—even in the client's home. Information can be stored, sent to your agency computer or directly to a printer. You can update your client's records including history, your assessment, the

BOX 26-1	Use of Wireless (Wi-Fi-Enabled) Handheld Devices

Advantages

- Improve the flow of communication, as well as work flow
- Easily portable; can be used at the point of care (client's bedside, in the home, etc.)
- Quick charting when nurse enters information by tapping menu selections
- Can contain reference resources about treatment, for medication dosage, and so forth, if uploaded
- Assists with customized decision making, reminders about standards of care, sends alerts
- Instant communication (e.g., nurse is signaled by beep regarding receipt of new information)
- Provide quick access to client records
- Provide clients with self-management tools
- Build support networks
- Provide a method of connecting with hard-to-reach clients

Disadvantages

- Possible threats to client's legal privacy rights.
- Nurse does not have a printed copy of information (until downloaded to agency printer).
- Small screen does not allow view of entire page of information.
- Technical problem may result in dysfunction and/or downtime.

problem list, or update other data and nursing notes. Your wireless handheld device can also be used to track information such as a client's medications and dosages or laboratory test results in a flow sheet format. For example, a nurse practitioner using a handheld device can call up a client's previous prescriptions, renew them at a touch, record this new information in the agency mainframe computer, correctly calculate the dosage of a new medication, write the order, and send this prescription to the client's pharmacy instantly— all without writing anything on paper.

Personal Digital Assistant

Personal digital assistant (PDA) is a generic term for any of several brands of small, handheld computerized electronic devices that fit in the palm of the nurse's hand. PDA apps can check for drug interactions, calculate dosages, analyze laboratory results, schedule procedures, order prescriptions, serve as a dictionary, or provide language translation, among other functions. It is easy to download reference sources, such as the latest medication information or disease treatment protocols.

PDAs can be taken to wherever the client is located. Most nurses seem to prefer use of **smartphones,** which do all of the above but also make phone calls.

Cellular Telephones

Ordinary cell phones can be used to locate clinicians, or verify and clarify information. Some hospitals are issuing mobile phones to staff nurses to use at work so they can directly contact physicians or other hospital departments from the client's bedside, give condition updates, or obtain verbal orders. Yet, other agencies continue to prohibit talking on cell phones. The major cost is not the actual phone device but the monthly service provider cost. Nurses working in the community use cellular phones to contact clients on the way to give home care. Phones provide easy access from the field back to the agency, to the client's primary physician, and to other resources. In the United Kingdom, nurses making home visits use mobile phones to improve communication with agencies and community services and to transmit client data (Blake, 2008a, 2008b). Cellular phones equipped with cameras and picture transmission capabilities have potential for long-distance diagnosis, a "snapshot" version of telehealth interactive video, and vocal transmissions.

Smartphones

Smartphones represent the convergence of cellular mobile phones and mobile computers. In addition to making telephone calls, these devices have other functions useful to nurses. They enable you to download and access PDA-type information resources; use health care apps; use quality response (QR) options to decode; provide Internet access to client information (new laboratory results or physician orders); and do instant messaging. Some downloaded apps provide alerts by beeping when there are new orders or newly available test results. In addition to housing downloaded reference programs such as those described for the PDA, smartphones with large enough memory may even house computer-assisted decision support systems. Downloadable apps such as Epocrates (www.epocrates.com), a free drug information program, not only provide drug information, but when you type in client information such as age, weight, and diagnosis, provide you with guidelines for correct dosage, contraindications, and side effects. New information alerts are sent to your device in a timely manner. National guidelines for best practice can also be downloaded. Smartphones are now outselling PDAs by a wide margin. Busis (2010) suggests a bar code reader as an add-on application for a smartphone, but newer ATTScanner apps might be more useful.

Laptop Computers and Tablets

Laptop computers are more powerful than tablets, yet both are still small and portable enough to be taken into the client's home. They are used to chart and transmit your client's care. If a device has Internet access, information can be sent or nursing documentation completed. Try Exercise 26-1.

Smart Cards

Until we achieve total interoperability between EHRs residing in "the cloud," all of a client's history can be carried on a **smart card** or a flash drive. When this client is admitted to a hospital with a fully integrated computer information system, the client's data is scanned into the electronic record. This can aid safe care. For example, an allergy to aspirin can be part of the information carried by your client. When the client travels outside the system, this information can be scanned into the new system's records.

ENHANCED WORK FLOW: REMOTE SITE MONITORING, DIAGNOSIS, TREATMENT, AND COMMUNICATION

Technological innovations can help make our care more efficient. Formerly, staff nurses in hospitals spent less than 40% of their day in actual client care and spent at least 25% of their time walking to answer phones, obtain charts, gather supplies, locate other staff, and so on. Nurses say it is about time that new technology systems help improve their work flow, are easily accessible, and allow them more time at the bedside! Technologic innovations are coming so fast we cannot be all inclusive. The following sections describe some examples of health care technologic innovations.

IN-HOSPITAL BIOMEDICAL MONITORING

When the point of care is at the client's hospital bedside, several of the technologies already mentioned, such as noninvasive automatic recording of vital signs and other wireless telemetry, can allow you to communicate with other team members, eliminating unnecessary travel. The use of "smart" beds with sensors transmits vital signs data wirelessly. Wireless technology extends into the client's home. Managing clinical care with help from the client in his or her home who transmits to your remote site is an example. A *Healthy People 2020* goal is to increase the proportion of people who communicate with their health care providers using the Internet (Healthy People 2020, HC/HIT-5-2).

E-VISITS AND TELEHOME HEALTH CARE

E-visits offer opportunities for diagnosis, treatment, and monitoring of client status via Internet portals. This makes care more affordable and convenient. Cook (2012) reports a 50% reduction in hospital admissions and an 80% reduction in home visits using telehome type technology, while Mehrotra and colleagues (2013) specifically report successful treatment of urinary infections just using technology to communicate. The client may sign onto a portal and access their secure health record and answer a series of questions about their condition. Within hours, their care provider makes a diagnosis, orders treatment, writes a progress note in the EHR, and replies to the client. In addition, a client may use intelligent vital monitoring products to obtain updates such as blood pressure, blood glucose levels, or current electrocardiogram strips. Your client then transmits this information to you, which you can assess without having to make a home visit (Hsu et al., 2011). E-visits are offered by numerous health systems and are reimbursable by insurance.

Case Example

The following case is an example of how this technology is designed to assist us to deliver better and safer nursing care more efficiently.

Gail Myer, RN, is assigned to Mrs. Sanchez as one of her eight clients on an obstetrical unit. Mrs. Sanchez is in preterm labor. Gail's clinical decision support

Continued

system (CDSS) automatically lists desired client outcomes based on her work assignment, lists "best practice" interventions, and then gives real-time feedback about client outcomes. Her handheld device receives electronic prompts to assist in clinical decision making. For example, the hospital's CDSS program calculates expected delivery date for Mrs. Sanchez and supplies the correct dose of the prescribed medication based on her weight. It alerts Gail if the prescribed dose she intends to administer exceeds maximum standard safety margins, and also cross-checks this new drug for potential drug interactions with the drugs Mrs. Sanchez is already taking. It pops up a screening tool for Gail to use to assess Mrs. Sanchez's current status and then alerts Gail if she should forget to document today's results.

TELECARE PROGRAMS

Telecare refers to **telemetry** that communicates client vital signs, monitors whether nurses wash hands, or signals you if a client falls and does not get up via sensors embedded in the hospital room or client's house. Families in the United States and England are using such sensors placed throughout the client's home to monitor for potential problems, such as stove burners left on, doors left open, a too cold house, or a client crisis, such as an epileptic seizure. In the literature this is referred to as "smart rooms," which is a form of automated medical technology.

RADIO FREQUENCY IDENTITY SMART TECHNOLOGY

Information can also be communicated to providers via data transmitted by **radio frequency identity (RFID)** chips inside our identification cards that we wear, or even from implanted chips.

If we need to locate a member of our team, such chips assist in tracking that doctor or other team member. Lots of us have chips implanted into our pets so they can be located if lost. Is it ethical to implant similar devices into Alzheimer clients or others who are unable to function without supervision?

Staff nurses walk hundreds of miles a year trying to locate and gather equipment and supplies they need to carry out their bedside care. RFID technology could instantly locate equipment, such as a needed infusion pump stored in the supply room. Perhaps robots will then deliver needed supplies to you! In a large review of this topic, Ajami and Rajabzadeh (2013) concluded that RFID technology needs to be integrated into an agency's HIT to best reduce clinical and medication errors.

TELEHEALTH

Telehealth is also called telemedicine, telenursing, or eHealth (in England). It is an umbrella term for services that use communications technology, defined as any real-time interactive use of the Internet for delivery of health care from a distance using telecommunications technologies. It has high-definition visual and audio two-way communication, allowing the telehealth nurse to see, monitor, and remotely interact with clients using their own devices (American Telemedicine Organization, n.d.).

Information is exchanged across geographic distances and is often used for specialist consultations. The consultant can manipulate ophthalmoscope or stethoscope attachments to assess retinas or breath sounds. Use of this communication technology is increasing exponentially (Marcin et al., 2012). Several studies show telehealth decision making and diagnosing of strokes are just as effective and may be more cost effective (Rubin and Demaerschalk, 2014; Silva et al., 2012). Use is becoming more commonplace. In Silva's study, 100% of participating emergency departments used this technology for evaluation of stroke clients.

Telehealth allows experts to be accessed remotely to diagnose and treat illness, provide preventive health care, or provide medical consultation. It initially was used to provide care to clients in rural areas but is now also used in urban areas. At first it originated at health facilities, now telehealth often originates from the client's home. The company iSelectMD (http://iselectmd.com/) is one example: the employer's health insurance charges a minimal additional health premium fee monthly, and then each employee has 24/7 access to a physician via telemedicine by signing onto a web site, entering symptoms, and paying a "visit" fee. The physician on call reviews the client's medical history and current symptoms, makes a diagnosis, and e-mails in a prescription if needed. A follow-up call is made 2 days later to determine whether the health issue was resolved. Obviously, only minor conditions such as urinary tract infections or respiratory illness can be treated in this remote technology fashion.

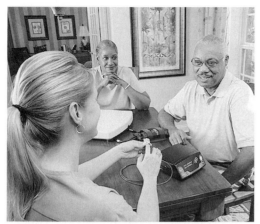

Home-based telehealth monitoring unit. *(Used with permission from Honeywell HomMed).*

Outcomes

Many studies show use of this technology reduces hospitalizations, increases quality of care and client satisfaction, decreases emergency department visits, and decreases health care costs. Barriers are legal and financial and include privacy concerns, interstate licensure or insurance coverage, and problems with insurance reimbursement.

CAMERAS EMBEDDED IN WIRELESS DEVICES

Smartphones and tablets offer opportunities to transmit pictures for consultation or to document pathology such as a skin lesion, biopsy site, and so forth. One suggestion made in the *American Family Physician* journal is using the client's own phone to capture a picture, which he or she can then display at a future visit for comparison ("Practice Pearls," 2013).

VOICE-ACTIVATED COMMUNICATION

Voice communication systems use wearable, hands-free devices that use the existing wireless network to support instant voice communication and messaging among staff within an agency. The nurse wears a small, lightweight badge that permits one-button voice access to other users of the system. It also will connect to the telephone system. One example is Vocera. It is said to reduce the time for key communications, such as looking for the medication keys, looking for others (a 45% reduction), paging doctors, or walking to the nursing station telephone (a 25% reduction). Nurses report that voice-activated communication facilitates

communication results in fewer interruptions, promotes better continuity of care, and improves their work flow.

COMPUTERIZED CLINICAL DECISION SUPPORT SYSTEMS

DECISION SUPPORT SYSTEM INFORMATION TO ASSIST CRITICAL THINKING AND DECISION MAKING

An important asset of HIT adoption is the provision of computerized **clinical decision support systems (CDSS)**. These systems assist you with clinical care by efficiently providing you with access to digital information, which helps you improve your decision making with specific clients. By doing so, they enhance the quality of your client care as well as its safety. CDSS is often integrated with order entry systems in the hospital, but versions can be available to nurses working in the community (Ranji et al., 2013). Key CDSS issues are speed and ease of access. CDSSs are useful but, of course, do not take the place of your own clinical critical thinking.

Case Example

Jim Dakota, age 69 years, runs Eagleview, a bed and breakfast business, in rural South Dakota. He recently was discharged after bowel surgery in a hospital 3 hours away. Because broadband fiberoptic cable recently made telehomecare possible in his home area, for his follow-up care, instead of closing his business and traveling a long distance, he is able to self-manage his wound healing with his remote accessed nurse's guidance. She also even can detect complications remotely.

The more sophisticated CDSS systems give interactive advice after comparing entries of your client data with a computerized knowledge base. The information offered to you is personalized to your client's condition (filtered) and is offered at appropriate times in your workday.

Since IOM and the Canadian Institutes of Health Research began advocating CDSS programs or supporting research into CDSS effect on client care, the suggested types of data in the CDSS system have come to include:

- Diagnosis and care information displays with care management priorities listed.
- It is a method for communication, that is, for order entry and for entering client data (system

offers prompts so you enter complete data; offers smart or model forms).

- Automatic checks for drug-drug, drug-allergy, and drug-formulary interactions are made.
- It is able to send reminders to clients according to their stated preference.
- Medication reconciliations and client summary of care at transitions of client care are made.
- It is able to send you electronic alerts or prompts if problems occur or you have not acknowledged receipt of information, such as the client's laboratory test results.

The hardware can be a computer terminal on your hospital unit or wireless handheld device. A software database can be information residing in the agency server or a central repository such as a disease registry or government database.

For the nurse, some CDSS software can generate specific information for your client care including assessment guidelines and forms, analyses of their laboratory test results, and use of best practice protocols to make specific recommendations for safe care. Ideally, this is integrated into the EHR system your agency is using. Ease of use is crucial. Studies continue to show that the majority of time, staff nurses still prefer to rely on colleagues to validate their decisions (Marshall et al., 2011).

Based on input about the current condition of your client (coded data), the CDSS is programmed to provide you with appropriate reminders or prompts. For example, after you complete care for your first assigned client, specific information is presented to you if you have not yet documented a needed intervention. This assists you in preventing treatment errors or omissions and helps improve your documentation. Blaser and colleagues (2007) demonstrated that their CDSS could speed up the time to intervention. More timely interventions should lead to fewer client complications. As an example, Levy and Heyes (2012) describe a system used in England that gives evidence-based information to support the nurse's choice of interventions, which can improve care of the client with atrial fibrillation who is consequently at risk for stroke. Our central focus remains patient-centered care, so we include our client's preferences in our clinical decisions.

CDSS technology is slowly being adopted. Early systems were stand-alone, but technology is rapidly advancing, leading to more user-friendly systems integrated into HIT to provide timely, relevant content. Because the system stores your information about your activity, you can, for example, obtain reports about your overall compliance with standards of care or provide data for research.

OUTCOMES OF COMPUTERIZED CLINICAL DECISION SUPPORT SYSTEMS

In Chapter 4 we noted that IOM attributed over 70% of health care errors to poor communication. Constant improvements to our electronic health care technologies are geared to improving the flow of communication, increasing safety, and improving the quality of our care. As an example, Fogel (2013) reported critically ill clients had significantly better blood glucose control when providers used a CDSS. In fact, reviewers who analyzed more than 15,000 articles concluded that the evidence is *strong* that CDSS use effectively improves health outcomes on a range of measures for clients in diverse settings (Agency for Healthcare Research and Quality [AHRQ], 2012). In another report of a comprehensive review of research study findings, AHRQ (2009) concluded that evidence is limited as to effect of CDSS on nurses' work flow.

Alerts

The literature shows mixed results when reminders or alerts are sent. Nurses have been found to be more likely to chart when an electronic reminder is received. Clients have been shown to respond much more positively to reminders and to CDSS coaching about their self-care and even to express a willingness to pay for text messaging health reminders (Cocosila et al., 2008; Finkelstein et al., 2012).

Clinical Practice Guidelines: Access to Online Information

By standardizing interventions based on outcome evidence, practice guidelines promote quality and safety. Nurses have the opportunity to search databases when they need information, using computers or smartphones. Clinical practice guidelines need to be easily accessible, usable in your daily practice, with content from trusted, credible sources. Clinical guideline databases should allow input from you about your client, then provide customized clinical decision guidance. Clinical databases have been systematically developed to provide appropriate care recommendations for your specific client's diagnoses based on available research evidence.

Among many free, downloadable apps and guides for care, one example is *The Guide to Clinical Preventive Services*. You can search by age, sex, and risk factors (U.S. Preventive Services Task Force: www.epss.ahrq.gov). Many other protocols are available from AHRQ (www.ahrq.gov), from professional organizations such as the American Nurses Association (ANA) (www.nursingworld.com/ce), and from free or subscribed data bases such as Mosby's Nursing Consult where you click on the diagnosis of interest. Many national and regional nurse associations also have or soon will have such databases. There are multiple private for-profit companies that would also supply you with such information for a subscription fee. Most hospitals and larger agencies have resident experts, such as medical librarians or clinical nurse specialists, to help staff nurses access information about evidence-based care guidelines.

CLIENT ENGAGEMENT
ELECTRONIC HEALTH CARE COMMUNICATION AMONG PROVIDERS AND CLIENTS

Mobile technology has not only changed the way we document, it now provides unlimited resources we can use for client education (Manning et al., 2013). Consumers will have the ability to view, download, and transmit their health information (Kennedy, 2014). Many health care systems use secure Internet portals to allow their clients access to communicate both with physicians and nurses, or to obtain information. Insurance and pharmaceutical companies have portals that provide consumer and health care provider access to drug information. Other technology consumers are using include the following.

E-mail

E-mail can be a convenient, rapid, inexpensive method of communicating between providers and clients. Yet, while most clients express a desire to communicate with their health care providers via e-mail, only about 72% of physicians in large medical centers reported using this method of communication (Bradley et al., 2011). Barriers include concern about lack of income generation, confidentiality, malpractice, and time factors.

Office nurses use e-mail for scheduling appointments, posting test results, providing prescription refills, and other health reminders. Nurses also use e-mail for education or follow-up, for example, in tracking the response of clients who are on new medication, instead of waiting until their next office appointment. American Medical Association (AMA) guidelines (2004) suggest that electronic or paper copies be made of e-mail messages sent to clients.

Secure Instant Messaging and Texting

Text instant messaging (IM) is commonly used in daily life. On average a typical American sends or receives more than 700 messages each month. So most team members and clients will be familiar with texting; *secure IMs* can be used to improve communications between members of the health team or between clients and providers. IM can be used when the nurse wants to request an additional pain medication for an assigned client from the resident on call, although the nurse is not supposed to accept texted orders back. IM can be used by clients to communicate self-monitored information to their care provider. The provider can also text message reminders to the client. Nurses provide personalized IM to clients as one intervention in preventive or chronic care, such as weight management, smoking cessation, or drug rehabilitation. IMs are also used as interventions with clients managing their cancer, asthma, diabetes, or other chronic diseases. However, The Joint Commission (TJC) has said "it is NOT acceptable for the physician or licensed independent practitioner to text orders for patients to the hospital…" (TJC, 2011). The rationale is that you cannot verify who is actually sending the order. How is this different from faxed orders or verbal orders?

E-referrals and Consultations

With computerization and the Internet, making electronic referrals is easy as long as clients sign privacy waivers. Technology offers great potential for nurses, nurse-practitioners, and physician assistants, especially those who comprise a significant portion of the rural health care labor force. Rural populations comprise 20% in the United States and tend to be poorer and medically underserved. Use of HIT as discussed in this chapter can increase resources available to rural providers.

TECHNOLOGY FOR CLIENT HEALTH SELF-MANAGEMENT

Digital devices are perfect for anytime, anywhere learning. Clients can access health articles, professional portals, participate in social media or podcasts, webinars or videoconferencing.

CONSUMER HEALTH INFORMATION ON THE INTERNET FOR DISEASE MANAGEMENT

There is a major push for health consumer activism via the use of technology to communicate. AHRQ (n.d.) encourages clients to ask questions by advertisements, such as "Open Up and Say Anything" or "Questions Are the Answer," basically urging clients to assertively communicate with care providers, including nurses. People are willing to access the Internet for self-education or support to meet their health care needs. For example, a survey of senior citizens showed they want to be able to request prescription renewals online (American Health Information Management Association [AHIMA], 2014). Online learning has been found to be as effective as traditional learning (Pilcher and Bradley, 2013). Most people have searched the Internet for health information, using one of the many consumer health information sites. There is strong potential for improved health learning associated with interactive computer teaching programs.

Clients may also increase direct access to health care. Companies such as Teladoc, provide access to a physician's advice or treatment by telephone to its members for a nominal annual fee. Entrepreneurs are greatly expanding sites that provide disease information and support about diseases, sometimes for a fee. Examples include: Crohnology for those with Crohn disease; TalkSession for mental health problems; or DermLink for skin conditions.

Lifestyle Management

Not only do these educational programs increase client knowledge about their disease and their role in health promotion and disease management, but computerized information about health conditions has been shown to positively impact client outcomes. Support and reminders about health self-management have already been described. Many Internet sites provide interactive management. Others provide access to client support groups, such as the National Institutes of Health. Nurses frequently recommend Internet sites to clients.

Client Alerts

Using the Internet, you can send electronic alerts to your clients who need medication renewals, screening examinations, or other health services. A 2009 Kaiser Permanente study showed a marked decrease in primary care office visits after implementation of an electronic system with intensive provider-client communication via a secure Internet portal. According to Kaiser, 85% of users report that being able to communicate electronically with their physicians improved their ability to manage their own health. A personalized Internet site can be used by an agency for far broader functions than providing business hours or travel directions. Nearly all health care organizations have their own sites. Such sites can include health assessment tools and allow clients to schedule appointments. Another primary function is to provide health information. Internet sites can have hyperlinks embedded that clients can use to access general information about their condition, medications, or treatment. They can also contain an e-mail link so that clients can directly contact the nurse responsible for patient education.

Group E-support: Communication via Internet Chat Rooms

Computers are used to mediate support groups for families and clients with various health problems. These formal Internet groups provide information, but they also importantly have been shown to provide improved social support for the ill client. Rains and Young's 2009 analysis of 28 research studies showed Internet group participants report less depression, increases in quality of life, as well as improved ability to manage their disease condition. Technologies associated with providing support include e-mail, instant (text) messaging, chat rooms, and discussion forums. The chat rooms are usually synchronous, in real time, providing immediate feedback. Usually discussion forums are asynchronous with time delays between postings and responses, allowing for more reflection before posting. Communication with group members over the Internet has been shown to be associated with lower levels of reported stress, especially in older adults. More studies are needed before we can specify the needed frequency, duration, or quality of content for optimal client support.

OUTCOMES OF TECHNOLOGY USE

Nursing communication. For nurses, technology is said to improve work flow, provide safer care, provide automatic monitoring and documentation of some client data, allow more nurse independence, and improve communications among team members. Acute care providers quickly adopted wireless devices at the bedside for communication (Manning et al., 2013). Evidence continues to present mixed findings about the effects of technology. There is an expectation that it will decrease long-term costs. Generally it seems to improve the flow of communications. But some negative outcomes include perceptions that electronic communication damages the team interpersonal relationships (Wu et al., 2011). Does new technology assist or impede work flow? Evidence is just beginning to be analyzed. In an example, nurses caring for ventilator-dependent clients began to use wireless devices to access communication tools for clients (Improving Communication, 2014). We know that nurses are assuming increased responsibilities for interpretation of transmitted data and for instituting interventions.

Client-provider communication. Care may be less labor intensive and easier if delivered remotely via smartphones to clients. Technology is said to facilitate self-monitoring, improve self-management, improve cognitive functioning, reduce time spent in physician offices, provide needed information, provide support, decrease rehospitalization, increase markers of quality of life, and improve timely communication with health providers (Marcin et al., 2012). Smartphone apps are effective methods for teaching preventive care. In an example, apps such as "Call the Shots" or texting reminders have been shown to increase compliance with immunization (Peck, 2014). It may be the preferred modality for clients, especially younger generations.

The Agency for Healthcare Research and Quality's analysis of 146 studies of the impact of computer health modules on client outcomes found that these programs succeeded in engaging client attention, but more significantly they improved client clinical health (AHRQ, 2009). Just as studies have documented positive health outcomes after telephone support from nurses, contact with providers using interactive computer programs for client health education using webcam technology real-time (synchronous) communication between nurse and client can deliver health maintenance information, provide answers to illness-related questions, and lead to positive health outcomes.

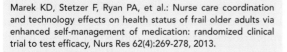

Developing an Evidence-Based Practice

Marek KD, Stetzer F, Ryan PA, et al.: Nurse care coordination and technology effects on health status of frail older adults via enhanced self-management of medication: randomized clinical trial to test efficacy, Nurs Res 62(4):269-278, 2013.

Purpose: This study was designed to evaluate health status outcomes over the course of 1 year for 456 frail adults, age 60 years or older, who had chronic illnesses and were self-managing their conditions including self-administration of their medications. Random assignment was done to four groups. Nurses did a pharmacy screening for all subjects at baseline. The control group received no interventions. Other groups had periodic visits from a nurse care coordinator, with one group also using a medication planner, while the fourth group used a medication dispensing machine (nurses refilled machines periodically).

Results: All the nurse care–coordinated groups showed significant improvement in outcomes measures: positive effects on cognitive functioning, functional status and quality of life measures, with decreases in depressive symptoms. In the technology aspect of the evaluation, the group using the medication planner, but not the group using the medication dispensing machine, showed significant results.

Application to Your Practice: Maintaining ill older adults in their homes longer may be possible if nurses make care coordination visits, especially if clients use medication planners for medication self-administration. Would the cost savings of maintaining folks in their own homes offset the cost of nurses making home visits?

QSEN defines evidence-based practice (EBP) as "integrating the best current evidence with clinical expertise and patient/family preferences and values for delivery of optimal health care" (www.qsen.org). Try using one or more apps to find EBP guidelines and then mark which of your next nursing care plan's listed interventions are evidence-based. Some suggested sites are:

Apple store health apps
Pepid Primary Care Plus (PCP) Suite:
    www.pepid.com
Epocrates: www.epocrates.com
National Guideline Clearinghouse (NCG):
    www.guideline.gov
Skyscape Medical Library: www.skyscape.com
Electronic preventive services selector (ePSS):
    http://epss.ahrq.gov/PDA/index.jsp

APPLICATIONS

TECHNOLOGY USE

Technology cannot replace your accumulated knowledge and expertise in making a decision, but it can provide supplementary tools to help make these decisions. Competency in HIT use has broadly been cited by national nursing organizations, accrediting agencies, government agencies, and policy organizations as an essential of basic nursing practice. Use of Informatics is a QSEN expected competency for new nurse graduates. Under this competency, *Knowledge* objectives include ability to identify information available in a common database to support care. *Skills* include ability to respond appropriately to clinical decision-making supports and alerts. Students are expected to demonstrate an *Attitude,* which values use of technology for making decisions, preventing errors, and coordinating care.

In addition to employers, regulatory agencies, professional agencies, and academic agencies, we, as professional nurses, are each responsible for maintaining this competency (ANA, 2008).

Standards of care are applicable to electronic nursing just as to bedside care. General standards are discussed in Chapter 2. More specific standards may be available from nursing organizations such as ANA or the American Academy of Ambulatory Care Nursing.

In electronic care, as in all our care, we need to be aware of our client's preferences. For example, maybe only one-third of our clients will say they prefer digital reminders be sent to them.

POINT OF CARE

Wireless entry of data at the point of care can increase your access to and use of evidence-based resources in your practice. If smartphones are used for personal business, as well as in work situations, secure separate e-mail and/or messaging accounts would be needed. Handheld devices at point of care provide timely access to client information, are convenient, and are cost-effective in the long run. Their prompts should help you provide safer, more comprehensive care. Many organizations offer access to databases that give you information specific to your current client's current health problem.

INFECTION CONTROL

Prevention of device contamination is a concern. When we are giving hands-on care or setting our device down in a client's space, we need to avoid contamination by disinfecting before and after. Some suggest using an inexpensive plastic bag to encase our device. Certainly hand hygiene is crucial. Some reports describe use of hand hygiene sensors. In studies, an amazing 40% to 70% of providers failed to disinfect, although the known presence of sensors does improve compliance (Miskelly, 2013).

WIRELESS HANDHELD COMPUTER USE

New mobile devices with Internet access offer amazing ways for us to engage our clients in their care. Clients who see us using a mobile device and to whom we recommend a health monitoring app are more likely to use theirs to manage their condition. This is particularly true if they have a chronic condition (AHIMA, 2014).

ELECTRONIC MAIL

Guidelines are available for physician use of e-mail to communicate with clients (AMA, 2004); these guidelines are also appropriate for nurses. No one knows how many nurses are accustomed to using wireless technology devices in their care of clients. Guidelines for their use in giving client care still need to be developed.

SMARTPHONES AND PERSONAL DIGITAL ASSISTANTS

Although just about every nursing student has seen or used a wireless or cellular telephone, not everyone has used them as an aid to giving client care. There are still hospitals that prohibit nurses from using cell phones, even though studies show these devices can save time, decrease errors, and simplify information retrieval at the point of care. Nursing is just beginning to deal with guidelines. Ethically, you do not use electronic devices in your workplace for personal, nonprofessional use. All information needs to be Health Insurance Portability and Accountability Act (HIPAA) secure.

E-MESSAGING AND TEXTING

Electronic provider-client IM can be used to communicate simple data. Texts are used to remind clients of appointments, services, or to take a medication or perform self-monitoring care. This may promote better quality care and improved client utilization. Multiple articles in the literature describe the efficacy of using personalized IM for helping clients manage their conditions. In one example, your hypertensive client taking a new medication could text message his blood pressures to you today after self-monitoring, or your diabetic client could send today's glucose results after testing her blood sugar. Remember, however, that most IM sites are not HIPAA secure so TJC has forbidden providers from texting patient orders (TJC, 2011).

USE OF SOCIAL MEDIA

Social media sites are powerful communication platforms, using the Internet-based venues to communicate, strengthen interpersonal relationships, and even disseminate information for education. According to Desai (2013), social media and portable devices with downloadable apps will revolutionize health information systems and our communication (with clients) in ways we do not yet realize. Among multiple platforms are video-hosting sites, social networking sites, social tagging, and blogging sites. Just as social media is transforming the way people interact, it has potential to transform traditional nurse-client relationships. Use of social media may improve our nursing practice by increasing our access to information and support. It allows us to instantly communicate with hundreds of people simultaneously. It gives us instant feedback and immediate access to information about treatment. Some hospitals are using social media sites such as Twitter or Facebook for public relations purposes. Meanwhile, professional organizations are using the same media sites to send alerts or tips about new care information (Siwek and Lin, 2013).

Nurses' common use of social media, however, may blur the lines between social and professional behavior. We are so accustomed to using social media in our personal lives, sometime we fail to differentiate what would be acceptable in our professional relationships. Consider the following case of Cassie.

Case Example

Cassie takes great pleasure in her semester-long home visit assignment caring for Clyde, age 4, who has severe cerebral palsy. She feels this is a great learning experience and that she is contributing to Clyde's progress. Today she snaps a really cute photo of him enjoying his first ice cream and then texts it to her friends, later posting it on Facebook.

What about this is inappropriate from a professional nursing viewpoint? According to the National Council of State Boards of Nursing (NCSBN) and HIPAA, nurses breach client privacy when they post photos or videos or comment about clients in enough detail that the client could be identified, or when degrading messages are posted (NCSBN, 2011). Refer to Table 26-1.

Nurses using social medial are bound by professional code or standards of practice and are subject to HIPAA regulations to guard the privacy of clients. Duffy (2011) cautions us not to name our employing agency, unless we be perceived as a representative speaking for that agency.

TABLE 26-1	Online Guidelines for Nurses Using Social Media	
Principles	**Actions**
Posts are bound by confidentiality and privacy laws, such as the Health Insurance Portability and Accountability Act (HIPAA).	Refrain from posting identifiable client information, especially photos and videos, or even naming the medications your client is taking.
Professional ethical standards need to be followed.	Separate personal and professional content (use two separate sites).
	Observe nurse-client boundaries: avoid crossing into social friendship.
Social media sites are public forums.	Any disparaging comments are considered as lateral violence or "cyberbullying."
	Use privacy settings and be aware of changes.
	Understand that colleagues, employers, and clients may read your posts.
Libel laws and nursing ethical codes apply to online information. State Boards of Nursing act on complaints.	Understand that social media is powerful and permanent, so be aware of possible impact.
	Civil, criminal, and professional penalties can apply.

Adapted from the American Medical Association (AMA), American Nurses Association (ANA), National Council of State Boards of Nursing (NCSBN), National Student Nurses' Association (NSNA), 2014.

We need to differentiate between the general open-to-all social sites, such as Twitter, from secure sites with restricted access, such as those created by hospitals as internal professional staff social networks.

CLINICAL DECISION SUPPORT SYSTEMS

CDSSs include knowledge management, triage systems, assessment forms, prescribing systems, or systems for test ordering and analysis. We use CDSS as another tool to manage our nursing care. It never eliminates the need for us to use our critical thinking skills. This is most likely to occur when the CDSS is integrated into existing EHR systems and automatically provides care recommendations. CDSSs align your clinical decisions for your specific client with best practice guidelines and evidence-based practices at the point of care.

USE

Use of CDSS primarily helps us improve client care, but it also helps us justify our decisions (Desai, 2013). The "active" or automatic provision of suggestions that prompts nurses and supports their clinical decisions is more effective than "passive" systems, which wait for the user to request data.

For example, a CDSS may offer you reminders or alerts about a certain client when you access his electronic record or when you access a medication order on his EHR. You would be given information about whether there would be any possible harmful interactions with other medications your client is already taking. CDSS "reminders" integrated with your work flow gives you suggestions about interventions that are based on researched best practice. Perhaps the CDSS offers you a suggested alternative to the intervention you plan. In another example, nurses working with pediatric cancer clients have long used calculators to determine correct fractional dosage based on the child's weight. Now instead, they can use this automated support system because it automatically predetermines the correct doses.

ALARM FATIGUE

A common problem is that the CDSS might send you so many alerts that you ignore them. **Alarm fatigue** is a commonly reported problem. This is particularly true for drug-drug interactions. Studies suggest that as many as 90% of alarm alerts are overridden (Phansalkar, 2013). Customizing alerts to your client assignment or gradating the warning into low-priority (warning but no alarm) and high-priority (audible alarm) might overcome this problem of alarm fatigue. A number of studies show positive results, especially in areas of drug-dosing alerts or reminders about preventive care. More studies are needed to examine effects of CDSS on communication, but data suggest a positive effect. In Canada, nurses use PDAs to access the Registered Nurses' Association of Ontario best-practice guidelines to receive timely information specific to their assigned clients.

COST

Cost and usability are the main issues in adopting technology. Does your agency provide devices and access to software programs? Access needs to be user friendly, integrated into your work flow, relevant to your care, and provide information quickly at times that really fit into your existing work flow. Reflect on whether technology integrated into the student learning experience is more likely to be used after graduation.

APPLICATION OF CLINICAL GUIDELINES TO PRACTICE

Access at the point of care to databases containing evidence-based guidelines for care, means you have resources specifically tailored to suggest interventions for a specific client.

CRITERIA FOR DOWNLOADABLE CLINICAL PRACTICE GUIDELINES

- They are evidence-based.
- They are easily accessible on your wireless device.
- They allow you to enter client data to customize the interventions (data from EHR).
- They contain hotlinks to allow you to obtain and print more information.

mHEALTH: TECHNOLOGY FOR CLIENT ENGAGEMENT

TECHNOLOGY TO ASSIST CLIENTS TO SELF-MANAGE

New technologies are changing the way clients exchange health information and communicate interactively.

Mobile health care (mHealth) can mean any use of a wireless mobile device and the apps designed for use on them independent of location to achieve a health goal (Morrissey, 2014). Portable devices with downloadable apps give clients hugely expanded opportunities to communicate with providers, seek advice, gain knowledge about their health concerns, and access online information databases and resources to manage their own health care needs. High-quality care can be ensured when providers use technology to give information, offer self-care instruction and reminders, or recommend links to Internet resources (HealthIT.gov, n.d.). Johnson envisions nurses who empower client use of social network sites to promote health and manage disease (Johnson, 2013).

Use of Portals

Various providers and agencies have increased ease of consumer access via use of Internet portals. Clients sign on and click on various menu bars to access some areas of their EHRs or access other information. This not only decreases use of staff time to answer phone calls and so on, but it also records that the client accessed and received certain information (HealthIT.gov, n.d.). For example, your client can obtain laboratory test results, request medication refills, and so forth. There are Internet sites that allow consumers to rate hospitals and individual care providers by name, such as the Hospital Compare web site (www.medicare.gov/hospitalcompare).

Use of Health and Lifestyle Monitoring Apps

Of course, use of apps is not quite as easy as it sounds, requiring us to develop skills. Currently clients may download many apps that assist them in tracking their self-assessment. Examples include Glucose Buddy, which is an iPhone app that allows clients to enter glucose testing results and record carbohydrate consumption and other parameters. This information can then be viewed online. Another app is uChek, which is a digital log of urinalysis testing results with data entered using the smartphone camera to record urine dip stick results. New devices, such as smart watches, fitness bands, and so forth, make use of wellness and diagnostic apps even easier to use. Currently most are not regulated.

Outcomes of mHEALTH

One goal of *Healthy People 2020* is to achieve an increase in the proportion of persons who use electronic personal health management tools. Nurses can recommend sites, preferably interactive ones, on the Internet that clients can use to have a positive impact on their health. Laptops, notebooks, and smartphones can be used for anywhere, anytime learning. Online learning has been repeatedly shown to be as effective or superior to traditional forms of learning (Pilcher and Bradley, 2013). Have you used podcasts? Webinars?

Cyber Health Education for Health Promotion

There is considerable evidence about the efficacy of providing health care education and information online. Limited areas of the client's EHR can be accessed for information. Clients could sign on and obtain results of laboratory tests. One advantage is that this information would be available at all times, rather than just during office hours. See Chapter 14 for discussion of health promotion concepts.

Cyber Education for Client Disease Management

Disease self-management using computers will greatly change the way nurses deliver health education. Health information about preventive health or about controlling their chronic disease conditions can be provided to clients effectively, quickly, and inexpensively via the Internet. Nurse-provided information, often to their client's mobile device, allows clients to make better self-management decisions. Actively engaging and giving decision support is another way to provide patient-centered care, shifting the focus to self-care in their own home. One problem for clients accessing Internet health information is that not all online information is accurate or easy for the user to verify in measurable *outcomes*; Internet-based education programs have been shown to lead to better understanding and to greater disease control. See Chapter 15 for health teaching concepts.

In the United States, documentation of each client education session must contain:

- The topic discussed
- The time spent
- Your mutual behavioral goal
- Your assessment of client's readiness to learn
- Your observations about the client's level of understanding of his or her disease

Cyber Support for Clients

Caregivers or clients with chronic conditions can use Internet support groups, chat rooms, e-mail, or direct communication with care providers to gain support. Also, nurses can gain insight and better understand the "lived experiences" of their clients by participating in these Internet opportunities. Clients are accustomed to accessing support from friends when they use Facebook, Twitter, and so on. Because support via telephone has been shown to be a cost-effective method for improving functioning and quality of life for diabetic clients, the same effects need to be documented for cyber support. For example, use of cyber support opportunities has been shown to empower asthma caregivers (Sullivan, 2008). Client use of CDSS programs that provide information about treatment options and the benefits and risks for each option can help them clarify their choice and can improve nurse-client communication.

ISSUES

COMMUNICATION TECHNOLOGY ACCESS

Internationally the number of individuals without access to the Internet is shrinking, as are the number who have yet to develop computer skills. Cautions or barriers to application of new technologies include user resistance and literacy issues. The transition to use of eHealth technology in nursing implies a learning curve. Some providers cite problems such as the time involved in learning how to use, cost, equipment design limitations, access issues, interference with work flow, and fears about losing handheld devices. In all cases, our communication needs to be tailored to the needs and literacy level of our client.

Guidelines for professional relationships apply to use of electronic media. Caution is advised in communicating with clients outside the professional relationship. Online contact with clients or former clients blurs the relationship boundary.

Liability Issues

Use of the Internet presents many questions about how to maximize its communication potential with an increasingly diverse population. Liability and regulatory statutes are outmoded, relevant to the century gone by. For example, if transmission (and treatment) crosses state lines, in which region does the provider need to be licensed? If malpractice occurs, in which region or state would legal action occur?

Privacy Issues

Separate organizations providing care to the same client need to share information securely. Any information you learn during the course of treatment must be safeguarded. With any computer use, we are concerned about maintaining this *security*. Many surveys of consumer concerns cite breach of privacy as their biggest concern. As HIT systems become more sophisticated and accessibility is a top priority, mechanisms and regulations to ensure privacy become more complex.

Security experts recommend data encryption and always using a required login password, which is changed periodically. Legally, the federal government has laws that protect client privacy. Refer to Chapter 2 for discussion of HIPAA privacy rules. This is why you have sign-on passcodes for portable computer terminals or automatic screen saver modes to darken screens, preventing visitors from reading client records.

Professionally, there are also rules for privacy protection. Except for sharing information with other health team members, a nurse can reveal client information only in very limited, specific situations: when failure to disclose would result in significant harm or when legally required to do so. One example would be if you recognize signs of physical abuse in a child.

Refer to Table 26-1 for a useful guideline. NCSBN states that in the majority of times, complaints result in disciplinary action by the State Board.

Ethically, rules for disclosure are less concrete, but an example might be a client who tells you he is going to commit suicide or murder. In professional relationships, clients are usually advised upfront that such comments are not bound by rules of confidentially. Reflect on the Ethical Dilemma box at the end of this chapter.

PROFESSIONAL ONLINE NURSING EDUCATION

Many organizations provide useful resources for your own continuing education, such as the ANA (www.nursingworld.org) or AHRQ (www.ahrq.gov). Some nursing programs are offered entirely online, but most have incorporated at least some computer-enhanced courses in response to student demand. Students say they prefer asynchronous (not in real time) courses that they can access at their convenience.

As professionals we are responsible for maintaining our continuing education. Information is expanding exponentially. We know we will be required to seek lifelong learning sources. Technology provides access to continuing education for credit via webinars, podcasts, and so forth. With handheld devices, you can learn anytime, anyplace. After graduation, would

---

EXERCISE 26-2 | **Critique of an Internet Nursing Resource Database**

Purpose: To encourage students to gain familiarity with Internet resources.

Procedure
As an out-of-class assignment, access any nursing resource database, preferably using a handheld wireless device. Many sites are listed in the online references.
   Write a one-paragraph critique; rate the web site from 0 = useless to 10 = excellent.

1. How quickly were you able to find a specific piece of information?
2. How applicable to your clinical practice?
3. To what degree was the information evidence-based?

Discussion
Use results as a basis for a general in-class discussion.

---

you prefer this method to earn continuing education credits as required for your relicensure or recertification? How about for work-related meetings? Try Exercise 26-2 as practice.

SUMMARY

HIT is an emerging force transforming the way nurses communicate with other professionals, clients, and data. HIT provides nurses with new tools to deliver nursing at the client's point of care. Moreover, it is anticipated that use of HIT will improve the quality of care. Tools discussed in this chapter include CDSS programs, messaging, telehealth, and remote monitoring. HIT gives clients new ways to educate themselves, to manage their health, and to communicate with health care professionals.

ETHICAL DILEMMA   What Would You Do?

"One of the staff nurses you work with "friends" you on Facebook allowing you to read postings sent to her by a student nurse assigned to her unit. The student has posted information about a 17 year old former client who threatens to commit suicide. You do not personally know either the student nurse or the client.
1. Since this information is openly available on the Internet, what ethical responsibility do you have to intervene?
2. Did the student nurse violate the client's legal right to privacy?
3. If you were the student, what steps would you take as soon as you receive this information?"

DISCUSSION QUESTIONS

1. Reflect on how you would determine if an Internet site is providing reliable information.
2. How likely is it that you would access one of the AHRQ sites described in this chapter? Would registering with them to receive periodic-emails or "tweets" increase your use?
3. For what future professional uses can you envision using social media sites?

REFERENCES

Kass-Bartelmes BL, Ortiz E, Rutherford MK: *Using informatics for better and safer health care. Rockville (MD): Agency for Healthcare Research and Quality*, 2002. 2002. Research in Action Issue 6. AHRQ Pub. No. 02–0031.

Agency for Healthcare Research and Quality (AHRQ): Healthcare decisionmaking. . Pub. No. 12-E0001-EF [Pub.no.12-E0001-EF]. Accessed August 14, 2014 www.ahrq.gov/research/findings/evidence-based-reports/er203-abstract.html, 2012.

Agency for Healthcare Research and Quality (AHRQ): *Impact of consumer health informatics applications*, Evidence Report, Publication No.10–E019 . Accessed July 8, 2014 www.ahrq.gov/clinic/tp/chiapptp.htm, 2009.

Agency for Healthcare Research and Quality (AHRQ) (n.d.). Questions to ask your doctor: Questions are the answer: your health depends on good communication. www.ahrq.gov/questionsaretheanswer.

American Health Information Management Association (AHIMA): Seniors want their health IT [addendum], *J AHIMA* 85(2):78, 2014.

Ajami S, Rajabzadeh A: Radio frequency identification [RFID] technology and patient safety, *J Res Med Sci* 18(9):809–813, 2013.

American Academy of Colleges of Nursing (AACN): *The Essentials of Baccalaureate Education for Professional Nursing Practice*, Washington, DC, 2008, Author.

Practice pearls: [advertisement] *Am Fam Physician* 87(12):890, 2013.

American Medical Association (AMA): *Guidelines for physician patient electronic communication*, Report in response to AMA Resolution 810(A-99) bot2a00.rtf Accessed August 14, 2014 www.ama-assn.org, 2004.

American Nurses Association (ANA): *Position Statement 'Professional Role Competence'*, Accessed August 18, 2014 www.nursingworld.org/MainMenuCategories/Policy-Advocacy/Positions-and-Resolutions/ANAPositionStatements/Position-Statements-alphabetically/Professional-Role-Competence.html, May 28, 2008.

American Telemedicine Organization (n.d.). www.Americantelemed.org/about-telemedicine/what-is-telemedicine Accessed August 13, 2014.

Barnsteiner J, Disch J, Johnson J, McGuinn, et al.: Diffusing QSEN competencies across schools of nursing: The AACN/RWJF Faculty Development Institutes, *J Prof Nurs* 29(2):68–74, 2013.

Blake H: mobile phone technology in patient care, *Br J Community Nurs*, 2008a. Innovation in practice 13(4):160–162–165.

Blake H: Mobile phone technology in chronic disease management, *Nurs Stand* 23(12):43–46, 2008b.

Blaser R, Schnabel M, Biber C, et al.: Improving pathway compliance and clinician performance by using information technology, *Int J Med Inform* 76:151–156, 2007.

Bolton LB, Gassert CA, Cipriano PF: Technology solutions can make nursing care safer and more efficient, *J Healthc Inf Manag* 22(4):24–30, 2008.

Bradley LJ, Hendricks B, Lock R, Whiting PP, et al.: E-mail communication: Issues for mental health counselors, *J Ment Health Counsel* 33(1):1–3, 2011.

Busis N: Mobile phones to improve the practice of neurology, *Neurol Clin* 28:395–410, 2010.

Carter LM, Rukholm E: A study of critical thinking, teacher-student interaction, and discipline-specific writing in an online educational setting for registered nurses, *J Contin Educ Nurs* 39(3):133–138, 2008.

Cipriano PF, Bowles K, Dailey M, Dykes P, et al.: The importance of health information technology in care coordination and transitional care, *Nurs Outlook* 61:475–489, 2013.

Department of Health & Human Services: Center for Medicare and Medicaid Services (CMS), *MLN Matters, no. SE1409*, August 13, 2004. accessed August 14, 2014 www.cms.gov/.

Cocosila M, Archer N, Yuan Y: *Would people pay for text messaging health reminders? Telemed J E Health* 14(10):1091–1095, 2008.

Cook R: Exploring the benefits and challenges of telehealth, *Nurs Times* 108(24):16–17, 2012.

Crawford M: Making data sweet, *J AHIMA* 85(2):24–27, 2014.

Desai A: Focus of the Future: Environmental scan illuminates the path ahead for HIM, *J AHIMA* 84(8):48–52, 2013.

Duffy M: iNurse: Facebook, Twitter, and LinkedIn, Oh my!, *Am J Nurs* 111(4):56–59, 2011.

Drenkard K: MAGNET Perspectives: Patient engagement: Essential partnerships to improve outcomes, *J Nurs Admin* 44(1):3–4, 2014.

Finkelstein J, Knight A, Marinopoulos S, et al.: Enabling patient-centered care through health information technology, *Evid Rep Technol Assess (Full Rep)* 206:1–1531, 2012. Accessed January 4, 2014.

Fogel SL: Effects of computerized decision support systems on blood glucose regulation in critically ill surgical patients, *J Am Coll Surg* 216(4):1–2, 2013.

Forester DA, Fowler S, Gaidemak H, Alves F: Voice communications technology: healthcare provider perceptions and satisfaction, *Am Nurse Today* 6(2):1–5, 2011.

HealthIT.gov. (n.d.) Benefits of EHRs: Patient participation. www.healthit.gov/providers-professionals/patient-participation/. Accessed January 13, 2014.

U.S. Department of Health and Human Services. (n.d.) *Healthy People 2020*. Health Communication and Health Technology. HealthyPeople.gov/2020/topicsobjectives2020/overview.aspx?topicid=18. Accessed August 16, 2014.

HealthIT.gov: Health IT Legislation and Regulations: Health IT Legislation: HITECH Act. Acccessed August 12, 2014 www.healthit.gov/, 2009.

Hsu C, Tseng KC, Chuang Y: Predictors of future use of tele-homecare health services by middle-aged people in Taiwan, *Soc Behav Pers* 39(9):1251–1261, 2011, http://dx.doi.org/10.224/sbp.2011.39.9.1251.

Improving communication to improve patient care in intensive care units: *Robert Wood Johnson Foundation*. Accessed January 3, 2014 www.rejf.org/en/about-rwjf/newsroom/newsroom-content/2014/101/improving-communication-to-improve-patient-care-in-intensive-car.html, January 23, 2014.

Johnson J: *Module Four—Informatics*. www.QSEN.org/, 2013.

The Joint Commission (TJC): *Standards FAQ Details: texting orders.* Accessed September 29, 2013 http://www.jointcommission.org/standards_information/jcfaqdetails.aspx?StandardsFaqId=401&ProgramId=47, 2011.

Mobile health is here today: not tomorrow [addendum] *J AHIMA* 85(1):80, 2014.

Healthy People, 2020. U.S. Department of Health and Human Services. www.Healthypeople.gov/2020/

Kennedy A: Looking back and moving forward: The journey to consumer-driven healthcare continues, *J AHIMA* 85(1):10, 2014.

Levy S, Heyes B: Information systems that support effective clinical decision making, *Nurs Manag* 19(7):20–22, 2012.

Manning ML, Davis J, Sparnon E, Ballard RM: iPads, droids, and bugs: Infection prevention for mobile handheld devices at the point of care, *Am J Infect Control* 41(11):1–6, 2013.

Marcin JP, Sadorra C, Dharmar M: The role of telemedicine in treating the critically ill, *ICU Director* 4(3):70–74, 2012.

Marek KD, Stetzer F, Ryan PA, Bub LD, et al.: Nurse care coordination and technology effects on health status of frail older adults via enhanced self-management of medication, *Nursing Research* 62(4):269–278, 2013.

Marshall AP, West SH, Aitkin LM: Preferred information sources for clinical decision making: critical care nurses' perceptions of information accessibility and usefulness, *Worldviews Evid Based Nurs* 8(4):224–235, 2011, http://dx.doi.org/10.1111/j.1741.6787.2011.x. Epub June 7, 2011.

Mehrotra A, Paone S, Marrtich GD, Albert SM, et al.: A comparison of care at E-Visits and physician office visit for sinusitis and urinary tract infection, *JAMA Intern Med* 173(1):72–74, 2013.

Miskelly F: Application of a novel smart-sensor technology to achieve accurate hand hygiene monitoring and sustained compliance, without disruption to work flow, *Am J Infect Contr* 41(6):1–2, 2013.

Morrissey J: Connecting the continuum: connecting clinicians and patients who are just "a wall away.", *Hosp Health Netw* 88(1):18–19, 2014.

National Council of State Boards of Nursing (NCSBN): *White Paper: A Nurse's Guide to the Use of Social Media*. Accessed October 1, 2013 https://www.ncsbn.org/Social_Media.pdf, 2011.

Peck JL: Smartphone preventive healthcare: Parental use of an immunization reminder system, *J Pediatr Health Care* 28(1):35–42, 2014.

Phansalkar S, van der Sijs H, Tucker AD, Bell AA, et al.: Drug-drug interactions that should be non-interruptive in order to reduce alert fatigue in electronic health records, *J Am Med Inform Assoc* 20:489–493, 2013.

Pilcher J, Bradley DA: Best practices for learning with technology, *J Nurs Prof Dev* 29(3):133–137, 2013.

QSEN. www.QSEN.org/Pre-licensure competency.

Rains SA, Young V: A meta-analysis of research on formal computer-mediated support groups: examining group characteristics and health outcomes, *Hum Commun Res* 35:309–336, 2009.

Ranji SR, Rennke S, Wachter RM: Computerized Provider Order Entry with Clinical Decision Support Systems: A brief update. Evidence Reports/Technology Assessments No. 211 In Health Care Safer Making, editor: *An Updated Critical Analysis of the Evidence for Patient Safety Practices*, Rockville, MD, 2013, Agency for Healthcare Research and Quality (AHRQ). II Chapter 41 www.ncbi.nlm.nih.gov/pubmedhealth/PMH0055944/.

Rubin MN, Demaerschalk BM: The use of telemedicine in the management of acute stroke, *Neurosurg Focus* 36(1):e4, 2014.

Schickedanz A, Huang D, Lopez A, Cheung E, et al.: Access, interest, and attitudes toward electronic communication for health care among patients in the medical safety net, *J Gen Intern Med* 28(7):914–920, 2013.

Silva GS, Farrell S, Shandra E, Viswanathan A, et al.: The status of telestroke in the United States: A survey of currently active stroke telemedicine programs, *Stroke* 43:2078–2085, 2012.

Siwek J, Lin KW: Choosing wisely: More good clinical recommendations to improve health care quality and reduce harm, *Am Fam Physician* 88(3):164–168, 2013.

Sullivan CF: Cybersupport: empowering asthma caregivers, *Pediatr Nurs* 34(3):217–224, 2008.

Wu R, Rossos P, Quan S, Reeves S, et al.: An evaluation of the use of smartphones to communicate between clinicians: a mixed-methods study, *J Med Internet Res* 13(3):e59, 2011.

Zadvinskis IM, Chipps E, Yen P: Exploring nurses' confirmed expectations regarding health IT: A phenomenological study, *Inter J Med Inform* 83(2):89–98, 2014.

GLOSSARY

Accommodation A desire to smooth over a conflict through cooperative but nonassertive responses. (ch. 13)

Acculturation Describes how a person from a different culture initially learns the behavior norms and values of the dominant culture, and begins to adopt its behaviors and language patterns. (ch. 7)

Active listening Refers to listening with full attention on the client for the purpose of developing and understanding collaboratively constructed meanings. (ch. 5)

Acute grief Refers to somatic distress that occurs in waves with feelings of tightness in the throat, shortness of breath, an empty feeling in the abdomen, a sense of heaviness and lack of muscular power, and intense mental pain. (ch. 9)

Advance directive A legal document, executed by a competent client or legal proxy, specifically identifying individual preferences for level of treatment at end of life, should the client become unable to make valid decisions at that time. (chs. 3, 7, 21)

Advance organizers Sometimes called a mnemonic, is a teaching strategy that uses cue words, phrases, or letters related to more complex data to help people remember important concepts. (ch. 15)

Advanced practice nurses Registered nurses with a baccalaureate degree in nursing and an advanced degree in a selected clinical specialty with relevant clinical experience. (chs. 1, 22)

Advocacy Interceding or acting on behalf of the clients to provide the highest quality of care obtainable. (chs. 7, 19, 24)

Affective domain The learning domain concerned with emotional attitudes related to acceptance, compliance, and taking personal responsibility for health care. (ch. 15)

Affordable Care Act (Patient Protection and Affordable Care Act (PPCA) A federal law, which requires US citizens and legal immigrants to have a basic level of health care insurance. (ch. 1)

Aggregated data Compilation of multiple bits of factual information into large groupings allowing analysis. (ch. 25)

Aggressive behavior A response in which the individual acts to defend the self and to deflect the emotional impact of the perceived threat to the self through personal attack, blaming, or an extreme reaction to a tangential issue. (ch. 13)

Aging A universal life process of advancing through the life cycle, beginning at birth and ending at death. (ch. 19)

Active Aging An empowerment process of optimizing opportunities for health, participation, and security in order to enhance quality of life as people age. (ch. 19)

Andragogy Art and science of helping adults learn. (ch. 15)

Anticipatory grief An emotional response that occurs before the actual death around a family member with a degenerative or terminal disorder. (ch. 21)

Anticipatory guidance A proactive provider strategy to help clients cope effectively with stressful situations, thereby helping clients reduce unnecessary stress. (ch. 16)

Anxiety A vague, persistent feeling of impending doom. (ch. 11)

Aphasia A neurological linguistic deficit that is most commonly associated with neurological trauma to the brain. (ch. 17)

Apraxia The loss of ability or the inability to take purposeful action even when the muscles, senses, and vocabulary seem intact. (ch. 19)

Art of nursing A seamless interactive process in which nurses blend their knowledge, skills, and scientific understandings with their individualized knowledge of each client as a unique human being. (ch. 1)

Assertive behavior Setting goals, acting on those goals in a clear, consistent manner, and taking responsibility for the consequences of those actions. (ch. 13)

Assimilation A person's full adoption of the behaviors, customs, values, and language of the mainstream culture. (ch. 7)

Authenticity The capacity to be true to one's personality, spirit, and character in interacting with clients and others in the nurse-client relationship. (ch. 10)

Authoritarian Group Leadership A leadership style in which leaders take full responsibility for group direction and control group interaction. (ch. 8)

Autonomy The client's right to self-determination. (chs. 3, 19)

Avoidance A withdrawal from conflict. (ch. 13)

Beneficence Ethical principle guiding decisions, based on doing the greatest good for the greatest number and avoiding malfeasance. (ch. 3)

Behavioral emergency Refers to when a crisis escalates to the point that the situation requires immediate intervention to avoid injury or death. (ch. 20)

Best practice Nursing interventions derived from research evidence demonstrating successful outcome for client. (chs. 4, 23, 25)

Biofeedback Immediate and continuous information about a person's physiological responses; auditory and visual signals that increase one's response to external events. (ch. 16)

Body image The physical dimension of self-concept. (ch. 9)

Body language (also kinesics) Involving the conscious or unconscious body positioning or actions of the communicator. (chs. 5, 6)

Boundaries Represent invisible structures imposed by legal, ethical, and professional standards of nursing that respect nurse and client rights, and protect the functional integrity of the alliance between nurse and client. (chs. 1, 5, 12, 24)

Boundary violations Boundary violations take advantage of the client's vulnerability and represent a conflict of interest that usually is harmful to the goals of the therapeutic relationship. (ch. 10)

Briefing Oral statement of roles and responsibilities prior to activity. (ch. 4)

Burnout A state of fatigue or frustration brought about by devotion to a cause, way of life, or relationship that failed to produce an expected reward. (chs. 13, 16, 20)

Callouts The team reviews the situation aloud. (ch. 4)

Caring An intentional human action characterized by commitment and a sufficient level of knowledge and skill to allow the nurse to support the basic integrity of the client. (chs. 6, 11)

Case management A collaborative process of assessment, planning, facilitation, and advocacy for options and services to meet an individual's health needs that is used to promote quality cost-effective outcomes. (ch. 24)

Catastrophic reactions Emotional overreactions to situations, which look like temper tantrums; these are usually associated with dementia. (ch. 19)

Channels of communication Refers to one or more of the five senses through which a person receives messages: sight, hearing, taste, touch, and smell. (ch. 1)

Charting by exception A type of charting in which normal data are charted using check marks on flow sheets, with only abnormal or significant findings, called *exceptions*, being charted in a descriptive format. (ch. 25)

Chronic Health Conditions Refers to health problems that require ongoing self-management over a period of years or decades.

Chronic sorrow A normal grief response associated with an ongoing living loss that is permanent, progressive, recurring, and cyclic in nature. (ch. 21)

Circular questions Questions that focus on family interrelationships and the effect of a serious health alteration on individual family members and the equilibrium of the family system. (ch. 12)

Civil laws Developed through court decisions, which are created through precedents, rather than written statutes. (ch. 2)

Clarification A therapeutic active listening strategy designed to aid in understanding the message of the client by asking for more information or for elaboration on a point. (ch. 5)

Client Centered Care Care that is respectful of and responsive to individual patient preferences, needs, and values Care considers the impact of an illness or injury on a person physiologically, mentally, spiritually, and socially. (chs. 1, 5, 7, 10, 14, 24)

Clinical Decision Support System [CDSS] Software programs that input specific information about your client, analyze it, and make recommendations based on best practice outcomes as established by research (ch. 26)

Client (patient) education A set of planned educational activities, resulting in changes in health-related behaviors and attitudes as well as knowledge. (ch. 15)

Clinical pathway (also critical pathway) A documentation tool based on standardized plans of care for a specific health condition, usually demonstrating predefined progress toward recovery. (chs. 4, 25)

Clinical practice guidelines Protocols listing standardized recommended care. (ch. 26)

Clinical preceptor An experienced nurse, chosen for clinical competence, and charged with supporting, guiding, and participating in the evaluation of student clinical competence. (ch. 22)

Close-Ended Questions Question format which requires a yes or no or single phase response; they are used in emergency situations to quickly gather information.

Cloud, the Supercomputers storing client health data that can be accessed remotely by a variety of providers with client permission. (ch. 25)

Coaching An effective supportive teaching strategy nurses use to teach self-management and problem-solving skills to clients and families experiencing unfamiliar tasks and procedures.

Coding systems Alphanumerics assigned to label each type of health care intervention, making computerization possible. (ch. 25)

Cognition Refers to the thinking processes people use to make sense of their perceptions.

Cognitive dissonance The holding of two or more conflicting values at the same time. (ch. 3)

Cognitive distortions Faulty or negative thinking that causes a person to interpret neutral situations in an unrealistic, exaggerated, or negative way. (ch. 16)

Cognitive domain The domain of learning focus when the client has a knowledge deficit. (ch. 15)

Cohesion (Group) An essential curative factor in therapeutic groups defined as the value a group holds for its members and underscores the level of member commitment to the group. (ch. 8)

Collaborative Health Care Team A health care team refers to a coordinated group of professionals with complementary skills, who are mutually committed to specific performance goals, with shared accountability for goal achievement. (chs. 4, 8, 22, 23)

Co-Leadership A form of shared leadership found in therapy groups.

Commendations The practice of noticing, drawing forth, and highlighting previously unobserved, forgotten, or unspoken family strengths, competencies, or resources. (ch. 12)

Communication A combination of verbal and nonverbal behaviors integrated for the purpose of sharing information. (chs. 1, 5, 6, 14)

Communication disability Includes any client who has any impairment in body structure or function that interferes with communication. (ch. 17)

Community Any group of citizens that have either a geographic, population-based, or self-defined relationship and whose health may be improved by a health promotion approach.

Compassion fatigue A syndrome associated with serious spiritual, physical, and emotional depletion related to caring for clients that can affect the nurse's ability to care for seriously ill clients. (ch. 21)

Compassionate witnessing Defined as noticing and feeling empathy for others, which helps to support and broaden a client's perspective.

Competency a set of capabilities, skills, aptitude, and experience.

Competition A response style characterized by domination. (ch. 13)

Complicated grieving Represents a form of grief, distinguished by being unusually intense, significantly longer in duration and emotionally incapacitating. (ch. 21)

Computerized Provider Entry Systems [CPOE] Part of the health information system which allows providers to order tests and treatments. (ch. 25)

Concrete operations period Piaget's developmental stage in which a child can play cooperatively and employ complex rules. (ch. 18)

Confidentiality The respect for another's privacy that involves holding and not divulging information given in confidence except in case of suspected abuse, commission of a crime, or threat of harm to self or others. (chs. 2, 11, 25)

Conflict A mental struggle, either conscious or unconscious, resulting from the simultaneous presence of opposing or incompatible thoughts, or disharmony between individuals. (chs. 13, 23)

Connotation A more personalized meaning of the word or phrase. (ch. 6)

Continuity of Care Describes a multidimensional longitudinal construct in health care, which emphasizes seamless provision and coordination of client-centered quality care across clinical settings. (ch. 24)

Coping Any response to external life strains that serves to prevent, avoid, or control emotional distress (ch. 21)

Countertransference Feelings representing unconscious attitudes or exaggerated feelings a nurse may develop toward a client. (ch. 10)

Criminal laws Reserved for cases in which there was intentional misconduct and/or the action taken by the health care provider represents a serious violation of professional standards of care. (ch. 2)

Crisis A crisis describes a stressful life event, which overwhelms an individual's ability to cope effectively in the face of a perceived challenge or threat. (ch. 20)

Crisis intervention The systematic application of problem-solving techniques, based on crisis theory, designed to help the client move through the crisis process as swiftly and painlessly as possible with a return to an individual's pre-crisis functional level. (ch. 20)

Crisis state An acute normal human response to severely abnormal circumstances; it is not a mental illness. (ch. 20)

Critical incident debriefing Strategy used to help a group of people who have witnessed or experienced a mass trauma crisis event externalize and process its meaning (chs. 4, 20, 23)

Critical thinking An analytical process in which you purposefully use specific thinking skills to make complex clinical decisions. (chs. 3, 26)

Cultural competence A set of cultural behaviors and attitudes integrated into the practice methods of a system, agency, or its professionals, which enables them to work effectively in cross-cultural situations. (ch. 7)

Culture A complex social concept that encompasses the entirety of socially transmitted communication styles, family customs, political systems, and ethnic identity held by a particular group of people. (ch. 7)

Cultural Competence Cultural behaviors and attitudes integrated into the practice methods of a system, agency, or its professionals, enabling them to work effectively in cross-cultural situations. (ch. 7)

Cultural diversity Variations among cultural groups. (ch. 7)

Cultural relativism The belief that each culture is unique and should be judged only on the basis of its own values and standards. (ch. 7)

Cultural sensitivity The ability to be appropriately responsive to the attitudes, feelings, or circumstances of groups of people that share a common and distinctive racial, national, religious, linguistic, or cultural heritage. (ch. 7)

Decentralized access A nurse can use Internet devices to view or document client information even when in the community or in the client's home. (ch. 26)

Delegation The transfer of responsibility for the performance of an activity from one individual to another while retaining accountability for the outcome. (ch. 23)

Democratic Group Leadership A group leadership style in which the leader involves members in active open discussion and shared decision making. (ch. 8)

Denial An unconscious refusal to allow painful facts, feelings, and perceptions into conscious awareness. (ch. 20)

Denotation The generalized meaning assigned to a word. (ch. 6)

Deontologic model (also duty-based model) A duty-based model for making ethical decisions. (ch. 3)

Dependent nursing interventions Interventions that require an oral or a written order from a physician to implement. (ch. 2)

Disaster A calamitous event of slow or rapid onset that results in large-scale physical destruction of property, social infrastructure, and human life. (ch. 20)

Discharge planning A process of concentration, coordination, and technology integration, through the cooperation of health care professionals, clients, and their families, to ensure that all patients receive continuing care after being discharged. (ch. 24)

Discipline of Nursing Nursing is a "practice" discipline, which combines specialized knowledge and skills with prudent clinical judgment to meet client, family, and community health care needs. (chs. 1, 22)

Discrimination A legal statute refers to actions in which a person is denied a legitimate opportunity offered to others because of prejudice. (ch. 11)

Disease prevention A concept concerned with identifying modifiable risk and protective factors associated with diseases and disorders. (ch. 14)

Disruptive behavior Conduct that interferes with safe client care by negatively affecting the ability of the team to work together, such as bullying, harassment, blaming, etc. (ch. 23)

Distress A negative stress causes a higher level of anxiety and is perceived as exceeding the person's coping abilities. (ch. 21)

Documentation The process of obtaining, organizing, and conveying client health information to others in print or electronic format. (ch. 25)

Dysfunctional conflict Conflict in which information is withheld, feelings are expressed too strongly, the problem is obscured by a double message, or feelings are denied or projected onto others. (ch. 13)

Ecomap A sociogram, illustrating the shared relationships between family members and the external environment. (ch. 12)

Ego defense mechanisms Conscious and unconscious coping methods used by people to change the meaning of a situation in their minds. (ch. 16)

Ego integrity Relates to the capacity of older adults to look back on their lives with satisfaction and few regrets. (ch. 19)

Electronic health record (EHR) Various types of computerized client health records. (ch. 25)

Emancipated minors Mentally competent adolescents younger than age 18 years, who petition the courts for adult status. (ch. 2)

Emotional cutoff A person's withdrawal from other family members as a means of avoiding family issues that create anxiety. (ch. 12)

Emotion-focused coping Strategies focused on the person and designed to distance the person from stress. (ch. 16)

Empathy The ability to be sensitive to and communicate understanding of the client's feelings. (chs. 4, 5, 10, 11)

Empowerment Helping a person become a self-advocate; an interpersonal process of providing the appropriate tools, resources, and environment to build, develop, and increase the ability of others to set and reach goals. (chs. 11, 14, 16,19)

End-of-life (EOL) decision making The process that health care providers, patients, and patients' families go through when considering what treatments will or will not be used to treat a life-threatening illness. (ch. 21)

Environment The internal and external context of the client, as it shapes and is affected by a client's health care situation. (ch. 1)

Ethical dilemma (also moral dilemma) The conflict of two or more moral issues; a situation in which there are two or more conflicting ways of looking at a situation. (ch. 3)

E-prescribing Prescriptions typed into the health record and transmitted as hardcopy and electronically. (ch. 26)

Ethnicity Personal awareness of a shared cultural heritage with others based on common racial, geographic, ancestral, religious or historical bonds. (ch. 7)

Ethnocentrism The belief that one's own culture should be the norm and has the right to impose its standards of "correct" behavior and values on another because it is better or more enlightened than others. (ch. 7)

Eustress A short-term mild level of stress. (ch. 16)

Facial expression Facial configurations convey feelings without words. Facial expression either reinforces or modifies the message the listener hears. (chs. 8, 10)

Evidence Based Nursing Practice Refers to the blending of extensive clinical experience with sound clinical research and professional judgment in real-time client situations. (ch. 1)

Familismo Refers to having a strong family loyalty with corresponding responsibilities for ensuring the family stability; Particularly strong value in Hispanic/Latino communities (ch. 7)

Family A self-identified group of two more or individuals whose association is characterized by special terms, who may or may not be related by bloodlines or law, but who function in such a way that they consider themselves to be a family. (ch. 12)

Family projection process An unconscious casting of unresolved family emotional issues or attributes people in the past from the past onto a child. (ch. 12)

Feedback A message given by the nurse to the client in response to a message or observed behavior. (chs. 1, 5, 10, 16)

Flow sheets Charting on sheets with client's progress in preprinted categories of information. (ch. 25)

Formal operations period Piaget's developmental stage in which abstract reality and logical thought processes emerge and independent decisions can be made. (ch. 18)

Focused Questions Refer to questions needing a specific short response rather than a yes or no answer. They help clients describe specific details about an illness.

Functional similarity A term used to describe group members who are similar enough—intellectually, emotionally, and experientially to interact with each other in a meaningful way.

Functional status A broad range of purposeful abilities related to physical health maintenance, role performance, cognitive or intellectual abilities, social activities, and level of emotional functioning. (ch. 19)

Gender Describes socially constructed and enacted roles and behaviors that occur in a historical and cultural context, and that vary across societies and over time related to male and female characteristics

Genogram A standardized set of connections to graphically record basic information about family members and their relationships over three generations. (ch. 12)

"Good" death A death that is free from unavoidable distress and suffering for patients, families, and caregivers; in general accord with patients and families' wishes; and reasonably consistent with clinical, cultural, and ethical standards. (ch. 21)

Grief Represents a holistic, adaptive process that a person goes through following a significant loss (ch. 21)

Group A human communication system composed of three or more individuals, interacting for the achievement of some common goal(s) who influence and are influenced by each other (ch. 8)

Group dynamics A term used to describe the communication processes and behaviors occurring during the life of the group. (ch. 8)

Group norms Refer to the unwritten behavioral rules of conduct expected of group members. Norms can be universal (present in all groups) and group specific referring to those constructed by group members (ch. 8)

Group process Refers to the structural development of small group relationships (forming, storming, performing and adjourning. (ch. 8)

Group think Occurs when the approval of other group members becomes so important that group members support a decision they fundamentally do not agree with, just for the sake of harmony (ch. 8)

Handheld wireless communication devices Any small portable computer that uses the Internet to transmit client information. (ch. 26)

Handoffs (also handovers) Transfer process taking place when clients are reassigned to another team of health care providers. (chs. 2, 4)

Health A multidimensional concept, having physical, psychological, sociocultural, developmental, and spiritual characteristics that is used to describe an individual's state of well-being and level of functioning. (chs. 1, 14, 15)

Collaborative Health Care Team A health care team refers to a coordinated group of professionals with complementary skills, who are mutually committed to specific performance goals, with shared accountability for goal achievement. (chs. 8, 22)

Health disparity A particular type of health difference that is closely linked with social, economic, and/or environmental disadvantage. (chs. 7, 14)

Health Insurance Portability and Accountability Act (HIPAA) Federal privacy standards enacted in 2003, designed to protect client records and other health information provided to health plans and other health care providers. (chs. 1, 2, 25)

Health information technology (HIT) Creation of a whole new electronic interactive system designed to support the multiple information needs required by today's complex client care. (chs. 1, 25, 26)

Health literacy The degree to which people have the capacity to obtain, process, and understand basic health information and services needed to make appropriate health decisions. (chs. 7, 14, 16, 19)

Health promotion An educational support process that enables people to take control over their health. (ch. 14)

Health teaching A specialized form of teaching, defined as a focused, creative, interpersonal nursing intervention in which the nurse provides information, emotional support, and health-related skill training. (chs. 14, 15)

Hearing screening Includes testing for receptive acuity, pitch, and tone perception via use of whisper, tuning fork or an audiometry machine. (ch. 17)

Homeostasis (also dynamic equilibrium) A person's sense of personal security and balance. (chs. 16, 20)

Hospitalist A physician or nurse practitioner employed by the hospital to clinically manage a client's medical care; this provider assumes *full* responsibility for coordinating care.

Huddle Brief health team gathering to decided on a course of action (ch. 4)

Human rights-based model Based on the belief that each client has basic rights. (ch. 3)

Independent nursing interventions Interventions that nurses can provide without a physician's order or direction from another health professional. (ch. 2)

Inference An educated guess about the meaning of a behavior or statement. (ch. 5)

Informed consent A focused communication process in which the professional nurse or physician discloses all relevant information related to a procedure or treatment, with full opportunity for dialogue, questions, and expressions of concern, prior to asking for the client's signed permission. (chs. 2, 7, 15)

Informational Continuity Refers to data exchanges between providers, provider systems and clients for the purpose of providing coordinated care. (ch. 24)

Interagency accessibility Transmission and availability of client information across departments in a health care agency. (ch. 25)

Intercultural communication Conversations between people from different cultures that embrace differences in perceptions, language, and nonverbal behaviors, and recognition of different interpretative contexts. (ch.7)

Interpersonal communication A transactional, reciprocal, interactive and dynamic process, with value, cultural, and cognitive variables influencing its transmission and reception. It is multidimensional and irreversible. (chs. 1, 5)

Interpersonal competence The ability to interpret the content of a message from the point of view of each of the participants and the ability to use language and nonverbal behaviors strategically to achieve the goals of the interaction. (ch. 6)

Interprofessional education Occasions when two or more professions learn from and about each other to improve collaboration and the quality of care. (ch. 22)

Interprofessional Health Team A small number of providers with complementary skills who are committed to a common purpose, performance goals, and approach for which they are mutually accountable in client centered health care situations. (ch. 22)

Intrapersonal communication Takes place within the self in the form of inner thoughts; beliefs are colored by feelings and influence behavior. (ch. 1)

Justice Ethical principle guiding decision making. Justice is actually a legal term; however, in ethics it refers to being fair or impartial. (ch. 3)

Laissez-faire Group Leadership Style A disengaged form of leadership style in which the leader avoids decision making and is minimally available to group members. (ch. 8)

Leadership Refers to Interpersonal influence that is exercised in situations and directed through the communication process toward attainment of a specified goal or goals. (chs. 8, 22)

Learning readiness A person's mind-set and openness to engage in a learning or counseling process for the purpose of adopting new behaviors. (ch. 15)

Lifestyle Patterns of choices made from the alternatives that are available to people according to their socioeconomic circumstances and the ease with which they are able to choose certain ones over others. (ch. 14)

Longitudinal Plan of Care [LPC] Electronic multidisciplinary care plan used across sites to improve continuity of care. (ch. 25)

Linear communication model Simplest communication model through which people communicate, consisting of sender, message, receiver and context.

Magnet Recognition Program A unique national program that recognizes quality patient care and nursing excellence in health care institutions and agencies by identifying them as work environments that act as a "magnet" for professional nurses desiring to work there because of their excellence. (ch. 22)

Management Continuity Management strategy of developing pathways and aligning resources to encourage timely effective information flow between all entities involved in facilitating client centered care.

Medical home A medical home is a place that serves as a central first contact point in primary care and provides regular, accessible, comprehensive primary care services for designated clients and families within a single familiar setting. (ch. 24)

Mentoring A special type of professional relationship in which an experienced nurse or clinician (mentor) assumes a role responsibility for guiding the professional growth and advancement of a less-experienced person (protégé). (ch. 22)

Message Consists of the transmitted verbal or nonverbal expression of thoughts and feelings. (ch. 1)

Message competency The ability to use language and nonverbal behaviors strategically in the intervention phase of the nursing process to achieve the goals of the interaction. (ch. 6)

Metacommunication A broad term which describes all of the verbal and nonverbal factors used to enhance or negate the meaning of words. (chs. 1, 5, 6)

Minimal cues The simple, encouraging phrases, body actions, or words that communicate interest and encourage clients to continue with their story. (ch. 5)

Modeling A behavioral strategy that describes learning by observing another person performing a behavior. (ch. 15)

Moral distress A feeling that occurs when one knows what is "right" but feels bound to do otherwise because of legal or institutional constraints. (ch. 2)

Moral uncertainty A difficulty in deciding which moral rules (e.g. values or beliefs) apply to a given situation. (ch. 3)

Motivation The forces that activate behavior and direct it toward one goal instead of another. (chs. 14, 15)

Multiculturalism A term to describe a heterogeneous society in which diverse cultural worldviews can coexist with some general characteristics shared by all cultural groups and some perspectives that are unique to each group. (chs. 7, 11)

Multigenerational transmission The emotional transmission of behavioral patterns, roles, and communication response styles from generation to generation. (chs. 7, 12)

Mutuality An agreement on problems and the means for resolving them; a commitment by both parties to enhance well-being. (ch. 11)

NNN Abbreviation designating the combination of North American Nursing Diagnosis Association (NANDA), Nursing Interventions Classification (NIC), and Nursing Outcomes Classification (NOC). (ch. 25)

Nonverbal communication Refers to physical expressions and behaviors not expressed in words, which help clinicians understand the emotional meanings of messages. (ch. 5)

Noise Noise factors refer to *any* distraction that interferes with either the nurse or client being able to pay full attention to the discussion. (chs. 1, 5)

Nonmaleficence Avoiding actions that bring harm to another person. (ch. 3)

Nonverbal gesture A body movement that conveys a message without words. (ch. 6)

North American Nursing Diagnosis Association International (NANDA-I) A professional organization of registered nurses that promotes accepted nursing diagnoses. (chs. 2, 25)

Nuclear family emotional system The way family members relate to one another within their immediate family, when stressed. (ch. 12)

Numeracy The ability to understand and use numbers in daily life, for example in medication dosages.

Nurse Practice Acts Legal documents that communicate professional nursing's scope of practice, and outline nurses' rights, responsibilities, and licensing requirements in providing care to individual clients, families, and communities. (ch. 2)

Nursing Interventions Classification (NIC) A standardized language describing direct and indirect care that nurses perform. NIC and Nursing Outcomes Classification (NOC) attempt to quantify nursing care so that it becomes visible and defines professional practice. (ch. 25)

Nursing's Metaparadigm Identifies the central constructs of professional nursing practice found in all theories and models: person, environment, health, and nursing.

Nursing Outcomes Classification (NOC) The measure of how nursing care affects client outcomes. NOC and Nursing Interventions Classifications (NIC) attempt to quantify nursing care so that it becomes visible and defines professional practice. (ch. 25)

Objective data Data that are directly observable or verifiable through physical examination or tests. (ch. 2)

Omaha System A comprehensive computerized information management system for documentation at the point of care (i.e., the client's location). (ch. 25)

Open-ended questions A question format designed to help clients express health problems and needs in their own words. Open ended questions are open to interpretation and cannot be answered by yes, no, or another one-word response. (chs. 5, 9, 10, 11)

Pager Converts voice mail into e-mail that can be read. (ch. 4)

Palliative care a comprehensive philosophy of care aimed at primarily relieving symptoms associated with terminal illness and providing support for seriously ill patients and their families. (ch. 21)

Paralanguage The oral delivery of a verbal message expressed through tone of voice and inflection, sighing, or crying. (ch. 6)

Paraphrasing Transforming the client's words into the nurse's words, while keeping the meaning intact. (ch. 5)

Patterns of knowing Multiple integrated knowledge data patterns: empirical, personal, aesthetic, ethical that nurses use to provide effective, efficient and compassionate care based on client needs, individuality, complexity and situational contexts. (ch. 1)

Pedagogy The processes used to help children learn. (ch. 15)

Perception A cognitive process by which a person transforms external sensory data into personalized images of reality. (ch. 9)

Person A unitary concept that includes physiological, psychological, spiritual, and social elements. (ch. 1)

Personal digital assistant (PDA) A wireless electronic device containing databases that may also have the potential for electronic message transfer. (ch. 26)

Personal identity An intrapersonal psychological process consisting of a person's perceptions or images of personal abilities, characteristics, and potential growth potential. (ch. 9)

Personal medical identification number A unique series of digits assigned to each client, used by every health agent and agency. (This would replace use of identifying numbers such as social security number, which were not intended to be used for health care.) (ch. 25)

Personal space The invisible and changing boundary around an individual that provides a sense of comfort and protection to a person and that is defined by past experiences and culture. (ch. 11)

Point of care Whatever location the nurse is in to provide care to the client, whether at the bedside in the hospital room, in an outpatient clinic, or even in the client's own home. (ch. 26)

Point-of-care information Client information and reference material that is updated via wireless Internet devices at any location. (ch. 26)

Portals – see WEB portals

Possible selves Used to explain the future-oriented component of self-concept. (ch. 9)

Prejudices Stereotypes based on strong emotions. (ch. 11)

Premack principle Term used in behavior modification to choosing reinforcers that have meaning and value to the individual learner. (ch. 15)

Preoperational period Piaget's developmental stage in which learning by the toddler is developed through concrete experiences and devices and the child is markedly egocentric. (ch. 18)

Presbycusis Decrease in hearing associated with aging. (ch. 17)

Presbyopia Decrease in visual adjustments associated with aging. (ch. 17)

Primary prevention Actions taken to preclude illness or to prevent the natural course of illness from occurring; Strategies target modifiable risk factors with health education to promote a healthy lifestyle. (ch. 14)

Primary care Refers to a wide range of integrated ambulatory health care services delivered in community-based settings. (ch. 24)

Privacy A client's right to have control over personal information, whereas confidentiality refers to the obligation not to divulge anything said in a nurse-client relationship. (ch. 2)

Problem-oriented record (POR) A chart containing four basic sections: (1) a database, (2) a list of the client's identified problems, (3) a treatment plan, and (4) progress notes. (ch. 25)

Professional boundaries The invisible structures imposed by legal, ethical, and professional standards of nursing that respect nurse and client rights and protect the functional integrity of the alliance between nurse and client. (ch. 10)

Professional networking Establishing and using contacts for information, support, and other assistance in order to achieve career goals. (ch. 22)

Professional performance standards A competent level of professional role behavior related to quality of care, practice evaluation, continuing education, collegiality, collaboration, ethics, research, resource utilization, and leadership. (ch. 2)

Professional standards of practice The knowledge and clinical skills required of nurses to practice competently and safely. (ch. 2)

Protective Factors Behavioral activities or conditions delay the emergence of chronic disease or lessen its impact.

Proxemics The study of an individual's use of space. (chs. 6, 11)

Psychomotor domain Domain of learning focused on learning a skill through hands-on practice. (ch. 15)

QSEN Quality and Safety Education for Nurses (QSEN) nursing competencies considered fundamental to providing client-centered care and team collaboration in clinical practice (chs. 1, 2, 5)

Quality improvement (QI) the combined efforts of healthcare professionals, patients and their families, researchers, payers, planners and educators—to make changes resulting in better clinical outcomes (health) care and system performance. (chs. 1, 22)

Quality of life A personal experience of subjective well-being and general satisfaction with life that includes, but is not limited to, physical health. (chs. 8, 19)

QSEN competencies [Quality and Safety Education for Nurses] Any of six clinical practice behaviors, attitudes, knowledge, and skills, expected of nurses, as defined by the QSEN organization. (all chapters)

Radio Frequency Identity Chips [RFID] Small computerized discs that can be located remotely. (ch. 26)

Receiver The recipient of the message. (ch. 1)

Reflection A listening response focused on the emotional implications of a message used to help clients clarify important feelings related to message content.

Reframing Changing the frame in which a person perceives events in order to change the meaning. (ch. 5)

Reinforcement Refers to establishing consequences for performing targeted behaviors; positive reinforcement increases the probability of a response, and negative reinforcement decreases the probability of a response. (ch. 15)

Relational continuity A shared enterprise of therapeutic care delivery relationships across multiple systems, characterized by client centeredness, collaboration and coordination. (ch. 24)

Resilience Strength in the midst of change and stressful life events; the power of springing back or recovering readily from adversity. (chs. 14, 16)

Role A multidimensional psychosocial concept defined as a traditional pattern of behavior and self-expression, performed by or expected of an individual within a given society. (ch. 22)

Safety The minimization of risk of harm to clients and to providers; the avoidance of adverse outcomes or injuries stemming from the health care process. (chs. 4, 25)

SBAR (situation, background, assessment, recommendation) A standardized communication format, used in handoffs and discharge or transfer of clients to communicate critical information about a client. (chs. 2, 4, 23)

Scope of practice A broad term referring to the legal and ethical boundaries of practice for professional nurses established by each state; it is defined in written state statutes. (ch. 2)

Secondary prevention Interventions designed to promote early diagnosis of symptoms through health screening or timely treatment after the onset of the disease, thus minimizing their effects on a person's life. (ch. 14)

Self-concept A term describing peoples' complex understanding of their cultural heritage, their environment, their upbringing and education, their basic personality traits, and cumulative life experiences. (ch. 9)

Self-differentiation A person's capacity to define him- or herself within the family system as an individual having legitimate needs and wants. (ch. 12)

Self-disclosure Intentional revealing of personal experiences or feelings that are similar to or different from those of the client. (ch. 10)

Self-efficacy A term which refers to a person's perceptual belief that he or she has the capability to perform general or specific life tasks successfully. (chs. 9, 14, 15)

Self-esteem The emotional value a person places on his or her personal self-concept and the degree to which people approve of themselves in relation to others and the environment. (ch. 9)

Self-reflection Developing mindfulness of personal behaviors and values, which allows nurses to recognize the effects their words and behaviors have on the communication process in client centered relationships. (ch. 9)

Self-talk A cognitive process people can use to lessen cognitive distortions. (ch. 9)

Sender The source or initiator of the message. (ch. 1)

Sensorimotor period Piaget's developmental stage in which the infant explores its own body as a source of information about the world. (ch. 18)

Shaping The reinforcement of successive approximations of the target behavior. (ch. 15)

Sibling position A belief that sibling positions shape relationships and influence a person's expression of behavioral characteristics. (ch. 12)

Smart phone Handheld mobile phones with internet capability. (ch. 26)

Social cognitive competency The ability to interpret message content within interactions from the point of view of each of the participants. (ch. 6)

Social Determinants of Health A term used to identify a wide range of contextual factors influencing the health and well-being of individuals, and communities. (ch. 14)

Social media Any of multiple internet platforms allowing users to post information or pictures that can be accessed by the public (ch. 26)

Social support A person's "integration within a social network," and "the perceived availability of support" when it is needed (chs. 19, 24)

Societal emotional process Parallels that Bowen found between the family system and the emotional system operating at the institutional level in society. (ch. 12)

Speech amplifiers Devices to assist hearing. (ch. 17)

Speech-generating devices Laptop computers, fax machines, and personal device assistants (PDAs). (ch. 17)

Spirituality A unified concept, closely linked to a person's worldview, providing a foundation for a personal belief system about the nature of God or a Higher Power, moral-ethical conduct, and reality. (chs. 7, 9, 16, 19, 21)

Standard communication tools Uniformly used formats for communication of client information among all care providers, such as situation, background, assessment, recommendation (SBAR). (chs. 4, 23)

Statutory laws Legislated laws, drafted and enacted at federal or state levels. (ch. 2)

Stereotyping The process of attributing characteristics to a group of people as though all persons in the identified group possessed them. (ch. 11)

Stress A natural physiologic, psychological, and spiritual response to the presence of a stressor. (ch. 16)

Stressor A demand, situation, internal stimulus, or circumstance that threatens a person's personal security or self-integrity. (ch. 16)

Subculture A smaller group of people living within the dominant culture who have adopted a cultural lifestyle distinct from that of the mainstream population. (ch. 7)

Subsystems Member unit relationships within the family such as spousal, sibling, and child-parent subsystems. (ch. 12)

Sundowning Episodic agitated behavior occurring later in the day with clients with dementia. (ch. 19)

Summarization An active listening skill used to pull several ideas and feelings together, either from one interaction, or a series of interactions, into a few succinct sentences.

Taxonomy A hierarchical method of classifying vocabulary. (ch. 25)

TCAB An acronym for the program Transforming Care At the Bedside, which empowers nurses to make changes which improve client safety. (chs. 4, 26)

Teach back Method A teaching strategy used in patient education to evaluate and verify a client's understanding of health teaching and/or ability to execute self-management skills by asking the client to demonstrate requisite knowledge and skills. (ch. 15)

TeamSTEPPS A program (Team Strategies and Tools to Enhance Performance and Patient Safety), which emphasizes improving client outcomes by improving communication. (chs. 4, 23)

Telehealth Any use of Internet-transmitted visualization for health care diagnosis or treatment. Also known as telemedicine, telenursing, eHealth. (chs. 1, 2, 5, 25, 26)

Tertiary prevention Rehabilitation strategies designed to minimize the handicapping effects of a disease or injury, once it occurs. (ch. 14)

Theme The underlying emotions and interpretations associated with concrete verbal facts a client presents. (ch. 5)

Therapeutic communication A goal directed form of communication used in health care to achieve goals that promote client health and well-being. (chs. 1, 5)

Therapeutic relationship A professional interpersonal alliance in which the nurse and client join together for a defined period of time to achieve health-related treatment goals. (ch. 10)

Timeout A tool used by teams to stop and review a situation. (ch. 4)

Touch A communication strategy designed to provide comfort and communication through purposeful contact. (ch. 19)

Transference Projecting irrational attitudes and feelings from the past onto people in the present. (ch. 8)

Transactional communication models Communication models that employ systems concepts to describe communication context, feedback loops and validation; each person influences the other and is both a sender and receiver simultaneously within the interaction. (ch. 1)

Transitional care A set of actions designed to ensure the coordination and continuity of health care as patients transfer between different locations or different levels of care within the same location. (ch. 24)

Triage A tem used to describe how health workers sort out the severity of client needs and determine the priority of client treatments in a mass emergency or disaster situation. (ch. 20)

Triangles A defensive way of reducing, neutralizing, or defusing heightened anxiety between two family members by drawing a third person or object into the relationship. (ch. 12)

Trust A dynamic relational process, that involves the deepest needs and vulnerabilities of individuals. (chs. 5, 6, 10, 11, 23)

Uniform standards Guidelines of accepted practice. (chs. 5, 25)

Utilitarian or goal-based model A framework for making ethical decisions in which the rights of the client and the duties of the nurse are determined by what will achieve maximum welfare. (ch. 3)

Validation A focused form of feedback involving verbal and nonverbal confirmation that both participants have the same basic understanding of a message. Feedback loops validate information, or allow the human system to correct its original information. (chs. 1, 7, 10)

Values A set of personal beliefs and attitudes about truth, beauty, and the worth of any thought, object, or behavior. Attitudes, beliefs, feelings, worries, or convictions that have not been clearly established are called value indicators. (ch. 3)

Values acquisitions The conscious assumption of a new value. (ch. 3)

Values clarification A process that encourages one to clarify one's own values by sorting them through, analyzing them, and setting priorities. (ch. 3)

Verbal communication Refers to language communication consisting of the spoken words people use to communicate with each other. (ch. 5)

Violence A mental health emergency, which can create a critical challenge to the safety, well-being, and health of the clients and others in their environment. (chs. 13, 20)

Web portal An agency web site that provides opportunities for consumers to use hyperlinks to access a variety of information, receive cyber support, or even make appointments. (chs. 25, 26)

Well-being A person's subjective experience of satisfaction about his or her life related to six personal dimensions: intellectual, physical, emotional, social, occupational, and spiritual. (ch. 14)

Wireless text communication Texting or instant messaging. (chs. 17, 26)

Wisdom The virtue associated with Erikson's final stage of ego development represents an integrated system of "knowing" about the meaning and conduct of life. (chs. 9, 19)

Worldview The way people tend to look out upon their world or their universe to form a picture or value stance about life or the world around them. (chs. 1, 9)

PHOTOGRAPH CREDITS

Chapter 1
Courtesy University of Maryland School of Nursing

Chapter 2
Courtesy of the University of Maryland School of Nursing

Chapter 4
Courtesy Endur ID Incorporated, Hampton, NH

Chapter 5
Courtesy University of Maryland School of Nursing.
From Harkreader H: Fundamentals of nursing: caring and clinical judgment, Philadelphia, 2000, WB Saunders

Chapter 6
From deWit, SE: Fundamental concepts and skills for nursing, Philadelphia, 2001, Saunders

Chapter 9
Courtesy of Thomas Kenney and Father Joseph Freeman

Chapter 10
Potter PA, Perry AG: Basic Nursing, ed. 7, St. Louis, 2011, Mosby

Chapter 11
Courtesy Adam Boggs

Chapter 12
Yoder-Wise PS: Leading and Managing in Nursing, ed. 5, St. Louis, 2011, Mosby

Chapter 13
Courtesy Elizabeth Arnold

Chapter 14
From Amanda Mills, 2011, Atlanta, GA, CDC.

Chapter 15
From Amanda Mills, 2011, Atlanta, GA, CDC.

Chapter 17
From deWit, SE: Fundamental concepts and skills for nursing, Philadelphia, 2001, Saunders

Chapter 19
Leake P: Community/Public Health Nursing Online for Stanhope and Lancaster Foundations of Nursing in the Community, ed. 3, St. Louis, 2010, Mosby.

Chapter 26
Courtesy Honeywell, Inc.

INDEX

Note: Page numbers followed by *f* indicate figures; *t*, tables; *b*, boxes.